HANDBOOK OF FUNCTIONAL NEUROIMAGING OF COGNITION

Cognitive Neuroscience
Michael Gazzaniga, editor

Gary Lynch, *Synapses, Circuits and the Beginning of Memory*

Barry E. Stein and M. Alex Meredith, *The Merging of the Senses*

Richard B. Ivry and Lynn C. Robertson, *The Two Sides of Perception*

Steven J. Luck, *An Introduction to the Event-Related Potential Technique*

Roberto Cabeza and Alan Kingstone, eds., *Handbook of Functional Neuroimaging of Cognition*

HANDBOOK OF FUNCTIONAL NEUROIMAGING OF COGNITION

Second Edition

edited by Roberto Cabeza and Alan Kingstone

A Bradford Book
The MIT Press
Cambridge, Massachusetts
London, England

This book was set in Times Roman by SNP Best-set Typesetter Ltd., Hong Kong.

Library of Congress Cataloging-in-Publication Data

Handbook of function neuroimaging of cognition/editor by Roberto Cabeza and Alan Kingstone.—2nd ed.
    p. cm.
Includes bibliographical references and index.
ISBN 978-0-262-03344-2 (hc), 978-0-262-55279-0 (pb)
1. Cognitive neuroscience—Handbooks, manuals, etc. 2. Brain—Tomography—Handbooks, manuals, etc. 3. Brain—magnetic resonance imaging—Handbooks, manuals, etc. I. Cabeza, Roberto. II. Kingstone, Alan.
QP360.5H36   2005   612.8′2′028–dc22   2005052049

To our families

Contents

Preface

These are changing times—rapidly changing times—for those many people who want to understand what makes human beings tick. What brain changes are responsible for our ability to think, feel, and remember? How are scientists able to pursue these questions? What answers are they finding now? And what are the "big questions" for the next five or ten years?

The new edition of *Handbook of Functional Neuroimaging of Cognition* presents fourteen concisely written chapters that manage to capture and explain not only what *has happened* and what *is happening* in a broad range of the most important cognitive domains in science (e.g., attention, memory, language, emotion, development, skill learning, and aging), but also what *will happen* in these domains in the future.

This book was written with two types of readers in mind: senior undergraduate and graduate students (and instructors) who want to learn how the rapidly expanding field of cognitive functional neuroimaging is changing the very face of cognitive research; and postdoctoral as well as more established cognitive and social neuroscientists who are experts in a particular domain of cognition who wish to learn both what leading scientists in their research domain see as the current and emerging issues in their field, and who also seek to broaden their understanding across a range of cognitive domains and brain systems.

To facilitate the use by undergraduate and graduate students and instructors, the writing is exceedingly accessible and the chapters have been kept to a length that would be manageable for coverage in one or two lectures. In addition, new chapters on the history of imaging, the physics of functional neuroimaging, and its methodology have been incorporated. For more senior researchers, the chapters in the core cognitive domains have been completely updated from the previous edition to reflect the many new developments that have emerged in the last four to five years; moreover, a number of new chapters have been added to reflect the rapid expansion of functional neuroimaging into a number of new domains, such as skill learning, emotions, and human development.

Most important, the new book has maintained the two fundamental features that made it such a success originally. First, each chapter is written by one or more recognized world leaders in the field. Second, each chapter is divided into three key sections: a background section that introduces the domain being considered, a section that provides a comprehensive examination of what is currently occurring in the research domain, and a final section that explores and considers the major issues that are arising in the area. Thus, both in its individual parts of high-caliber science and in its overall *gestalt*, the book manages to capture the inherent dynamism that both defines and fuels the field of functional neuroimaging of cognition.

I HISTORY AND METHODS

1 Functional Neuroimaging: A Historical and Physiological Perspective

Marcus E. Raichle

Introduction

Bridging the gap between descriptions of human behaviors and underlying neural events has been a dream of both psychologists and neuroscientists for quite some time. William James, in his monumental two-volume work *The Principles of Psychology*, devotes two insightful chapters to the brain and its relationship to behavior. The prescience of his remarks is particularly remarkable given the fact that they were written 1890. In a fashion typical of much of his writing, James clearly identifies the challenge: "A science of the mind must reduce ... complexities [of behavior] to their elements. A science of the brain must point out the functions of its elements. A science of the relations of mind and brain must show how the elementary ingredients of the former correspond to the elementary functions of the latter" (James, 1890, vol. 1, p. 28).

The importance of meeting this challenge was appreciated at about the same time by no less a neuroscientist than Sir Charles Sherrington, who wrote that "... physiology and psychology, instead of prosecuting their studies, as some now recommend, more strictly apart one from another than at present, will find it serviceable for each to give to the results achieved by the other even closer heed than has been customary hitherto" (Sherrington, 1906, p. 387). While it is clear that progress has been made from the time of James and Sherrington until the present through studies in experimental animals and in patients with various diseases afflicting the brain, the opportunity to relate normal behavior to normal brain function in humans was largely nonexistent until the latter part of the twentieth century.

None other than the great experimental physiologist (some might say biological psychologist) Ivan Pavlov envisioned what was needed: "If we could look through the skull into the brain of a consciously thinking person, and if the place of optimal excitability were luminous, then we should see playing over the cerebral surface, a bright spot with fantastic, waving borders constantly fluctuating in size and form, surrounded by a darkness more or less deep, covering the rest of the hemispheres (1928; for translation, see Brugger, 1997). For many years such a vision seemed mere fantasy.

It was the introduction of modern brain imaging techniques in the 1970s, particularly positron emission tomography (PET) and magnetic resonance imaging (MRI), that permitted us to realize Pavlov's vision of monitoring human brain function in a safe yet increasingly detailed and quantitative way. Using strategies to map local changes in *brain circulation and metabolism* associated with changes in brain cellular activity, these brain imaging techniques initiated a revolution in the relationship between neuroscience and cognitive science that resulted in the birth of cognitive neuroscience (for a review, see Posner & Raichle, 1994).

Cognitive neuroscience has combined with surprising success the experimental strategies of cognitive psychology with brain imaging techniques to actually examine how brain function supports mental activities. The number of papers reporting the results of such studies is increasing at an exponential rate (Illes et al., 2003), as is the investment in brain imaging centers worldwide (many now in psychology departments) devoted to the study of brain-behavior relationships (Raichle, 2003a). Unheard-of in the late 1980s, when the James S. McDonnell Foundation and the Pew Charitable Trusts initiated their program in cognitive neuroscience, were faculty positions in psychology departments for cognitive neuroscientists. They are now common, and young scientists with combined qualifications in imaging and psychology are eagerly sought. Additionally, the research areas included are rapidly expanding into a domain now increasingly referred to as social neuroscience (Cacioppo et al., 2002).

The recent prominence of functional imaging in the scientific literature as well in as the popular press makes it easy to conclude that much of the work leading to the current state of research has evolved since the mid-1990s. Actually, work relevant to the development of these tools has been evolving for more than a century. In order to place current work in its proper perspective, a brief historical review is presented in this chapter along with a brief look at current trends and future directions.

Functional Neuroimaging: A Historical and Physiological Perspective

Historical Background: The Antecedents of Imaging

The quest for an understanding of the functional organization of the normal human brain, using techniques to assess changes in brain circulation and metabolism, as modern functional brain imaging techniques do, has occupied mankind for more than a century. One has only to consult William James again (James, 1890, vol. 1, p. 97) to find reference to changes in brain blood flow during mental activities. He references primarily the work of the Italian physiologist Angelo Mosso (Mosso, 1881), who recorded the pulsation of the human cortex in patients with skull defects following neurosurgical procedures. Mosso showed, in what must arguably be the first cognitive activation ever performed, that these pulsation increased regionally during mental activity (specifically, mental arithmetic). Mosso concluded—correctly, we now know—that brain circulation changes selectively with neuronal activity.

Despite a promising beginning, including the seminal animal experimental observations of Roy and Sherrington (Roy & Sherrington, 1890) that suggested a link between brain circulation and metabolism, interest in this research virtually ceased during the first quarter of the twentieth century. Undoubtedly, this was due in part to a lack of tools sufficiently sophisticated to pursue this line of research. In addition, the work of Leonard Hill, Hunterian Professor of the Royal College of Surgeons in England, was very influential (Hill, 1896). His eminence as a physiologist overshadowed the inadequacy of his own experiments that led him to conclude that no relationship existed between brain function and brain circulation.

There was no serious challenge to Leonard Hill's views until a remarkable clinical study was reported by John Fulton in 1928, in the journal *Brain* (Fulton, 1928). At the time of the report Fulton was a neurosurgery resident under Harvey Cushing at the Peter Bent Brigham Hospital in Boston. A patient presented to Cushing's service with gradually decreasing vision due to an arteriovenous malformation of the occipital cortex. Surgical removal of the malformation was attempted but unsuccessful, leaving the patient with a bony defect over primary visual cortex. Fulton elicited a history of a cranial bruit audible to the patient whenever he engaged in a visual task. Based on this history, Fulton pursued a detailed investigation of the behavior of the bruit, which he could auscultate and record over occipital cortex. Remarkably consistent changes in the character of the bruit could be appreciated, depending upon the visual activities of the patient. While opening the eyes produced only modest increases in the intensity of the bruit, reading produced striking increases. The changes in cortical blood flow related to the complexity of the visual task and the attention of the subject to that task anticipated findings and concepts that have only recently been addressed with modern functional imaging techniques (for a recent review, see Corbetta & Shulman, 2002; Ress et al., 2000).

At the close of World War II, Seymour Kety and his colleagues opened the next chapter in studies of brain circulation and metabolism. Working with a then young Lou Sokoloff and others, Kety developed the first quantitative methods for measuring whole-brain blood flow and metabolism in humans. The introduction of an in vivo tissue autoradiographic measurement of regional blood flow in laboratory animals by Kety's group (Kety, 1960; Landau et al., 1955) provided the first glimpse of quantitative changes in regional blood flow in the brain related directly to brain function. Given the later importance of derivatives of this technique to functional brain imaging with both PET and fMRI, it is interesting to note the (dis)regard the developers had for this technique as a means of assessing brain functional organization. Quoting from the comments of William Landau to the members of the American Neurological Association meeting in Atlantic City (Landau et al., 1955): "Of course we recognize that this is a very secondhand way of determining physiological activity; it is rather like trying to measure what a factory does by measuring the intake of water and the output of sewage. This is only a problem of plumbing and only secondary inferences can be made about function. We would not suggest that this is a substitute for electrical recording in terms of easy evaluation of what is going on." With the introduction of the deoxyglucose technique for the regional measurement of glucose metabolism in laboratory animals (Sokoloff et al., 1977) and its later adaptation for PET (Reivich et al., 1979), enthusiasm was much greater for the potential of metabolism as well as blood flow measurements to enhance our knowledge of brain function (Raichle, 1987).

Soon after Kety and his colleagues introduced their quantitative methods for measuring whole-brain blood flow and metabolism in humans, David Ingvar, Neils Lassen, and their Scandinavian colleagues introduced methods applicable to man that permitted regional blood flow measurements to be made using scintillation detectors arrayed like a helmet over the head (Lassen et al., 1963). They demonstrated directly in normal human subjects that blood flow changes regionally during changes in brain functional activity. The first study of functionally induced regional changes in blood flow using these techniques in normal humans was reported by Ingvar and Risberg at an early meeting on brain blood flow and metabolism (Ingvar & Risberg, 1965) and was greeted with cautious enthusiasm and a clear sense of its potential importance for studies of human brain function in this way by Seymour Kety (Kety, 1965). However, despite many studies of functionally induced changes in regional cerebral blood that followed (for reviews, see Lassen et al., 1978; Raichle, 1987), this approach was not embraced by most neuroscientists or cognitive scientists. It is interesting to note that this indifference disappeared almost completely in the 1980s, a subject to which I shall return shortly.

X-ray Computed Tomography and the Introduction of Imaging

In 1973 Godfrey Hounsfield (Hounsfield, 1973) introduced X-ray computed tomography (CT), a technique based upon principles presented in 1963 by Alan Cormack (Cormack, 1963, 1973; Kevles, 1997; Webb, 1990). Overnight the way in which we look at the human brain changed. Immediately, researchers envisioned another type of tomography, positron emission tomography (PET), which created in vivo autoradioagraphs of brain function (Phelps et al., 1976; Ter-Pogossian et al., 1975). A new era of functional brain mapping began. The autoradiographic techniques for the measurement of blood flow (Landau et al., 1955) and glucose metabolism (Sokoloff et al., 1977) in laboratory animals could now be performed safely in humans (Raichle et al., 1983; Reivich et al., 1979). Additionally, quantitative techniques were developed (Frackowiak et al., 1980; Mintun et al., 1984) and, importantly, validated (Altman et al., 1991; Mintun et al., 1984) for the measurement of oxygen consumption.

As a result of collaboration among neuroscientists, imaging scientists, and cognitive psychologists, a distinct behavioral strategy for the functional mapping of neuronal activity emerged in early days of functional brain imaging with PET. This strategy had three important components. First, while measurements of changes in brain function could be accomplished with measurements of blood flow or metabolism (Raichle, 1987), blood flow became the favored technique because it could be measured quickly (<1 min as compared with 30–40 min for metabolism) by using an easily produced radiopharmaceutical ($H_2^{15}O$) with a short half-life (123 sec), which allowed many repeat measurements in the same subject.

Second, brain blood flow measurements were averaged across individuals to improve the signal-to-noise properties of the resulting imaging data (ref Fox, Mintun et al., 1988). An early worry was that individual differences would be sufficiently great that attempts to average imaging data across individuals to improve signals and diminish noise would be doomed to failure. Those fears were quickly put to rest by the very first attempts to average functional imaging data across individuals. The results were stunning (Fox, Mintun et al., 1988). Researchers immediately appreciated a remarkable increase in the signal-to-noise ratio in their images (for a historical review of these interesting and important developments, see Raichle, 2000, p. 57). The approach of averaging data across individuals into a standardized anatomical space (Fox, Perlmutter et al., 1985) has since dominated the field of cognitive neuroscience with great success.

Third, brain blood flow measurements with PET were combined with a strategy first enunciated by the Dutch physiologist Franciscus C. Donders in 1868 (repr. in Donders, 1969) and later expanded during the cognitive revolution of the 1950s (for an elegant summary of this important work, see Posner, 1978). Donders proposed a general method to measure thought processes based on a simple logic. He subtracted the time needed to respond to a light (say, by pressing a key) from the time needed to respond to a particular color of light. He found that discriminating color required about 50 msec. In this way, Donders isolated and measured a mental process for the first time by subtracting a control state (i.e., responding to a light with a key press) from a task state (i.e., discriminating the color of the light). The application of this strategy of cognitive subtraction to imaging first appeared in a pair of papers on the cortical anatomy of single word processing (Petersen et al., 1988; Petersen et al., 1989) that incorporated image averaging with task subtraction to isolate putative brain systems associated with particular mental operations. It may well have been this combination of cognitive science, systems neuroscience, and brain imaging that lifted functional studies of brain circulation and metabolism in humans from a state of indifference in the neuroscience community in the 1970s to its current role of exceptional prominence.

The Introduction of Functional Magnetic Resonance Imaging

To understand the introduction of MRI into functional brain imaging, it is first important to review a bit of what was being learned about the relationship between brain function and brain circulation and metabolism in the 1970s and 1980s. Recall that the signal being used in positron emission tomography (PET) functional brain imaging was blood flow change. This was based on the fact that changes in the cellular activity of the brain of normal, awake humans and unanesthetized laboratory animals had invariably been observed to be accompanied by changes in local blood flow (for a review, see Raichle, 1987). This robust, empirical relationship had fascinated scientists for well over a hundred years and it seemed likely to most (e.g., see Siesjo, 1978) that it simply reflected increased need of the brain for oxygen during an increase in cellular activity. It was, therefore, quite surprising when it was demonstrated that while these changes in blood flow were accompanied by equivalent changes in glucose consumption (glucose is the primary fuel for metabolism in the brain), the changes in oxygen consumption were significantly smaller than those in either the blood flow or the glucose consumption (Fox & Raichle, 1986; Fox, Raichle et al., 1988).

In effect, during periods of increased functional activity the brain appears to shift its strategy for energy production from oxidative phosphorylation (i.e., burning glucose to carbon dioxide and water) to glycolysis (i.e., breaking down glucose to lactic acid without the use of oxygen). In doing so, it appears that a trade-off is made between a highly efficient but slowly changing source of energy (oxidative phosphorylation) and a less efficient but rapidly adapting one (glycolysis) to meet the need to accommodate rapidly changing aspects of neuronal function. The practical result this fascinating bit of physiology is that the oxygen content of the vasculature increases at the site of an increase in brain activity (i.e., supply exceeds demand). When brain activity decreases, the opposite occurs (Shmuel et al., 2003; G. L. Shulman et al., 1997).

These brain activity-associated changes in blood oxygenation provided an opening for MRI in functional brain imaging. By combining this observation with a much earlier observation by Pauling and Coryell (Pauling & Coryell, 1936) that changing the amount of oxygen carried by hemoglobin changes the degree to which hemoglobin disturbs a magnetic field, Ogawa et al. (Ogawa, Lee et al., 1990) were able to demonstrate that in vivo changes in blood oxygenation could be detected with MRI. The MRI signal (technically known as T2* or "tee-two-star") arising from this unique combination of brain physiology (Fox & Raichle, 1986) and nuclear magnetic resonance physics (Pauling & Coryell, 1936; Thulborn et al., 1982) became known as the blood oxygen level-dependent or BOLD signal (Ogawa, Lee et al., 1990). There quickly followed several demonstrations of BOLD signal changes in normal humans during functional brain activation (Bandettini et al., 1992; Frahm et al., 1992; Kwong et al., 1992; Ogawa, Tank et al., 1992), giving birth to functional MRI (fMRI). fMRI has dominated functional brain imaging research ever since.

A final comment about the changes in brain circulation and metabolism we observe in functional imaging studies should be made. As noted above, changes in blood flow appear to be accompanied by changes in glucose utilization that exceed the increase in oxygen consumption (Blomqvist et al., 1994; Fox, Raichle et al., 1988; Ueki et al., 1988; Woolsey et al., 1996). Thus, glycolysis appears to provide an increased proportion of the energy needed for transient changes in brain activity. This observation has stimulated experiments on the cellular processes responsible for the imaging signals. These studies have focused on the excitatory neurotransmitter glutamate and how it is removed from the synapse and recycled (Chatton et al., 2003; Kasischke et al., 2004; Magistretti et al., 1999; Pellerin & Magistretti, 1994). It has been demonstrated that glutamate is removed from the synapse by an energy-dependent process involving its uptake by astrocytes and its conversion to glutamine. The energy required for both steps in this process appears to be supplied by aerobic glycolysis. As a result, one interpretation of brain imaging signals (in particular the BOLD signal) is that they reflect changes in excitatory neurotransmission. How inhibitory processes influence imaging signals, particularly GABA, the brain's main inhibitory neurotransmitter, remains to be determined, but they appear not to involve glycolysis-dependent processes in astrocytes (Chatton et al., 2003). Therefore, the contribution of inhibitory processes to the brain's energy consumption and their role in the signals we observe with functional imaging remain a significant gap in our knowledge.

The Current State of Functional Imaging

Despite all of the progress that has been made and the apparent success that functional brain imaging has achieved, interpretations frequently stated or implied about functional imaging data (e.g., see Nichols & Newsome, 1999; Uttal, 2001) suggest that, if one is not careful, brain imaging could be viewed as no more than a modern and extraordinarily expensive version of nineteenth-century phrenology (for alternative views, see Posner, 2003; Raichle, 2003a). In this regard, it is worth noting that functional imaging researchers themselves have occasionally unwittingly perpetuated this notion. Data presentations in journal articles, at meetings, and in lay publications have focused on specific areas of the brain, frequently without presenting the entire data set for inspection. These areas are then discussed in terms of complex mental functions. This risks bringing us full circle and discussing the relationship between brain areas and mental functions in a manner akin to phrenology.

It was Korbinian Brodmann, one of the pioneers in studying the organization of the human brain from both a micro- and a macroscopic point of view, whose perspective I find appealing even though it was written well in advance of the discovery of modern imaging technology (1909 to be exact; Brodmann, 1909). He said, "Indeed, recently theories have abounded which, like phrenology, attempt to localize complex mental activity such as memory, will, fantasy, intelligence or spatial qualities such as appreciation of shape and position to circumscribed cortical zones." He continued, "These mental faculties are notions used to designate extraordinarily involved complexes of mental functions. . . . One cannot think of their taking place in any other way than through an infinitely complex and involved interaction and cooperation of numerous elementary activities. . . . in each particular case [these] supposed elementary functional loci are active in differing numbers, in differing degrees and in differing combinations. . . . Such activities are . . . always the result . . . of the function of a large number of suborgans distributed more or less widely over the cortical surface" (for these English translations, see Garey, 1994, pp. 254–255).

With this prescient admonition in mind, the task of functional brain imaging would seem to be clear. First, identify the network of regions of the brain and their relationship to the performance of a well-designed task. This is a process that is well under way in the functional imaging community and is complemented by a long history of lesion behavior work from the neuropsychology community and, in some instances, neurophysiological and neuroanatomical studies in laboratory animals as well as humans. Second, and definitely more challenging, identify the elementary operations performed within such a network and relate these operations to the task of interest. This agenda has progressed in interesting ways.

Functional brain imaging studies have clearly and, not surprisingly, revealed that networks of brain areas rather than single areas are associated with the performance of tasks. Probably of even greater interest is the fact that elements of these networks can be seen across many different tasks, suggesting the presence of elementary operations that are common across tasks. While some might view this as evidence for a lack of specificity in functional imaging data, others, including myself, see this as an important clue to the manner in which the brain allocates its finite processing resources to the accomplishment of an infinite range of behaviors. A model of how one might think about this observation comes from studies in invertebrate neurobiology where ensembles of neurons have been observed to reconfigure their relationships depending upon the task at hand, thus multiplying the potential of finite resources to serve the needs of the organism (Marder & Weimann, 1991; Prinz et al., 2004). It would not be too surprising if this rather sensible strategy had been conserved in an expanded version in the vertebrate brain. Obviously, success in pursuing information of this type will require very careful task analysis, with particular attention to the presence of common elements in tasks that might superficially seem quite different.

In pursuit of these ideas, debate has arisen about the level of representation that might be expected in particular areas (i.e., how "elementary" is elementary when seeking the operations performed in a particular area?). This is exemplified in the interesting results and discussions about the specificity of face perception in the human brain (for contrasting views, see Duchaine et al., 2004; Grill-Spector et al., 2004; Hanson et al., 2004; Haxby et al., 2001). We must be careful in adjudicating such a debate until we have a more complete understanding of the detailed anatomy of the area under consideration. For the putative face area of the medial temporal lobe of humans we lack such detailed information. A contrasting example exists in the ventral medial prefrontal cortex, where processes related to emotion have been suspected (Bush et al., 2000; Drevets et al., 1997; Mayberg et al., 1999; Simpson et al., 2001). Recent extension of detailed cytoarchitectonics maps from monkey to man (Gusnard et al., 2003; Ongur et al., 2003) illustrates the type of information that will lay the foundation for a more complete understanding of exactly what is going on.

Future Directions

Integration Across Levels of Analysis

Nowhere has the integration of levels of analysis been more important to the functional imaging agenda than in a recent pioneering group of studies that have sought to provide an understanding of the relationship between the neurophysiological activity of cells within the brain and the circulatory and metabolic signals that are observed with functional imaging techniques (Lauritzen, 2001; Logothetis, 2003; Logothetis et al., 2001). To put this work in perspective, it is important to note that for the neurophysiologists, task-induced changes in brain activity are traditionally recorded as changes in the firing rate or spiking activity of individual neurons (usually large "principal" cells), which reflects their output to cells elsewhere in the brain. For neurophysiologists, spiking has been the gold standard. They have most often ignored the signals associated with the input to cells that are reflected in very complex electrical signals (often called "local field potentials") generated by millions of tiny but very important cell processes (i.e., dendrites and axon terminals together, occasionally referred to as the neuropil). The new data directly correlating neurophysiology with imaging signals (Lauritzen, 2001; Logothetis et al., 2001) reveal that imaging signals reflect changes in the neuropil and not spiking. As is the case in so much of science, these findings were clearly anticipated by others (Creutzfeldt, 1975; Schwartz et al., 1979).

Thus, for neurophysiologists and cognitive neuroscientists to communicate, they must first realize that the aspects of brain function they routinely measure are different. While they may at times correlate nicely, they are not causally related in any simple manner (see Raichle, 2003a for recent discussions). As a result, both the neurophysiologists and the cognitive neuroscientists have necessary but not sufficient information to obtain a complete picture of events critical to an ultimate understanding of the function of the brain at a system level. A balanced perspective without claims to a privileged access to the complete truth will be most helpful as we seek to understand these issues. Cognitive neuroscientists who remain informed on this evolving dialogue will be able to draw much more from the work they do.

Individual Differences

Another issue likely to be of increasing importance to our future understanding of human brain function is the matter of individual differences. As noted earlier in this chapter, the success of image averaging was so impressive that it quickly blinded us, with few exceptions (e.g., see Canli et al., 2001; Gusnard et al., 2003; Simpson et al., 2001), to the potential richness of individual differences in our imaging data. Only recently has this begun to change. For all who have carefully examined recent data (particularly high-quality fMRI data), the existence of individual differences begins to emerge with exciting prospects for an even deeper understanding of human behavior (e.g., see Gusnard et al., 2003). Coupled with a long-standing interest in and techniques for the characterization of personality differences from psychology and psychiatry, we are poised to make major advances in this area in the coming years.

The Brain's "Dark Energy"

Finally, in the work ahead it will be critically important to maintain a sense of proportion when it comes to viewing functional imaging signals. In the average adult human, the brain represents about 2% of the total body weight but accounts for about 20% of the energy consumed, 10 times that predicted by its weight alone (Clark & Sokoloff, 1999). In relation to this very high rate of ongoing or "basal" metabolism (usually measured while one is resting quietly but awake with eyes closed), regional imaging signals are remarkably small. Thus, regional changes in absolute blood flow are rarely more than 5–10% of the resting blood flow of the brain in the areas typically affected by cognitive tasks. These are modest modulations in ongoing circulatory activity and often do not appreciably affect the overall rate of brain blood flow during even the most vigorous sensory and motor activity (Fox et al., 1987; Fox et al., 1985; Sokoloff et al., 1955). (For interesting exceptions related to more demanding cognitive tasks, see Friston et al., 1990; Lennox, 1931; Madsen et al., 1995; Roland et al., 1987).

Faced with the above observations, it is important to ask just what this enormous energy budget of our brain supports. Recent work in magnetic resonance spectroscopy (Hyder et al., 2002; R. G. Shulman et al., 2001; Sibson et al., 1997; Sibson et al., 1998), as well as estimates based on known costs of the cellular processes associated with excitatory neurotransmission (Ames, 2000; Attwell & Laughlin, 2001; Lennie, 2003), suggest that well more than 50% of this energy (estimates range as high as 80%) support the ongoing activity of neurotransmitters. This remarkable fact should alert all who do functional brain imaging and neurophysiology as well to the fact that much of what the brain is actually doing is being ignored. It is a challenging problem much like that faced by astronomers and cosmologists who have long recognized the presence of "dark energy" in the universe.

The above "cost analysis" of human brain function calls to mind the view, long espoused but little noticed (e.g., see Brown, 1911; Brown, 1915; Llinás, 1974; Llinás, 1988), that the brain operates intrinsically with sensory information, often in an impoverished form, modulating rather than informing the system. As William James observed many years ago, "Whilst part of what we perceive comes through our senses from the object before us, another part (and it may be the larger part) always comes . . . out of our own head" (James, 1890, vol. 2, p. 103). This view has led many to posit that the brain operates as a Bayesian inference machine (Kording & Wolpert, 2004; Olshausen, 2003), maintaining a state of "priors" related both to experience and to our genetic endowment. Beautiful reminders of the latter have recently appeared (Kuhl, 2003; Meltzoff & Decety, 2003). As well, a recently published experiment in the cat visual cortex is a direct demonstration of the phenomenon I am describing. In the absence of any sensory input the cat visual cortex appeared to be creating, in its spontaneous activity, representations of anticipated visual stimuli (Kenet et al., 2003). These and other observations have led me to endorse the general view that the brain develops and maintains a probabilistic model of anticipated events and that the majority of ongoing neuronal activity is an internal representation of that model against which sensory information is compared. As cognitive neuroscience contemplates its agenda, appreciating this perspective will be crucial.

Conclusions

Since the 1970s members of the medical and scientific communities have witnessed a truly remarkable transformation in the way we are able to examine the human brain through imaging. The results of this work provide a strong incentive for continued development of new imaging methods. Because of the dramatic nature of much of this imaging work and its intuitive appeal, highly creative people from a wide variety of disciplines are increasingly involved. Such people have a choice of many questions on which they can fruitfully spend their time. It remains important to detect subatomic particles, to probe the cosmos, and to exploit the sequencing of the genomes of various species including humans, but to this list we can now add the goal of observing and understanding the human brain at work.

In such a rapidly evolving field it is difficult to make long-range predictions about advances in imaging over the next decade. Functional MRI will play a dominant role in the day-to-day mapping of the brain. The ability to trace single cognitive events in individual subjects (see above) is just one of a number of innovations that make fMRI such a powerful and appealing tool for this work. Combining fMRI with traditional electrophysiological techniques applicable to humans such as the electroencephalogram (EEG) both alone (e.g., see Laufs et al., 2003) and in the detection of event-related potentials (ERP) will likely provide the spatial and temporal information necessary to understand information processing in the human brain.

As well, it appears that the promise of MRI-based techniques to map the fiber pathways in the human brain (often referred to as "diffusion tensor imaging") will soon be realized. While much slower to develop than many of us anticipated at the time of its introduction (Conturo et al., 1999), refined techniques based on the in vivo diffusion of water along fiber pathways in the human brain now offer exciting prospects for near-term advances (e.g., see Catani et al., 2004; McKinstry et al., 2002).

PET was obviously a pivotal technique in establishing functional brain imaging. Some might consider its role now only of historical interest, but that is unlikely to be the case. PET remains our gold standard for the measurement of many critical variables of physiological interest in the brain—blood flow, oxygen consumption, and glucose utilization to name the most obvious. We have much left to learn about the signals that give rise to fMRI (Raichle, 1998). With so much at stake, understanding these signals must be a high priority item on our agenda. PET will play a significant role in this work.

Functional imaging of the future will undoubtedly involve more than measurements directly related to moment-to-moment changes in neuronal activity (e.g., changes in BOLD contrast). Also of importance will be changes in neurotransmitter and neuromodulator release involving diffuse projecting systems for dopamine, norepinephrine and serotonin. Such changes are probably involved in learning, reinforcement of behavior, attention, and sensorimotor integration. Here PET is presently in almost sole possession of the agenda. A recent behavioral study with PET demonstrating the release of dopamine in the human brain during the performance of a goal-directed motor task is illustrative of what is in store (Koepp et al., 1998).

Finally, one cannot help being impressed by the expanding domain of functional brain imaging studies. In the past several years they have moved from sophisticated studies in classical areas of psychology, such as memory, attention, language, and emotion, to studies of human social behaviors such as economic (McClure et al., 2004) and moral decisions (Greene et al., 2001; Moll et al., 2002). At the moment much of this is clearly a work in progress that is immensely interesting to many of us because it offers the potential of extending the relationship of brain science to a broad range of important and exciting issues.

Taking a lesson from the immense success of cognitive neuroscience, those interested in this broader agenda, which some have dubbed social neuroscience (Cacioppo et al., 2002), need to focus on the training of a new generation of social scientists who understand and can use effectively the new tools of neuroscience such as functional brain imaging (Raichle, 2003b). These new researchers must understand not only the important questions to be asked but also how relevant information on brain function can be obtained to help in their quest for answers. The challenge will be to understand how best to integrate the potential of tools such as brain imaging with the fascinating yet complex issues of interest to social scientists. We will all be the beneficiaries of the success of this venture.

Acknowledgments

I would like to acknowledge many years of generous support from NINDS, NHLBI, the McDonnell Center for Studies of Higher Brain Function at Washington University, the John D. and Katherine T. MacArthur Foundation, and the Charles A. Dana Foundation.

References

Altman, D. I., Lich, L. L., & Powers, W. J. (1991). Brief inhalation method to measure cerebral oxygen extraction fraction with PET: Accuracy determination under pathological conditions. *Journal of Nuclear Medicine* 32, 1738–1741.

Ames, A. I. (2000). CNS energy metabolism as related to function. *Brain Research Reviews* 34, 42–68.

Attwell, D., & Laughlin, S. B. (2001). An energy budget for signaling in the grey matter of the brain. *Journal of Cerebral Blood Flow and Metabolism* 21, 1133–1145.

Bandettini, P. A., Wong, E. C., Hinks, R. S., Tikofsky, R. S., & Hyde, J. S. (1992). Time course EPI of human brain function during task activation. *Magnetic Resonance in Medicine* 25, 390–397.

Blomqvist, G., Seitz, R. J., Sjogren, I., Halldin, C., Stone-Elander, S., Widen, L., and Haaparanta, M. (1994). Regional cerebral oxidative and total glucose consumption during rest and activation studied with positron emission tomography. *Acta Physiologica Scandinavica* 151, 29–43.

Brodmann, K. (1909). *Vergleichende Lokalisationlehre der Grosshirnrinde*. Leipzig: J. A. Barth.

Brown, T. G. (1911). The intrinsic factors in the act of progression in the mammal. *Proceedings of the Royal Society of London* B84, 308–319.

Brown, T. G. (1915). On the nature of the fundamental activity of the nervous centres: Together with an analysis of the conditioning of rhythmic activity in progression, and a theory of the evolution of function in the nervous system. *Journal of Physiology* 48, 18–46.

Brugger, P. (1997). Pavlov on neuroimaging. *Journal of Neurology, Neurosurgery and Psychiatry* 62, 636.

Bush, G., Luu, P., & Posner, M. I. (2000). Cognitive and emotional influences in anterior cingulate cortex. *Trends in Cognitive Sciences* 4(6), 215–222.

Cacioppo, J. T., Berntson, G. G., Adolphs, R., Carter, C. S., Davidson, R. J., McClintock, M. K., et al. (Eds.). (2002). *Foundations in Social Neuroscience.* Cambridge, MA.: MIT Press.

Canli, T., Zhao, Z., Kang, E., Gross, J., Desmond, J. E., & Gabrieli, J. D. E. (2001). An fMRI study of personality influences on brain reactivity to emotional stimuli. *Behavioral Neuroscience* 115, 33–42.

Catani, M., Jones, D. K., & Ffytche, D. H. (2004). Perisylvian language networks of the human brain. *Annals of Neurology* 57, 8–16.

Chatton, J.-Y., Pellerin, L., & Magistretti, P. J. (2003). GABA uptake into astrocytes is not associated with significant metabolic cost: Implications for brain imaging of inhibitory transmission. *Proceedings of the National Academy of Sciences USA* 100, 12456–12461.

Clark, D. D., & Sokoloff, L. (1999). Circulation and energy metabolism of the brain. In G. J. Siegel, B. W. Agranoff, R. W. Albers, S. K. Fisher & M. D. Uhler (Eds.), *Basic Neurochemistry: Molecular, Cellular and Medical Aspects*, 6th ed., 637–670. Philadelphia: Lippincott-Raven.

Conturo, T. E., Lori, N. F., Cull, T. S., Akbudak, E., Snyder, A. Z., Shimony, J. S., et al. (1999). Tracking neuronal fiber pathways in the living human brain. *Proceedings of the National Academy of Sciences USA* 96, 10422–10427.

Corbetta, M., & Shulman, G. L. (2002). Control of goal-directed and stimulus-driven attention in the brain. *Nature Reviews Neuroscience* 3, 201–215.

Cormack, A. M. (1963). Representation of a function by its line integrals, with some radiological physics. *Journal of Applied Physics* 34, 2722–2727.

Cormack, A. M. (1973). Reconstruction of densities from their projections, with applications in radiological physics. *Physics in Medicine and Biology* 18(2), 195–207.

Creutzfeldt, O. D. (1975). Neurophysiological correlates of different functional states of the brain. In D. H. Ingvar & N. A. Lassen (Eds.), *Brain Work: The Coupling of Function, Metabolism and Blood Flow in the Brain*, (21–46). Copenhagen: Munksgaard.

Donders, F. C. (1868; 1969). On the speed of mental processes. *Acta Psychologia* 30, 412–431.

Drevets, W. C., Price, J. L., Simpson, J. R., Jr., Todd, R. D., Reich, T., Vannier, M. W., et al. (1997). Subgenual prefrontal cortex abnormalities in mood disorders. *Nature* 386, 824–827.

Duchaine, B. C., Dingle, K., Butterworth, E., & Nakayama, K. (2004). Normal greeble learning in a severe case of developmental prosopagnosia. *Neuron* 43, 469–473.

Fox, P. T., Burton, H., & Raichle, M. E. (1987). Mapping human somatosensory cortex with positron emission tomography. *Journal of Neurosurgery* 67, 34–43.

Fox, P. T., Fox, J. M., Raichle, M. E., & Burde, R. M. (1985). The role of cerebral cortex in the generation of voluntary saccades: A positron emission tomographic study. *Journal of Neurophysiology* 54(2), 348–369.

Fox, P. T., Mintun, M. A., Rieman, E. M., & Raichle, M. E. (1988). Enhanced detection of focal brain responses using intersubject averaging and change-distribution analysis of subtracted PET images. *Journal of Cerebral Blood Flow and Metabolism* 8, 642–653.

Fox, P. T., Perlmutter, J. S., & Raichle, M. E. (1985). A stereotactic method of anatomical localization for positron emission tomography. *Journal of Computer Assisted Tomography* 9(1), 141–153.

Fox, P. T., & Raichle, M. E. (1986). Focal physiological uncoupling of cerebral blood flow and oxidative metabolism during somatosensory stimulation in human subjects. *Proceedings of the National Academy of Sciences USA* 83, 1140–1144.

Fox, P. T., Raichle, M. E., Mintun, M. A., & Dence, C. (1988). Nonoxidative glucose consumption during focal physiologic neural activity. *Science* 241, 462–464.

Frackowiak, R. S. J., Lenzi, G. L., L., Jones, T., & Heather, J. D. (1980). Quantitative measurement of regional cerebral blood flow and oxygen metabolism in man using ^{15}O and positron emission tomography: Theory, procedure, and normal values. *Journal of Assisted Computed Tomography* 4(6), 727–736.

Frahm, J., Bruhn, H., Merboldt, K. D., & Hanicke, W. (1992). Dynamic MR imaging of human brain oxygenation during rest and photic stimulation. *Journal of Magnetic Resonance Imaging* 2(5), 501–505.

Friston, K. J., Frith, C. D., Liddle, P. F., Dolan, R. J., Lammertsma, A. A., & Frackowiak, R. S. J. (1990). The relationship between global and local changes in PET scans. *Journal of Cerebral Blood Flow and Metabolism* 10, 458–466.

Fulton, J. F. (1928). Observations upon the vascularity of the human occipital lobe during visual activity. *Brain* 51, 310–320.

Garey, L. J. (1994). *Brodmann's "Localization in the Cerebral Cortex"* (L. J. Garey, Trans.). London: Smith-Gordon.

Greene, J. D., Sommerville, R. B., Nystrom, L. E., Darley, J. M., & Cohen, J. D. (2001). An fMRI Investigation of Emotional Engagement in Moral Judgment. *Science* 293, 2105–2108.

Grill-Spector, K., Knouf, N., & Kanwisher, N. (2004). The fusiform face area subserves face perception, not generic within-category indentification. *Nature Neuroscience* 7, 555–562.

Gusnard, D. A., Ollinger, J. M., Shulman, G. L., Cloninger, C. R., Price, J. L., Van Essen, D. C., et al. (2003). Persistence and brain circuitry. *Proceedings of the National Academy of Sciences USA* 100, 3479–3484.

Hanson, S. J., Matsuka, T., & Haxby, J. V. (2004). Combinatorial codes in ventral temporal lobe for object recognition: Haxby (2001) revisited: Is there a "face" area? *NeuroImage* 23, 156–166.

Haxby, J. V., Gobbini, M. I., Furey, M. L., Ishai, A., Schouten, J. L., & Pietrini, P. (2001). Distributed and overlapping representations of faces and objects in ventral temporal cortex. *Science* 293, 2425–2430.

Hill, L. (1896). *The Physiology and Pathology of the Cerebral Circulation: An Experimental Research.* London: J. & A. Churchill.

Hounsfield, G. N. (1973). Computerized transverse axial scanning (tomography): Part I. Description of system. *British Journal of Radiology* 46, 1016–1022.

Hyder, F., Rothman, D. L., & Shulman, R. G. (2002). Total neuroenergetics support localized brain activity: Implications for the interpretation of fMRI. *Proceedings of the National Academy of Sciences USA* 99, 10771–10776.

Illes, J., Krischen, M. P., & Gabrieli, J. D. E. (2003). From neuroimaging to neuroethics. *Nature Neuroscience* 6, 205.

Ingvar, D. H., & Risberg, J. (1965). Influence of mental activity upon regional cerebral blood flow in man. *Acta Neurological Scandinavica* supp. 14, 183–186.

James, W. (1890). *Principles of Psychology.* 2 vols. New York: Henry Holt.

Kasischke, K. A., Vishwasrao, H. D., Fisher, P. J., Zipfel, W. R., & Webb, W. W. (2004). Neural activity triggers neuronal oxidative metabolism followed by astrocytic glycolysis. *Science* 305, 99–103.

Kenet, T., Bibitchkov, D., Tsodyks, M., Grinvald, A., & Ariell, A. (2003). Spontaneously emerging cortical representations of visual attributes. *Nature* 425, 954–956.

Kety, S. (1960). Measurement of local blood flow by the exchange on an inert diffusible substance. *Methods of Medical Research* 8, 228–236.

Kety, S. (1965). Closing comments. *Acta Neurological Scandinavica* supp. 14, 197.

Kevles, B. H. (1997). *Naked to the Bone: Medical Imaging in the Twentieth Century.* New Brunswick, NJ: Rutgers University Press.

Koepp, M. J., Gunn, R. N., Lawrence, A. D., Cunningham, V. J., Dagher, A., Jones, T., et al. (1998). Evidence for striatal dopamine release during a video game. *Nature* 393(May 21), 266–268.

Kording, K. P., & Wolpert, D. M. (2004). Bayesian integration in sensorimotor learning. *Nature* 427, 244–247.

Kuhl, P. K. (2003). Human speech and birdsong: Communication and the social brain. *Proceedings of the National Academy of Sciences USA* 100, 9645–9646.

Kwong, K. K., Belliveau, J. W., Chesler, D. A., Goldberg, I. E., Weiskoff, R. M., Poncelet, B. P., et al. (1992). Dynamic magnetic resonance imaging of human brain activity during primary sensory stimulation. *Proceedings of the National Academy of Sciences USA* 89, 5675–5679.

Landau, W. M., Freygang, W. H. J., Roland, L. P., Sokoloff, L., & Kety, S. S. (1955). The local circulation of the living brain: Values in the unanesthetized and anesthetized cat. *Transactions of the American Neurology Association* 80, 125–129.

Lassen, N. A., Hoedt-Rasmussen, K., Sorensen, S. C., Skinhoj, E., Cronquist, B., Bodforss, E., & Ingvar, D. H. (1963). Regional cerebral blood flow in man determined by Krypton-85. *Neurology* 13, 719–727.

Lassen, N. A., Ingvar, D. H., & Skinhoj, E. (1978). Brain function and blood flow. *Scientific American* 239, 62–71.

Laufs, H., Krakow, K., Sterzer, P., Egger, E., Beyerle, A., Salek-Haddadi, A., et al. (2003). Electroencephalographic signatures of attentional and cogntive default modes in spontaneous brain activity fluctuations at rest. *Proceedings of the National Academy of Sciences USA* 100, 11053–11058.

Lauritzen, M. (2001). Relationship of spikes, synaptic activity, and local changes of cerebral blood flow. *Journal of Cerebral Blood Flow and Metabolism* 21(12), 1367–1383.

Lennie, P. (2003). The cost of cortical computation. *Current Biology* 13, 493–497.

Lennox, W. G. (1931). The cerebral circulation: XV. Effect of mental work. *Archives of Neurology and Psychiatry* 26, 725–730.

Llinás, R. (1974). La Forme et la fonction des cellules nerveuses. *La Recherche* 5, 232–240.

Llinás, R. (1988). The intrinsic electrophysiological properties of mammalian neurons: Insights into central nervous system function. *Science* 242, 1654–1664.

Logothetis, N. K. (2003). The underpinnings of the BOLD functional magnetic resonance imaging signal. *Journal of Neuroscience* 23, 3963–3971.

Logothetis, N. K., Pauls, J., Augath, M., Trinath, T., & Oeltermann, A. (2001). Neurophysiological investigation of the basis of the fMRI signal. *Nature* 412, 150–157.

Madsen, P. L., Hasselbalch, S. G., Hagemann, L. P., Olsen, K. S., Bulow, J., Holm, S., et al. (1995). Persistent resetting of the cerebral oxygen/glucose uptake ratio by brain activation: Evidence obtained with the Kety-Schmidt technique. *Journal of Cerebral Blood Flow and Metabolism* 15, 485–491.

Magistretti, P. J., Pellerin, L., Rothman, D. L., & Shulman, R. G. (1999). Energy on demand. *Science* 283, 496–497.

Marder, E., & Weimann, J. M. (1991). Modulatory control of multiple task processing in the stomatogastric nervous system. In J. Kien, C. McCrohan, & B. Winlow (Eds.), *Neurobiology of Motor Program Selection: New Approaches to Mechanisms of Behavioral Choice*, 3–19. Manchester, UK: Manchester University Press.

Mayberg, H. S., Liotti, M., Brannan, S. K., McGinnis, S., Mahurin, R. K., Jerabek, P. A., et al. (1999). Reciprocal limbic-cortical function and negative mood: Converging PET findings in depression and normal sadness. *American Journal of Psychiatry* 156, 675–682.

McClure, S. M., Laibson, D. I., Loewenstein, G., & Cohen, J. D. (2004). Separate neural systems value immediate and delayed monetary rewards. *Science* 306, 503–507.

McKinstry, R. C., Mathur, A., Miller, J. H., Ozcan, A., Snyder, A. Z., Schefft, G. L., et al. (2002). Radial organization of developing preterm human cerebral cortex revealed by non-invasive water diffusion anisotropy MRI. *Cerebral Cortex* 12, 1237–1243.

Meltzoff, A. N., & Decety, J. (2003). What imitation tells us about social cognition: A rapprochement between developmental psychology and cognitive neuroscience. *Philosophical Transactions of the Royal Society of London* B 358, 491–500.

Mintun, M. A., Raichle, M. E., Martin, W. R., & Herscovitch, P. (1984). Brain oxygen utilization measured with O-15 radiotracers and positron emission tomography. *Journal of Nuclear Medicine* 25(2), 177–187.

Moll, J., de Oliveira-Souza, R., Eslinger, P. J., Bramati, I. E., Mourao-Miranda, J., Andreiuolo, P. A., et al. (2002). The neural correlates of moral sensitivity: A functional magnetic resonance imaging investigation of basic and moral emotions. *Journal of Neuroscience* 22, 2730–2736.

Mosso, A. (1881). *Ueber den Kreislauf des Blutes im menschlichen Gehirn*. Leipzig: Verlag von Veit.

Nichols, M. J., & Newsome, W. T. (1999). The neurobiology of cognition. *Nature* 402, C35–C38.

Ogawa, S., Lee, T. M., Kay, A. R., & Tank, D. W. (1990). Brain magnetic resonance imaging with contrast depedent on blood oxygenation. *Proceedings of the National Academy of Sciences USA* 87, 9868–9872.

Ogawa, S., Tank, D. W., Menon, R., Ellermann, J. M., Kim, S. G., Merkle, H., & Ubergil, K. (1992). Instrinsic signal changes accompanying sensory stimulation: Functional brain mapping with magnetic resonance imaging. *Proceedings of the National Academy of Sciences USA* 89, 5951–5955.

Olshausen, B. A. (2003). Principles of image representation in visual cortex. In L. M. Chalupa & J. S. Werner (Eds.), *The Visual Neurosciences*, 1603–1615. Cambridge, MA: MIT Press.

Öngür, D., Ferry, A. T., & Price, J. L. (2003). Architectonic subdivisions of the human orbital and medial prefontal cortex. *Journal of Comparative Neurology* 460, 425–449.

Pauling, L., & Coryell, C. D. (1936). The magnetic properties and structure of hemoglobin, oxyhemoglobin and carbonmonoxyhemoglobin. *Proceedings of the National Academy of Sciences USA* 22, 210–216.

Pellerin, L., & Magistretti, P. J. (1994). Glutamate uptake into astrocytes stimulates aerobic glycolysis: A mechanism coupling neuronal activity to glucose utilization. *Proceedings of the National Academy of Sciences USA* 91, 10625–10629.

Petersen, S. E., Fox, P. T., Posner, M. I., Mintun, M., & Raichle, M. E. (1988). Positron emission tomographic studies of the cortical anatomy of single-word processing. *Nature* 331, 585–589.

Petersen, S. E., Fox, P. T., Posner, M. I., Mintun, M. A., & Raichle, M. E. (1989). Positron emission tomographic studies of the processing of single words. *Journal of Cognitive Neuroscience* 1, 153–170.

Phelps, M. E., Hoffman, E. J., Coleman, R. E., Welch, M. J., Raichle, M. E., Weiss, E. S., et al. (1976). Tomographic images of blood pool and perfusion in brain and heart. *Journal of Nuclear Medicine* 17(7), 603–612.

Posner, M. I. (1978). *Chronometric Explorations of Mind*. Englewood Cliffs, NJ: Lawrence Erlbaum Associates.

Posner, M. I. (2003). Imaging a science of mind. *Trends in Cognitive Sciences* 7, 450–453.

Posner, M. I., & Raichle, M. E. (1994). *Images of Mind*. New York: W.H. Freeman.

Prinz, A. A., Bucher, D., & Marder, E. (2004). Similar network activity from disparate circuit parameters. *Nature Neuroscience* 7, 1345–1352.

Raichle, M. E. (1987). Circulatory and metabolic correlates of brain function in normal humans. In F. Plum (Ed.), *Handbook of Physiology: The Nervous System*. Vol. 5, *Higher Functions of the Brain*, 643–674. Bethesda, MD: American Physiological Society.

Raichle, M. E. (1998). Behind the sceues of functional brain imaging: A historical and physiological perspective. *Proceedings of the National Academy of Sciences USA* 95, 765–772.

Raichle, M. E. (2000). A brief history of human functional brain mapping. In A. W. Toga & J. C. Mazziotta (Eds.), *Brain Mapping: The Systems*, 33–75. San Diego: Academic Press.

Raichle, M. E. (2003a). Functional brain imaging and human brain function (miniseries). *Journal of Neuroscience* 23, 3959–3962.

Raichle, M. E. (2003b). Social neuroscience: A role for brain imaging. *Political Psychology* 24, 759–764.

Raichle, M. E., Martin, W. R., Herscovitch, P., Mintun, M. A., & Markham, J. (1983). Brain blood flow measured with intravenous $H_2^{15}O$. II. Implementation and validation. *Journal of Nuclear Medicine* 24(9), 790–798.

Reivich, M., Kuhl, D., Wolf, A., Greenberg, J., Phelps, M., Ido, T., et al. (1979). The [^{18}F] fluorodeoxyglucose method for the measurement of local cerebral glucose utilization in man. *Circulation Research* 44, 127–137.

Ress, D., Backus, B. T., & Heeger, D. J. (2000). Activity in primary visual cortex predicts performance in a visual detection task. *Nature Neuroscience* 3, 940–945.

Roland, P. E., Eriksson, L., Stone-Elander, S., & Widen, L. (1987). Does mental activity change the oxidative metabolism of the brain? *Journal of Neuroscience* 7, 2373–2389.

Roy, C. S., & Sherrington, C. S. (1890). On the regulation of the blood supply of the brain. *Journal of Physiology* London, 11, 85–108.

Schwartz, W. J., Smith, C. B., Davidsen, L., Savaki, H., Sokoloff, L., Mata, M., et al. (1979). Metabolic mapping of functional activity in the hypothalamo-neurohypophysial system of the rat. *Science* 205, 723–725.

Sherrington, C. (1906). *The Integrative Action of the Nervous System.* New Haven: Yale University Press.

Shmuel, A., Augath, M., Oeltermann, A., Pauls, J., Murayama, Y., & Logothetis, N. K. (2003). *The negative BOLD response in monkey V1 is associated with decreases in neuronal activity.* Paper presented at the Organization for Human Brain Mapping, New York City.

Shulman, G. L., Fiez, J. A., Corbetta, M., Buckner, R. L., Miezin, F. M., Raichle, M. E., & Petersen, S. E. (1997). Common blood flow changes across visual tasks: II. Decreases in cerebral cortex. *Journal of Cognitive Neuroscience* 9, 648–663.

Shulman, R. G., Hyder, F., & Rothman, D. L. (2001). Cerebral energetics and the glycogen shunt: Neurochemical basis of functional imaging. *Proceedings of the National Academy of Sciences USA* 98, 6417–6422.

Sibson, N. R., Dhankhar, A., Mason, G. F., Behar, K. L., Rothman, D. L., & Shulman, R. G. (1997). In vivo ^{13}C NMR measurements of cerebral glutamate synthesis as evidence for glutamate-glutamine cycling. *Proceedings of the National Academy of Sciences USA* 94, 2699–2704.

Sibson, N. R., Dhankhar, A., Mason, G. F., Rothman, D. L., Behar, K. L., & Shulman, R. G. (1998). Stoichiometric coupling of brain glucose metabolism and glutamatergic neuronal activity. *Proceedings of the National Academy of Sciences USA* 95, 316–321.

Siesjo, B. K. (1978). *Brain Energy Metabolism.* New York: Wiley.

Simpson, J. R. J., Drevets, W. C., Snyder, A. Z., Gusnard, D. A., & Raichle, M. E. (2001). Emotion-induced changes in human medial prefrontal cortex: II. During anticipatory anxiety. *Proceedings of the National Academy of Sciences USA* 98, 688–691.

Sokoloff, L., Mangold, R., Wechsler, R., Kennedy, C., & Kety, S. S. (1955). The effect of mental arithmetic on cerebral circulation and metabolism. *Journal of Clinical Investigation* 34, 1101–1108.

Sokoloff, L., Reivich, M., Kennedy, C., Des Rosiers, M. H., Patlak, C. S., Pettigrew, K. D., et al. (1977). The [^{14}C]deoxyglucose method for the measurement of local glucose utilization: Theory, procedure and normal values in the conscious and anesthetized albino rat. *Journal of Neurochemistry* 28, 897–916.

Ter-Pogossian, M. M., Phelps, M. E., Hoffman, E. J., & Mullani, N. A. (1975). A positron-emission tomography for nuclear imaging (PET). *Radiology* 114, 89–98.

Thulborn, K. R., Waterton, J. C., Matthews, P. M., & Radda, G. K. (1982). Oxygenation dependence of the transverse relaxation time of water protons in whole blood at high field. *Biochimica et Biophysica Acta* 714, 265–270.

Ueki, M., Linn, F., & Hossmann, K.-A. (1988). Functional activation of cerebral blood flow and metabolism before and after global ischemia of rat brain. *Journal of Cerebral Blood Flow and Metabolism* 8, 486–494.

Uttal, W. R. (2001). *The New Phrenology.* Cambridge, MA: MIT Press.

Webb, S. (1990). *From the watching of Shadows.* New York: Adam Hilger.

Woolsey, T. A., Rovainen, C. M., Cox, S. B., Henegar, M. H., Liang, G. E., Liu, D., et al. (1996). Neuronal units linked to microvascular modules in cerebral cortex: Response elements for imaging the brain. *Cerebral Cortex* 6(5), 647–660.

2   Functional Neuroimaging: Basic Principles of Functional MRI

Allen W. Song, Scott A. Huettel, and Gregory McCarthy

Introduction

An understanding of the physical and physiological origins of functional magnetic resonance imaging (fMRI) is critical for the effective design and analysis of experiments. The origins of fMRI, like those of MRI itself, rest on the twin foundations of nuclear magnetic resonance and image formation. But, for images to provide information about *function*, there must be a physiological marker of neuronal activity that is measurable by MRI. Such a marker was identified in 1990 with the discovery that the signal intensity of some forms of MR images was decreased in the presence of paramagnetic deoxygenated blood. This phenomenon, now known as blood-oxygenation-level-dependent (BOLD) contrast, forms the basis for nearly all fMRI studies.

In this chapter, we will first discuss how the MRI signal is generated, using a combination of strong static magnetic fields and brief electromagnetic pulses, followed by how that signal is modulated across space, using magnetic field gradients. Then, we will consider how neuronal activity evokes local metabolic demands that in turn alter the amount of deoxygenated hemoglobin present in nearby blood vessels. We will integrate the physics and physiology by describing the changes in BOLD contrast measurable on T_2*-weighted MR images and the pulse sequences used to collect those images.

Following the introduction of these core concepts, we will turn to a set of key topics that guide much current research into fMRI methodology. In many ways, the idea of fMRI as a single technique is misleading: there are almost as many approaches to the collection of fMRI data as there are researchers in the field. And, as improvements are made in scanner hardware, pulse sequences, and experimental design, even the most central concepts may change. We therefore highlight selected advances, both well-established and speculative, that promise to allow new research questions to be addressed by fMRI.

Basic Principles of Functional MRI

Principles of fMRI

Consider one atom of hydrogen, which consists of a single proton. Under normal conditions, thermal energy causes the proton to spin about itself. Because the proton carries a positive charge, its spinning motion generates a current, which in turn induces a magnetic field and, subsequently, a magnetic moment. Because the proton has an odd atomic mass, its spinning also generates angular momentum. Both a magnetic moment and angular momentum, as present in ^{1}H, ^{13}C, ^{19}F, ^{23}Na, and ^{31}P, are necessary for a nucleus to be measurable using MRI. Such nuclei are commonly known as spins, and a collection of them in a volume is known as a spin system. However, nearly all MRI measures characteristics of hydrogen nuclei, which are by far the most common in the human body, and we will restrict our discussion to single protons of hydrogen (typically in water molecules) hereafter.

Typical clinical MRI scanners have magnetic fields of about 1.5 to 3 Tesla (i.e., 30,000 to 60,000 times as strong as the earth's magnetic field), and newer scanners dedicated to human fMRI can have field strengths of 7 Tesla or higher (figure 2.1). In the absence of any strong magnetic field, hydrogen spins within the body are oriented randomly, and their magnetic moments and angular momenta tend to cancel each other out. However, in the presence of the strong magnetic field of the scanner (figure 2.2), spins will align either parallel to that field (i.e., in a low-energy state) or anti-parallel to that field (i.e., in a high-energy state). Because slightly more spins align in the low-energy state, there is greater magnetization in the parallel direction than in the antiparallel direction. This small but significant difference results in a net magnetization (M) parallel to the main magnetic field of the scanner.

We can think of the net magnetization as a vector with two components: a longitudinal component parallel to the magnetic field and a transverse component perpendicular to the magnetic field. The longitudinal component of the net magnetization depends upon the difference between the number of the spins in the parallel and anti-parallel states, which reflects several factors, most importantly the strength of the external magnetic field (B).

To understand the transverse component of the net magnetization, it is important to recognize that spins in a spin system are not static. Instead, they undergo a gyroscopic motion known as precession, as shown in figure 2.1. To understand precession, imagine a spinning top on a desk. The top does not spin perfectly upright; instead,

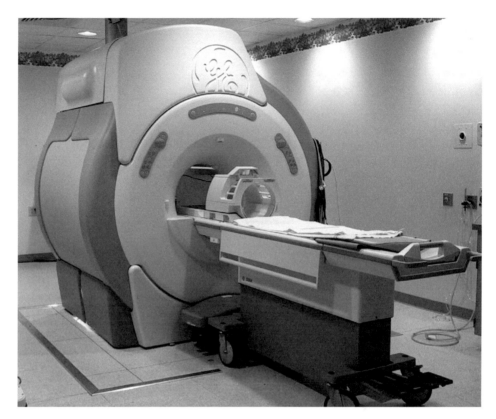

Figure 2.1
A modern MRI scanner. The main magnetic field of the scanner shown is 1.5 Tesla, about 30,000 times the strength of the earth's magnetic field. The subject lies on the table at the front of the scanner, with the head inside the volume coil at the center of the image. The table then moves into the bore of the scanner until the head is positioned at the very center.

its axis of rotation traces a circle perpendicular to the earth's gravitational field. At any moment in time the top is tilted from the vertical, but it does not fall. Why does the top spin at an angle? Spinning objects respond to applied forces by moving their axes in a direction perpendicular to the applied force. A bicycle, for example, is very stable at high speeds because of the gyroscopic effects of its spinning wheels, and resists falling over. In fact, if a rider leans to one side, the moving bicycle will not fall, but will instead turn in that direction. Similarly, a spinning top turns its axis of rotation at an angle perpendicular to the force exerted by gravity, so that the top precesses in a circle around a vertical axis.

Protons in a magnetic field behave analogously to spinning tops in a gravitational field, precessing about the axis of the magnetic field, with the angle determined by

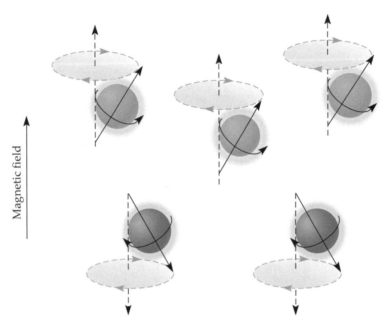

Magnetic field

Figure 2.2
Protons precessing in high and low energy states. Protons in an external magnetic field assume one of two possible states: the parallel state (light), which has a lower energy level, and the antiparallel state (dark), which has a higher energy level. There always will be more protons in the parallel state than in the antiparallel state. Regardless of state, protons precess around the main axis of the magnetic field at a frequency determined by the field strength.

their angular momentum and the frequency determined by the strength of the magnetic field. Because of the enormous number of spins with even the smallest volume, under normal conditions the transverse components are evenly distributed and cancel out, so that only the longitudinal components are present. However, if energy is applied to the spins so that they precess in synchrony, their individual transverse components will not cancel, and the net magnetization of the entire spin system will precess around the main axis of the magnetic field. This concept, known as spin excitation, has important consequences for MRI.

Spin Excitation

While the main magnet of the MRI scanner is necessary to create the net magnetization, a second component—an excitation/reception coil—is required to measure changes in the net magnetization. Because spins within a magnetic field can take either high or low energy states, changes between those states involve the absorption or emission of energy (figure 2.3). To cause spins to change from low to high energy

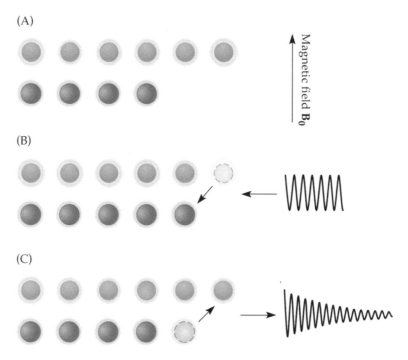

Figure 2.3
Change between states due to absorption or transmission of energy. When spins are placed in an external magnetic field (*A*), more will be at the low energy state (light) than at the high energy state (dark). During excitation, the MRI scanner applies a magnetic field that oscillates at the precession frequency of the spins of interest (as shown at right in *B*). This field is known as an excitation pulse or a radiofrequency pulse, because the precession frequency is in the radio range of the electromagnetic spectrum. Because of the match between pulse frequency and spin frequency, some spins will absorb energy from the excitation pulse and jump to the higher energy state (*B*). But after the excitation pulse ceases, some of the spins in the higher energy state will return to the lower energy state (*C*). When they do so, they release the absorbed energy as a radio frequency wave that decays over time.

states, coils within the scanner irradiate the spin system with electromagnetic fields (i.e., collections of photons) whose frequency is calibrated to the energy difference between the states. This process is known as excitation, and the energy delivery is known as an excitation pulse. Because excitation disrupts the thermal equilibrium of a spin system, when the irradiation ceases, the excess nuclei at the higher energy state return to the lower energy state by releasing electromagnetic energy. The resulting MR signal can be measured as a change in voltage in the same electromagnetic coils, in a process known as reception. Because the emitted and absorbed electromagnetic fields oscillate in the radio frequency range, the generating equipment is often called radiofrequency coils.

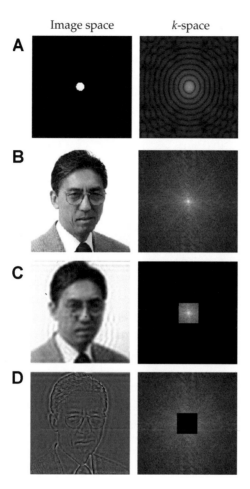

Figure 2.4
Image space and k-space. In (A) a single circle at the center of image space and the representation of that circle in k-space are shown. The k-space representation follows a *sinc* function, with greatest intensity at the center and intensity bands of decreasing amplitude toward the edges of k-space. Any image, no matter how complex, can be represented in the spatial frequency domain of k-space (B). Different portions of k-space contribute differently to the resulting image. The center of k-space contains most of the image intensity, in the form of low-frequency components. Thus, using only the center of k-space would result in a blurred version of the image (C). In contrast, the periphery of k-space contains high-frequency components (D).

Image Formation

After the generation of MR signal, the next critical step is to use that signal to differentiate between tissues that have different characteristics. In the context of MRI, an *image* is a map that illustrates the spatial distribution of some spin property within the sample. To create images, a third component of the MRI scanner is required: coils to generate magnetic field gradients. As first demonstrated by the Nobel laureate Paul Lauterbur, the superimposition of a magnetic field that varies linearly across space will cause spins at different locations to precess at different frequencies in a controlled fashion (Lauterbur, 1973). By measuring changes in magnetization as a function of precession frequency, the total MR signal can be parsed into components associated with different frequencies.

A primary use of magnetic field gradients is slice selection. If a magnetic field gradient is activated perpendicular to the plane of the slices (e.g., for axial slices, a vertical or z-direction gradient is required), spins will show a corresponding gradient in their precession frequencies. For example, a positive gradient parallel to the main magnetic field will cause spins near the top of the brain to precess more rapidly than those near the bottom of the brain. One can then tailor an excitation pulse to the band of frequencies that correspond to a specific slice in space. It is important to note that all spins within a slice are excited simultaneously, so that they all contribute to the MR signal.

Magnetic field gradients are also used to distinguish the contributions of spins from different spatial locations within a slice. To do so, gradient magnetic fields that vary in two dimensions are applied. These fields change the strength of the magnetic field at different locations, so that some spins precess at a faster rate and others at a slower rate. The MR signal collected in this way can be reorganized into a coordinate system known as k-space.

Despite its importance, k-space is one of the most difficult-to-grasp concepts in MRI, and thus we will introduce it first by analogy. Imagine listening to the sound of a tuning fork after it is struck. The sound you hear comes from rapid changes in air pressure that cause your eardrum to vibrate at a fixed frequency. For example, if the tuning fork was at "middle A" you would hear a note with fundamental frequency of 440 Hz. If we wanted to represent this sound graphically, we could do so in two ways. One way is to plot the air pressure at your eardrum over time, resulting in a sine wave that oscillates at 440 Hz. A second approach would be to plot the frequencies contained within the sound, showing that it has power at 440 Hz but not at any other frequency. While this example is purposefully simplified, it conveys the key idea that any time-varying signal (e.g., a sound) can be expressed as a collection of frequencies, and vice versa. To convert a signal from its frequency expression to its time expression, a mathematical technique known as the Fourier transform is required, and to convert it back from time to frequency, one must use an inverse Fourier transform.

This equivalence can be extended into two dimensions as well, so that images can be represented by sets of *spatial* frequencies. Just as power at a temporal frequency is given by a sine wave that oscillates in time, power at a spatial frequency is given by a sine grating that oscillates across space. By adding together gratings of different frequency (and phase and intensity), we can construct any image, no matter how complex, using a two-dimensional inverse fourier transform (figure 2.4). Now, why is this fact important for fMRI? Recall that the application of magnetic gradients, as used in fMRI, causes the phase of the precessing spins within a slice to vary over space. Spins that experience a strong additive gradient increase their precession speed more than spins that experience a weak gradient. The results of applying linear gradients, therefore, are grating patterns of spin phase across space—perfect building blocks for constructing an image via an inverse fourier transform. These building blocks (and thus the associated gradients) are represented mathematically in k-space. As will be discussed later in the chapter, the order in which different parts of k-space are sampled has important consequences for fMRI studies.

Image Contrast: T_1, T_2, T_2*

By placing spins in a strong magnetic field to generate net magnetization, tipping the net magnetization using excitation pulses, and introducing gradient magnetic fields to change precession frequency over space, one can generate an image of MR signal intensity. For that signal to be interpretable, however, the images must be made sensitive to a particular form of contrast. In the terminology of MRI, *contrast* refers to how well we can make distinctions between substances with different properties. The power of MRI is that it can be used to collect images using an extraordinarily wide range of contrasts compared with other methods for neuroimaging (figure 2.5). For anatomical MRI, images can be collected that have contrast based upon the type, number, and/or relaxation properties (e.g., T_1, T_2) of atomic nuclei within a voxel. For most fMRI imaging, images are collected that are sensitive to T_2* contrast (which was introduced earlier in the chapter).

To change the form of contrast to which our images are sensitive, we can alter two aspects of the data collection process: the interval between successive excitation pulses (repetition time, or TR) and the interval between the excitation pulse and data acquisition (echo time, or TE). These parameters have important effects on the amount of MR signal recorded. If we make TR very short (e.g., much less than T_1 for a given tissue), there will be relatively little recovery of the longitudinal magnetization, but if we make TR very long, there will be full longitudinal recovery.

(A)   (B)

(C)   (D)

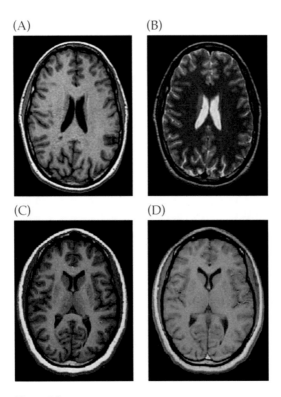

Figure 2.5
Contrast and contrast-to-noise in MR images. Shown at top are images sensitive to two different contrast types. At top left (A) is an image sensitive to T_1 contrast, and at top right (B) is an image sensitive to T_2 contrast. Note that although much of the same brain structure is present in both images, the relative intensities of different tissue types are very different. At bottom are two images with the same contrast type but different contrast-to-noise ratios. The image at bottom left (C) has very high contrast to noise, and significant detail can be seen in the image. The image at bottom right (D) has lower contrast to noise, and some distinctions, such as the boundary between gray and white matter, are more difficult to identify.

Similarly, TE influences the amount of transverse decay that occurs between excitation and data acquisition.

By varying the TR or TE under which images are collected, the image intensity at each point in space can be made more or less sensitive to T_1 or T_2 differences among tissues. For example, if we collect an image with an intermediate TR and a very short TE, then tissues with smaller T_1 values (e.g., white matter) will recover more than tissues with longer T_1 values (e.g., gray matter), and thus their intensity will be brighter on the image. But because TE is very short, there will be little time for decay of transverse magnetization, and T_2 differences between tissues would not affect the images. Conversely, if a long TR and medium TE are used, the longitudinal magnetization will recover fully for all tissues (so that T_1 values will not affect the images), but differences in T_2 will influence the rate at which transverse magnetization is lost. Such images would be sensitive to T_2 but not T_1.

While T_1 and T_2 are important parameters for anatomical MRI, a third parameter called T_2* is most critical for functional MRI. Like T_2, T_2* expresses the rate of change of transverse magnetization. However, it includes an additional factor associated with inhomogeneities in the local magnetic field that cause changes in spin precession frequency. Quantitatively, the relationship between T_2 and T_2* is given by $1/T_2* = 1/T_2 + 1/T_2'$, where T_2' reflects the field inhomogeneity effect. As will be discussed in the next section, the homogeneity of the local magnetic field within a brain voxel is influenced by the amount of deoxygenated hemoglobin present, so T_2* imaging is of particular importance for fMRI.

Discovery of BOLD Contrast

To a first approximation, information processing within the brain depends upon the electrical activity of neurons. Thus, to assess changes in brain function, we must use a measure that indexes neuronal activity. One possible approach is to measure this activity directly, using electrodes that can measure changes in voltage in neurons' axons or dendrites. Direct measurements by placing electrodes in or adjacent to individual neurons are called single-unit recordings, and have been invaluable for mapping cognitive processes in nonhuman animals for more than a century. However, implanting electrodes inside the brain is obviously an invasive procedure, so it has been limited in humans to individuals with clinical needs for the electrodes (e.g., to measure epileptiform activity). For most human electrophysiological studies, therefore, electrical or electromagnetic activity is measured by using detectors outside the surface of the scalp, resulting in severe limitations on spatial resolution.

Because of the limitations of direct electrical measurement, scientists have adopted a second approach, namely to assess neuronal activity *indirectly* by measuring its metabolic correlates. For example, positron emission tomography (PET), which became prominent in the 1980s and was the first imaging technique that could be used in normal human subjects, measures the local quantities of radioactively labeled glucose, oxygen, or other metabolites. Though not requiring implantation of electrodes, PET is still considered an invasive technique because compounds that emit ionizing radiation must be injected into the body before each scan. Of great interest to researchers, therefore, would be metabolic changes in the brain that could be measured without such invasive procedures.

One such metabolic change was suggested in 1936 by the chemists Linus Pauling and Charles Coryell, who studied the magnetic properties of hemoglobin, the oxygen-carrying molecule within red blood cells (Pauling & Coryell, 1936). They found that oxygenated hemoglobin is diamagnetic, meaning that it does not affect the strength of the surrounding magnetic field. However, deoxygenated hemoglobin was found to be paramagnetic, so that it distorts local magnetic fields. This reduces T_2^* values, as demonstrated decades later by Thulborn and colleagues (Thulborn et al., 1982). Thus, if blood oxygenation varies spatially according to brain function, then that spatial variation should be measurable using MRI.

This idea was tested experimentally by Seiji Ogawa and colleagues, who scanned anesthetized rodents using high field MRI (Ogawa et al., 1990). To manipulate blood oxygenation, they changed the proportion of oxygen that the rodent breathed. When the rodents were breathing 100% oxygen, T_2^* images of their brains showed structural differences but few blood vessels. But as the proportion of oxygen was reduced, the images took on a very different character. Thin, dark lines became visible throughout the cerebral cortex, usually perpendicular to its surface. To verify that these changes in the brain resulted from effects of magnetic field inhomogeneities, Ogawa et al. filled test tubes with oxygenated or deoxygenated blood, placed them in a saline-filled container, and took T_2^*-weighted images. The image of the oxygenated blood was a black circle of the tube's diameter, because the blood had a shorter T_2^* than the surrounding saline. However, the image of the deoxygenated blood had a much larger area of signal loss that extended well into the surrounding saline.

Ogawa and colleagues speculated that this finding, which would come to be called blood-oxygenation-level-dependent (BOLD) contrast, could enable measurement of functional changes in brain activity. Although it seems reasonable that increased neuronal activity would result in increased oxygen consumption, and thus decreased BOLD signal, as Ogawa and colleagues originally hypothesized, the opposite actually occurs. To understand why neuronal activity results in this paradoxical increase in deoxygenated blood, we must next consider the physiological changes that link neuronal activity to vascular changes in the brain.

Physiological Basis for BOLD Contrast

The energy that supports neuronal activity comes from oxygen and glucose. One might expect that the vascular supply of these metabolites is tightly coupled to their demand, such that oxygen and glucose metabolism is proportional to neuronal activity. This coupling was tested in an influential series of PET experiments by Fox, Raichle, and their colleagues (Fox et al., 1988), who measured cerebral blood flow (CBF), cerebral metabolic rate for glucose (CMR_{glu}), and cerebral metabolic rate for oxygen ($CMRO_2$) during rest and during visual stimulation. They found that when subjects were exposed to prolonged visual stimulation, presumably resulting in increased neuronal activity, CBF in visual cortex increased by 50% and CMR_{glu} increased by 51%. However, $CMRO_2$ increased by only a few percent. A number of subsequent studies have found similar uncoupling between glucose metabolism and oxygen consumption, although the disparity has not always been quite as dramatic.

But while there is general agreement on these facts, their interpretation is still controversial. One potential consequence of reduced $CMRO_2$ compared with CMR_{glu} is that some of the increase in glucose metabolism could be achieved through nonoxidative means; that is, through anaerobic glycolysis. Though rapid, anaerobic glycolysis is extremely inefficient compared with aerobic glycolysis and produces much less energy from each molecule of glucose. Support for this interpretation has come from studies by two groups which suggest that increased release of glutamate by active neurons stimulates rapid anaerobic glycolysis in adjacent astrocytes (Shulman & Rothman, 1998; Magistretti & Pellerin, 1999; Shulman et al., 2001). The energy generated by this process removes the glutamate from the extracellular space near synapses, preventing its potentially toxic effects upon postsynaptic membranes.

Another possible (and nonexclusive) interpretation is that the changes in metabolism accompanying neuronal activity reflect a different form of decoupling, such that blood flow is poorly matched to neuronal demands. To test this idea, Malonek, Grinvald, and their colleagues have used high-resolution optical imaging methods in which the surface of visual cortex in the cat is exposed to a light source, and the reflected light is analyzed (Malonek & Grinvald, 1996). Then, by stimulating visual cortex using line gratings of particular orientations, the concentrations of oxygenated and deoxygenated hemoglobin could be measured. Not surprisingly, the concentration of deoxygenated hemoglobin increased for the first several seconds, and then decreased thereafter, reflecting the initial demands of neuronal activity. More striking were the changes in oxygenated hemoglobin, for which there was a large and spatially extensive increase in concentration. These results indicate, somewhat paradoxically, that neuronal activity evokes a coarse vascular response that overcompensates for metabolic demands. In a sense, even if only a small region is active for a short time period, the vascular system supplies oxygen to a larger surrounding region for a longer period of time.

This latter finding, combined with demonstrations that following stimulation, blood flow increases more than blood volume (Mandeville et al., 1999), provides a clear account of BOLD fMRI hemodynamics. As the excess oxygenated blood flows through active regions, it flushes the deoxygenated hemoglobin from the capillaries supporting the active neural tissue and from the downstream venules. Thus, an increase in BOLD signal following neuronal activity occurs not because the oxygenated hemoglobin increases the MR signal, but because it displaces the deoxygenated hemoglobin that had been suppressing the MR signal (figure 2.6, plate 1). When neuronal activity and the corresponding metabolic demand cease, blood flow

(A)

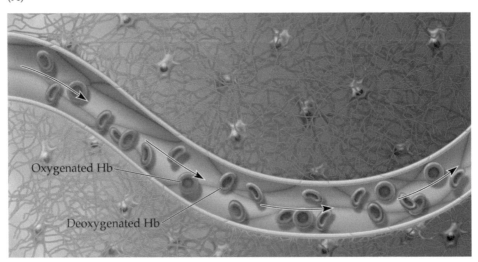

(B)

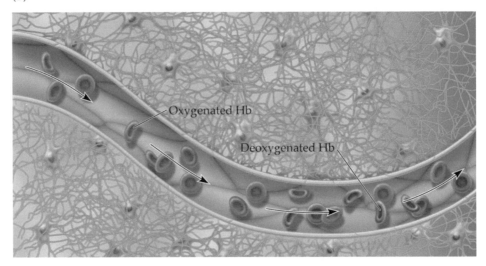

Figure 2.6
Summary of BOLD signal generation. Under normal conditions, oxygenated hemoglobin is converted to deoxygenated hemoglobin at a constant rate within the capillary bed (*A*). However, when neurons become active, there is an increase in the supply of oxygenated hemoglobin above that needed by the neurons. This results in a relative decrease in the amount of deoxygenated hemoglobin (*B*) and a corresponding decrease in the signal loss due to T_2^* effects. The fMRI signal thus increases in areas of neuronal activity. See plate 1 for color version.

decreases more rapidly than blood volume. While blood flow is near normal levels but blood volume remains elevated, more deoxygenated hemoglobin will be present in a given brain region. Thus, the overall fMRI signal will be reduced below baseline levels, in what is known as the poststimulus undershoot.

Pulse Sequences

So far, we have described a physiological phenomenon, changes in amount of deoxygenated hemoglobin, that can be measured using T_2* MRI. To measure efficiently, researchers must employ pulse sequences (i.e., sets of instructions for the MRI scanner) that can measure T_2* changes with appropriate spatial and temporal resolution. For comparison, the first human MR images were collected using an extraordinarily slow process in which each voxel was collected individually by moving the subject. This rate is far too slow for even anatomical imaging, in that a single low-resolution image could take many hours to acquire, and thus early researchers investigated new methods for collecting clinical MRI data. Peter Mansfield, who shared the 2003 Nobel Prize in medicine with Paul Lauterbur, led the development of a technique called echo-planar imaging or EPI (Mansfield and Maudsley, 1977). In EPI an entire slice is collected using rapid gradient switching following a single excitation. It is worth noting that although EPI was intended to solve a clinical problem, it has been relatively unimportant for clinical MRI but critical for the development of functional MRI.

The basic EPI pulse sequence has changed little since its development by Mansfield (figure 2.7a, b; plate 2). To discuss the properties of EPI—or any type of pulse sequence—we must return to the idea of k-space introduced briefly earlier in this chapter. To collect an image, therefore, one must manipulate the scanner's gradients to collect points throughout k-space (e.g., spatial frequency gratings that can be used to build an image). One strategy for doing this is to excite a slice, then collect a few k-space points, excite the slice again, collect a few more points, and so on, incrementally building an image. Mansfield's insight was that all of the k-space data could be collected following a single excitation pulse. In the EPI framework he devised, k-space data is collected in a back-and-forth pattern that rapidly cycles the directions of the scanner's gradient coils. A single EPI image could be acquired within only a few tens of milliseconds. This speed of acquisition stimulated the growth of fMRI two decades later, since it allowed researchers to balance spatial coverage with temporal resolution: data from the entire brain could be collected every few seconds.

While still enormously important for fMRI, EPI does have some disadvantages. Its back-and-forth approach heavily taxes the gradient hardware, since different sets of gradients must be cycled on and off to enable the 90° turns in the k-space. It is

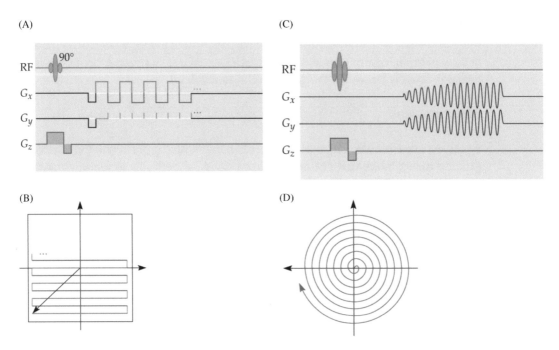

Figure 2.7
Pulse sequences used in fMRI. Most common for fMRI are pulse sequences using echo-planar imaging (EPI). In an EPI pulse sequence (*A*), the spatial gradients are rapidly cycled on and off in a stair-step pattern following the initial excitation pulse. This results in a back-and-forth trajectory through *k*-space (*B*). Pulse sequences used in fMRI. Recently developed spiral imaging sequences use sinusoidally changing gradients (*C*) to generate a curving path through *k*-space (*B*). See plate 2 for color version.

also inefficient, in that data collected while transitioning from one line of *k*-space to another is not used in the image creation process. To overcome these limitations, researchers have developed a new family of spiral pulse sequences that utilize a very different trajectory in *k*-space (figure 2.7c, d). Spiral pulse sequences use sinusoidal changes in the gradients to trace a corkscrew path through *k*-space, typically beginning at the center and winding outward to the periphery. Because there are no right angles in the *k*-space path, spiral imaging can be much less taxing on a gradient system and can reduce the time needed to collect an image. Furthermore, all points sampled along the spiral trajectory are used for reconstructing the final image, improving the efficiency of the acquisition. A disadvantage of spiral imaging is that the *k*-space data do not follow a Cartesian grid. This necessitates an additional step in which the acquired data points are resampled back onto a Cartesian grid, so that a Fourier transform can be used to reconstruct the image. A variant known as inverse spiral imaging begins at the periphery of *k*-space and winds inward to the center, which can further improve the throughput (i.e., number of slices acquired per second).

To summarize what has been discussed so far, we have outlined the basic principles of fMRI through a small set of key concepts. For collection of MR images, three things are necessary: a strong static magnet to align spins (e.g., protons) and generate net magnetization due to their common precession, an excitation/reception coil to send energy (electromagnetic waves) into the sample (e.g., the brain) and measure the return of that energy over time, and weaker magnetic gradients to change the precession frequency across space and gather spatial information. One type of image, T_2* contrast, is sensitive to differences in magnetic field homogeneity, allowing physiological properties that alter magnetic homogeneity to be measured. Such a property is the amount of deoxygenated hemoglobin, which is an indirect measure of neuronal activity. Finally, by using pulse sequences that permit rapid collection of images, researchers can measure changes in deoxygenated hemoglobin rapidly enough to enable inferences about brain function.

Issues

While fMRI is maturing as a technique, several important areas remain for future research. In general, these can be grouped into three main areas. The first, and most noticeable, reflects the desire to improve the fidelity of our fMRI data to the underlying neuronal activity. As fidelity improves, both spatially and temporally, we will be better equipped to answer outstanding questions about brain function. However, other developments hold promise not simply for better answering existing questions but also for creating new questions to be asked. A second area of research, therefore, lies in the development of new experimental designs for fMRI. Finally, many laboratories are experimenting with alternatives to the traditional BOLD contrast described above. These range from improved targeting of particular vascular compartments, through measures of other properties of the vascular system such as blood perfusion, all the way to direct measurement of neuronal activity. Despite the rapid pace of all three of these areas of research, there is no optimal technique to which all should aspire. Different forms of fMRI provide different information about brain function, so the primary challenge for the next generation of researchers will be the integration of information from multiple techniques (both within fMRI itself and across other modalities) to address a single research question from converging perspectives.

The Relation Between BOLD and Neuronal Activity

Permeating all fMRI research is the rarely articulated assumption that the BOLD signal provides a faithful representation of neuronal activity. As discussed earlier in this chapter, substantial empirical evidence has demonstrated that neuronal activity is associated with the sorts of physiological changes necessary to evoke a BOLD response. And literally thousands of fMRI studies have provided operational evidence through fMRI results that match previous electrophysiological evidence (e.g., mapping of visual, motor, and language systems; presurgical planning; etc.). Yet, even if the gross correspondence of BOLD with neuronal activity is well established, the fine details of the causal mechanism are not.

Consider what it would mean if we knew that the BOLD response had a different time course across brain regions, due to variations in neuronal timing or the vascular system. If that were true, then standard analysis techniques would risk identifying some regions of activity while missing others. Or imagine that the BOLD response to a given pattern of neuronal firing were different, depending on the previous activity of the vascular system. Would we be able to make inferences about neuronal activity if all we knew was the BOLD signal? As a last challenge, reflect upon the link between neuronal activity and the BOLD response. What if the BOLD response did not depend simply upon the amount of neuronal activity, but instead upon the synchronicity of neuronal activity across space or upon the particular firing pattern in time? What, then, would we be able to conclude from a colored blob on a fMRI activation map?

We pose these questions not just as rhetorical devices, but as examples of the sorts of challenges considered by many researchers. Each of these hypothetical scenarios (and likely, all of them) may be closer to the truth than the canonical assumptions of current fMRI practice. In this section, we evaluate recent research that investigates the relation between BOLD and neuronal activity, and we continue our discussion of fidelity in the following sections on temporal and spatial resolution and on high-field fMRI.

It is seemingly straightforward to validate the relation between neuronal and BOLD activity by comparing data of the measures. However, such comparisons face daunting technical challenges. In a landmark study, Logothetis and colleagues simultaneously recorded both fMRI and electrophysiological data within the primary visual cortex of the monkey (Logothetis et al., 2001). The monkeys viewed a rotating visual checkerboard stimulus while being scanned in a 4.7-T scanner using gradient-echo echoplanar imaging, during which time concurrent single-unit, multiunit, and local field potential data were recorded. When the visual stimulus was presented, there was a transient increase in BOLD signal that persisted until its offset. This pattern of activity was also present in the local field potential data (i.e., the summation of integrative activity in dendrites), but was only weakly or not at all evident in the multi- or single-unit activity (i.e., the axonal firings of individual neurons). Converging evidence has been advanced by studies of cerebellar cortex that compared multiunit activity, local field potentials, and blood flow via laser Doppler (Lauritzen, 2001). Stimulation of two inputs to Purkinje cells, excitatory climbing fibers and inhibitory parallel fibers, increases local field potential activity without causing action potentials. Under such conditions, blood flow varies proportionally to changes in local field potentials, even when no action potentials occur. Thus, the BOLD contrast mechanism seems to reflect the dendritic inputs and intracortical processing in a given area, rather than its axonal outputs associated with action potential firing.

This result is consistent with analyses of the energy budget of the brain and how that budget is met through increased vascular supply of metabolites. Results from rodent studies indicate that the vast majority of energy required by the brain goes to support axonal (47%) and dendritic (34%) activity (Attwell & Laughlin, 2001). Because the primate brain has a much higher synaptic density, it has been estimated that dendritic activity consumes about three-quarters of its energy (Attwell & Laughlin, 2001), and thus by inference the BOLD activity within a region should reflect the amount and timing of dendritic activity.

But, as argued by Attwell and Iadecola, this finding (in conjunction with demonstrations of neuronal and neurotransmitter control of blood flow changes) has broader implications for BOLD fMRI (Attwell & Iadecola, 2002). They suggest that the BOLD effect should not be considered a consequence of total energy utilization, but instead reflects neuronal signaling within a brain region. That is, deficits in available oxygen or glucose within a region do not directly regulate the supply of oxygenated hemoglobin. Instead, blood flow seems to be controlled by neurotransmitter action, the firing of particular classes of cells within brain regions, and/or the activity of large-scale systems of fibers that ascend from midbrain nuclei. Thus, changes in the form of neuronal firing, but not in the total metabolic demand, could evoke BOLD activity, while changes in metabolic demand that do not trigger vascular control systems might not evoke any BOLD response.

Despite the many advances in recent years in the understanding of the BOLD signal, much work remains. Key challenges include extension of studies like those described above from primates performing simple visual tasks to human higher cognition. If the conjecture of Attwell and Iadecola is correct, for example, then one might expect the coupling between these measures to depend on the form of information processing in a region. We have compared these BOLD fMRI and electrophysiological measures in human subjects (Huettel, McKeown, et al., 2004). Changes in local field potentials were measured in patients awaiting neurosurgery who had implanted electrodes, while BOLD changes were measured in neurologically normal volunteers. As in the Logothetis study described above, there was a strong correspondence between the amplitude and duration of local field potentials and the duration of the BOLD response in brain regions around primary visual cortex. However, in other visual cortical regions, this relation was less clear. In the lateral occipitotemporal cortex, neither the field potentials nor the BOLD response was systematically altered by stimulus duration. In contrast, within the fusiform gyrus, there was a clear dissociation between the measures: as stimulus duration increased, the BOLD response increased but field potential activity did not. Such results suggest that other aspects of neuronal activity, such as the synchronicity across neurons within a region, may contribute to the BOLD response. Future studies directly comparing fMRI and electrophysiological measures will be necessary to extend the results discussed in this section to additional brain regions, stimulus conditions, and subject populations.

Spatial and Temporal Resolution

Improving the spatial and temporal resolution of fMRI will require more than just collecting smaller voxels and sampling the MR signal more frequently. While such improvements are likely, especially with advances in hardware quality, real improvements in resolution will require fundamental changes in data collection techniques. Images must be collected using pulse sequences that more closely map fMRI signal changes to neuronal activity, both in space and in time. Distortions caused by magnetic inhomogeneities must be corrected. And, as will be discussed later in this chapter, additional forms of contrast must be developed and validated to overcome key limitations of BOLD fMRI.

While spatial resolution has long been considered to be a strength of fMRI, especially compared with PET imaging, its resolution is actually quite coarse compared with what can be obtained using anatomical MRI. Recent demonstrations of ultrahigh-resolution MRI, also known as MR microscopy, have created images of rodent brains with voxels less than 1/20 of a millimeter on a side (Johnson et al., 2002). To put this achievement in perspective, approximately 700,000 of these voxels could fit into a single voxel that was collected at the resolution typical of human fMRI studies. Unfortunately, the experimental techniques used in ultrahigh-resolution MRI do not easily adapt to fMRI studies. Very strong field strengths are used (often 9 T or greater); while homogeneous fields of that strength can be readily generated using MR scanners with small bore sizes that fit rodents, they are very difficult to generate in scanners large enough to fit the human head. Very long acquisition times are also used in ultrahigh-resolution MRT, such that a single animal (anesthetized or euthanized to prevent motion) might remain in the scanner for 24 hours.

Setting aside increases in field strength or imaging time for the moment, one effective and less costly way to increase spatial and temporal resolution is to collect data more rapidly, using a technique known as parallel imaging. In parallel imaging, several detector coils are used to simultaneously sample the brain; this can used to increase the amount of data sampled per unit time and to improve spatial resolution, or to reduce the amount of data sampled per coil and improve temporal resolution.

To understand how parallel imaging can improve spatial resolution, assume that normally a single coil is used to acquire a single image. Using four coils, one could collect four images with overlapping fields of view and larger coverage in k-space to reach higher resolution. The k-space data are subsampled for individual coils, resulting in severely aliased images. These aliased images must be corrected either in image space (in the case of SENSE, or *sen*sitivity *e*ncoding) or in k-space (in the case of SMASH, or *si*multaneous *a*cquisition of *s*patial *h*armonics), restoring original image quality (Sodickson & Manning, 1997; Pruessmann et al., 1999). By incorporating sensitivity maps from individual coils and using an iterative reconstruction process to remove aliasing artifacts, a final image with uniform spatial coverage and high spatial resolution can be achieved. The relation between the number of coils and the matrix size can be expressed more generally in the following way. Assuming the number of receiver coils is M, the number of sampling points for each coil is P, and the number of voxels desired in the final reconstructed image is N^2, we must use enough coils so that $M \times P > N^2$. Thus, as M coils are used, the matrix size could increases by a factor up to $\sqrt{M}$ for a given acquisition time. In addition to increasing spatial resolution, parallel imaging can also increase the raw signal–noise ratio by targeting multiple coils at the same brain region. One common approach for doing this is the use of a four-channel phased-array coil targeted at human visual cortex. This allows better segmentation of gray and white matter in anatomical images and improved estimation of BOLD changes in functional images.

Likewise, parallel imaging can have salutary effects upon temporal resolution. If there are M receiver coils each sampling P points, the requirement for redundancy means that there must be more samples than voxels in the image: $M \times P > N^2$. Thus, temporal resolution decreases proportionally to the number of receiver coils used; that is, by a factor of M. This improvement is in image acquisition time only, and does not affect problems with insufficient recovery time or the delay introduced by the hemodynamic response. As we discussed earlier in this chapter, the net magnetization of voxels within an image requires time to recover between successive excitations, so that the signal-to-noise ratio can be reduced dramatically at very short TRs. Note that parallel imaging has slightly different effects on spatial resolution and temporal resolution. Because spatial resolution is measured in squared units within a slice (mm^2), it improves with the square root of the number of coils. But temporal resolution is measured in linear units (s), and it improves linearly with the number of coils.

Another area of research in which important advances have been made is the correction for magnetic susceptibility artifacts, or signal losses or spatial distortions in ventral brain areas that are near interfaces between air and brain tissue (figure 2.8a). Susceptibility artifacts are present on any T$_2$* weighted image, and are exacerbated by fast imaging methods, long TEs, and high-field scanning. The areas of

(A)   (B)

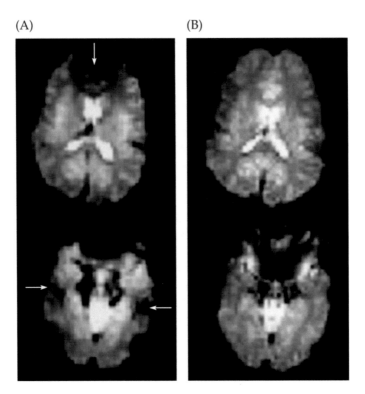

Figure 2.8
Susceptibility artifacts and their compensation. Shown in (*A*) are two representative axial slices acquired using gradient-echo echo-planar imaging. Visible is the typical pattern of susceptibility-induced signal losses in frontal and inferior temporal regions (indicated by arrows). In (*B*) the same slices are shown; they were acquired using a single-shot susceptibility compensation sequence. Much greater signal is present in the regions of susceptibility artifact, and anatomical details are clearly visible within those regions. Both pairs of images were collected at 4 T from the same subject.

most common distortion include the ventral frontal lobe and the lateral inferior temporal lobe; the former is immediately above the sphenoid sinus, and the latter is above the auditory canals. Susceptibility artifacts have had a significant impact upon functional brain mapping. Because no fMRI signal can be measured from these regions, they are often excluded from characterization of functional brain systems. Nevertheless, evidence from other modalities has shown that these areas are important for many cognitive and perceptive processes, including memory, emotion, attention, language, and olfaction. It is thus critically important to develop methods for recovering the fMRI signal from these regions.

Several research groups have developed methods for minimizing susceptibility artifacts. One approach is to use thinner slices (i.e., <1.5 mm) to reduce the field change through the slice. This approach ameliorates but does not eliminate the artifacts, while reducing both SNR and spatial coverage to levels that are not practical for most fMRI studies. Thus, it is not commonly used. A second approach, known as a "z-shim technique," is to use multiple linear gradients to compensate for the susceptibility-induced field distortions (Frahm et al., 1988). Despite its effectiveness in recovering signal, this approach is not feasible for most fMRI experiments because it requires multiple excitations (as many as 16) to collect a single image, greatly increasing the effective TR of the experiment. More efficient susceptibility compensation methods have been implemented that use higher-order gradients to correct for field inhomogeneities, reducing the number of needed gradients to a more tolerable level. For example, early work by Cho and colleagues used an excitation pulse with a quadratic profile to better match real field inhomogeneities (Cho & Ro, 1992). This development reduced the number of excitations to two: a quadratic profile, for regions with signal loss; and a standard uniform profile, for regions without signal loss. More recently implemented single-shot methods provide much-improved signal recovery (figure 2.8b) with minimal cost to temporal resolution, as implemented by Song for EPI and Glover and colleagues for spiral imaging (Glover & Law, 2001; Song, 2001).

High-Field Scanning

Since fMRI's beginnings about 1990, the field strength at which images have been collected has steadily increased. The 1.5 T scanner is no longer considered a high-field platform, but is now a standard workhorse machine. As institutions install machines of 4 T, 7 T, and even 9 T, it is important to consider the advantages and disadvantages of high-field scanning. What do such scanners offer that would engender such enthusiasm among researchers despite the sometimes prohibitively high cost?

The primary advantage of high-field scanning comes from increased signal. As the scanner field strength increases, a greater proportion of spins will align parallel with the static field, and thus net magnetization will increase. This increase in raw MR signal is quadratic with field strength; that is, as field strength doubles, the raw signal recorded by the scanner quadruples. Mitigating this advantage, however, is a corresponding increase in thermal noise, which increases linearly with field strength. The signal-to-noise ratio (or SNR) thus increases linearly (i.e., a quadratic increase divided by a linear increase equals a linear increase) with increasing field strength. In principle, the increased SNR can allow the image to be parceled into smaller voxels while maintaining sufficient SNR within each, improving spatial resolution. For example, studies of ocular dominance columns, which are approximately 1 millimeter in width, have been carried out at 4 T (Cheng et al., 2001).

It is important to recognize that the quality of fMRI data depends not just upon net magnetization and thermal noise; it also depends upon physiological and neural variability, which are collectively called physiological noise. The strength of the static field has different effects upon thermal noise and physiological noise (figure 2.9). While thermal noise increases linearly with increasing field strength, physiological noise increases quadratically with field strength (Kruger & Glover, 2001). So, as field strength increases from 1.5*T to 3 T, raw signal will quadruple, thermal noise will double, and physiological noise will quadruple. Thus, at very high field strengths, physiological noise may become dominant, and thus the improvements associated with increasing field strength may be considerably less than linear (i.e., smaller than for raw SNR). Although there have been theoretical suggestions that there may be an asymptotic upper limit for effective field strength in fMRI (Kruger & Glover, 2001), those suggestions have yet to be tested because of the current paucity of very high-field scanners.

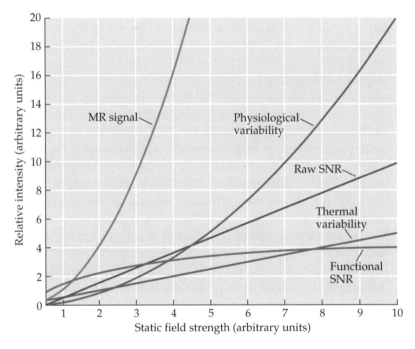

Figure 2.9
Changes in signal and noise with increasing static field strength. MR signal increases with the square of the field strength, whereas thermal noise increases linearly with field strength. The ratio of these quantities, raw SNR, thus increases linearly with field strength. However, because physiological noise increases with the square of field strength, functional SNR (which is dependent on both thermal and physiological noise) may asymptote at high fields. Note that here the field strength is indicated in arbitrary units; the field strength beyond which such an asymptote would occur is not yet established.

A direct consequence of increased SNR for fMRI studies is the increased spatial extent of activation (i.e., number of active voxels within a region). As functional SNR increases within a voxel, the probability of that voxel passing a threshold for statistical significance also increases (Huettel & McCarthy, 2001). Yang and colleagues measured activity within sensorimotor cortex while subjects performed a blocked-design finger-tapping task at either 1.5*T or 4 T (Yang et al., 1999). Under optimal TR and TE parameters, there were approximately 70% more active voxels within the region at 4 T, suggesting that detection power throughout the brain improves with increasing field strength. Increased field strength also affects the relaxation parameters T_1 and T_2*, each of which influences the signal recorded in fMRI experiments. The parameter T_1 increases with field strength (by about 30% from 1.5 T to 3 T), reducing the effective recovery of the MR signal at short TR values. The parameter T_2* decreases with field strength (by about 25% in gray matter from 1.5 T to 3 T), causing the MR signal to decay more rapidly and thus reducing the time available for its acquisition. Finally, just as the BOLD signal (which results from local magnetic field inhomogeneities) increases with field strength, so do susceptibility artifacts resulting from inhomogeneities near air–tissue boundaries. Techniques like those described in the previous section become even more critical at higher field strengths.

Improved Experimental Design

Although improvements in scanner hardware are important, they are hardly panaceas for the many challenges faced by fMRI studies. Even more valuable, in our view, are advances in experimental design, which not only improve the ability to answer experimental questions but also allow novel questions to be posed.

A simple method to improve the temporal resolution of fMRI data is to introduce jitter into the sampling of the hemodynamic response, in a method known as interleaved stimulus presentation. By staggering the presentation of events of interest relative to TR onset, the effective sampling rate can be increased. Imagine that you can collect data from the entire brain with a TR of 2 sec. To improve temporal resolution within this design, you could present some of the stimuli at the onset of the TR, some at 500 ms following TR onset, some 1000 ms following TR onset, and some 1500 ms following TR onset. By combining data across all of these timing conditions, the effective sampling rate is reduced to 500 ms. However, the TR itself remains long, so a large number of slices can be collected and substantial TR recovery can occur between successive excitations. The primary disadvantage of this approach is that the number of trials within each timing condition are greatly reduced (i.e., in the above example, by a factor of 4). Thus, to maintain the estimation power for each timing condition, the experiment length must be increased considerably.

A lesser disadvantage lies in the need for careful adjustments for slice acquisition timing during preprocessing, since each stimulus is presented at a different point in the TR and thus at a different point in the slice acquisition series.

Although with interleaved acquisition the effective TR could be arbitrarily short, in practice, temporal resolution would still be limited by the intrinsic delay and dispersion in the hemodynamic response. That is, the temporal uncertainty introduced by the fMRI hemodynamic response function will undermine any attempt to make millisecond-level assessments of the underlying neuronal activity. To overcome this problem in the study of one brain system, Ogawa and colleagues have developed a technique that induces either excitatory or inhibitory neural interactions by presenting consecutive stimuli (to the forepaw of a rat) separated by very short intervals, on the order of tens of milliseconds. By manipulating the interstimulus interval, the research team was able to detect the inhibition due to neuronal refractoriness on the response to the second stimulus (Ogawa et al., 2000). Such an inhibition effect is subsequently manifested in the BOLD signal. With such a clever manipulation, one can achieve improved temporal resolution without physically increasing the sampling interval, since neuronal interactions on the order of milliseconds can lead to very different hemodynamic responses.

A number of groups have used the conceptually similar approach of analyzing the effects of previous stimuli upon the characteristics of the fMRI hemodynamic response. Early studies demonstrated that the amplitude of the hemodynamic response was roughly proportional to the duration and number of presented stimuli (Boynton et al., 1996; Dale & Buckner, 1997). That is, given the hemodynamic response of a 6 sec. duration stimulus, one could estimate the response to a 12 sec. stimulus by adding together two 6 sec. responses (Boynton et al., 1996). Similarly, when two stimuli were presented in rapid succession, the combined response was roughly equivalent to the summation of two responses to a single stimulus in isolation (Dale & Buckner, 1997). However, even in these first studies there was evidence that this simple picture was not entirely correct, and a number of subsequent studies confirmed that the fMRI hemodynamic response attenuates with repeated activation of a brain region (Friston et al., 1998; Robson et al., 1998; Vazquez & Noll, 1998; Huettel & McCarthy, 2000).

While this refractory effect poses challenges for some analyses, it has turned out to be important for a new class of experimental designs that use stimulus adaptation. Studies by Grill-Spector, Malach, and colleagues have investigated whether individual regions of visual cortex are sensitive to changes in higher-order properties of objects (Grill-Spector & Malach, 2001). Their designs compare two types of conditions: one in which the same stimulus is presented repeatedly within a block, and another in which some aspect of the stimulus changes continually over time. For example, an "identical face" block might show the same view of the same person's face over and over, while a "size changing" block might present the same face in a variety of sizes on the display. They found that activity in the fusiform gyrus, for example, was greatly reduced to repeated presentations of identical, size-varying, or position-varying faces, compared with repeated presentations of different people's faces. In contrast, variation in direction of illumination or viewpoint caused a recovery from adaptation. From these results, they concluded that the fusiform gyrus recognizes facial identity over size or position manipulations, but not over illumination or viewpoint manipulations. This approach has since been used by other groups and with other stimulus domains to investigate the attribute specificity of the fMRI hemodynamic response (Boynton & Finney, 2003; Soon et al., 2003; Huettel, Obeme, et al., 2004).

Finally, new classes of experimental designs take into account the dynamic properties of fMRI time courses. As described in the following chapter, most fMRI studies use either blocked designs in which events are concentrated in time or event-related designs that seek to separate consecutive events by extended (or random) intervals. Recent theoretical advances have demonstrated that designs with characteristics of both blocked and event-related approaches provide substantial improvements in both detection power and estimation efficiency (Liu et al., 2001; Birn et al., 2002; Liu, 2004). In semirandom designs, stimulus probability varies systematically over time so that there are some time periods in which many events occur and other time periods in which few occur. However, the timing of individual events is still staggered in a way that allows estimation of the fMRI time course.

Non-BOLD Contrasts

While nearly all fMRI studies have used (and continue to use) BOLD contrast, a number of potential alternative measures have been developed. Most are intended to overcome one limitation of BOLD imaging: that oxygenation changes following activity are present in a wide range (both in type and in space) of vascular tissues, from capillaries that are near active neurons to veins that drain large anatomical regions. During brain activation, local control of oxygen delivery is facilitated through microvascular dilatation and constriction, and thus techniques that are sensitive to MR signal from capillaries should be more localized to the true neuronal activity. Three such techniques are perfusion imaging, vascular-space-occupancy (VASO) imaging, and diffusion-weighted imaging.

By using arterial spin labeling (ASL), images can be collected that are sensitive to blood flow from upstream arterial networks into the local vascular system around an area of function. This flow is known as perfusion. Perfusion imaging is sensitive to capillary activity, where oxygen exchange takes place, but is less sensitive to changes in large veins because of T_1 recovery effects. Therefore, optimized perfusion contrast is believed to have better functional resolution than BOLD contrast (Luh et al., 2000; Duong et al., 2001). In VASO imaging, signal from within blood vessels is eliminated, so that images are sensitive only to changes in extravascular signal (Lu et al., 2003). Such images can be used to measure blood volume changes (without having to inject contrast agents), which are greater in smaller vessels like capillaries than in larger vessels like veins. A third approach, diffusion-weighted imaging, collects images that are sensitive to the amount of motion of spins across space. Since spins (i.e., protons within water molecules) diffuse more quickly through large vessels, diffusion weighting can be used to selectively attenuate large vessel contributions to the BOLD signal. In addition, measurement of differences in the apparent diffusion coefficient (ADC) across space can provide information about capillary activity (Song et al., 2002).

One of the most recent advances is among the most intriguing: the use of fMRI to image neuronal activity, so that a more direct measure of information processing can be obtained. This will be challenging, at best, due to the transience, weakness, and inhomogeneity of the electrical activity of neurons. As an example, an early study used spin-echo imaging to measure changes in spin phase associated with the field perturbations of electrical currents in human nerves (Joy et al., 1989). However, these results have not been confirmed by further studies, and the application of this technique to neurons in the brain may be more challenging than to peripheral nerves. Another approach involves the measurement of Lorentz forces, which arise from the movement of charged particles through a magnetic field. As the particles move through the field, they experience a force that is perpendicular to both the local magnetic field and the particles' direction of motion. This force acts to displace the particles; if the particles are within a conductor, it will be displaced within the external medium (figure 2.10). Proof-of-concept results have been reported for wires within gel phantoms at $10\,\mu m$ accuracy (Song & Takahashi, 2001), and similar effects may be observable in the axons of active neurons.

Recognizing that rapidly changing magnetic fields may indicate electrical activity of neurons, Bodurka and Bandettini attempted to selectively detect rapidly changing magnetic fields while suppressing slowly changing magnetic fields (Bodurka & Bandettini, 2002). The initial concept was tested on a phantom with implanted wires. The timing of transient currents in the wires was modulated relative to a 180° excitation pulse. Very small phase differences were detected, demonstrating the feasibility of the approach. To illustrate the potential importance of this effect, the magnetic field changes measured were as short as only 40 ms in duration and as small as only $2 \times 10^{-10}\,T$ (200 pT). These magnetic changes are about 10 billion times smaller than typical static field strengths, illustrating the profound technical requirements of direct neuronal imaging.

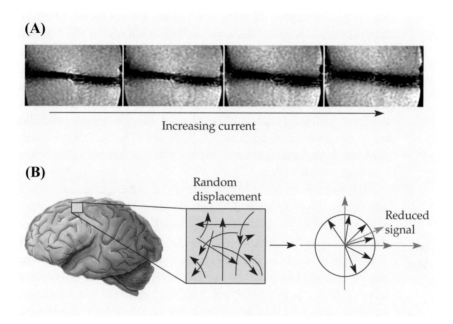

Figure 2.10
Lorentz effect imaging. Any linear current-carrying object (e.g., a wire, a neuronal axon) will be subject to a lateral force when placed in a magnetic field. This force is known as the Lorentz force, and the resulting displacement can be measured in principle using MRI. Shown in (*A*) are results from a phantom containing a wire carrying different amounts of charge; from left, $0\,\mu A$, $100\,\mu A$, $200\,\mu A$, and $500\,\mu A$. The magnitude of the MRI distortion increases with increasing current. The potential application of Lorentz effect imaging to fMRI is shown in (*B*). Within a cortical voxel, the electrical currents will be largely randomly oriented, so that Lorentz effects in different directions will cause signal loss due to reduced phase coherence (i.e., analogous to T_2^* effects). As activity increases within that voxel, there will be increasing phase incoherence, and thus decreasing MR signal. Thus, Lorentz effect imaging (and similar techniques) have the potential for facilitating direct measurement of neuronal activity using MRI.

Summary

Functional magnetic resonance imaging uses standard clinical MRI hardware to collect information about changes in brain metabolism that are associated with neuronal activity. As in standard MRI, fMRI signal is recorded from hydrogen protons in water molecules. These protons (or "spins") exhibit rapid gyroscopic precession when placed in the strong magnetic field of an MRI scanner. The axis around which they precess is known as the longitudinal direction, and the plane in which they precess is known as the transverse plane. Each spin adopts either a lower or a higher energy state, parallel or anti-parallel to the magnetic field, respectively. Since slightly more spins adopt the lower-energy parallel state, the net magnetization across all spins is a vector parallel to the static magnetic field. By applying an electromagnetic pulse that oscillates at the resonant (Larmor) frequency of the spins, a process known as excitation, the net magnetization vector is tipped from the longitudinal direction into the transverse plane, where it generates MR signal that can be measured in an external detector coil. After the excitation pulse ends, the net magnetization's longitudinal component recovers according to the time constant T_1, while its transverse component magnetization decays according to the time constant T_2 or T_2*. Also after the excitation, spatially varying magnetic field gradients are used for selecting image slices and for encoding spatial locations within a slice.

Different sets of scanner instructions, or pulse sequences, apply excitation pulses and magnetic gradients in different patterns to allow different forms of image collection. In fMRI experiments, high-speed gradient-echo pulse sequences are typically used to collect images sensitive to distortions in the local magnetic field (e.g., T_2* effects) that result from the presence of paramagnetic deoxygenated hemoglobin. As neuronal activity and the resulting demand for oxygen increase, there is an increase in the supply of oxygenated hemoglobin beyond that needed by the active neurons. This increased supply has the effect of reducing local concentrations of deoxygenated hemoglobin in areas of neuronal activity, thus increasing the amount of MR signal measured on T_2* images. This results in blood-oxygenation-level-dependent (BOLD) contrast. As the technique of fMRI matures, researchers are investigating the physiological origins of the BOLD signal and how to improve its spatial and temporal fidelity to the neuronal activity of interest. Also of considerable interest will be the study of alternative, non-BOLD techniques for directly imaging neuronal activity using fMRI.

Note

The first two authors made equal contributions to this chapter, and their order of authorship was determined arbitrarily. Portions of this chapter and its figures are excerpted with permission from our textbook *Functional Magnetic Resonance Imaging*, published by Sinauer Associates (Huettel et al., 2004a).

References

Attwell, D., & Laughlin, S. B. (2001). An energy budget for signaling in the grey matter of the brain. *Journal of Cerebral Blood Flow and Metabolism* 21, 1133–1145.

Attwell, D., & Iadecola, C. (2002). The neural basis of functional brain imaging signals. *Trends in Neurosciences* 25, 621–625.

Birn, R. M., Cox, R. W., & Bandettini, P. A. (2002). Detection versus estimation in event-related fMRI: Choosing the optimal stimulus timing. *NeuroImage* 15, 252–264.

Bodurka, J., & Bandettini, P. A. (2002). Toward direct mapping of neuronal activity: MRI detection of ultraweak, transient magnetic field changes. *Magnetic Resonance in Medicine* 47, 1052–1058.

Boynton, G. M., Engel, S. A., Glover, G. H., & Heeger, D. J. (1996). Linear systems analysis of functional magnetic resonance imaging in human V1. *Journal of Neuroscience* 16, 4207–4221.

Boynton, G. M., & Finney, E. M. (2003). Orientation-specific adaptation in human visual cortex. *Journal of Neuroscience* 23, 8781–8787.

Cheng, K., Waggoner, R. A., & Tanaka, K. (2001). Human ocular dominance columns as revealed by high-field functional magnetic resonance imaging. *Neuron* 32, 359–374.

Cho, Z. H., & Ro, Y. M. (1992). Reduction of susceptibility artifact in gradient-echo imaging. *Magnetic Resonance in Medicine* 23, 193–200.

Dale, A. M., & Buckner, R. L. (1997). Selective averaging of rapidly presented individual trials using fMRI. *Human Brain Mapping* 5, 329–340.

Duong, T. Q., Kim, D. S., Ugurbil, K., & Kim, S. G. (2001). Localized cerebral blood flow response at submillimeter columnar resolution. *Proceedings of the National Academy of Sciences USA*, 98, 10904–10909.

Fox, P. T., Raichle, M. E., Mintun, M. A., & Dence, C. (1988). Nonoxidative glucose consumption during focal physiologic neural activity. *Science* 241, 462–464.

Frahm, J., Merboldt, K. D., & Hanicke, W. (1988). Direct FLASH MR imaging of magnetic field inhomogeneities by gradient compensation. *Magnetic Resonance in Medicine* 6, 474–480.

Friston, K. J., Josephs, O., Rees, G., & Turner, R. (1998). Nonlinear event-related responses in fMRI. *Magnetic Resonance in Medicine* 39, 41–52.

Glover, G. H., & Law, C. S. (2001). Spiral-in/out BOLD fMRI for increased SNR and reduced susceptibility artifacts. *Magnetic Resonance in Medicine* 46, 515–522.

Grill-Spector, K., & Malach, R. (2001). fMR-adaptation: A tool for studying the functional properties of human cortical neurons. *Acta Psychologica* (Amsterdam) 107, 293–321.

Huettel, S. A., & McCarthy, G. (2000). Evidence for a refractory period in the hemodynamic response to visual stimuli as measured by MRI. *NeuroImage* 11, 547–553.

Huettel, S. A., & McCarthy, G. (2001). The effects of single-trial averaging upon the spatial extent of fMRI activation. *NeuroReport* 12, 2411–2416.

Huettel, S. A., McKeown, M. J., Song, A. W., Hart, S., Spencer, D. D., Allison, T., & McCarthy, G. (2004). Linking hemodynamic and electrophysiological measures of brain activity: Evidence from functional MRI and intracranial field potentials. *NeuroReport* 14, 165–173.

Huettel, S. A., Obembe, J., Song, A., & Woldorff, M. (2004). The BOLD fMRI refractory effect is specific to stimulus attributes: Evidence from a visual motion paradigm. *NeuroImage* 21, 402–408.

Huettel, S. A., Song, A. W., & McCarthy, G. (2004). *Functional Magnetic Resonance Imaging.* Sunderland, MA: Sinauer.

Johnson, G. A., Cofer, G. P., Gewalt, S. L., & Hedlund, L. W. (2002). Morphologic phenotyping with MR microscopy: The visible mouse. *Radiology* 222, 789–793.

Joy, M., Scott, G., & Henkelman, M. (1989). In vivo detection of applied electric currents by magnetic resonance imaging. *Magnetic Resonance Imaging* 7, 89–94.

Kruger, G., & Glover, G. H. (2001). Physiological noise in oxygenation-sensitive magnetic resonance imaging. *Magnetic Resonance in Medicine* 46, 631–637.

Lauritzen, M. (2001). Relationship of spikes, synaptic activity, and local changes of cerebral blood flow. *Journal of Cerebral Blood Flow and Metabolism* 21(12), 1367–1383.

Lauterbur, P. C. (1973). Image formation by induced local interactions: Examples employing nuclear magnetic resonance. *Nature* 242, 190–191.

Liu, T. T. (2004). Efficiency, power, and entropy in event-related fMRI with multiple trial types. Part II: Design of experiments. *NeuroImage* 21, 401–413.

Liu, T. T., Frank, L. R., Wong, E. C., & Buxton, R. B. (2001). Detection power, estimation efficiency, and predictability in event-related fMRI. *NeuroImage* 13, 759–773.

Logothetis, N. K., Pauls, J., Augath, M., Trinath, T., & Oeltermann, A. (2001). Neurophysiological investigation of the basis of the fMRI signal. *Nature* 412, 150–157.

The central concept of magnetic resonance is that both the emitted excitation pulse and the received MR signal are electromagnetic waves that oscillate at the precession frequency of the targeted spins. To understand this, imagine that you are pushing someone on a swing. If you want to make the person swing higher, you must transfer kinetic energy to him or her. The most efficient way of doing so is to given a small push each time the person swings by; that is, to push the person at the same rate as the natural frequency of the swing. Analogously, the optimal way to change the net magnetization of a spin system is for the excitation/reception coil to provide energy at the spins' precession frequency (e.g., for hydrogen at 1.5 T, 63.87 MHz). In most forms of MRI, the effect of excitation is to tip the net magnetization from the longitudinal direction into the transverse plane, where it rotates at its precession frequency. The resulting magnetic field change over time induces a voltage change in the excitation/reception coil that also oscillates at the precession frequency; the measurement of this signal forms the basis of all MRI.

The effects of the excitation pulse upon the net magnetization can be characterized in simple equations. After the cessation of the excitation pulse, the amplitudes of the longitudinal (M_z) and transverse (M_{xy}) components of the net magnetization begin to change over time (figure 2.4). The longitudinal component experiences an exponential recovery as spins return to the parallel state from the antiparallel state. The rate at which this recovery occurs for a given substance depends on a time constant known as T_1. That is, substances with a very long T_1 value (e.g., cerebrospinal fluid, which has a T_1 value of 4000 ms at 1.5 T) will recover net magnetization very slowly, while substances with a shorter T_1 value (e.g., white matter, with T_1 of 600 ms at 1.5 T) will recover net magnetization much more rapidly.

However, the transverse component of the net magnetization experiences an exponential decay due to the loss of phase coherence (or synchrony) among the spins. Even though spins may have the same phase following excitation, two factors reduce coherence over time. First, the spins exert effects on each other (i.e., spin-spin interactions) that cause some to precess more rapidly and some to precess more slowly. The rate of transverse decay caused by these spin-spin interactions is governed by a time constant known as T_2. The second contributor to the loss of phase coherence is local inhomogeneity in the magnetic field. Since the precession frequency of a spin is determined by the magnetic field it experiences, small differences in magnetic field intensity across space will cause some spins to precess more rapidly and some more slowly. The combined effects of both factors, spin-spin interactions and local magnetic inhomogeneities, are described by the decay constant T_2^*. We will reconsider these recovery and decay processes later in this chapter, because T_1 and T_2 are critical for anatomical MRI and T_2^* forms the basis for nearly all forms of functional MRI.

Lu, H., Golay, X., Pekar, J. J., & Van Zijl, P. C. (2003). Functional magnetic resonance imaging based on changes in vascular space occupancy. *Magnetic Resonance in Medicine* 50, 263–274.

Magistretti, P. J., & Pellerin, L. (1999). Cellular mechanisms of brain energy metabolism and their relevance to functional brain imaging. *Philosophical Transactions of the Royal Society of London* B354, 1155–1163.

Malonek, D., & Grinvald, A. (1996). Interactions between electrical activity and cortical microcirculation revealed by imaging spectroscopy: Implications for functional brain mapping. *Science* 272, 551–554.

Mandeville, J. B., Marota, J. J., Ayata, C., Moskowitz, M. A., Weisskoff, R. M., & Rosen, B. R. (1999). MRI measurement of the temporal evolution of relative CMRO(2) during rat forepaw stimulation. *Magnetic Resonance in Medicine* 42, 944–951.

Mansfield, P., & Maudsley, A. A. (1977). Medical imaging by NMR. *British Journal of Radiology* 50, 188–194.

Ogawa, S., Lee, T. M., Nayak, A. S., & Glynn, P. (1990). Oxygenation-sensitive contrast in magnetic resonance image of rodent brain at high magnetic fields. *Magnetic Resonance in Medicine* 14, 68–78.

Ogawa, S., Lee, T. M., Stepnoski, R., Chen, W., Zhu, X. H., & Ugurbil, K. (2000). An approach to probe some neural systems interaction by functional MRI at neural time scale down to milliseconds. *Proceedings of the National Academy of Sciences USA* 97, 11026–11031.

Pauling, L., & Coryell, C. D. (1936). The magnetic properties and structure of hemoglobin, oxyhemoglobin, and carbonmonoxyhemoglobin. *Proceedings of the National Academy of Sciences USA* 22, 210–236.

Pruessmann, K. P., Weiger, M., Scheidegger, M. B., & Boesiger, P. (1999). SENSE: Sensitivity encoding for fast MRI. *Magnetic Resonance in Medicine* 42, 952–962.

Robson, M. D., Dorosz, J. L., & Gore, J. C. (1998). Measurements of the temporal fMRI response of the human auditory cortex to trains of tones. *NeuroImage* 7, 185–198.

Shulman, R. G., & Rothman, D. L. (1998). Interpreting functional imaging studies in terms of neurotransmitter cycling. *Proceedings of the National Academy of Sciences USA* 95, 11993–11998.

Shulman, R. G., Hyder, F., & Rothman, D. L. (2001). Cerebral energetics and the glycogen shunt: Neurochemical basis of functional imaging. *Proceedings of the National Academy of Sciences USA* 98, 6417–6422.

Sodickson, D. K., & Manning, W. J. (1997). Simultaneous acquisition of spatial harmonics (SMASH): Fast imaging with radiofrequency coil arrays. *Magnetic Resonance in Medicine* 38, 591–603.

Song, A. W. (2001). Single-shot EPI with signal recovery from the susceptibility-induced losses. *Magnetic Resonance in Medicine* 46, 2.

Song, A. W., & Takahashi, A. M. (2001). Lorentz effect imaging. *Magnetic Resonance Imaging* 19, 763–767.

Song, A. W., Woldorff, M. G., Gangstead, S., Mangun, G. R., & McCarthy, G. (2002). Enhanced spatial localization of neuronal activation using simultaneous apparent-diffusion-coefficient and blood-oxygenation functional magnetic resonance imaging. *Neuroimage* 17, 742–750.

Soon, C.-S., Venkatraman, V., & Chee, M. W. L. (2003). Stimulus repetition and hemodynamic response refractoriness in event-related fMRI. *Human Brain Mapping* 20, 1–12.

Thulborn, K. R., Waterton, J. C., Matthews, P. M., & Radda, G. K. (1982). Oxygenation dependence of the transverse relaxation time of water protons in whole blood at high field. *Biochimica et Biophysica Acta* 714, 265–270.

Vazquez, A. L., & Noll, D. C. (1998). Nonlinear aspects of the BOLD response in functional MRI. *NeuroImage* 7, 108–118.

Yang, Y., Wen, H., Mattay, V. S., Balaban, R. S., Frank, J. A., & Duyn, J. H. (1999). Comparison of 3D BOLD functional MRI with spiral acquisition at 1.5 and 4.0T. *NeuroImage* 9, 446–451.

3 Functional Neuroimaging: Experimental Design and Analysis

Jody C. Culham

> ... *the single most critical piece of equipment is still the researcher's own brain. All the equipment in the world will not help us if we do not know how to use it properly, which requires more than just knowing how to operate it. Aristotle would not necessarily have been more profound had he owned a laptop and known how to program. What is badly needed now, with all these scanners whirring away, is an understanding of exactly what we are observing, and seeing, and measuring, and wondering about.*
> —Endel Tulving, interview in *Cognitive Neuroscience* (Gazzaniga, Ivry, & Mangun eds. [New York: Norton, 2002], 323)

Introduction

With the advent of positron emission tomography (PET) in the 1980s (Fox et al., 1986) and functional magnetic resonance imaging (fMRI) in the 1990s (Kwong et al., 1992; Ogawa et al., 1992), neuroimaging became a keystone for the growing field of cognitive neuroscience. Historically, our knowledge of the human brain has been far more limited than for brains of other species (Crick & Jones, 1993), primarily due to the restriction against using invasive techniques, such as single neuron recording, in humans. Although human neuropsychological studies have been very enlightening, newer noninvasive neuroimaging methods, particularly fMRI, enable exploration of the normal rather than the disordered human brain and allow resolution at a fine spatial scale that lesions rarely provide (Savoy, 2001). These new imaging methods have identified dozens of functionally specific areas in the human brain, some of which seem comparable with areas in other species, particularly the macaque monkey, and some of which may be uniquely human (Culham & Kanwisher, 2001; Duncan & Owen, 2000; Grill-Spector & Malach, 2004; Tootell et al., 1998). Within numerous human regions that have been identified, detailed explorations have revealed the underlying computational processes (e.g., Wandell, 1999).

The growth of neuroimaging has been phenomenal. Neuroimaging publications continue to increase exponentially (Fox, 1997), with recent estimates of four published papers each day (Tootell et al., 2003). The caliber of imaging papers has improved considerably with the growth of the field, primarily due to the theory-driven approaches and high standards of experimental design expected in other disciplines. However, for many newcomers, fMRI methodology can seem overwhelmingly complex, leading to an increasing demand for resources to learn neuroimaging techniques. Numerous resources have suggested *how* neuroimaging experiments should be designed, but show limited consideration of the philosophy behind experimental design. One exception is an article by Steve Kosslyn, whose clever title posed the question "*If neuroimaging is the answer, what is the question?*" (Kosslyn, 1999). Another exception is William Uttal's book *The New Phrenology* (Uttal, 2001), which poses numerous pessimistic criticisms of the entire brain imaging enterprise (for a rebuttal, see Donaldson, 2004).

Here I intend to present a brief overview of neuroimaging design principles, followed by a somewhat opinionated review of my thoughts regarding the types of questions for which neuroimaging is (and is not) suited. As well, I will outline some of the principles that can lead to better questions and better experimental designs. The emphasis will be on fMRI, but many of the same principles apply to studies performed with PET. Space does not permit detailed recommendations for design issues, but the reader will find many useful resources in print (Aguirre & D'Esposito, 1999; Buckner & Logan, 2001; Chein & Schneider, 2003; Huettel et al., 2004; Jezzard et al., 2001) and online (such as my Web site, *fMRI for Dummies*, http://defiant.ssc. uwo.ca/Jody_web/fmri4dummies.htm). By no means do I intend to present a cynical view of the brain imaging enterprise. Rather, I hope to prompt newcomers to the field to think carefully about their approaches and the caveats, so that their contribution to the enterprise will become more fruitful.

Functional Neuroimaging: Experimental Design and Analysis

In neuroimaging, brain activation levels must always be considered relative to another condition. The signal strength in a particular area depends on many factors, such as inherent metabolic rate and location with respect to the coil (particularly true for surface coils that sample some regions of the brain with a higher signal-to-noise ratio, or SNR, than other areas). Thus the absolute level of signal is relatively meaningless on its own. As a consequence, all neuroimaging experiments rely on *subtraction logic* to make sense of the data.

Subtraction logic was developed in the nineteenth century for the study of reaction times to infer differences in cognitive processing (Donders, 1868; repr. in Donders, 1969). In subtraction logic, one compares two events that putatively differ by only one factor. For example, consider two reaction times.[1] In condition A, the subject must press a button whenever a light of any color turns on. In condition B, the subject must press a button whenever a red light turns on. Assuming that condition B differs from A only in the need to discriminate the color of the light, a subtraction of the reaction time for A from that for B should reveal the cognitive processing time required to make the discrimination (with components common to both tasks, say visual processing time, being "subtracted out"). Subtraction logic relies on the *assumption of pure insertion*, the belief that two conditions differ in *one and only one* critical component. If this assumption is false, and multiple differences exist, then it is impossible to distinguish between them.

Subtraction logic forms the basis for all neuroimaging experiments. The neuroimager must choose the best baseline condition that will subtract out all activation other than the process of interest. At first, this can be harder than it seems. The final section of this chapter will consider some of the issues involved in choosing appropriate baselines and some alternative designs (such as parametric designs) that are less vulnerable to the problems of subtraction logic.

The vast majority of neuroimaging experiments are considered *hypothesis-driven*. That is, the researcher plans the experiment with certain expectations regarding what types of differences will be observed between critical conditions. Statistical tests are then performed to determine whether such differences exist and are unlikely to be due to chance. In recent years, an alternative has been provided in the form of *data-driven* approaches that make no a priori assumptions about the expected patterns in the data. Newer approaches use sophisticated statistical techniques, such as independent component analysis (ICA), to extract the patterns that account for the most variability within the data (e.g., Biswal & Ulmer, 1999; McKeown et al., 1998). Such techniques have advantages in that they require fewer assumptions about the data and they may discover sources of variability unexpected by the experimenter. They have the potential to be useful for generating new hypotheses about processing; however, to date, data-driven approaches have been quite limited, and in the vast majority of studies the experimenters have definitive hypotheses to test. Thus the remainder of this chapter will focus on standard hypothesis-driven approaches.

Among hypothesis-driven analyses, there are two main approaches, the *voxelwise approach* and the *region of interest (ROI) approach*. In the voxelwise approach, the experimenter performs a statistical comparison between two (or more) conditions of interest on a voxel-by-voxel basis. No prior assumptions are needed regarding which specific brain areas will be differentially activated. Based on statistical evaluation, a list of areas in which significant activation differences were observed can be generated. This approach requires that every subject's data be transformed into a standard space that enables averaging across different brains, The two most common stereotaxic systems are the Talairach atlas (Talairach & Tournoux, 1988) and the Montreal Neurological Institute (MNI) space (Evans et al., 1993). This is a powerful approach in that it enables the researcher to investigate the whole brain (or as much of the volume as can be scanned, given other constraints), without the need for detailed hypotheses regarding expected loci of activation. Because the approach is highly contingent on solid statistical methods, it is essential for the user to be quite savvy about the statistics that are employed and to have access to an analysis package that offers the appropriate statistics and corrections.

The alternative ROI approach focuses on the role of previously described regions in a novel experiment. ROIs may be defined on the basis of anatomical criteria. For example, in a memory study, regions of the hippocampus may be identified and selected on the basis of the anatomical slice data. More commonly, ROIs are well-established areas defined by their functional responses. For example, in vision science, common ROIs include the middle temporal complex (MT+), which responds more to motion than to still images (Culham, He, et al., 2001); the fusiform face area (FFA), which responds more to faces than to other categories of objects (Kanwisher et al., 1997); and striate and extrastriate visual areas defined by boundaries in retinotopic maps (Wandell, 1999). In the ROI approach, regions are first identified using a *localizer* based on prior studies that have reported reliable activation for a particular comparison. Activation in these ROIs is then evaluated in an independent line of experiments designed to test a new hypothesis. For example, a localizer for MT+ would compare activation during visual motion against a stationary state, possibly at low contrast, to isolate the MT+ complex from other motion-related areas (Tootell, Reppas, Kwong, et al., 1995). After the ROI has been identified in each subject, the activation time courses are extracted and analyzed statistically to determine whether there are significant differences in the comparison for the new experimental task. For example, one study investigated whether area MT+, as defined by a standard localizer, was more activated with static images that implied motion than those that did not (Kourtzi & Kanwisher, 2000a).

The standards for appropriate neuroimaging statistics (used in both voxelwise and ROI approaches) have been evolving over the years. Many statistical developments have become more commonplace with their introduction into standard statistical packages for neuroimaging data. In the early days of brain imaging, simple statistics such as t-tests and correlations were applied to data, sometimes without preprocessing, and statistical thresholds were determined either arbitrarily or with conservative corrections for the problem that one was simultaneously examining tens of thousands of individual voxels (the Bonferroni correction for multiple comparisons). Currently, standard procedures often include preprocessing (such as correcting for motion of the subject's head, spatial filtering, and temporal filtering), corrections for serial correlations (to correct the false assumption that activation at one point in time is unrelated to activation at the preceding and following points in time), less conservative corrections for multiple comparisons (such as false discovery rate corrections; Genovese et al., 2002), and random effects analyses that allow generalization from the group of tested subjects to the population as a whole. In addition, many statistical packages now include general linear model analyses. General linear models can decompose the data into various factors, both *predictors of interest* to the experimenter (such as the differences between two conditions) and *predictors of no interest* that account for known sources of noise in the data (such as head movements that may be spuriously correlated with the signal).

One of the most useful advances in neuroimaging has been the development of event-related designs (Buckner & Braver, 1999; Donaldson & Buckner, 2001). In PET, and in the early years of fMRI, researchers used only block designs with long continuous periods (typically 10–30 sec) for each condition. Even when individual trials were brief, many trials of the same type were presented sequentially because researchers believed that the slow rise and fall of the hemodynamic response would prevent the resolution of individual events. Several key breakthroughs in the mid-1990s challenged this assumption and led to the development of event-related designs (Blamire et al., 1992; Buckner et al., 1996; Dale & Buckner, 1997). Unlike block designs, event-related designs allow the presentation of trials in an unpredictable order. In slow event-related designs, trials are widely separated in time (ideally 12–14 sec or longer) to ensure that the signal returns to baseline between events (Bandettini & Cox, 2000). The trials can be subjected to time-locked averaging to extract the common signal change related to the event while smoothing out the noise. In rapid event-related designs (Dale & Buckner, 1997), trials of various types can be intermixed and presented rapidly (e.g., every 2 sec). The analysis of rapid event-related designs is more complex and requires either careful counterbalancing of trial sequences or deconvolution of the fMRI signal, using "jittered" designs with irregular intervals.

Although event-related designs have a somewhat lesser statistical power to detect activation than block designs, they offer many valuable advantages. They make it possible to see the unfolding of sequential processes, for example, in paradigms with a delay interval interposed between stimulus and response. The randomized and unpredictable sequences of events prevents subjects from locking into a mental set. Trials can also be categorized by subjects' performances, for example, into correct and incorrect trials. Particularly in domains such as memory research, event-related approaches have opened many possibilities for elegant designs. Mixed designs, which incorporate blocks of variable trials, also hold promise for distinguishing between transient and sustained processing (Donaldson, 2004).

Although standard fMRI designs allow the experimenter to evaluate only the responses of an entire population of neurons within an imaging voxel, recently developed fMRI adaptation techniques hold excellent potential for evaluating the nature of the mental representations within an area (Grill-Spector et al., 1999; Grill-Spector & Malach, 2001). While behavioral adaptation has been called the "psycho-physicist's microelectrode" (Frisby, 1979), fMR adaptation may become the "neuroimager's microelectrode." Both behavioral and fMRI adaptation work on the same principle: with continued stimulation, neurons show reduced responses. These reduced responses can be used to determine the dimensions to which a neuron (or neuronal subpopulation or voxel or ROI) is sensitive.

For example, in object-selective cortex, including the lateral occipital cortex and the FFA, the response is lower for prolonged exposure to repeated images of the same face than for images of different faces. Grill-Spector and colleagues (1999) investigated whether neurons within the FFA are sensitive to viewpoint by comparing (1) the response to images of *different faces* seen from the *same viewpoint*; (2) the responses to repeated images of the *same face* seen from the *same viewpoint*; and (3) the response to repeated images of the *same face* seen from *different viewpoints*. A basic adaptation effect was observed as indicated by a reduced response to condition 2 (same face, same viewpoint) relative to condition 1 (different faces, same viewpoint). The experiments also tested whether object-selective regions were viewpoint-dependent or viewpoint-invariant. If the regions were selective for viewpoint, the same faces viewed from different viewpoints would be processed by different subpopulations of neurons, and thus adaptation would be weak. If the regions were invariant to viewpoint, the same faces viewed from different viewpoints would be processed by the same subpopulation of neurons. Adaptation would then be strong, and activation levels would be expected to drop by a comparable amount for conditions 2 and 3 relative to condition 1. Object-selective regions showed little adaptation to condition 3, suggesting viewpoint dependence.

Regardless of the exact design selected (data-driven vs. hypothesis-driven, voxel-wise vs. ROI, block vs. event-related, adaptation), it is essential to optimize the imaging parameters for the question being asked (for extended discussion, see Huettel et al., 2004). The experimenter has many decisions to make regarding the type of coil to employ (surface coil for high regional signal-to-noise ratio [SNR] vs. head coil for moderate global SNR vs. phased array coils for high global SNR) and trade-offs between high spatial resolution (up to 1 mm), high temporal resolution (up to 100s of ms) and the number of slices covered (Menon & Goodyear, 2001). The experimenter must also decide how many subjects to test and the number of runs and their duration, using assumptions about how large the difference between conditions is likely to be. The order of conditions within a run must be decided and is often constrained by counterbalancing issues. Some experiments are best suited to the statistical power of block designs whereas others can benefit from the elegance of event-related paradigms. Even for event-related designs, there is the choice between slow and rapid trial presentation. Once the design has been established, many more analysis decisions follow—preprocessing (motion correction, spatial smoothing, temporal filtering), statistical analysis (correlations, t-tests, general linear models, Fourier analysis, parametric vs. nonparametric statistics), group analysis vs. single subject analysis, brain presentation (2-D slice data, 3-D volumetric data, or cortical surface rendering), and—the biggest bugaboo—statistical thresholds and the application of corrections for inappropriate assumptions (multiple comparisons, serial correlations, fixed vs. random effects). It is not possible to recommend a single optimal design because the decisions will strongly depend on the priorities of the given experiment and the overall approach (voxelwise vs. ROI).

Issues

In ten years of doing neuroimaging and teaching others how to design successful experiments, I have noticed many common mistakes that I made myself and now see other newcomers frequently making. In some ways, it may be easier to explain how NOT to do an imaging experiment, based on some of the common pitfalls, than it is to explain how to do an imaging experiment well. Perhaps the most common mistake of newcomers to brain imaging is to take a well-established paradigm that has been used with other techniques (e.g., cognitive psychology or neurophysiology) and simply to run *exactly* the same paradigm in the scanner, without optimizing the design or considering whether the possible outcomes can enlighten theories about the process in question. In the worst examples, the experimenter does not consider changing any of the parameters that may be critical in neuroimaging designs, such as event timing. In the simplest experiments, two conditions are compared and lists (sometimes gigantic ones) of activation foci are published, followed by a post hoc "just so story" about why the task recruits the "subcortico-occipito-parieto-temporo-frontal network" (known to laypeople as "the brain"). Often, the areas that are activated are likely to include numerous parietal and frontal cortical areas that seem to be activated across a whopping variety of heterogeneous tasks from visuomotor control (Culham & Kanwisher, 2001) to meditation (e.g., Lazar et al., 2000) to gum-chewing (e.g., Takada & Miyamoto, 2004). Alternatively, poorly considered experiments may fail to find any meaningful activation. For instance, newcomers are often tempted to examine very subtle behavioral effects in brain areas where more robust effects have not yet been established. In such cases, there is little hope of an enlightening result.

Here, I make the case that careful consideration of the reasons and methods for doing neuroimaging can lead to more successful imaging experiments, making more valuable contributions to the field of cognitive neuroscience. I suggest consideration of the following points prior to starting new neuroimaging projects.

Do the Thought Experiment First

The cost of neuroimaging is exorbitant, with scan time typically costing between U.S.$200 and $1000 per hour, not including additional expenses such as subject fees, equipment, and staff salaries. In an environment with limited resources, particularly grant funds, it becomes critical to plan effective studies with a high probability of generating meaningful conclusions. Thought experiments are essentially free, and can save considerable wasted effort in real experiments.

The first question that should be asked in a thought experiment is whether the information about the anatomical foci that are activated during a particular comparison would constrain theories about the mechanisms involved. With the exception of rare dualists, most cognitive neuroscientists today believe that all behaviors have some neural correlate in the brain. The question, then, is whether knowing something about the *particular* neural correlate constrains possible theories of cognitive function. Certainly, in clinical research, such as presurgical planning, localization is very valuable; however, in cognitive neuroscience, localization is valuable only insofar as it informs theories of cognitive function.

There is no single good reason for doing an imaging study; nevertheless, I would like to suggest certain types of studies in which neuroimaging can make a unique contribution above and beyond what can be learned from other techniques. Where possible, I have provided specific examples, often taken from my own domain, vision and visual cognition.

Comparisons of Activation Across Multiple Tasks

It can be quite informative to investigate whether two tasks involve similar or different networks of areas. As one example, there has been much debate about whether subjects can pay attention to locations other than where they are directly looking (Klein, 1980; Rizzolatti et al., 1994). An elegant study by Maurizio Corbetta and colleagues (1998) demonstrated that attention and eye movements evoke activation in nearly equivalent brain networks. This fMRI experiment did not definitively resolve whether the two functions can be dissociated (as behavioral evidence suggests they can), but it certainly supported a close linkage between them. Comparisons can also provide interesting dissociations, or even double dissociations, based on the same logic used in neuropsychological studies. For example, theories about dissociations between vision for perception and vision for action (Milner & Goodale, 1995) have received some support from neuroimaging (Culham et al., 2003; James et al., 2003).

Characterization of a Single ROI's Responses

Neuroimaging can be used to identify one particular ROI and then to systematically investigate the stimuli and tasks that drive that region. Excellent examples come from seminal studies that identified key areas in the recognition of faces (Kanwisher et al., 1997) and other categories of objects (Malach et al., 1995). Subsequent experiments have categorized the activation of these regions across a wide range of stimuli and tasks (for a review, see Kanwisher et al., 2001), and have led to much more detailed hypotheses about face and object processing in the normal and the disordered human brain (e.g., Hadjikhani et al., 2004; Hasson, Avidan, et al., 2003).

Correlation Between Brain and Behavior

Studies that acquire concurrent behavioral data with the imaging acquisitions have the ability to examine the neural correlates of human behavior. Such neural correlates have been investigated in other species (e.g., Logothetis & Schall, 1989), but it is more challenging to infer subjective states in other species and the results may not generalize to humans. Numerous interesting experiments have investigated the relationship between a particular neural response in an area and conscious awareness (Rees, 2001; Ress & Heeger, 2003; Tong et al., 1998), performance, or subsequent memory for items (e.g., Brewer et al., 1998; Wagner et al., 1998).

Evaluation of the Role of Experience

Studies of subjects with different levels of training can help distinguish the degree of innate hardwiring versus experience-driven plasticity in an area. Due to the noninvasiveness of fMRI, subjects can be scanned multiple times with an intervening training period (e.g., Gauthier et al., 1999). Alternatively, activation patterns can be compared between experts and novices (e.g., Gauthier et al., 2000; Maguire et al., 1997).

Comparisons Between Species

Cognitive neuroscience has a wealth of information about brain processing in other species, particularly macaque monkeys, and tends to assume that similar mechanisms exist in the human brain; neuroimaging allows us to test this assumption. In some cases, there are strong cases for homologies between species, such as in early visual areas (Tootell et al., 1998). In other cases, discrepancies have been reported (Tootell et al., 1997). In higher-order cognitive areas, there are some speculative suggestions for homologies (e.g., Culham, 2003; Rizzolatti & Arbib, 1998).

Exploration of Uniquely Human Functions

Many functions may be considerably more developed in humans than other species, and thus cannot be explored using comparative techniques. Neuroimaging has been used to investigate topics including mathematical cognition (e.g., Naccache & Dehaene, 2001), theory of mind (e.g., Saxe et al., 2004), and tool usage (e.g., Chao & Martin, 2000). The rising new field of social cognitive neuroscience uses neuroimaging to investigate the links between human social behavior and brain mechanisms (Blakemore et al., 2004; Ochsner, 2004).

Derivation of General Organizational Principles

The ability of neuroimaging studies to investigate activation across many stimuli and tasks may provide some insight into the organization of the human brain. For example, there has been debate about whether object-selective regions of the temporal lobe have discrete or distributed representations of object categories (Ishai et al., 1999). One group has proposed an interesting theory that accounts for why category-selective subregions would exist in the arrangement that is observed across numerous fMRI studies (Hasson, Harel, et al., 2003).

Examination of Irregular Brain Function

Neuroimaging offers the opportunity to study the disordered human brain in action. In addition to using anatomical scans to determine lesion foci, functional neuroimaging can reveal which brain areas are impaired and which areas remain intact (e.g., Hasson, Avidan, et al., 2003; James et al., 2003; Steeves et al., 2004). This can elucidate which brain areas may be necessary or sufficient for a particular cognitive function. In addition, neuroimaging may be able to determine how connectivity has been affected by lesions (Maguire et al., 2001). Neuroimaging studies may also help explain the unusual functioning of patient populations. One fascinating study found activation of the auditory cortex in schizophrenic patients when they heard voices (Dierks et al., 1999). Neuroimaging may become increasingly useful in diagnosing and treating brain disorders (Matthews & Jezzard, 2004).

Assuming that an interesting question does exist, one might consider whether neuroimaging is the best approach and whether other techniques might be able to address the same issue in a better way. Other techniques may offer benefits such as better temporal resolution (as with event-related potentials or transcranial magnetic stimulation) or may be more cost-effective (as with behavioral studies). In my opinion, neuroimaging experiments are most successful when they are based on a strong foundation of research from other domains, particularly behavioral studies. For instance, neuroimaging of human visual function has been quite successful (as reviewed in Wandell, 1999), likely because it is based on over a century of psychophysics, as well as considerable neurophysiology, neuropsychology, and modeling. Neuroimaging of poorly understood phenomena may be largely futile.

Assuming that the neural substrates subserving some aspect of cognition form an interesting question, the next step should be to generate plausible hypotheses (including the null hypothesis) and the conclusions that would be derived if those hypotheses were true. A worthwhile experiment demands more than one plausible hypothesis. If all theories predict the same outcome, there's no point in doing the experiment. For each hypothesis, the experimenter should consider the likelihood of that hypothesis being supported. Even with a potentially groundbreaking hypothesis, the experiment may not be worth doing if that outcome is highly improbable. The best experiments are the ones in which several possible hypotheses (including the null hypothesis) would each lead to interesting and publishable results. The results of a study should be worthy of at least one "publicon" (one unknown scientist's name for "the smallest unit of publishable matter") that advances the existing knowledge in the field. It's worth thinking in advance about what the headline of that publicon might be and whether it would be worth the time, effort, and funding required.

Considering the expense of brain imaging, it is not always recommended to go straight from the thought experiment to the full data set. Often, it is worth running several iterations of pilot experiments and fine-tuning the design as necessary. Many newcomers plan to test hypotheses based on very subtle effects from other paradigms that are based on a complex series of assumptions. Sometimes, it may be worthwhile to establish basic effects and validate assumptions before moving on to subtleties. The temptation is always to include as many conditions as possible to provide the most stringent controls. Often, however, for the optimal statistical power during pilot testing, it is best to run a couple of subjects with the maximum number of trials in only the critical comparison conditions. The pilot results can be used to evaluate the minimum amount of data necessary to extract the basic effect. If the basic effect requires intensive data, it may be better to add control conditions in separate sessions.

Another issue worth considering is the acquisition of behavioral data. It may be beneficial to obtain behavioral data during pilot testing and/or during the actual scan session itself. Behavioral data such as response times, accuracy measures, and eye movement monitoring can be useful in interpreting neuroimaging data. Often, it is desirable to have such measures equated across conditions, in which case, behavioral piloting can be very important. In other cases, the protocol used in basic behavioral testing may need to be modified to optimize neuroimaging designs. Here it is critical to ensure that the basic effect still holds, despite any changes to the paradigm. In event-related designs, behavioral data can provide additional information that can be correlated with brain activation on a trial-by-trial basis.

Consider the Pros and Cons of Voxelwise vs. ROI Approaches When Deciding How to Design Your Experiment

Surprisingly in brain imaging, scientists tend to exclusively follow either the voxelwise approach or the ROI approach, sometimes fervently. Often the choice is made not by careful thought, but rather by the experimenter's field (with the voxelwise approach more common from groups with a background in PET and the ROI approach more common from groups who have utilized only fMRI), geographical area (with the voxelwise approach more common in Europe and the ROI approach more common in North America), and statistical package (some of which facilitate one approach over the other).

Each approach has its pros and cons. Voxelwise approaches are very useful during an initial foray into the neural substrates of a behavior, whereas ROI approaches are useful for characterizing a broad range of responses of a given area. Voxelwise approaches are useful when one has few hypotheses or very general hypotheses (e.g., Task X will activate Lobe Y), whereas ROI approaches force one to generate specific hypotheses about known areas. Voxelwise approaches can lead to short experiments that focus on the contrasts of interest, whereas experiments that use functionally defined ROIs require that time be spent on localizer runs. Users of voxelwise approaches must be very knowledgeable about the current and ever-changing norms for statistics, and may need to employ overly conservative corrections, whereas users of ROI approaches can use very basic statistics and more liberal thresholds because the hypotheses and regions are very limited. Voxelwise approaches are useful for large areas of activation that are relatively consistent between individual subjects. When anatomical foci are large and overlap well between subjects, voxelwise approaches make it easier to observe overall patterns of activity across the group without the confusion of intersubject variability. However, ROI approaches are preferable for areas that are small, are adjacent to other distinct areas, or require precise functional localization (e.g., retinotopic cortex). ROI approaches allow regions to be tailored to individual neuroanatomy. This can be quite important, given that activation tends to be more consistent with respect to sulcal landmarks than to stereotaxic coordinates (Watson et al., 1993) and sulci can vary considerably between subjects (Ono et al., 1990). A compromise between the two approaches may become more feasible with the development of algorithms that use sulcal landmarks and/or functionally defined foci to constrain intersubject averaging (Fischl et al., 1999).

The two approaches are not mutually exclusive, and there may be benefits to combining them. An ROI approach forces the experimenter to consider full hypotheses for at least one area. ROI approaches can be invaluable for establishing the role of critical regions across many variants of tasks and stimuli. However, overdependence on the ROI approach can lead scientists to overlook other regions that may also play a critical role. As an example, the vast majority of studies on motion perception have focused on the most robust "motion area," the middle temporal complex (MT+), despite the fact that more than a dozen other areas have been implicated in motion processing (Sunaert et al., 1999). Neuroimaging has an advantage over single-neuron recording by being able to easily investigate multiple regions simultaneously; yet many researchers ignore all but the clearest activations. In fact, it's not unheard-of for experimenters to deliberately exclude regions whose activations they can't understand or that may detract from the areas they are interested in (with the cerebellum being a very common target for exclusion!). ROI approaches have an advantage in being able to facilitate cross-talk between laboratories. With stereotaxic coordinates, it's never certain whether two labs that report coordinates in the same vicinity are actually studying the same area. Monkey neurophysiology suggests that the human cortex may consist of a mosaic of small, closely packed regions finer than the resolution of group-averaged data. With ROI approaches, groups that use the same localizers and contrasts within individual subjects can be more confident that they are evaluating the same functional area. One approach that can be very useful is the development of a functional brain bank for a pool of commonly scanned subjects. Using modern analysis packages, each individual subject's data from each session can be aligned to a standard anatomical image from that subject. That way, data from that subject can be compared across many subjects, each with numerous localizers. This approach has been quite successful in many labs that utilize retinotopic mapping in which the localizers are very time-intensive to collect (e.g., Tootell et al., 1998).

Think Carefully About Subtraction Logic

As described earlier, neuroimaging studies must rely on subtraction logic to measure *differences* in activation rather than absolute levels of activation per se. The assumption of pure insertion requires that the two critical conditions being compared differ in only one important aspect. Ideally, the two conditions to be compared should differ either in the stimulus or in the task, but not both. Stimulus manipulations are best for cognitive processes that are largely automatic (e.g., visual processing, face perception), and task manipulations are better for controlled processes (e.g., attention).

Even "simple" baselines may not be simple (Gusnard & Raichle, 2001). Early PET studies often used a passive rest condition as a baseline, but even at rest, the brain is still active. Indeed, this has posed problems in domains, such as memory research, where the ongoing mental processes during rest may actually lead to higher activation than active memory tasks. Some suggest that other active baseline tasks which distract the subject from memory encoding and retrieval may be preferable (Stark & Squire, 2001). Deactivations observed across many diverse tasks (Shulman et al., 1997) have been attributed to a "default mode network" that is activated when the subject is at rest (Raichle, 2001).

The assumption of pure insertion is likely often false because components may not summate with simple addition. Consider an example of measuring the neural activation for saccadic (i.e., rapid and sudden) eye movements to targets. The experimental condition may consist of eye movements to briefly flashed targets. Two control conditions are possible. In the most common design for a saccade system localizer, the control condition would be fixation on a central point. When subtracting fixation from saccades, the assumption is that the purely inserted component is the eye movement. Of course, in reality, other components are also being inserted. The flash of the target provokes a visual transient and draws attention. An alternative control condition would be to have fixation of a central point with target flashes that are ignored. Superficially, in the subtraction of this control from saccades, target transients and stimulus-driven attention would subtract out, leaving "purely inserted" saccades. The situation may not be so simple, however. Some neurons in saccade areas may respond both to stimulus-driven attention and to eye movements (e.g., Colby et al., 1996) such that the activation during the experimental condition depends on whether these components summate and whether they do so using straightforward (linear) addition. There may be other differences between the components of the tasks. Fixation during flashing targets may involve preparation and suppression of saccades and could in fact yield more signal than pure saccades.

More sophisticated designs can sometimes reduce the problems of selecting the correct baseline. One particularly attractive design is the parametric study, developed in cognitive psychology to avoid some of the similar problems with subtraction logic that occur with reaction time experiments (Sternberg, 1969). Parametric imaging studies search for brain activation that scales with the *amount* of a particular component that is added rather than searching for brain activation that increases with the first addition of that component. In our example of saccadic eye movements, an example would be to compare conditions with saccades at different rates (e.g., 2 vs. 1 vs. 0.5 saccades per second), on the assumption that areas involved in saccades would respond in proportion to saccade frequency (Beauchamp et al., 2000). Even with parametric designs, there may be reasons to expect nonlinear relationships between the stimulus manipulation and brain activation that can be used to address important theoretical issues (e.g., Culham, Cavanagh et al., 2001; Price et al., 1994).

Another approach is the factorial design, where at least two factors are manipulated in the same experiment to evaluate main effects and interactions (Price & Friston, 1997). In our example of a saccade task, we could have a 2×2 design with one manipulation being saccades vs. fixation, and the other being the use of static or flashed targets. That would lead to four conditions: (1) fixation on a point with only static targets present; (2) saccades between static targets; (3) fixation on a point with flashed targets; and (4) saccades between flashed targets. A region with a role in saccadic eye movements would be expected to show a main effect of eye movements (saccades vs. fixation, collapsed across flashing and static events). A region with a role in stimulus-driven attention would be expected to show a main effect of stimulus transience (flashed vs. static, collapsed across saccade and fixation events). More complex regions might show interactions (e.g., a much bigger response for saccades to flashed targets than would be predicted from the two main effects alone). Because factorial designs include comparisons across multiple conditions, they are less subject to the problems of a single subtraction between just two conditions.

Variations in task difficulty or in the degree of attention required to do the task frequently violate the assumption of pure insertion. Many studies have demonstrated that brain activation is strongly modulated by the degree of attention devoted to the task (e.g., O'Craven et al., 1997). Attention is a common confound in many neuroimaging studies and may account for the fact that a surprising number of very diverse studies seem to find activation in the network of areas that subserves attention—including a large extent of the intraparietal sulcus as well as the frontal eye fields (Corbetta et al., 1998; Culham & Kanwisher, 2001; Wojciulik & Kanwisher, 1999).

The common wisdom to avoid confounding differences in attention is to equate stimuli for attentional salience and to equate tasks for attentional performance. This is often easier in theory than in practice. Many stimuli are inherently more interesting than their control condition counterparts. A common solution is to introduce a task that demands attention for all stimuli, such as a *1-back task*, where the subject must press a button whenever the same stimulus appears twice in a row. This technique works well when the 1-back task has comparable difficulty in all conditions. Unfortunately, that isn't always the case. For example, 1-back tasks are common in localizers for object-selective visual areas in which objects and scrambled objects are compared. The 1-back task is easier for objects, and subjects may use different strategies for objects (e.g., remembering semantic labels) than scrambled objects (e.g., attending to spatial relationships). The 1-back approach works well in temporal cortex, but not so well in parietal cortex, where object-selective areas may also be involved in attention and spatial processing.

In other cases, attention may be a fundamental aspect of neuronal function. For example, much debate has been sparked regarding the relationship between attention and awareness. In studies of awareness, then, would it be appropriate even to try to control for attention? Such issues have been raised in the context of motion illusions that have been suggested to relate to the perception of motion (Culham et al., 1999; He et al., 1998; Tootell, Reppas, Dale, et al., 1995) vs. attention to motion (Huk et al., 2001). Given that the strength of the perceived motion is strongly related to the degree of attention directed to the motion (e.g., Beauchamp et al., 1997; Rees et al., 1997), the dichotomy may not be so straightforward.

Be Aware of the Caveats of Neuroimaging

fMRI has been an invaluable tool in cognitive neuroscience, but the technique is still so new that the underlying mechanisms are quite poorly understood. It is well established that the blood-oxygenation-level dependent (BOLD) signal, measured by fMRI, indirectly reflects neuronal activity levels. What remains poorly understood is the relationship between various aspects of neuronal processing and the changes in BOLD activity. Much recent research has addressed this relationship and is well summarized elsewhere (chapter 2 in this volume) (Logothetis & Wandell, 2004).

At present, the predominant hypothesis, proposed by Logothetis and colleagues (2001), is that BOLD activation may reflect synaptic inputs and local processing within an area more than action potentials. This may help to account for some discrepancies between the results from human fMRI studies and monkey neurophysiology studies. For instance, human fMRI results indicate that attention modulates activity in primary visual cortex (e.g., Gandhi et al., 1999), in contrast to monkey neurophysiology, where negligible attentional effects have been reported (e.g., Luck et al., 1997). This difference could arise from the different mechanisms of BOLD vs. action potentials or from the reduced spatial resolution of fMRI, which cannot disentangle feedforward vs. feedback signals. Furthermore, both neurophysiology and BOLD imaging have inherent biases. Neurophysiological recordings are biased toward selecting larger neurons (such as pyramidal cells in cortex) while bypassing smaller neurons (Logothetis & Wandell, 2004). BOLD imaging depends on vascular density, which is correlated with the number of synapses rather than the number of neurons, in an area and varies considerably between brain areas (Duvernoy et al., 1981). For instance, primary visual cortex (V1) has more dense vascularization than adjacent extrastriate cortex (namely V2). Some have suggested that it may be easier to observe BOLD activation in some regions compared with others because of differences in vasculature (Harrison et al., 2002). This may account for why some regions—for example, in frontal cortex (Duncan & Owen, 2000)—are notoriously hard to activate, while others, such as the intraparietal sulcus, seem to be activated by practically anything (Culham & Kanwisher, 2001).

Cognitive neuroscientists tend to assume that neuronal action potentials measured by single-neuron recording are the gold standard in interpreting brain processes; however, the BOLD signal may provide information about additional mechanisms beyond the action potential that are a fundamental component of neural processing. Given the biases of each technique, multiple approaches may provide a more complete picture.

In addition to the uncertainty regarding the relationship between neuronal spikes and BOLD activity, there are problems in using single-neuron activity to predict the response of the population that will be measured by neuroimaging. Scannell and Young (1999) provide an excellent exposition of these issues. They used computational models of single-unit activity in the MT+ motion complex to predict the population response that would be recorded with BOLD. They found cases in which it was possible to observe a subpopulation of neurons that responded vigorously to a stimulus without a corresponding difference in BOLD signal. The population response was a function of several factors, including baseline firing rate, the modulation of the firing rate, the tuning function for each attribute, and the number of attributes encoded. Their models suggested that effects which induce small changes in the firing rates of large numbers of neurons, specifically attention, have a much greater population result than effects that induce large changes in a small number of neurons. They also suggested that as experience leads to narrowing of tuning functions, BOLD population response differences become smaller.

Other problems arise in the actual modeling of the BOLD signal. Although the hemodynamic response profile has been well-characterized, data suggest that it can vary considerably from subject to subject (Aguirre et al., 1998) and from area to area. Thus many of the models employed may be accurate on average but subject to error for an individual case.

The paradigm of fMR adaptation holds great promise for expanding the types of questions that can be addressed with fMRI; however, it remains poorly understood and may be far more complex than it appears to be on the surface. The many names for the phenomenon, ranging from repetition suppression (Henson & Rugg, 2003) to adaptation (Grill-Spector & Malach, 2001) to priming (Henson, 2003), illustrate the confusion regarding possible mechanisms. In some brain regions, particularly the object-selective lateral occipital complex, the technique has been very successful (e.g., Grill-Spector et al., 1999; James et al., 2002; Kourtzi & Kanwisher, 2000b). In other regions however, even those where adaptation is known to occur from psychophysical techniques, some experimenters have failed to find it with fMRI (Boynton & Finney, 2003; Murray & Wojciulik, 2004).

At this point, it is not clear why some paradigms produce better fMR adaptation than others. Differences may depend on the time scale of adaptation (Henson et al., 2000; Henson, 2003). Although some have suggested that the adaptation approach avoids the problem of attentional confounds that occur with regular paradigms (Huk et al., 2001), priming does indeed appear to be highly dependent on attention (Eger et al., 2004; Murray & Wojciulik, 2004). Just as with regular fMRI, the specificity of adaptation is subject to differences in the mechanisms of blood supply across brain regions, and the technique may be particularly sensitive to synaptic inputs and local processing rather than to outgoing action potentials (Tolias et al., 2001). Finally, the correspondence of such repetition effects with behavioral measures of priming is often incomplete (Henson, 2003; Henson & Rugg, 2003; Thiel et al., 2001). Given these concerns, while fMR adaptation remains an exciting tool for neuroimagers, a better understanding is necessary to make sense of the results it produces.

Look at the Data and Understand What the Preprocessing and Statistics Are Doing

Since the advent of neuroimaging, many sophisticated analysis packages for neuroimaging data have been developed. Many of these packages offer a bewildering array of options to the novice neuroimager. The temptation can be simply to follow the standard recipe to "see what blobs light up," without ever looking at the raw data. This can be risky, particularly with temperamental fMRI magnets; days of "dysfunctional" MRI are not uncommon. Even simple exploration, such as *voxel-surfing*—viewing the time courses of voxels selected at random—can be enlightening. For example, some data sets may have spikes in the data that can lead to spurious activation or can prevent real activation from passing the statistical threshold.

In my opinion (and I realize large camps of neuroimagers would disagree), the ability to view time course data easily, either for random voxels or for regions of interest, is an underrated tool in statistical analysis packages. Voxel-surfing (or region-surfing) can be a very effective way to flag problems in the data and violations of statistical assumptions. Viewing of movies of the brain over subsequent points in time can also reveal possible problems with the data (e.g., spikes may appear as a brightening of the entire image) or with the subject (e.g., head motion will appear as shifts in the movie). Movie viewing *following* motion correction can sometimes reveal residual problems that remain. Analysis of single subjects and/or single runs can sometimes indicate problematic data that should be removed from the final analysis (of course, this should be done only when there is a valid objective reason for doing so, not simply because a subject's data are inconsistent with the hypothesis).

It is often worth analyzing data in several different ways to evaluate the effect of various manipulations. In the case of robust data, the conclusions will be the same, regardless of the specific analysis. However, in some cases, different analyses may produce different results, and the reasons for the differences may themselves be enlightening. For example, one might want to evaluate an effect with both an ROI approach and a voxelwise approach. If the two approaches lead to similar conclusions, there is no problem. If they lead to different conclusions, the underlying reasons may be interesting. If a result is significant in an ROI approach but not a voxelwise approach, it may indicate that the effect is weak and the voxelwise approach is too stringent. If a voxelwise analysis shows activation within a subregion of the ROI, it may be that functional subdivisions exist within the region. I am *not* advocating an approach of trying every possible combination of analyses to find *something* that reaches significance. It's still important to have an a priori plan about how best to proceed, and to maintain standards of acceptable data analysis.

Some neuroimaging statistics packages offer formulaic steps for data analysis that, although seemingly simple, warrant careful consideration. One excellent example is the application of motion correction algorithms. There is a tendency to assume that these algorithms are a panacea for possible head motion artifacts, and that as long as the algorithms are run as a default, concerns about motion have been sufficiently addressed. This is not always true, and in some cases, motion correction can induce artifacts that were not present in the original data (Freire & Mangin, 2001). In my experience, the success of these algorithms is quite limited and often does not suffice to fix all motion-related problems, particularly ones with large, abrupt movements. The algorithms assume that the head can move with six degrees of freedom (three translations and three rotations), and that as long as the shifted position of the head is reset to the starting point, the problem will have been fixed.

There are several problems with this approach. First, the data must be resampled, so information is lost because it is unavailable (particularly in the top and bottom slices) or because it has been interpolated. Prospective motion correction, in which slices are replanned on the fly, with each volume adjusted on the basis of detected motion, is now being provided by some scanner manufacturers and appears to provide output superior to traditional post hoc corrections (Lee et al., 1996). Second, although adjustment of six parameters works well with PET data, the situation is more complex in fMRI. Unfortunately, in fMRI, when the head moves, it changes its position not only relative to the frame of the image but also relative to the magnetic field. In an inhomogeneous field, this means that the overall signal level can remain distorted when the head is returned to its original position in the image (Jezzard & Clare, 1999). A procedure known as *shimming* attempts to make the magnetic field as homogeneous as possible, but it is never completely successful. The pattern of inhomogeneities is dependent on the distribution of mass in the bore. With movement of the head, this distribution changes such that not only is the head in a different part of the field, but the field itself may be different (and thus signal levels throughout the volume may be affected). Simple coregistration of volumes over time ignores this problem. Furthermore, field distortions can arise due to the changing distribution of mass from body parts other than the head.

In cases where movements are correlated with the paradigm (e.g., studies of speech, swallowing, or grasping), slow, event-related paradigms can be used to dissociate the artifacts (which occur with no lag) from brain activation (which occurs with the appropriate hemodynamic lag; Birn et al., 1999). Figure 3.1 (see plate 3) illustrates a case where movement of mass within the field leads to profound artifacts that in turn lead to faulty motion detection and correction. Such artifacts occur whenever any mass moves in the field, and are worst for movements closest to the head (as in head movements themselves but also movements of the tongue, throat, and jaw, as in swallowing artifacts, and with movements of the chest during respiration). New subjects are always instructed not to move the head; however, much better results are obtained with more detailed instructions that discourage swallowing and changes to mouth and body posture during functional scans. (Breathing, however, is encouraged.) Although motion correction algorithms may sometimes improve data quality, nothing works as well as *preventing* motion in the first place. Although the development of high-field strength and impressive new technology (e.g., phased array coils) has greatly improved signal-to-noise, so-called *physiological noise* (of which motion is a large component) remains a major limiting factor in data quality.

The researcher should be aware of common fallacies in statistical logic and the representation of statistical data. Here are three examples.

One very common mistake is the indirect comparison. The researcher assumes that if a particular region responds more in one condition than the control state, but not more in a second condition than the control state, then the activation must be higher in the first state than the second. To understand why this logic is false, recall that statistical significance depends not only on the size of the effect but also on the threshold selected and the variability in the data. As shown in figure 3.2, one contrast may be more significant than another because of a larger effect size or, alternatively, because of small differences in statistical significance or because of reduced variability. In sum, "Differences in significance do not necessarily indicate significant differences" (as succinctly stated by Nancy Kanwisher, personal communication). The straightforward solution is to perform *direct* comparisons between critical conditions.

Another common mistake is to misinterpret interactions in factorial designs. An interaction occurs whenever a manipulation has different effect sizes depending on the status of another manipulation. When graphing factorial effects, an interaction can be seen by any pair (or more) of lines that do not run parallel to one another. Consider a hypothesis that attention to a stimulus will amplify activity in brain areas known to process that stimulus, but not other areas. ROIs selective for faces (FFA) and scenes (parahippocampal place area, or PPA) could be identified using a localizer scan. Subjects could then be shown photographs of either faces or places (main

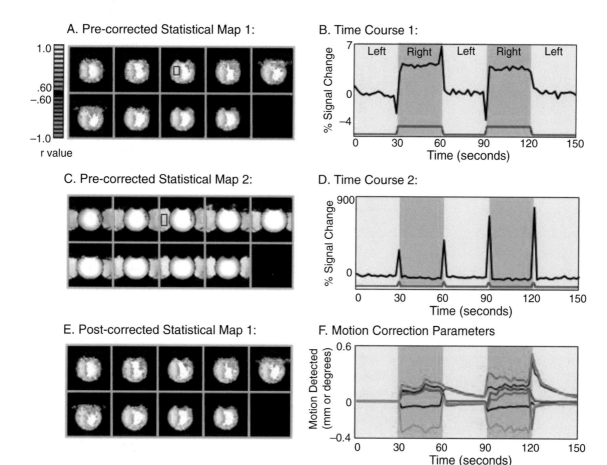

Figure 3.1
Experiment illustrating the contamination of data by the movement of mass within the magnetic field. A spherical phantom remained completely stationary during a series of T2*-weighted scans. Four 1-kg bags of saline solution were mounted on a wooden pole to approximate the mass of a human arm. Every 30 sec, the mass moved between the left and right side of the phantom and then remained stationary for the remainder of the interval. (*A*) A comparison between the signal when the mass was to the right versus the left of the phantom illustrates widespread false "activation." (*B*) The time course within a region denoted by the black box in the third slice of (*A*) is shown by the black line. Note the changes in overall signal level and the brief spikes whenever the external mass changed position. The reference time course used to generate the map in (*A*) is indicated by the blue line. (*C*) A statistical map showing regions where spiking occurred at the time of movement. (*D*) The time course within the region indicated by the black box in the third slice of (*C*) is shown by the black line. The reference time course used to generate the map in (*C*) is indicated by the blue line. (*E*) The comparison between the signal with the mass at each position is shown after motion correction was applied. There is no reduction of false activation. (*F*) Output of a motion detection and correction algorithm (in Brain Voyager, with similar results from Statistical Parametric Mapping software). The resulting three translation parameters are shown by blue lines, and the three rotation parameters are shown by red lines. Note that although there was no movement whatsoever in the phantom, the algorithm detected and falsely attempted to correct for spurious motion created by the moving external mass. See plate 3 for color version.

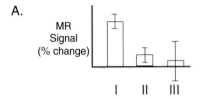

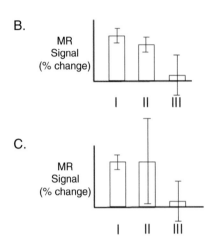

Figure 3.2
Schematic illustration of faulty statistical logic regarding differences of significance. In all three hypothetical data sets, the statistics indicate that condition I is *significantly* different from condition III and condition II is *not significantly* different from condition III. Is it therefore true that condition I is different from condition II in all cases? (*A*) The difference in significance between the two comparisons (I vs. III and II vs. III) occurs primarily because of differences in the magnitude of activation. (*B*) The difference in significance also occurs because of differences in the magnitude of activation, but may or may not be present, depending on the statistical threshold chosen. (*C*) The difference in significance occurs primarily because of differences in the variability of activation. Error bars indicate 95% confidence intervals.

effect of object category) and asked to attend to the stimulus or to an irrelevant attribute (e.g., the color of the fixation point). The hypothesis leads to the prediction that in the FFA, the difference between attending vs. not attending to the stimulus will be higher for faces than for places (figure 3.3). Conversely, the hypothesis predicts that in the PPA, the difference between attending vs. not attending to the stimulus will be higher for places than for faces. For simplicity, let's consider only the FFA. The obvious way to test whether the hypothesis holds true would be to perform a voxelwise 2×2 factorial analysis (stimulus category $\times$ attentional state) and to look for a significant interaction. If an interaction is found, is the hypothesis correct? Not necessarily. Just as in conventional statistics, interactions can occur for many reasons. To phrase it another way, in the graphs for a factorial design, the

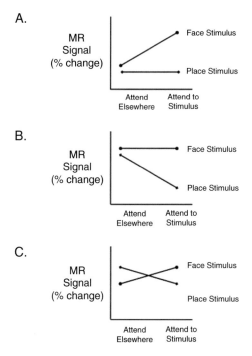

Figure 3.3
Schematic illustration of faulty statistical logic regarding interactions. Graphs show hypothetical activation in the fusiform face area when the subject attends to a particular stimulus (a face or a place) or attends to a central fixation point. A reasonable hypothesis may be that attention will enhance activation for the preferred stimulus category (faces) but not for other categories (e.g., places). In (*A*), the interaction appears consistent with the hypothesis. In (*B*) and (*C*), similar interactions occur but are not consistent with the hypothesis. This example illustrates that the interaction term alone is not sufficient to understand the outcome of a factorial design.

lines can be nonparallel for several reasons. Post hoc t-tests would help confirm the pattern (e.g., attend stimulus vs. attend elsewhere should be significant for faces but not places).

A third common problem is that of "proving the obvious" in ROI approaches. When you use statistics to select a region, that region must of necessity demonstrate the effect indicated in the statistics. For example, if you identify the motion complex, MT+, by contrasting moving vs. stationary images and then do a post hoc test to compare moving minus stationary conditions, it should come as little surprise that they differ significantly. This seems obvious, but it is not uncommon to see manuscripts that comment on significant differences within an area defined by a statistical test of that difference. In cases where post hoc analyses are performed on the same comparison used to localize a region, it should be clarified whether they would of necessity be significant or whether the analysis adds new information.

Future Directions

Neuroimaging is a very young science experiencing a combination of enthusiasm, cynicism, and growing pains. Progress since the 1980s has been phenomenal. Basic scanning techniques have improved considerably, and many recent capabilities of fMRI, such as event-related designs and fMR adaptation, were unanticipated in the early years. Recent developments hold much promise for solutions to many of the problems described here, and for adding powerful new techniques to the cognitive neuroscientist's toolbox. Some of the most promising recent developments include (1) the use of diffusion tensor imaging (e.g., Basser et al., 2000) and functional connectivity studies (Friston et al., 1997; McIntosh, 1999) to determine the wiring of functional brain areas; (2) the use of mental chronometry to push the temporal resolution of fMRI (Formisano & Goebel, 2003); (3) the development of imaging genomics to correlate genetic markers, brain activation, and behavior (Hariri & Weinberger, 2003); (4) the combination of neuroimaging with other techniques such as event-related potentials (ERPs), magnetoencephalography (MEG) and or transcranial magnetic stimulation (TMS) to benefit from the combined strengths of each technique (Paus et al., 1997); and (5) the combination of monkey physiology, monkey neuroimaging, and human neuroimaging to better understand differences between techniques and between species (Logothetis et al., 1999; Orban et al., 2004).

Acknowledgments

I would like to thank many colleagues over the years who have provided stimulating discussions and debates about experimental design. In particular, I would like to thank Nancy Kanwisher, who first gave me the opportunity to become involved in brain imaging and shared many valuable insights into experimental design, some of which I have included here. I thank my assistant, Ken Valyear, for comments, for assistance with the preparation of figure 3.1, and for valuable discussion of fMR adaptation caveats. I also thank Matt Brown, Christine Carter, Cristiana Cavina Pratesi, Stefan Kohler, Mary Ellen Large, Anthony Singhal, and an anonymous reviewer for comments on the manuscript. Any interpretations, omissions, or errors are my own. This work was supported by the Canadian Institutes for Health Research and the National Sciences and Engineering Research Council of Canada.

Note

1. Although some authors differentiate between reaction times and response times, for simplicity I will use the single term "reaction time" to indicate the time between initial stimulus presentation and the pressing of a response key.

Culham, J. C., Cavanagh, P., & Kanwisher, N. G. (2001). Attention response functions. Characterizing brain areas using fMRI activation during parametric variations of attentional load. *Neuron* 32, 737–745.

Culham, J. C., Danckert, S. L., DeSouza, J. F., Gati, J. S., Menon, R. S., & Goodale, M. A. (2003). Visually guided grasping produces fMRI activation in dorsal but not ventral stream brain areas. *Experimental Brain Research* 153, 180–189.

Culham, J. C., Dukelow, S. P., Vilis, T., Hassard, F. A., Gati, J. S., Menon, R. S., et al. (1999). Recovery of fMRI activation in motion area MT following storage of the motion aftereffect. *Journal of Neurophysiology* 81, 388–393.

Culham, J. C., & Kanwisher, N. G. (2001). Neuroimaging of cognitive functions in human parietal cortex. *Current Opinion in Neurobiology* 11, 157–163.

Dale, A. M., & Buckner, R. L. (1997). Selective averaging of rapidly presented individual trials using fMRI. *Human Brain Mapping* 5, 329–340.

Dierks, T., Linden, D. E., Jandl, M., Formisano, E., Goebel, R., Lanfermann, H., et al. (1999). Activation of Heschl's gyrus during auditory hallucinations. *Neuron* 22, 615–621.

Donaldson, D. I. (2004). Parsing brain activity with fMRI and mixed designs: What kind of a state is neuroimaging in? *Trends in Neurosciences* 27, 442–444.

Donaldson, D. I., & Buckner, R. L. (2001). Effective paradigm design. In P. Jezzard, P. M. Matthews, & S. M. Smith (Eds.), *Functional MRI: An Introduction to Methods*, 177–195. Oxford: Oxford University Press.

Donders, F. C. (1868). Die Schnelligkeit psychischer Prozesse. *Archiv für Anatomie und Physiologie und wissenschaftliche Medizin*, 657–681.

Donders, F. C. (1969). On the speed of mental processes. *Acta Psychologica* 30, 412–431.

Duncan, J., & Owen, A. M. (2000). Common regions of the human frontal lobe recruited by diverse cognitive demands. *Trends in Neurosciences* 23, 475–483.

Duvernoy, H. M., Delon, S., & Vannson, J. L. (1981). Cortical blood vessels of the human brain. *Brain Research Bulletin* 7, 519–579.

Eger, E., Henson, R. N., Driver, J., & Dolan, R. J. (2004). BOLD repetition decreases in object-responsive ventral visual areas depend on spatial attention. *Journal of Neurophysiology* 92, 1241–1247.

Evans, A. C., Collins, D. L., Mills, S. R., Brown, E. D., Kelly, R. L., & Peters, T. M. (1993). 3D statistical neuroanatomical models from 305 MRI volumes. *Proceedings of the IEEE-Nuclear Science Symposium and Medical Imaging Conference*, 1813–1817.

Fischl, B., Sereno, M. I., Tootell, R. B., & Dale, A. M. (1999). High-resolution intersubject averaging and a coordinate system for the cortical surface. *Human Brain Mapping* 8, 272–284.

Formisano, E., & Goebel, R. (2003). Tracking cognitive processes with functional MRI mental chronometry. *Current Opinion in Neurobiology* 13, 174–181.

Fox, P. T. (1997). The growth of human brain mapping. *Human Brain Mapping* 5, 1–2.

Fox, P. T., Mintun, M. A., Raichle, M. E., Miezin, F. M., Allman, J. M., & Van Essen, D. C. (1986). Mapping human visual cortex with positron emission tomography. *Nature* 323, 806–809.

Freire, L., & Mangin, J. F. (2001). Motion correction algorithms may create spurious brain activations in the absence of subject motion. *NeuroImage* 14, 709–722.

Frisby, J. P. (1979). *Seeing: Illusion, Brain, and Mind.* Oxford: Oxford University Press.

Friston, K. J., Buechel, C., Fink, G. R., Morris, J., Rolls, E., & Dolan, R. J. (1997). Psychophysiological and modulatory interactions in neuroimaging. *NeuroImage* 6, 218–229.

Gandhi, S. P., Heeger, D. J., & Boynton, G. M. (1999). Spatial attention affects brain activity in human primary visual cortex. *Proceedings of the National Academy of Sciences USA* 96, 3314–3319.

Gauthier, I., Skudlarski, P., Gore, J. C., & Anderson, A. W. (2000). Expertise for cars and birds recruits brain areas involved in face recognition. *Nature Neuroscience* 3(2), 191–197.

Gauthier, I., Tarr, M. J., Anderson, A. W., Skudlarski, P., & Gore, J. C. (1999). Activation of the middle fusiform "face area" increases with expertise in recognizing novel objects. *Nature Neuroscience* 2(6), 568–573.

Genovese, C. R., Lazar, N. A., & Nichols, T. (2002). Thresholding of statistical maps in functional neuroimaging using the false discovery rate. *NeuroImage* 15, 870–878.

Grill-Spector, K., Kushnir, T., Edelman, S., Avidan, G., Itzchak, Y., & Malach, R. (1999). Differential processing of objects under various viewing conditions in the human lateral occipital complex. *Neuron* 24, 187–203.

Grill-Spector, K., & Malach, R. (2001). fMR-adaptation: A tool for studying the functional properties of human cortical neurons. *Acta Psychologica* (Amsterdam), 107, 293–321.

Grill-Spector, K., & Malach, R. (2004). The human visual cortex. *Annual Review of Neuroscience* 27, 649–677.

Gusnard, D. A., & Raichle, M. E. (2001). Searching for a baseline: Functional imaging and the resting human brain. *Nature Reviews Neuroscience* 2, 685–694.

Hadjikhani, N., Joseph, R. M., Snyder, J., Chabris, C. F., Clark, J., Steele, S., et al. (2004). Activation of the fusiform gyrus when individuals with autism spectrum disorder view faces. *NeuroImage* 22, 1141–1150.

Hariri, A. R., & Weinberger, D. R. (2003). Imaging genomics. *British Medical Bulletin* 65, 259–270.

Harrison, R. V., Harel, N., Panesar, J., & Mount, R. J. (2002). Blood capillary distribution correlates with hemodynamic-based functional imaging in cerebral cortex. *Cerebral Cortex* 12, 225–233.

Hasson, U., Avidan, G., Deouell, L. Y., Bentin, S., & Malach, R. (2003). Face-selective activation in a congenital prosopagnosic subject. *Journal of Cognitive Neuroscience* 15, 419–431.

Hasson, U., Harel, M., Levy, I., & Malach, R. (2003). Large-scale mirror-symmetry organization of human occipito-temporal object areas. *Neuron* 37, 1027–1041.

He, S., Cohen, E. R., & Hu, X. (1998). Close correlation between activity in brain area MT/V5 and the perception of a visual motion aftereffect. *Current Biology* 8, 1215–1218.

Henson, R., Shallice, T., & Dolan, R. (2000). Neuroimaging evidence for dissociable forms of repetition priming. *Science* 287, 1269–1272.

Henson, R. N. (2003). Neuroimaging studies of priming. *Progress in Neurobiology* 70, 53–81.

Henson, R. N., & Rugg, M. D. (2003). Neural response suppression, haemodynamic repetition effects, and behavioural priming. *Neuropsychologia* 41, 263–270.

Huettel, S. A., Song, A. W., & McCarthy, G. (2004). *Functional Magnetic Resonance Imaging.* Sunderland, MA: Sinauer.

Huk, A. C., Ress, D., & Heeger, D. J. (2001). Neuronal basis of the motion aftereffect reconsidered. *Neuron* 32, 161–172.

Ishai, A., Ungerleider, L. G., Martin, A., Schouten, J. L., & Haxby, J. V. (1999). Distributed representation of objects in the human ventral visual pathway. *Proceedings of the National Academy of Sciences USA* 96, 9379–9384.

James, T. W., Culham, J., Humphrey, G. K., Milner, A. D., & Goodale, M. A. (2003). Ventral occipital lesions impair object recognition but not object-directed grasping: An fMRI study. *Brain* 126, 2463–2475.

James, T. W., Humphrey, G. K., Gati, J. S., Servos, P., Menon, R. S., & Goodale, M. A. (2002). Haptic study of three-dimensional objects activates extrastriate visual areas. *Neuropsychologia* 40, 1706–1714.

Jezzard, P., & Clare, S. (1999). Sources of distortion in functional MRI data. *Human Brain Mapping* 8, 80–85.

Jezzard, P., Matthews, P. M., & Smith, S. M. (2001). *Functional MRI: An Introduction to Methods.* Oxford: Oxford University Press.

Kanwisher, N., Downing, P., Epstein, R., & Kourtzi, Z. (2001). Functional neuroimaging of visual recognition. In R. Cabeza & A. Kingstone (Eds.), *Handbook of Functional Neuroimaging of Cognition*, 109–152. Cambridge, MA: MIT Press.

Kanwisher, N., McDermott, J., & Chun, M. M. (1997). The fusiform face area: A module in human extrastriate cortex specialized for face perception. *Journal of Neuroscience* 17(11), 4302–4311.

Klein, R. M. (1980). Does oculomotor readiness mediate cognitive control of visual attention? In R. S. Nickerson (Ed.), *Attention and Performance VII*, 259–276. Hillsdale, NJ: Erlbaum.

Kosslyn, S. M. (1999). If neuroimaging is the answer, what is the question? *Philosophical Transactions of the Royal Societyof London* B354, 1283–1294.

Kourtzi, Z., & Kanwisher, N. (2000a). Activation in human MT/MST by static images with implied motion. *Journal of Cognitive Neuroscience* 12, 48–55.

Kourtzi, Z., & Kanwisher, N. (2000b). Cortical regions involved in perceiving object shape. *Journal of Neuroscience* 20, 3310–3318.

Kwong, K. K., Belliveau, J. W., Chesler, D. A., Goldberg, I. E., Weisskoff, R. M., Poncelet, B. P., et al. (1992). Dynamic magnetic resonance imaging of human brain activity during primary sensory stimulation. *Proceedings of the National Academy of Sciences USA* 89, 5675–5679.

Lazar, S. W., Bush, G., Gollub, R. L., Fricchione, G. L., Khalsa, G., & Benson, H. (2000). Functional brain mapping of the relaxation response and meditation. *NeuroReport* 11, 1581–1585.

Lee, C. C., Jack, C. R., Jr., Grimm, R. C., Rossman, P. J., Felmlee, J. P., Ehman, R. L., et al. (1996). Real-time adaptive motion correction in functional MRI. *Magnetic Resonance in Medicine* 36, 436–444.

Logothetis, N. K., Guggenberger, H., Peled, S., & Pauls, J. (1999). Functional imaging of the monkey brain. *Nature Neuroscience* 2, 555–562.

Logothetis, N. K., Pauls, J., Augath, M., Trinath, T., & Oeltermann, A. (2001). Neurophysiological investigation of the basis of the fMRI signal. *Nature* 412, 150–157.

Logothetis, N. K., & Schall, J. D. (1989). Neuronal correlates of subjective visual perception. *Science* 245, 761–763.

Logothetis, N. K., & Wandell, B. A. (2004). Interpreting the BOLD signal. *Annual Review of Physiology* 66, 735–769.

Luck, S. J., Chelazzi, L., Hillyard, S. A., & Desimone, R. (1997). Neural mechanisms of spatial selective attention in areas V1, V2, and V4 of macaque visual cortex. *Journal of Neurophysiology* 77, 24–42.

Maguire, E. A., Frackowiak, R. S. J., & Frith, C. D. (1997). Recalling routes around London: Activation of the right hippocampus in taxi drivers. *Journal of Neuroscience* 17, 7103–7110.

Maguire, E. A., Vargha-Khadem, F., & Mishkin, M. (2001). The effects of bilateral hippocampal damage on fMRI regional activations and interactions during memory retrieval. *Brain* 124, 1156–1170.

Malach, R., Reppas, J. B., Benson, R. R., Kwong, K. K., Jiang, H., Kennedy, W. A., et al. (1995). Object-related activity revealed by functional magnetic resonance imaging in human occipital cortex. *Proceedings of the National Academy of Sciences USA* 92, 8135–8139.

Matthews, P. M., & Jezzard, P. (2004). Functional magnetic resonance imaging. *Journal of Neurology, Neurosurgery and Psychiatry* 75, 6–12.

McIntosh, A. R. (1999). Mapping cognition to the brain through neural interactions. *Memory* 7, 523–548.

McKeown, M. J., Jung, T.-P., Makeig, S., Brown, G., Kinderman, S. S., Lee, T.-W., et al. (1998). Spatially independent activity patterns in functional magnetic resonance imaging data during the Stroop color-naming task. *Proceedings of the National Academy of Sciences USA* 95, 803–810.

Menon, R. S., & Goodyear, B. G. (2001). Spatial and temporal resolution in fMRI. In P. Jezzard, P. M. Matthews, & S. M. Smith (Eds.), *Functional MRI: An Introduction to Methods*, 145–158. Oxford: Oxford University Press.

Milner, A. D., & Goodale, M. A. (1995). *The Visual Brain in Action.* Oxford: Oxford University Press.

Murray, S. O., & Wojciulik, E. (2004). Attention increases neural selectivity in the human lateral occipital complex. *Nature Neuroscience* 7, 70–74.

Naccache, L., & Dehaene, S. (2001). The priming method: Imaging unconscious repetition priming reveals an abstract representation of number in the parietal lobes. *Cerebral Cortex* 11, 966–974.

Ochsner, K. N. (2004). Current directions in social cognitive neuroscience. *Current Opinion in Neurobiology* 14, 254–258.

O'Craven, K. M., Rosen, B. R., Kwong, K. K., Treisman, A., & Savoy, R. L. (1997). Voluntary attention modulates fMRI activity in human MT-MST. *Neuron* 18, 591–598.

Ogawa, S., Tank, D. W., Menon, R., Ellermann, J. M., Kim, S. G., Merkle, H., & Ugurbil, K. (1992). Intrinsic signal changes accompanying sensory stimulation: Functional brain mapping with magnetic resonance imaging. *Proceedings of the National Academy of Sciences USA* 89, 5951–5955.

Ono, M., Kubik, S., & Abernathey, C. D. (1990). *Atlas of the Cerebral Sulci.* Stuttgart: Thieme Medical Publishers.

Orban, G. A., Van Essen, D., & Vanduffel, W. (2004). Comparative mapping of higher visual areas in monkeys and humans. *Trends in Cognitive Sciences* 8, 315–324.

Paus, T., Jech, R., Thompson, C. J., Comeau, R., Peters, T., & Evans, A. C. (1997). Transcranial magnetic stimulation during positron emission tomography: A new method for studying connectivity of the human cerebral cortex. *Journal of Neuroscience* 17, 3178–3184.

Price, C. J., & Friston, K. J. (1997). Cognitive conjunction: A new approach to brain activation experiments. *NeuroImage* 5, 261–270.

Price, C. J., Wise, R. J., Watson, J. D., Patterson, K., Howard, D., & Frackowiak, R. S. (1994). Brain activity during reading. The effects of exposure duration and task. *Brain* 117(6), 1255–1269.

Raichle, M. E., MacLeod, A. M., Snyder, A. Z., Powers, W. J., Gusnard, D. A., & Shulman, G. L. (2001). A default mode of brain function. *Proceedings of the National Academy of Sciences USA* 98, 676–682.

Rees, G. (2001). Neuroimaging of visual awareness in patients and normal subjects. *Current Opinion in Neurobiology* 11, 150–156.

Rees, G., Frith, C. D., & Lavie, N. (1997). Modulating irrelevant motion perception by varying attentional load in an unrelated task. *Science* 278, 1616–1619.

Ress, D., & Heeger, D. J. (2003). Neuronal correlates of perception in early visual cortex. *Nature Neuroscience* 6, 414–420.

Rizzolatti, G., & Arbib, M. A. (1998). Language within our grasp. *Trends in Neurosciences* 21, 188–194.

Rizzolatti, G., Riggio, L., & Sheliga, B. M. (1994). Space and selective attention. In C. Umilta & M. Moscovitch (Eds.), *Attention and Performance XV*, 231–265. Cambridge, MA: MIT Press.

Savoy, R. (2001). History and future directions of human brain mapping. *Acta Psychologica* 107, 9–42.

Saxe, R., Carey, S., & Kanwisher, N. (2004). Understanding other minds: Linking developmental psychology and functional neuroimaging. *Annual Review of Psychology* 55, 87–124.

Scannell, J. W., & Young, M. P. (1999). Neuronal population activity and functional imaging. *Proceedings of the Royal Society of London* B266, 875–881.

Shulman, G. L., Fiez, J. A., Corbetta, M., Buckner, R. L., Miezin, F. M., Raichle, M. E., & Peterson, S. E. (1997). Common blood flow changes across visual tasks: II. Decreases in cerebral cortex. *Journal of Cognitive Neuroscience* 9, 648–663.

Stark, C. E., & Squire, L. R. (2001). When zero is not zero: The problem of ambiguous baseline conditions in fMRI. *Proceedings of the National Academy of Sciences USA* 98, 12760–12766.

Steeves, J. K. E., Humphrey, G. K., Culham, J. C., Menon, R. S., Milner, A. D., & Goodale, M. A. (2004). Behavioral and neuroimaging evidence for a contribution of color and texture information to scene classification in a patient with visual form agnosia. *Journal of Cognitive Neuroscience* 16, 955–965.

Sternberg, S. (1969). The discovery of processing stages: Extensions of Donders' method. *Acta Psychologica* 30, 276–315.

Sunaert, S., Van Hecke, P., Marchal, G., & Orban, G. A. (1999). Motion-responsive regions of the human brain. *Experimental Brain Research* 127, 355–370.

Takada, T., & Miyamoto, T. (2004). A fronto-parietal network for chewing of gum: A study on human subjects with functional magnetic resonance imaging. *Neuroscience Letters* 360, 137–140.

Talairach, J., & Tournoux, P. (1988). *Co-Planar Stereotaxic Atlas of the Human Brain.* New York: Thieme Medical Publishers.

Thiel, C. M., Henson, R. N., Morris, J. S., Friston, K. J., & Dolan, R. J. (2001). Pharmacological modulation of behavioral and neuronal correlates of repetition priming. *Journal of Neuroscience* 21, 6846–6852.

Tolias, A. S., Smirnakis, S. M., Augath, M. A., Trinath, T., & Logothetis, N. K. (2001). Motion processing in the macaque: revisited with functional magnetic resonance imaging. *Journal of Neuroscience* 21, 8594–8601.

Tong, F., Nakayama, K., Vaughan, J. T., & Kanwisher, N. (1998). Binocular rivalry and visual awareness in human extrastriate cortex. *Neuron* 21, 753–759.

Tootell, R. B., Tsao, D., & Vanduffel, W. (2003). Neuroimaging weighs in: Humans meet macaques in "primate" visual cortex. *Journal of Neuroscience* 23, 3981–3989.

Tootell, R. B. H., Hadjikhani, N. K., Mendola, J. D., Marrett, S., & Dale, A. M. (1998). From retinotopy to recognition: fMRI in visual cortex. *Trends in Cognitive Sciences* 2, 174–183.

Tootell, R. B. H., Mendola, J. D., Hadjikhani, N. K., Ledden, P. J., Lui, A. K., Reppas, J. B., et al. (1997). Functional analysis of V3A and related areas in human visual cortex. *Journal of Neuroscience* 17, 7060–7078.

Tootell, R. B. H., Reppas, J. B., Dale, A. M., Look, R. B., Sereno, M. I., Malach, R., et al. (1995). Visual motion aftereffect in human cortical area MT revealed by functional magnetic resonance imaging. *Nature* 375, 139–141.

Tootell, R. B. H., Reppas, J. B., Kwong, K. K., Malach, R., Born, R. T., Brady, T. J., et al. (1995). Functional analysis of human MT and related visual cortical areas using magnetic resonance imaging. *Journal of Neuroscience* 15, 3215–3230.

Uttal, W. R. (2001). *The New Phrenology: The Limits of Localizing Cognitive Processes in the Brain.* Cambridge, MA: MIT Press.

Wagner, A. D., Schacter, D. L., Rotte, M., Koutstaal, W., Maril, A., Dale, A. M., et al. (1998). Building memories: Remembering and forgetting of verbal experiences as predicted by brain activity. *Science* 281, 1188–1191.

Wandell, B. A. (1999). Computational neuroimaging of human visual cortex. *Annual Review of Neuroscience* 22, 145–173.

Watson, J. D. G., Myers, R., Frackowiak, R. S. J., Hajnal, J. V., Woods, R. P., Mazziotta, J. C., et al. (1993). Area V5 of the human brain: Evidence from a combined study using positron emission tomography and magnetic resonance imaging. *Cerebral Cortex* 3, 79–94.

Wojciulik, E., & Kanwisher, N. (1999). The generality of parietal involvement in visual attention. *Neuron* 23, 747–764.

II   COGNITIVE DOMAINS

4   Functional Neuroimaging of Attention

Barry Giesbrecht, Alan Kingstone, Todd C. Handy, Joseph B. Hopfinger, and George R. Mangun

Introduction

The empirical study of human brain function has advanced dramatically since the mid-1990s due to the advent of hemodynamic neuroimaging (e.g., Posner & Raichle, 1994). Methods such as positron emission tomography (PET) and functional magnetic resonance imaging (fMRI) hold the promise that variations in regional cerebral blood flow that are correlated with cognitive activity can be indexed with millimeter-level spatial resolution (e.g., Duong et al., 2001). In this chapter, we examine the use of these neuroimaging methods in relation to one of the central components of human cognition—*selective attention*.

We begin by introducing one form of selective visual attention, spatial attention, and then detail the role neuroimaging has played in furthering our understanding both of how selective attention functions at the cognitive level, and of how it is implemented at the neural level. In the second section of the chapter, we turn to a discussion of the ongoing efforts of attention researchers to understand the control of selective attention in terms of distributed neural networks that are composed of specific regions of the posterior parietal cortex and prefrontal cortex. In the conclusion of the chapter, we discuss how cutting-edge studies are investigating the role of attention in guiding interactions with the environment and a new research framework, called *cognitive ethology*, for studying the role of attention in the real world.

Functional Neuroimaging of Attention

At the most basic level, selective attention can be characterized as the "filtering" of sensory information, a process that is central to normal human function in that it allows us to rapidly isolate important input from the sensory environment for the highest levels of cognitive analysis (e.g., Broadbent, 1958). The empirical study of visual selective attention has focused on three general questions regarding such filtering: (1) Where in the afferent visual processing stream does attentional filtering or *"selection"* occur? (2) What neural mechanism(s) *controls* or mediates these selective effects of attention? and (3) What are the functional *consequences* of the selection process(es) for perception and performance? While the ultimate goal of this chapter is to provide an overview of some of the different ways in which neuroimaging techniques have been applied to the study of selective attention, we begin by reviewing the cognitive foundations of this critical mental ability.

From a cognitive perspective, selective attention may operate at different levels in visual processing, involving both "early" perceptual-level (e.g., Egly et al., 1994; Treisman & Gelade, 1980) and "later" postperceptual (e.g., Pashler, 1998; Shiu & Pashler, 1994; Sperling, 1984) processing operations. This suggests that selective attention has no unitary locus in the visual system. Rather, attention modulates stimulus processing at different stages of visual representation that correspond to the specific features being attended or ignored (e.g., color, shape, or spatial location) or as a consequence of other demands imposed by the specific task at hand (e.g., Johnston et al., 1995, 1996). In terms of attentional control, a general distinction is made at the cognitive level between stimulus-driven or *bottom-up* effects on attentional selection, and goal-driven or *top-down* influences (e.g., Desimone & Duncan, 1995; Yantis, 1998; Corbetta & Shulman, 2002). For example, the physical features of visual stimulation, such as the spatial arrangement or motion of objects in an array can affect what information is selected (e.g., Kingstone & Bischof, 1999; Driver, 1996; Folk et al., 1994; Prinzmetal, 1995). In turn, these bottom-up effects differ qualitatively from top-down attention effects, which involve voluntary mechanisms that are based upon the moment-to-moment requirements of task performance and are necessarily dependent on a host of higher-order processes, including working memory, long-term memory, decision processes, cognitive monitoring operations, and rule learning and implementation (e.g., Bunge, 2004; Shallice, 1994).

Given the breadth of factors affecting visual selective attention, when considering the neural substrates of the selection process, both the form of selection and the manner of its control must be made explicit. In this chapter, we emphasize one widely studied form of attentional selection in vision: spatial attention and its top-down control mechanisms.

Spatial Attention

As studied in the visual domain, spatial attention typically refers to a covert process whereby one's attention is directed to a location different from where the eyes are currently fixated. Although descriptions of spatial attention and its functional consequences can be traced back to James (1890) and his contemporaries, current research in visual spatial attention has its roots in two seminal, empirical studies that used behavioral measures to quantify attention. First, Eriksen and Hoffman (1972) measured vocal reaction times (RTs) to the onset of nonfoveal target letters that subjects were required to discriminate. Importantly, Eriksen and Hoffman found that if a target letter was presented simultaneously with a set of task-irrelevant noise (distractor) letters, the effect of the noise letters on target RTs depended on their spatial proximity to the target. When the noise letters were presented within 1 degree of visual angle from the target, target RTs were delayed relative to when no noise letters were present. However, this effect was eliminated when the noise letters were presented 1 degree or more from the target. This finding suggested that when attending to a nonfoveal location, the spatial extent of the attended region is restricted to about 1 degree of visual angle.

Second, Posner (1980) reported a number of experiments that measured manual RTs to nonfoveal targets as a function of whether the targets were presented in attended or unattended spatial locations. The critical manipulation in these studies was to inform subjects as to the most likely location of the target, typically via an arrow cue presented at fixation prior to target onset. Independent of whether the task involved detection or discrimination, Posner found that RTs were consistently faster when the targets were presented at the cued (or attended) location, relative to when the targets were presented at the uncued (or unattended) location. Whereas Eriksen and Hoffman (1972) had demonstrated the focal nature of spatial attention within the visual field, Posner's results indicated that focused spatial attention can directly alter the processing of stimulus inputs.

The Cognitive Model

The research inspired by Eriksen and Hoffman (1972) and Posner (1980) led to the suggestion that spatial attention is analogous to a mental spotlight or zoom lens that facilitates the processing of all stimuli falling within its focus (e.g., Eriksen & St. James, 1986; Posner, 1980; for a review, see Klein et al., 1992). In this manner, covertly orienting to a discrete location within the visual field operates as a mechanism of selective attention by conferring a processing "benefit" for attended-location stimuli, and a processing "cost" for unattended-location stimuli, relative to conditions where attention is distributed across all spatial locations (Posner, 1980). The general cognitive model thus posits that the attentional focus can be moved from location to location (e.g., Tsal, 1983), and any stimuli—independent of their physical properties—falling within this focus will receive measurable benefits in visual processing relative to stimuli falling outside the focus. Within this framework, the "spotlight" model has been refined further by data indicating that spatial attention can affect perceptual sensitivity (measured often as d-prime (d′); e.g., Downing, 1988; Müller & Humphreys, 1991; Hawkins et al., 1990). This body of work suggests that both the size of the focus and the rate at which processing benefits drop off from the focus of attention are dependent on the specific parameters of the task being performed, and that the attentional focus can be split, at least under certain stimulus conditions (e.g., Eriksen & Yeh, 1985; Handy et al., 1996; Kramer & Hahn, 1995).

The Neural Correlates

When considering the neural correlates of spatial attention, a distinction must be made between those brain areas that serve as the *source* of the attention effect and those brain areas that are the *site* of the attention effect (Posner, 1995; Posner & Petersen, 1990). The source includes those neural structures mediating top-down or executive control processes, such as deciding on which objects and locations in the visual field are currently important. In contrast, the attentional site involves those visuocortical areas that are primarily involved in stimulus processing, but whose functional activity can be modulated by spatial attention. For example, although spatial attention can affect perceptual sensitivity (e.g., Downing, 1988; Handy et al., 1996; Müller & Humphreys, 1991; Hawkins et al., 1990), these effects are manifest as modulations of processing operations that can proceed independent of attention. The sites at which selective attention can be observed have been demonstrated and fairly well characterized as increased neural activity in neuronal populations of retintopically organized visual cortex that represent the attended location in the visual field. These effects have been reviewed by others, including ourselves, and as a result will not be discussed here (Handy et al., 2001; Kanwisher & Wojciulik, 2000; Kastner & Ungerleider, 2000). Instead, we choose to focus on the sources of these attention effects, that is, we will review what is known of the neural mechanisms that control the orienting of selective spatial attention.

Control of Selection

Historically, the neuropsychological study of brain-lesioned patients has been a particularly effective technique for identifying the neural structures involved in attentional control (e.g., Driver, 1998; Mesulam, 1981; Rafal, 1996; Rafal & Henik, 1994). Much of the research in this domain has been premised on defining the act of attentional orienting as a three-step process (e.g., Posner et al., 1984; see Posner, 1995, for a review). According to this view, when a subject is cued to move his or her spatial attention to a new location, attention must first be *disengaged* from its current location within the visual field. Following disengagement, attention must then be *moved* from its initial location to the new location. Finally, once the attentional spotlight has been moved to the new location, attention must then be *engaged* with whatever stimuli are in the new location. Each of these three steps—disengage, move, and engage—involves an attention-specific operation associated with spotlight function, and the evidence from lesion studies has strongly suggested that these operations are performed by different neural structures.

For example, Posner et al. (1984) reported that when patients with unilateral damage to the parietal lobe oriented their attention to their ipsilesional visual field, they were greatly impaired in their ability to respond to targets presented in the contralesional visual field. Because patients showed no such impairments for contralesional targets when attention was pre-cued to the contralesional visual field, this was taken as evidence that the parietal lobe and temporal parietal junction are involved in mediating the act of disengaging attention from its current focus (see also Baynes et al., 1986; Friedrich et al., 1998; Morrow & Ratcliff, 1988; Posner et al., 1987).

In contrast, studies of patients with progressive supranuclear palsy—which results in degeneration of the superior colliculus and other midbrain structures involved in the control of saccadic eye movements—have shown that these patients are slowed in their ability to move their attentional focus (e.g., Posner et al., 1982; Posner et al., 1985). Specifically, if subjects have difficulty making saccades in a specific direction, their responses to nonfoveated targets are consistently delayed whenever they have to move their attention in the impaired direction in order to make the target response. These data thus suggest that the superior colliculus and related midbrain areas are responsible for the act of moving the attentional spotlight (see also Rafal, 1996).

Finally, the third component of attentional orienting—engaging stimuli at a new location—appears to be mediated by the pulvinar nucleus of the thalamus. Specifically, given sufficient time to orient their attention to a nonfoveal location, patients with unilateral damage to the pulvinar nucleus nevertheless showed selective delays in responding when the targets were in the contralesional visual field (see Posner, 1988). Because there were no similar delays in responding to targets in the ipsilesional visual field, and targets were occurring after attention had been moved, the delay in responding to targets in the contralesional field could be attributed to a selective impairment of the engagement operation—an effect on stimulus processing that is similar to that seen in patients with parietal-based visual neglect (e.g., Rafal, 1996; Rafal & Henik, 1994).

PET and fMRI Evidence

The question of what neural areas mediate the executive control of these orienting operations has brought together lesion and neuroimaging techniques. In a seminal

PET study, Corbetta, Miezin, Shulman, and Petersen (1993) compared sensory-evoked cortical activations as a function of whether attention was shifting to non-foveal locations in the visual field, or remained focused on fixation. In the shifting attention condition, subjects made voluntary attentional movements to the left or right of fixation throughout the scanning period while engaged in a target detection task. In the fixation condition, subjects were required to detect the onset of a target at fixation, while ignoring nonfoveal probe stimuli that matched the shifting attention condition in total peripheral stimulation. Corbetta et al. (1993) found activations in the superior parietal lobule (approximating Brodmann cytoarchitectural area [BA] 7) and superior frontal cortex (within BA 6) during the shifting attention condition relative to the fixation condition. That activity in both parietal and frontal regions was selective for movements of the attentional spotlight confirmed the findings from neuropsychological studies reviewed in the section "The Neural Correlates" (above).

However, comparing the parietal and frontal activations against a third condition—in which subjects passively viewed the peripheral probes while maintaining gaze at fixation—revealed that the parietal and frontal areas were involved in different aspects of the attention movement. In this third condition, the peripheral stimulation due to the probes was assumed to cause involuntary or *reflexive* shifts of spatial attention (see Posner & Cohen, 1984), shifts that did not occur during the fixation condition because attention was actively maintained at fixation. As a result, while the parietal areas were active during both voluntary and reflexive attentional movements, the frontal areas were active only during the voluntary movements. Consistent with the lesion data reviewed above, Corbetta et al. (1993) concluded that the parietal activations reflected processes associated with attentional movements, while the frontal activations selectively reflected the top-down executive control of voluntary movement.

Although the conclusion drawn by Corbetta et al. (1993) is entirely plausible, because of the experimental limitations of PET, in particular its blocked design, it is difficult to associate the pattern of PET results with a specific cognitive operation as the neural activity is integrated over relatively long periods of time (see chapter 1 in this volume). Event-related fMRI designs, however, do not suffer from the limitations inherent in blocked-design experiments (e.g., Buckner et al., 1996; Rosen et al., 1998; McCarthy et al., 1997; Burock et al., 1998). One of the most notable advantages of the event-related approach is the ability to examine not only the response to particular trials of interest, but also to specific within-trial events. This technique has been employed for years in human electrophysiology (i.e., electroencephalography, EEG) and animal neurophysiology (e.g., single-unit recordings) to study the component processes of attentional tasks (e.g., Chelazzi et al., 1993; Chelazzi et al., 1998; Luck et al., 1997; Hillyard and Münte, 1984; Hillyard et al.,

1985; Hillyard et al., 1995; Mangun and Hillyard, 1991; Mangun et al., 1993; Yamaguchi et al., 1994). Most notable is an EEG study of attentional control by Harter and his colleagues (1989).

Harter and colleagues (1989) were the first to decompose the cortical responses to within-trial events in the study of attentional control. They employed a traditional visual cuing paradigm (e.g., Posner, 1980), but unlike previous EEG experiments on spatial attention that focused on attention-related modulations of target-evoked activity, Harter et al. investigated the modulations of neural activity time-locked to the onset of the cue. The inferential logic of this approach is that because the cue represents the instruction to direct attention to a particular location in space, those areas which are activated in response to the cue should be those areas responsible for controlling directed attention. In response to the attention-directing spatial cues, Harter et al. found a large negative component over parietal sites contralateral to the attended location. Within about 500 ms after the cue, Harter et al. reported a positivity over occipital electrodes, again contralateral to the attended location.

Relating these events to cognitive processes, Harter et al. argued that the early negative component reflected the initiation of control processes, whereas the later positive component reflected the modulation of retinotopic visual areas corresponding to the location where the target was expected. These two components are consistent with the notion that top-down control involves parietal cortex mechanisms disengaging attention from its current focus soon after the cue is presented (e.g., Posner & Petersen, 1990) and maintenance of attention and/or control in lateral prefrontal cortex (e.g., Posner & Petersen, 1990; Desimone & Duncan, 1995), which in turn modulate acitivity in retinotopically organized visual areas as a way of priming the system for upcoming information (Mangun et al., 1993; Hillyard et al., 1995; Hillyard et al., 1998). The novel approach of measuring the neural activity evoked by the cue used by Harter et al. (1989) has proven to be a powerful tool in fMRI studies of attentional control and will be referred to as the "cue-related" approach.

Two noteworthy event-related fMRI studies have adopted the cue-related approach to isolating brain structures involved in the top-down control of attention (Hopfinger et al., 2000; Corbetta et al., 2000). These studies are noteworthy for three main reasons. First, they implicate the fronto-parietal network in the top-down control of attention. Second, they demonstrate the consequences of attention in two respects: (1) in terms of the impact of control systems on bottom-up sensory processing areas (Hopfinger et al., 2000); and (2) the adjustment of the system to breaches of expectation (Corbetta et al., 2000). Finally, although they are generally consistent in the patterns of activation, there are also key differences which indicate that the precise functions of the fronto-parietal network have yet to be clearly defined. These two studies are reviewed below.

Corbetta and his coworkers (2000) tested functional anatomical hypotheses regarding two component operations of the spotlight model of attentional orienting—cognitive operations often assumed to be at work in spatial attention tasks. The first is voluntary orienting to a spatial location, and the second is reorienting to stimuli presented at unattended locations. Based largely on the neuropsychological and PET data reviewed above, Corbetta et al. hypothesized that voluntary orienting to a location (i.e., directed attention) is mediated by posterior parietal cortex (PPC), particularly intraparietal sulcus (IPS). Reorienting to a new target location, on the other hand, was hypothesized to be mediated by the temporal-parietal junction (TPJ). These complementary hypotheses were tested using fMRI to measure the cortical response to visual cues that indicated the most likely location of the target. Consistent with the voluntary orienting hypothesis, Corbetta et al. found areas of ventral and anterior IPS active during the cue period, but before the target. Interestingly, this activity was protracted in time on a subset of trials in which the cue was followed by a delay and no target, suggesting the maintenance of top-down signals. Similarly, the activations revealed by the comparison of valid and invalid trials were consistent with the reorienting hypothesis, such that right TPJ exhibited the strongest validity effects in terms of blood-oxygenation-level-dependent (BOLD) activation and showed very little response to the attention-directing cue (see also Nobre et al., 1999). Corbetta et al. argued that their results dissociate voluntary orienting mechanisms from target detection mechanisms in parietal cortex, providing evidence converging with the neuropsychological literature implicating posterior parietal cortex as a key attentional control structure (e.g., Mesulam, 1981; Posner et al., 1987; Posner et al., 1984).

Where Corbetta et al. focused on parietal involvement in attentional control and breaches of cued expectation, Hopfinger et al. (2000) studied control structures and their effect on sensory processing mechanisms. In this study, subjects were presented with an arrow cue at fixation that instructed them to attend to right or left peripheral locations, and then to make a discrimination of a target at that location (i.e., the cue was 100% valid). Superior frontal, superior and inferior parietal, and superior temporal cortex were all activated in response to the cues. But, when compared directly with the target activations, only superior frontal, bilateral inferior parietal, superior temporal, and posterior cingulate areas were more active to the cues than to the targets. Hopfinger et al. assessed the impact of the fronto-parietal control system on retinotopically organized extrastriate visual areas (identified by retinotopic mapping; e.g., Sereno et al., 1995). These researchers found that in response to the centrally presented cue there were selective increases in activity in extrastriate areas VP and V4 (representing the peripheral target locations contralateral to the direction of attention) before the target was presented. This result suggests that top-down mechanisms serve to increase the excitability of neurons specialized for processing an upcoming target event (see also Kastner et al., 1999).

When considered together, the neuroimaging evidence provides evidence that dovetails extremely well with the pioneering neuropsychological work. Unlike the neuropsychological data studies, however, the event-related fMRI studies using the cue-related approach have specifically identified areas of frontal and parietal cortex as key areas that control the orienting of selective attention.

The Frontoparietal Attentional Control Network

Since the publication of the results of Corbetta et al. (2000) and Hopfinger et al. (2000), there has been a growing interest in understanding the cortical systems that mediate the control of attentional orienting. By and large these studies can be broken down into investigations of two complementary issues that concern (1) the generality of the attentional control network and (2) the specificity of the attentional control network.

The Generality of the Attentional Control Network

Considerable evidence demonstrates that in addition to spatial location, nonspatial attributes such as whole objects, or object features such as color and form, are key dimenions on which attentional control systems influence sensory processes (e.g., Duncan, 1984; Hillyard and Münte, 1984). Behavioral and PET studies have revealed that attending to nonspatial information (e.g., color, motion, form) leads to patterns of performance and neural activity that parallel those found in studies of spatial attention. Indeed, just as attending to a particular spatial location leads to improved performance for targets presented at the attended location and increased activity in neural populations that represent the attended location, attending to nonspatial features such as color, form, or motion can lead both to improved performance for targets consisting of the attended feature (e.g., Kingstone, 1992; Kingstone & Klein, 1991; Hillyard & Münte, 1984) and increased activity in areas of visual cortex that are selective for the attended feature (Corbetta et al., 1990; Chawla et al., 1999). The parallel effects of spatial and nonspatial attention extend beyond visual cortex and into parietal cortex; several studies have shown that areas of intraparietal cortex are activated in both spatial and nonspatial tasks (Wojciulik & Kanwisher, 1999; Le et al., 1998; McIntosh et al., 1994) as well as in spatial (Corbetta et al., 2000; Hopfinger et al., 2000) and nonspatial attention-directing cues (Shulman et al., 1999, 2002; Weissman et al., 2002; Liu et al., 2003). Thus, when one looks across studies, there is the suggestion that both spatial and nonspatial attention draw on a generalized network in frontal and parietal cortex that mediates top-down control.

Despite the compelling evidence that these studies provide for a generalized control system of attentional orienting, these studies either (a) used blocked designs or (b) did not include both nonspatial and spatial conditions. The studies that used blocked designs suffer from inferential limitations of attempting to associate a specific pattern of activation integrated over long periods of time with a single, specific cognitive operation. Those which used only a spatial or nonspatial task suffer from inferential limitations resulting from comparing across different subjects, paradigms, and studies. Thus, the suggestion of a generalized control network in frontal and parietal cortex based on these studies alone is constrained.

In an attempt to reconcile these inferential limitations, we recently reported the first within-subjects comparison of spatial and nonspatial attentional control systems using the cue-related approach (Giesbrecht et al., 2003). In this study, subjects were cued to attend to a spatial location or to a color. We found that when the two orienting conditions were tightly controlled for all operations except the attended dimension (i.e., location or color), location and color cues activated similar regions in parietal cortex. The overlap between the two conditions is shown in green in plate 4 (figure 4.1). The key areas that showed overlap include the IPS and areas of frontal cortex, including the precentral gyrus and frontal eye fields. These results provided

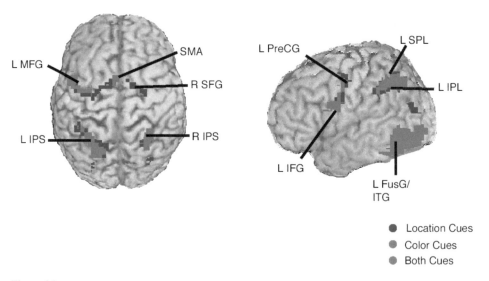

Figure 4.1
Cue-related activity. Group-averaged data for brain regions significantly activated to attention-directing cues, overlaid onto a brain rendered in 3D. Areas activated in response to location cues are shown in blue, to color cues are shown in red, and areas activated by both cues are shown in green. Maps are displayed using a height threshold of $p < 0.005$ (uncorrected) and an extent threshold of 10 contiguous voxels. See plate 4 for color version.

the first direct evidence that both spatial and nonspatial attention draw on similar control systems using the cue-related approach.

Although this initial evidence provides encouraging support for a generalized control network, successful isolation of attentional operations such as those involved in the location and color tasks within the cue-related approach is critically dependent not only on the appropriate choice of the orienting condition but also the reference condition. This is because attention-directing cues evoke a variety of cognitive operations that include (1) sensory processing of the cue, (2) extraction of an abstract/linguistic code from the cue symbol, (3) mapping of the code onto the task instruction (e.g., the arrow cue means to attend to the right), (4) covertly orienting to the relevant stimulus feature or location, (5) maintaining the task instruction during the cue-target interval, and (6) preparing to respond. Therefore, in order to understand the mechanisms that mediate voluntary orienting (i.e., stage 4) using the cue-related approach, one cannot simply measure activity evoked by the cue-related activity alone, but must dissociate orienting activity from activity that is related to other sensory, motor, and cognitive operations. The approach taken by most studies is to subtract the operations that are not of interest, using a reference condition that is assumed to have those operations in common with the condition of interest. In the Giesbrecht et al. study we included a sensory control condition that had exactly the same task structure, but the cues were meaningless. When the results of that condition were compared with the location and color cue conditions, it appeared that the overlap in occipitotemporal regions was likely due to similar sensory processing demands.

To further specify whether there were areas within frontal and parietal cortex that are generalized for orienting and not other cognitive operations (e.g., cue-symbol interpretation, working memory, and motor preparion), we conducted a meta-analysis of all the cue-related studies from our lab (Giesbrecht & Mangun, 2005). Using the simple framework of cue-evoked operations outlined above, cue-related activations were categorized into three types that differed in terms of their reference conditions. The categories were cue versus resting baseline condition, cue versus passive cue condition, and cue versus an alternative active cue condition. Based on the framework, each class of contrast differed with respect to the cognitive operations revealed. For example, a cue versus baseline contrast revealed areas involved in all six stages of processing (i.e., sensory processing, extraction of a linguistic code from the cue, mapping the code onto the task, orienting of attention, maintenance of attention, and motor preparation). A cue versus passive contrast, on the other hand, revealed orienting, maintenance, and preparatory operations because a passive cue condition also involves sensory processing, extraction, and code-mapping operations. Critically, the only cognitive operation that the three categories have in common is the involvement of voluntary orienting, either to a location or to a feature (e.g., color). We reasoned that if the only mental operation that these comparisons have in common is the involvement of voluntary orienting, then by overlaying the activations onto a single cortical representation, those areas which are activated in all of the studies should be those areas which are involved in the control of voluntary orienting of selective attention.

The results of the meta-analysis are shown in figure 4.2 (plate 5). Areas in white are the areas that the three contrasts had in common. These areas included posterior portions of the superior frontal sulcus (SFS) and portions of IPS bilaterally. Based on our logic, these results suggest that these areas are critically involved in the control of voluntary orienting of selective attention and none of the other cognitive operations evoked by the cue. Moreover, because the studies included in this meta-

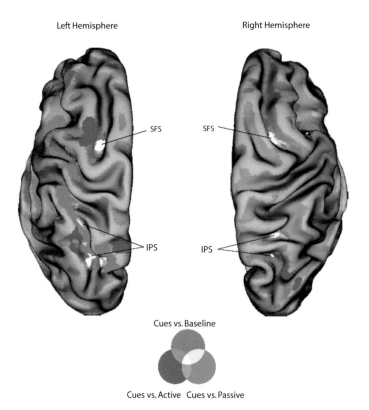

Figure 4.2
Anatomical overlap between the three categories of contrasts. Each focus was categorized into the Cue vs. Baseline (red), Cue vs. Passive (green), or Cue vs. Active (blue) group; projected onto the inflated brain; smoothed (8 mm); and painted onto the surface. White represents the intersection of all three categories. (Reprinted from *Neurobiology of Attention*, L. Itti, G. Rees, & J. Tsotsos (Eds). "Identifying the neural systems of top-down attentional control: A meta-analytic approach," pp. 63–68, Copyright 2005, with permission from Elsevier.) See plate 5 for color version.

analysis involved both spatial and nonspatial orienting, and yet overlap was still observed, the results are consistent with the notion that portions of the frontoparietal network are generalized with respect to the control of attentional orienting.

Specificity Within the Frontoparietal Network

A second key issue in the study of the control of attentional orienting is whether functional components of the frontoparietal control network can be specified more completely. The importance of this issue is brought into focus when one considers that the pattern of activations in studies of attentional control, such as those shown in figures 4.1 and 4.2, often covers large regions of frontal and parietal cortex that are known to be different in their cytoarchitectures and afferent and efferent connections, and are often observed in nonorienting tasks involving working memory, task-switching, and motor control (for reviews, see Cabeza & Nyberg, 1997, 2000). Thus, it seems plausible that while there may be some generalized components within the frontoparietal network (Shulman et al., 2002), it seems equally plausible that there is also specificity within the network. In this section, we present evidence which suggests that medial portions of intraparietal cortex and the frontal eye fields are specialized for the orienting of attention to spatial locations.

Clues to the specificity of the frontoparietal network come from the Giesbrecht et al. (2003) study of spatial and nonspatial attentional control described above. In that study, spatial and color cues were equated on all key respects except that in one condition, subjects oriented to one of two locations and in the other condition, subjects oriented to one of two colors. Applying standard subtraction logic, direct comparison of the cue-related activations should cancel all activations that are in common between the two conditions, leaving only areas that are selective to either spatial or color orienting. The results of one of these direct contrasts is shown in figure 4.3 (plate 6). Interestingly, superior frontal and superior parietal cortex were

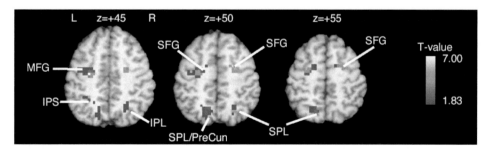

Figure 4.3
Group-average data for brain regions more active to location cues than color cues overlaid onto key slices of a single subject's anatomical image cutting through superior cortex ($z = 45, 50,$ and $55\,\mathrm{mm}$). See plate 6 for color version.

the only areas of the frontoparietal network that showed a cue-selective response: both of these areas were more active in response to location cues than to color cues. The organization of these spatial attention-selective activations is consistent with both the previous neuropsychological literature demonstrating that patients suffering from damage to either or both of these areas have severe difficulties in orienting attention in space (cf. Karnath et al., 2001; Mesulam, 1981; Mesulam, 1990; Posner et al., 1984) and the previous neuroimaging studies described above (as well as others not reviewed here) implicating a role for these areas in the control of covert orienting to spatial locations (e.g., Corbetta et al., 2000; Corbetta et al., 1993; Gitelman et al., 1999; Gitelman et al., 2000; Hopfinger et al., 2000; Kastner et al., 1999; Nobre et al., 1997; Yantis et al., 2002). Thus, as a complement to the generalized component of the frontoparietal network, the direct comparison between location and color cues suggests that subregions of the frontoparietal network are not merely involved in top-down control of attention in a generalized manner, but that they are *preferential*, and perhaps specific to, the control of covert orienting to spatial locations.

Consistent with this hypothesis, Woldorff et al. (2004) reported that portions of medial frontal and medial parietal cortex are involved in orienting to spatial locations. In their study, they reasoned that while parts of the frontoparietal network are likely responsible for interpreting the cue symbol, other parts were actually responsible for the shifting of attention to the cued location. To separate these different components, Woldorff et al. used the cue-related approach to measure the cortical response to spatial cues that directed subjects to attend to a particular location and the cortical response to passive cues that instructed subjects not to move attention. The addition of the passive cue condition was critical because the passive cues required many of the same cue-symbol interpretation and task-mapping operations as the attention-directing cues, but they did not require subjects to orient attention away from fixation. Thus, areas showing selective activation to the attention cues should be specifically involved in orienting, whereas areas not showing differential activation for the two types of cues should be involved in operations more related to cue-symbol interpretation. Woldorff et al. found that both passive and attention cues activated frontal and parietal cortex. In the lateral portions of the network, both types of cues evoked similar levels of activation. In the more medial areas of the network, including medial parietal cortex (precuneus and superior parietal cortex) and medial frontal cortex (superior frontal gyrus) there was more activity in response to the orienting cues relative to passive cues. Based on these results, Woldorff et al. concluded that the lateral areas were the part of the network that interpreted the cue symbol and mapped it onto the task instruction, whereas the more medial areas of the network were specific in their control of spatial orienting.

In a related study, Yantis et al. (2002) presented subjects with a rapid stream of items located on either side of fixation. Specific items within the streams acted as cues and instructed subjects either to hold attention at the current location or to shift attention to the other location. Yantis et al. directly compared the shift versus hold cues, reasoning that because both conditions were tightly controlled in all respects (including motor requirements) except that in one condition attention was moved and in the other attention was not moved, direct comparison of shift versus hold cues would reveal those areas which mediate the voluntary orienting of attention. Yantis et al. reported that superior parietal cortex was more active on shift trials than hold trials, showing a time course that was consistent with a transient burst of activity associated with the shift. The location of these activations was very similar to those spatially selective cue activations reported by Giesbrecht et al. (2003) and to the medial areas by Woldorff et al. (2004). Togther, these results suggest that medial parietal and frontal areas are specifically involved in the control of attentional orienting to spatial locations.

Summary

The results of the studies investigating these complementary issues paint a dynamic picture of frontoparietal involvement in attentional control. The results showing generality within the network suggests that it is flexible and amodal in the sense that they generalize across multiple aspects of the environment that are task-relevant (Shulman et al., 2002). The results showing that areas of frontal and parietal cortex are selective for covert spatial orienting are in line with the known role of these areas in eye movement control, suggesting a tight coupling of the oculomotor and spatial attention systems in these areas (Cabeza & Nyberg, 2000; Corbetta, 1998; see also Paus, 1996). When the issues are considered together, it appears that the generalized control areas may be able to recruit regions of superior frontal and parietal cortex that are specialized in the control of covert orienting to spatial locations because they are able to code behaviorally relevant locations in the visual field.

Issues

The foregoing discussion has centered on understanding spatial attention and, in particular, how functional neuroimaging has been used to help identify the neural systems involved in its control. What we have learned in this regard has indeed been impressive, yet many profound questions remain for research in attention. In this concluding section of the chapter, we turn to perhaps one of the most fundamental among these: If a mechanism of spatial selection exists in early visuocortical processing, what real-world perceptual challenges might this mechanism evolve to meet? The idea in raising this question is that not only does it help point us toward pursuing a more viable and accurate understanding of what spatial selection affords in visual processing, but it demands that we also consider the theoretical implications of bringing real-world constraints into laboratory-based cognitive research—implications that extend far beyond the domain of visual attention research. We discuss each of these issues in turn.

Spatial Selection and Visuomotor Processing

The effects of attending nonfoveally within the visual field have long been tied primarily—if not exclusively—to influences on visual perception. Indeed, attention improves signal detection performance (e.g., Bashinski & Bacharach, 1980; Downing, 1988; Handy et al., 1996), increases visual sensory gain (e.g., Heinze et al., 1994; Hillyard et al., 1998), and amplifies stimulus-evoked activity in object perception areas of the ventral visual processing stream (e.g., Wojciulik et al., 1998). However, a point rarely appreciated in the attention literature is that in the real world, visual perceptual goals are typically subserved by foveating an object of interest rather than covertly attending to it. While this does not question whether spatial attention can facilitate perception in the visual periphery, it does raise the very real issue of whether perceptual facilitation per se is the only—or even the primary—function of spatial selection.

For example, object-directed actions require transforming visual representations into object-specific motor programs, yet these acts are often performed in the absence of directly foveating the object in question. Hands are shaken while maintaining eye contact, coffee cups are grabbed while reading the newspaper, and doors are opened without looking down at the knob or handle. This suggests that the modulatory effects of spatial attention—long identified as enhancing stimulus processing in the ventral, perception-related visual pathway—may extend to visuomotor processes in the dorsal, action-related visual pathway (e.g., Milner & Goodale, 1995). In other words, the perceptual benefits of spatial attention may be a secondary consequence of a mechanism that evolved primarily to facilitate premotor planning (e.g., Rizzolatti et al., 1987; Rizzolatti et al., 1994).

To date, behavioral evidence suggesting that interactions exist between attention and visuomotor function have largely been predicated on examining how the activation of an object-specific motor program for a task-irrelevant object either facilitates or interferes with a target response. For example, manual reaction times to central targets are faster if the target is superimposed on an object that affords an action for the hand making a response, such as a pan with the handle oriented for a left- vs.

right-hand grasp (e.g., Tucker & Ellis, 1998). This suggests that the implicit processing of a single action-related object can selectively potentiate hand-specific responses. Conversely, when an overt movement is being made to an actual object, the speed of the movement is slowed if there are other graspable objects—or distractors—in the movement path (e.g., Pavese & Buxbaum, 2002; Tipper et al., 1992). Further, the slowing effect of the distractor is magnified if the distractor has an engagement characteristic that is incompatible with the terminal action requirement of the target, such as when the distractor is a knob designed for turning and the target is a knob designed for pulling (Weir et al., 2003). These data demonstrate that even under conditions where there is overt selection for and execution of an object-specific action, the action-related attributes of other, task-irrelevant objects will continue to be processed at an implicit level.

Neuroimaging data have directly extended these results by showing how the brain responds to a single action-related object. In particular, viewing tools, pictures of tools, and even the names of tools all lead to activation of motor-related regions of cortex independent of an observer's intention to act (e.g., Chao & Martin, 2000; Grafton et al., 1997; Grèzes & Decety, 2002; Grèzes et al., 2003; Jeannerod, 2001). This suggests that when a tool's representation is primed by visual input, the motor schema used for grasping that tool becomes primed as well (e.g., Craighero et al., 1999). Not only do these data agree with the notion that viewing a grabbable object will automatically lead to selection of that object's motor schema, but the data also demonstrate that there may be a direct neural marker of this implicit selection—object-specific activation of motor-related cortex, referred to as a visuomotor response (VMR). Building on this foundation, Handy and colleagues have conducted two studies using the VMR as a means to establish that covert visuospatial attention has reciprocal interactions with visuomotor processing.

The goal of an initial set of experiments was to examine whether visuospatial attention can be biased toward objects implicitly recognized as graspable (Handy et al., 2003). In their paradigm, participants viewed two task-irrelevant objects—one a "tool" and one a "non-tool"—while waiting for a target to be presented in one of the two object locations. Based on the prediction that the tool in the display would generate an implicit VMR, at issue was whether this would bias visuospatial attention toward the tool's location. Measuring the event-related brain potentials elicited by the targets as a function of their location (left visual field (LVF) vs. right visual field (RVF)) and the object over which they were superimposed (tool vs. non-tool), Handy et al. found that the magnitude of sensory gain increased at the tool's location, but only in the right visual hemifield, the lateral hemifield dominant for visuomotor processing. Using event-related fMRI, they confirmed that whether or not a tool generated a VMR was dependent on its visual field location in the bilateral display: a VMR was elicited by displays having a tool in the RVF location but not the LVF location. Not only were these data consistent with the hypothesis that object-specific visuomotor processes can bias covert visuospatial attention, but they revealed an important visual field asymmetry in the nature of attention-visuomotor interactions.

A central conclusion drawn from the results of Handy et al. (2003) is that visual attention may help to facilitate visuomotor processes. In a follow-up study, Handy et al. (2005) addressed this question directly. Participants again viewed a bilateral display containing one tool and one non-tool (e.g., a hammer and a cloud), but this time a manipulation of spatial attention was introduced such that participants were covertly attending to one of the two object locations at the time the objects were presented. Participants were instructed to wait for a target to be presented in the cued target location, and then discriminate whether the target was a square-wave grating with a low or high spatial frequency. Thus, the objects' locations were task-relevant but the objects themselves were task-irrelevant. In question was whether covertly attending to the tool's location would increase the VMR generated by that tool, relative to when the tool was in the same location but attention was oriented to the object in the contralateral visual hemifield. Handy et al. (2005) found that spatial attention did in fact modulate the VMR generated by the tool, but again the effect was restricted to tools in the RVF. In particular, when a tool was presented in the covertly attended RVF, it produced an increased fMRI BOLD response in the supplementary motor area (SMA) and left inferior parietal lobule (IPL). What the collective data suggest is that, in addition to facilitating visual perception, spatial attention can influence which object the motor system selects for a planned action.

In particular, Handy et al. (2005) found that selectively attending to the location of a tool in the RVF led to an increased fMRI response in left IPL and SMA, yet when the same object display was observed under divided attention conditions, an increased fMRI response was observed in bilateral IPL and just anterior to dorsal premotor cortex (prePMd) bilaterally (Handy et al., 2003). Given that the object display conditions remained constant between studies but the attention conditions varied, what this suggests is that the implicit processing of action-related objects will change with selective versus divided attention. For example, the results of Handy et al. (2003) are consistent with a situation where the motor system may implicitly recognize that one of the objects within the visual field has a motor affordance, but it has not yet engaged in the more selective process of planning the motor movements idiosyncratic to that object. Instead, that level of implicit motor planning may begin to occur only when visual attention is selectively oriented to the object's location and all other objects in the display fall outside of the attentional spotlight.

Theoretical Implications of Real-World Constraints.

As the above discussion highlights, consideration of the real-world perceptual challenges that spatial attention was designed to meet has led to an expanded model of its functions, which appear to include interactions with the visuomotor system. We now turn to the theoretical implications of bringing real-world constraints into laboratory-based cognitive research. In particular, functional neuroimaging—and cognitive science in general—is predicated on two fundamental assumptions. The first assumption is that human cognition in general, and selective human attention in particular, is subserved by dynamic processes that are stable across situations. Critically, this *assumption of stability* enables one to conduct a study in a laboratory environment and then propose that the process or processes being measured are the same as those expressed in everyday life, a point applicable to empirical science in general. The second assumption concerns experimental control. In short, given that processes are assumed to be stable across situations, it follows that one can reduce situational variability without compromising the nature of the process one is measuring (again, a point that is applicable to most experimental work),what we will refer to as the *assumption of control*. In the case of functional neuroimaging, a basic objective is to gain as much control over a situation as possible, so that any changes in brain activation can be attributed to the variable that is being manipulated.

As we have seen in this chapter, the assumptions of stability and control have been essential for developing our current understanding of the cortical systems underlying spatial selection in vision. However, these assumptions are not without their limitations (Kingstone et al., 2003; Kingstone et al., in press). For instance, the assumption of stability eliminates any need or obligation for the scientist to confirm that the processes being manipulated and measured in the lab actually express themselves in the real world. The field *does* check routinely that effects are stable within the lab environment, by the methodology of result replication. Unfortunately, a result that is stable within the lab is not necessarily stable outside the lab. Indeed, there are many examples in the field that even the most minor changes *within* a lab situation will compromise the replicability of an effect (Atchley & Kramer, 2001; Berry & Klein, 1993; Soto-Faraco et al., in press; Wolfe & Pokorny, 1990). And there are good reasons why this should be so. There is a large, well-established, and growing body of literature indicating that stability is tied intimately to the situations used to create it, with brain configurations changing across situations (e.g., see Duncan & Owen, 2000, for a review). Thus the risk is very real that the assumption of cognitive stability will often be invalid when a process is taken out of a lab situation.

Note that we are not saying that some functions and their neural correlates are not stable across situations. Rather, we are noting that such stability cannot be assumed to be the rule. Moreover, it is not clear that minimizing variance by applying the assumption of experimental control will reveal a complex stable system. General systems theory (see Ward, 2002; Weinberg, 1975) has established that while experimental control can be effective at revealing basic characteristics of simple linear systems, it is unlikely to be effective at revealing the characteristics of complex, nonlinear systems such as the human attention system. This is because certain characteristics of complex systems are revealed, or emerge, only when several variables vary together in highly specific ways. This is precisely what is not allowed to occur in highly controlled functional neuroimaging situations. Though controlled laboratory research may happen upon important constellations of variables that reveal critical characteristics of a complex system, such an approach clearly is extremely inefficient and certainly does not guarantee that important characteristics will ever be found.

Together, then, one finds that there are practical and principled reasons to question whether selecting tasks on the basis of assumptions of stability and control are likely to inform us about cognitive processes as they are expressed in real-life situations. What are researchers to do when posed with this difficult situation? Kingstone et al. (2003; see also Kingstone et al., in press; Kingstone et al., submitted; Smilek et al., in press) have argued that what is needed is to begin to study directly how people behave in complex environments. That is, rather than being locked into a laboratory paradigm with the a priori assumption that the paradigm and its associated tasks are tapping into processes that are expressed in everyday life situations, one might instead opt to explore how people behave as they function within the natural environment one ultimately intends to understand (i.e., the real world).

Kingstone and Smilek call this approach *cognitive* ethology. This research approach rejects the standard assumptions of stability and control, and aims instead to understand the situation and the variance within that situation. Description of people's attentional behavior in the real world is intrinsically valuable and meaningful because it is grounded in reality, and it is the main goal and subject matter of attentional research. By observing and measuring what people really do in their natural environments, one can begin to define the problem space in a manner that is tied to real-life situations and not contrived laboratory environments. This means that subsequent functional neuroimaging investigations can be protected from the pursuit of questions that are merely paradigm-driven and paradigm-specific. It also means that one is free to ask questions that are meaningful and relevant to real life rather than being constrained and limited to impoverished laboratory environments. Thus, the cognitive ethology research approach provides the opportunity to functional neuroimaging scientists to conduct research that will ultimately expand and deepen our understanding of human cognition and attention.

Acknowledgments

We would like to thank the following research agencies for their support of this chapter: BG—National Institute of Mental Health (NIMH), TCH, NIMH, and the Natural Sciences and Engineering Research Council of Canada (NSERC); JBH—NIMH (MH66034); GRM—NIMH; AK—NSERC, the Michael Smith Foundation for Health Research, the Hampton Fund, and the Human Early Learning Partnership.

References

Atchley, P., & Kramer, A. F. (2001). Object and space-based attentional selection in three-dimensional space. *Visual Cognition* 8, 1–32.

Bashinski, H. S., & Bacharach, V. R. (1980). Enhancement of perceptual sensitivity as the result of selectively attending to spatial locations. *Perception & Psychophysics* 28, 241–248.

Baynes, K., Holtzman, J. D., & Volpe, B. T. (1986). Components of visual attention: Alterations in response pattern to visual stimuli following parietal lobe infarction. *Brain* 109, 99–114.

Berry, G., & Klein, R. M. (1993) Motion-induced grouping may not modulate the flanker compatibility effect: A failure to replicate Driver & Baylis. *Canadian Journal of Experimental Psychology* 47, 714–729.

Broadbent, D. E. (1958). *Perception and Communication*. London: Pergamon.

Buckner, R. L., Bandettini, P. A., O'Craven, K. M., Savoy, R. L., Petersen, S. E., Raichle, M. E., & Rosen, B. R. (1996). Detection of cortical activation during averaged single trials of a cognitive task using functional magnetic resonance imaging. *Proceedings of the National Academy of Sciences USA*, 93, 14878–14883.

Bunge, S. A. (2004). How we use rules to select action: A review of evidence from cognitive neuroscience. *Cognitive, Affective, and Behavioral Neuroscience*.

Burock, M. A., Buckner, R. L., Woldorff, M. G., Rosen, B. R., & Dale, A. M. (1998). Randomized event-related experimental designs allow for extremely rapid presentation rates using functional MRI. *NeuroReport* 9, 3735–3739.

Cabeza, R., & Nyberg, L. (1997). Imaging cognition: An empirical review of PET studies with normal subjects. *Journal of Cognitive Neuroscience* 9, 1–26.

Cabeza, R., & Nyberg, L. (2000). Imaging cognition II: An empirical review of 275 PET and fMRI studies. *Journal of Cognitive Neuroscience* 12, 1–47.

Chao, L. L., & Martin, A. (2000). Representation of manipulable man-made objects in the dorsal stream. *NeuroImage* 12, 478–484.

Chawla, D., Rees, G., & Friston, K. J. (1999). The physiological basis of attentional modulation in extrastriate visual areas. *Nature Neuroscience* 2, 671–676.

Chelazzi, L., Duncan, J., Miller, E. K., & Desimone, R. (1998). Responses of neurons in inferior temporal cortex during memory-guided visual search. *Journal of Neurophysiology* 80, 2918–2940.

Chelazzi, L., Miller, E. K., Duncan, J., & Desimone, R. (1993). A neural basis for visual search in inferior temporal cortex. *Nature* 363, 345–347.

Corbetta, M. (1998). Frontoparietal cortical networks for directing attention and the eye to visual locations: Identical, independent, or overlapping neural systems? *Proceedings of the National Academy of Sciences USA* 95, 831–838.

Corbetta, M., Kincade, J. M., Ollinger, J. M., McAvoy, M. P., & Shulman, G. L. (2000). Voluntary orienting is dissociated from target detection in human posterior parietal cortex. *Nature Neuroscience* 3, 292–297.

Corbetta, M., Miezin, F. M., Shulman, G. L., & Petersen, S. E. (1993). A PET study of visuospatial attention. *Journal of Neuroscience* 13, 1202–1226.

Corbetta, M., Miezin, F. M., Dobmeyer, S., Shulman, G. L., & Petersen, S. E. (1990). Attentional modulation of neural processing of shape, color, and velocity in humans, *Science* 248, 1556–1559.

Corbetta, M., & Shulman, G. L. (2002). Control of goal-directed and stimulus-driven attention in the brain. *Nature Reviews Neuroscience* 3, 201–215.

Craighero, L., Fadiga, L., Rizzolatti, G., & Umiltà, C. (1999). Action for perception: A motor-visual attentional effect. *Journal of Experimental Psychology: Human Perception and Performance* 25, 1673–1692.

Desimone, R., & Duncan, J. (1995). Neural mechanisms of selective visual attention. *Annual Review of Neuroscience* 18, 193–222.

Downing, C. J. (1988). Expectancy and visuo-spatial attention: Effects on perceptual quality. *Journal of Experimental Psychology: Human Perception and Performance* 13, 228–241.

Driver, J. (1996). Attention and segmentation. *The Psychologist* 9, 119–123.

Driver, J. (1998). The neuropsychology of spatial attention. In H. Pashler (Ed.), *Attention*, 297–340. Hove, UK: Psychology Press.

Duncan, J. (1984). Selective attention and the organization of visual information. *Journal of Experimental Psychology: General* 113, 501–517.

Duncan, J. & Owen, A. M. (2000). Common regions of the human frontal lobe recruited by divers cognitive demands. *Trends in Neurosciences* 23, 475–483.

Duong, T. Q., Kim, D.-S., Ugurbil, K., & Kim, S.-G. (2001). Localized cerebral blood flow response at submillimeter columnar resolution. *Proceedings of the National Academy of Sciences USA* 98, 10904–10909.

Egly, R., Driver, J., & Rafal, R. D. (1994). Shifting visual attention between objects and locations: Evidence from normal and parietal lesion patients. *Journal of Experimental Psychology: General* 123 161–177.

Eriksen, C. W., & Hoffman, J. E. (1972). Temporal and spatial characteristics of selective encoding from visual displays. *Perception & Psychophysics* 12, 201–204.

Eriksen, C. W., & St. James, J. D. (1986). Visual attention within and around the field of focal attention: A zoom lens model. *Perception & Psychophysics* 40, 225–240.

Eriksen, C. W., & Yeh, Y.-Y. (1985). Allocation of attention in the visual field. *Journal of Experimental Psychology: Human Perception and Performance* 11, 583–597.

Folk, C. L., Remington, R. W., & Wright, J. H. (1994). The structure of attentional control: Contingent attentional capture by apparent motion, abrupt onset, and color. *Journal of Experimental Psychology: Human Perception and Performance* 20, 317–329.

Friedrich, F. J., Egly, R., Rafal, R. D., & Beck, D. (1998). Spatial attention deficits in humans: A comparison of superior parietal and temporal-parietal junction lesions. *Neuropsychology* 12, 193–207.

Giesbrecht, B., & Mangun, G. R. (2005). Identifying the neural systems of top-down attentional control: A meta-analytical approach. In L. Itti, G. Rees, & J. Tsotsos (Eds.), *Neurobiology of Attention*. New York: Academic Press/Elsevier.

Giesbrecht, B., Woldorff, M. G., Song, A. W., & Mangun, G. R. (2003). Neural mechanisms of top-down control during spatial and feature attention. *NeuroImage* 19, 496–512.

Gitelman, D. R., Nobre, A. C., Parrish, T. B., LaBar, K. S., Kim, Y. H., Meyer, J. R., & Mesulam, M. (1999). A large-scale distributed network for covert spatial attention: Further anatomical delineation based on stringent behavioural and cognitive controls. *Brain* 122, 1093–1106.

Gitelman, D. R., Parrish, T. B., LaBar, K. S., & Mesulam, M. M. (2000). Real-time monitoring of eye movements using infrared video-oculography during functional magnetic resonance imaging of the frontal eye fields. *NeuroImage* 11, 58–65.

Grafton, S. T., Fadiga, L., Arbib, M. A., & Rizzolatti, G. (1997). Premotor cortex activation during observation and naming of familiar tools. *NeuroImage* 6, 231–236.

Grèzes, J., & Decety, J. (2002). Does visual perception of object afford action? Evidence from a neuroimaging study. *Neuropsychologia* 40, 212–222.

Grèzes, J., Tucker, M., Armony, J., Ellis, R., & Passingham, R. E. (2003). Objects automatically potentiate action: An fMRI study of implicit processing. *European Journal of Neuroscience* 17, 2735–2740.

Grosbras, M.-H., & Paus, T. (2002). Transcranial magnetic stimulation of the human frontal eye field: Effects on visual perception and attention. *Journal of Cognitive Neuroscience* 14, 1109–1120.

Handy, T. C., Grafton, S. T., Shroff, N. M., Ketay, S. B., & Gazzaniga, M. S. (2003). Graspable objects grab attention when the potential for action is recognized. *Nature Neuroscience* 6, 421–427.

Handy, T. C., Hopfinger, J. B., & Mangun, G. R. (2001). Functional neuroimaging of attention. In R. Cabeza & A. Kingstone (Eds.), *The Handbook on Functional Neuroimaging of Cognition*. Cambridge, MA: MIT Press.

Handy, T. C., Kingstone, A., & Mangun, G. R. (1996). Spatial distribution of visual attention: Perceptual sensitivity and response latency. *Perception & Psychophysics* 58, 613–627.

Handy, T. C., Schaich Borg, J., Turk, D. J., Tipper, C., Grafton, S. T., & Gazzaniga, M. S. (Submitted). Placing a tool in the spotlight: Spatial attention modulates visuomotor responses in cortex. *NeuroImage* 26, 266–276.

Harter, M. R., Miller, S. L., Price, N. J., LaLonde, M. E., & Keyes, A. L. (1989). Neural processes involved in directing attention. *Journal of Cognitive Neuroscience* 1, 223–237.

Hawkins, H. L., Hillyard, S. A., Luck, S. J., Mouloua, M., Downing, C. J., & Woodward, D. P. (1990). Visual attention modulates signal detectability. *Journal of Experimental Psychology: Human Perception and Performance* 16, 802–811.

Heinze, H. J., Mangun, G. R., Burchert, W., Hinrichs, H., Scholz, M., Muente, T. F., et al. (1994). Combining spatial and temporal imaging of brain activity during visual selective attention in humans. *Nature* 372, 543–546.

Hillyard, S. A., Mangun, G. R., Woldorff, M. G., & Luck, S. J. (1995). Neural systems mediating selective attention. In M. S. Gazzaniga (Ed.), *The Cognitive Neurosciences*, 665–681. Cambridge, MA: MIT Press.

Hillyard, S. A., & Münte, T. F. (1984). Selective attention to color and location: An analysis with event-related brain potentials. *Perception & Psychophysics* 36, 185–198.

Hillyard, S. A., Münte, T. F., & Neville, H. J. (1985). Visual-spatial attention, orienting, and brain physiology. In M. I. Posner & O. S. M. Marin (Eds.), *Attention and Performance XI*. Hillsdale, NJ: Erlbaum.

Hillyard, S. A., Vogel, E. K., & Luck, S. J. (1998). Sensory gain control (amplification) as a mechanism of selective attention: Electrophysiological and neuroimaging evidence. *Philosophical Transactions of the Royal Society of London* B353, 1257–1270.

Hopf, J. M., & Mangun, G. R. (2000). Shifting visual attention in space: An electrophysiological analysis using high spatial resolution mapping. *Clinical Neurophysiology* 111, 1241–1257.

Hopfinger, J. B., Buonocore, M. H., & Mangun, G. R. (2000). The neural mechanisms of top-down attentional control. *Nature Neuroscience* 3, 284–291.

James, W. (1890; 1950). *The Principles of Psychology*. New York: Dover.

Jeannerod, M. (2001). Neural simulation of action: A unifying mechanism for motor cognition. *NeuroImage* 14, S103–S109.

Johnston, J. C., McCann, R. S., & Remington, R. W. (1995). Chronometric evidence for two types of attention. *Psychological Science* 6, 365–369.

Johnston, J. C., McCann, R. S., & Remington, R. W. (1996). Selective attention operates at two processing loci. In A. F. Kramer, M. G. H. Coles, & G. D. Logan (Eds.), *Converging Operations in the Study of Visual Selective Attention*. Washington, DC: American Psychological Association.

Kanwisher, N., & Wojciulik, E. (2000). Visual attention: Insights from brain imaging. *Nature Reviews Neuroscience* 1, 91–100.

Karnath, H. O., Ferber, S., & Himmelbach, M. (2001). Spatial awareness is a function of the temporal not the posterior parietal lobe. *Nature* 411, 950–953.

Kastner, S., Pinsk, M. A., De Weerd, P., Desimone, R., & Ungerleider, L. G. (1999). Increased activity in human visual cortex during directed attention in the absence of visual stimulation. *Neuron* 22, 751–761.

Kastner, S., & Ungerleider, L. G. (2000). Mechanisms of visual attention in the human cortex. *Annual Review of Neuroscience* 23, 315–341.

Kingstone, A. (1992). Combining expectancies. *Quarterly Journal of Experimental Psychology* 44A, 69–104.

Kingstone, A., & Bischof, W. F. (1999). Perceptual grouping and motion coherence in visual search. *Psychological Science* 10, 151–156

Kingstone, A., & Klein, R.M. (1991). Combining shape and position expectancies: Hierarchical processing and selective inhibition. *Journal of Experimental Psychology: Human Perception and Performance* 17, 512–519.

Kingstone, A., Smilek, D., Birmingham, E., Cameron, D., & Bischof, W. F. (In press). Cognitive ethology: Giving real life to attention research. In J. Duncan, L. Phillips, & P. McLeod (Eds.), *Speed, Control & Age: In Honour of Patrick Rabbitt.* Oxford: Oxford University Press.

Kingstone, A., Smilek. D., Eastwood, J. D., & Reynolds, M. (Submitted). Cognitive ethology: A new approach for studying human attention.

Kingstone, A., Smilek, D., Ristic, J., Friesen, C.K., & Eastword, J. D. (2003). Attention, Researchers! It is time to take a look at real world. *Current Directions in Psychological Science* 12, 176–180.

Klein, R., Kingstone, A., & Pontefract, A. (1992). Orienting of visual attention. In K. Rayner (Ed.), *Eye Movements and Visual Cognition: Scene Perception and Reading*, 46–65. New York: Springer-Verlag.

Kramer, A. F., & Hahn, S. (1995). Splitting the beam: Distribution of attention over noncontiguous regions of the visual field. *Psychological Science* 6, 381–386.

Le, T. H., Pardo, J. V., & Hu, X. (1998). 4 T-fMRI study of nonspatial shifting of selective attention: Cerebellar and parietal contributions. *Journal of Neurophysiology* 79, 1535–1548.

Liu, T., Slotnick, S. D., Serences, J. T., & Yantis, S. (2003). Cortical mechanisms of feature-based attentional control. *NeuroReport* 13, 1334–1343.

Luck, S. J., Chelazzi, L., Hillyard, S. A., Desimone, R. (1997). Neural mechanisms of spatial selective attention in areas V1, V2, and V4 of macaque visual cortex. *Journal of Neurophysiology* 77, 24–42.

Mangun, G. R. (1995). Neural mechanisms of visual selective attention. *Psychophysiology* 32, 4–18.

Mangun, G. R., & Hillyard, S. A. (1991). Modulation of sensory-evoked brain potentials provides evidence for changes in perceptual processing during visual-spatial priming. *Journal of Experimental Psychology: Human Perception and Performance* 17, 1057–1074.

Mangun, G. R., Hillyard, S. A., & Luck, S. J. (1993). Electrocortical substrates of visual selective attention. In D. Meyer & S. Kornblum (Eds.), *Attention and Performance XIV: Synergies in Experimental Psychology, Artificial Intelligence, and Cognitive Neuroscience*, 219–243. Cambridge, MA: MIT Press.

McCarthy, G., Luby, M., Gore, J., & Goldman-Rakic, P. (1997). Infrequent events transiently activate human prefrontal and parietal cortex as measured by functional MRI. *Journal of Neurophysiology* 77, 1630–1634.

McIntosh, A. R., Grady, C. L., Ungerleider, L. G., Haxby, J. V., Rapoport, S. I., & Horwitz, B. (1994). Network analysis of cortical visual pathways mapped with PET. *Journal of Neuroscience* 14, 655–666.

Mesulam, M.-M. (1981). A cortical network for directed attention and unilateral neglect. *Annals of Neurology* 10, 309–325.

Mesulam, M.-M. (1990). Large-scale neurocognitive networks and distributed processing for attention, memory, and language. *Annals of Neurology* 28, 597–613.

Milner, A. D., & Goodale, M. A. (1995). *The Visual Brain in Action.* New York: Oxford University Press.

Morrow, L. A., & Ratcliff, G. (1988). The disengagement of covert attention and the neglect syndrome. *Psychobiology* 16, 261–269.

Müller, H. J., & Humphreys, G. W. (1991). Luminance-increment detection: Capacity-limited or not? *Journal of Experimental Psychology: Human Perception and Performance* 17, 107–124.

Nobre, A. C., Coull, J. T., Frith, C. D., & Mesulam, M. M. (1999). Orbitofrontal cortex is activated during breaches of expectation in tasks of visual attention. *Nature Neuroscience* 2, 11–12.

Nobre, A. C., Sebestyen, G. N., Gitelman, D. R., Mesulam, M. M., Frackowiak, R. S. J., & Frith, C. D. (1997). Functional localization of the system for visuospatial attention using positron emission tomography. *Brain* 120, 515–533.

Pashler, H. E. (1998). *The Psychology of Attention.* Cambridge, MA: MIT Press.

Paus, T. (1996). Location and function of the human frontal eye field: A selective review. *Neuropsychologia* 34, 475–483.

Pavese, A., & Buxbaum, L. J. (2002). Action matters: The role of action plans and object affordances in selection for action. *Visual Cognition* 9, 559–590.

Posner, M. I. (1980). Orienting of attention. *Quarterly Journal of Experimental Psychology* 32, 3–25.

Posner, M. I. (1988). Structures and functions of selective attention. In T. Boll & B. Bryant (Eds.), *Master Lectures in Clinical Neuropsychology and Brain Function: Research, Measurement, and Practice*, 171–202. Washington, D.C.: American Psychological Association.

Posner, M. I. (1995). Attention in cognitive neuroscience: An overview. In M. S. Gazzaniga (Ed.), *The Cognitive Neurosciences*, 615–624. Cambridge, MA: MIT Press.

Posner, M. I., & Cohen, Y. (1984). Components of visual orienting. In H. Bouma & D. G. Bouwhuis (Eds.), *Attention and Performance X*, 531–556. Hillsdale, NJ: Erlbaum.

Posner, M. I., Cohen, Y., & Rafal, R. D. (1982). Neural systems control of spatial orienting. *Philosophical Transactions of the Royal Society of London* B298, 187–198.

Posner, M. I., & Petersen, S. E. (1990). The attention system of the human brain. *Annual Review of Neuroscience* 13, 25–42.

Posner, M. I., & Raichle, M. E. (1994). *Images of Mind.* New York: Scientific American Books.

Posner, M. I., Rafal, R. D., Choate, L., & Vaughn, J. (1985). Inhibition of return: Neural basis and function. *Cognitive Neuropsychology* 2, 211–228.

Posner, M. I., Walker, J. A., Friedrich, F. J., & Rafal, R. D. (1984). Effects of parietal injury on covert orienting of attention. *Journal of Neuroscience* 4, 1863–1874.

Posner, M. I., Walker, J. A., Friedrich, F. J., & Rafal, R. D. (1987). How do the parietal lobes direct covert attention? *Neuropsychologia* 25, 135–145.

Prinzmetal, W. (1995). Visual feature integration in a world of objects. *Current Directions in Psychological Science* 4, 90–94.

Rafal, R. D. (1996). Visual attention: Converging operations from neurology and psychology. In A. F. Kramer, M. G. H. Coles, & G. D. Logan (Eds.), *Converging Operations in the Study of Visual Selective Attention*, 139–192. Washington, DC: American Psychological Association.

Rafal, R. D., & Henik, A. (1994). The neurology of inhibition: Integrating controlled and automatic processes. In D. Dagenbach & T. H. Carr (Eds.), *Inhibitory Processes in Attention, Memory, and Language*, 1–52. San Diego: Academic Press.

Raichle, M. E. (2005). Functional brain imaging: An historical and physiological perspective. In R. Cabeza & A. Kingstone (Eds.), *Handbook of Functional Neuroimaging of Cognition*, vol. 2. Cambridge, MA: MIT Press.

Rizzolatti, G., Riggio, L., Dascola, I., & Umiltá, C. (1987). Reorienting attention across the horizontal and vertical meridians: Evidence in favor of a premotor theory of attention. *Neuropsychologia* 25, 31–40.

Rizzolatti, G., Riggio, L., & Sheliga, B. M. (1994). Space and selective attention. In C. Umiltà & M. Moscovitch (Eds.), *Attention and Performance XV*, 231–265. Cambridge, MA: MIT Press.

Rosen, B. R., Buckner, R. L., & Dale, A. M. (1998). Event-related functional MRI: Past, present, and future. *Proceedings of the National Academy of Sciences USA* 95, 773–780.

Sereno, M. I., Dale, A. M., Reppas, J. B., Kwong, K. K., Belliveau, J. W., Brady, T. J., Rosen, B. R., & Tootell, R. B. H. (1995). Borders of multiple visual areas in humans revealed by functional magnetic resonance imaging. *Science* 268, 889–893.

Shallice, T. (1994). Multiple levels of control processes. In C. Umiltà & M. Moscovitch (Eds.), *Attention and Performance XV*, 395–420. Cambridge, MA: MIT Press.

Shiu, L., & Pashler, H. (1994). Negligible effects of spatial precuing on identification of single digits. *Journal of Experimental Psychology: Human Perception & Performance* 20, 1037–1054.

Shulman, G. L., d'Avossa, G., Tansy, A. P., & Corbetta, M. (2002). Two attentional processes in the parietal lobe. *NeuroReport* 12, 1124–1131.

Shulman, G. L., Ollinger, J. M., Akbudak, E., Conturo, T. E., Snyder, A. Z., Petersen, S. E., & Corbetta, M. (1999). Areas involved in encoding and applying directional expectations to moving objects. *Journal of Neuroscience* 19, 9480–9496.

Smilek, D., Birmingham, E., Cameron, D., Bischof, W. F., & Kingstone, A. (In press). Cognitive ethology and exploring attention in real world scenes. *Cognitive Brain Research*.

Soto-Faraco, S., Morein-Zamir, S., & Kingstone, A. (In press). On audiovisual spatial synergy: The fragility of the phenomenon. *Perception & Psychophysics*.

Sperling, G. (1984). A unified theory of attention and signal detection. In R. Parasuraman & D. R. Davies (Eds.), *Varieties of Attention*, 103–181. Orlando, FL: Academic Press.

Tipper, S. P., Lortie, C., & Baylis, G. C. (1992). Selective reaching: Evidence for action-centered attention. *Journal of Experimental Psychology: Human Perception and Performance* 18, 891–905.

Treisman, A. M., & Gelade, G. (1980). A feature-integration theory of attention. *Cognitive Psychology* 12, 97–136.

Tsal, Y. (1983). Movements of attention across the visual field. *Journal of Experimental Psychology: Human Perception and Performance* 9, 523–530.

Tucker, M., & Ellis, R. (1998). On the relations between seen objects and components of potential actions. *Journal of Experimental Psychology: Human Perception and Performance* 24, 830–846.

Ward, L. M. (2002). *Dynamical Cognitive Science*. Cambridge, MA: MIT Press.

Weinberg, G. M. (1975). *An Introduction to General Systems Thinking*. New York: Wiley.

Weir, P. L., Weeks, D. J., Welsh, T. N., Elliott, D., Chua, R., Roy, E. A., & Lyons, J. (2003). Influence of terminal action requirements on action-centered distractor effects. *Experimental Brain Research* 149, 207–213.

Weissman, D. H., Woldorff, M. G., & Mangun, G. R. (2001). Neural correlates of voluntary orienting for global versus local processing. Poster presented at the 8th Annual Meeting of the Cognitive Neuroscience Society, New York, March.

Weissman, D. H., Woldorff, M. G., & Mangun, G. R. (2002). A role for top-down attentional orienting during interference between global and local aspects of hierarchical stimuli. *NeuroImage* 17, 1266–1276.

Wojciulik, E., & Kanwisher, N. (1999). The generality of parietal involvement in visual attention. *Neuron* 23, 747–764.

Wojciulik, E., Kanwisher, N., & Driver, J. (1998). Covert visual attention modulates face-specific activity in the human fusiform gyrus: fMRI study. *Journal of Neurophysiology* 79, 1574–1578.

Woldorff, M. G., Hazlett, C. J., Fichtenholtz, H. M., Weissman, D. H., Dale, A. M., & Song, A. W. (2004). Functional parcellation of attentional control regions of the brain. *Journal of Cognitive Neuorscience* 16(1), 149–165.

Wolfe, J. M., & Pokorny, C. W. (1990). Inhibitory tagging in visual search: A failure to replicate. *Perception & Psychophysics* 48, 357–362.

Yamaguchi, S., Tsuchiya, H., & Kobayashi, S. (1994). Electroencephalographic activity associated with shifts of visuospatial attention. *Brain* 117, 553–562.

Yantis, S. (1998). Control of visual attention. In H. Pashler (Ed.), *Attention*, 223–256. Hove, UK: Psychology Press.

Yantis, S., Schwarzbach, J., Serences, J. T., Carlson, R. L., Steinmetz, M. A., Pekar, J. J., & Courtney, S. M. (2002). Transient neural activity in human parietal cortex during spatial attention shifts. *Nature Neuroscience* 5, 995–1002.

5 Functional Neuroimaging of Skill Learning

Russell A. Poldrack and Daniel T. Willingham

Introduction

The concept of multiple memory systems has become one of the foundational constructs in cognitive neuroscience. First suggested by dissociations between different memory tasks in neuropsychological patients, the notion that memory is made up of a number of functionally and neurally distinct components has subsequently gained strong support from functional neuroimaging studies. The most prominent framework separates memory into a declarative system, which relies upon the medial temporal lobe (MTL), and a set of nondeclarative or procedural systems that rely upon brain systems other than the MTL (e.g., N. J. Cohen & Eichenbaum, 1993; Gabrieli, 1998; Squire, 1992). This framework has received substantial support from a wide range of techniques across human and nonhuman species, and has influenced much theoretical and empirical work in skill learning.

Some of the earliest evidence of dissociations between memory systems came from demonstrations that the patient H.M., though suffering from a dense amnesia for episodic information, was able to acquire motor skills in a normal manner (Corkin, 1968; Milner et al., 1968). Subsequent studies demonstrated that amnesic patients are also able to normally acquire a range of perceptual skills (N. J. Cohen & Squire, 1980) and cognitive skills (N. J. Cohen et al., 1985). These findings demonstrated that the MTL is not necessary for skill acquisition, but did not provide any clues as to which neural systems are involved in skill acquisition. Studies of patients with other disorders, particularly basal ganglia disorders such as Parkinson's disease (PD) and Huntington's disease (HD), have shown that the basal ganglia are involved in acquisition of a range of perceptual, cognitive, and motor skills (Heindel et al., 1989; Knowlton et al., 1996a). These findings have suggested to some researchers that the basal ganglia may serve as a general system for the acquisition of novel abilities across domains (e.g., Packard & Knowlton, 2002).

Functional Neuroimaging of Skill Learning

Neuroimaging of Skill Acquisition: Possibilities and Challenges

In the present chapter we review the insights that functional neuroimaging studies have provided into the neural systems that support skill acquisition. Neuroimaging is particularly useful for studying dynamic phenomena such as skill acquisition. Studies of patients with lesions can show whether or not a particular brain region is necessary to learn a particular skill, but cannot show how brain regions change as a function of training or when in the course of learning a region is involved. Thus, our review will focus on studies examining learning-related changes in brain activity. In many cases, however, it is also of interest to see what regions are engaged during skill acquisition even if they do not exhibit learning-related changes. This is particularly true for tasks where learning occurs quite rapidly, such that it is very difficult to image changes related to learning reliably. In these cases it may, however, be difficult to disentangle regions engaged in skill acquisition from those involved more generally in task performance.

Neuroimaging of skill learning involves a number of difficult conceptual and methodological issues that are not encountered in imaging of static performance on cognitive tasks. We have outlined these issues in detail elsewhere (Poldrack, 2000) and will only briefly discuss these issues in this chapter. In particular, it is important to highlight the fact that learning is almost invariably associated with changes in task performance (e.g., faster and more accurate responses). Because functional imaging signals are nonlinearly sensitive to time on task (Berns et al., 1999), it becomes difficult to determine whether changes in activation reflect the neural changes that result in skill learning or the neural effects of performance changes. Several strategies have been used to address this issue, and we highlight them throughout the discussion.

Skills are often heuristically divided into motor, perceptual, and cognitive domains, and we will adhere roughly to that classification here, focusing on classification learning in the cognitive domain. However, it is important to note that this taxonomy is largely one of convenience, since there is substantial diversity in the neural underpinnings of various tasks that fall within each of these categories, as well as commonalities across categories.

Imaging of Motor Skill Learning

A number of researchers have suggested that motor skill learning is supported by the same anatomic substrate that supports motor control: that is, there is plasticity in the structures underlying motor control, and learning occurs as these control processes adapt, with practice, to the particular constraints imposed by a task (Karni et al., 1995; Willingham, 1992). This hypothesis predicts that just as different brain regions support different aspects of control (e.g., calculation of force, trajectory, and timing), so will the anatomic basis of a motor skill vary, depending on the type of information required for improvement in the skill. Some skills may be mostly a matter of learning a spatial trajectory (e.g., a karate punch), whereas others might depend primarily on appropriate timing (e.g., batting in a video baseball game).

The prediction that different brain regions support skill depending on task demands is largely consistent with existing data, but a relatively narrow range of tasks has been tested. In this section, we review different types of skills segregated by the type of information that must be learned: sequencing of very simple motor movements either implicitly or explicitly, and learning new relationships between visual stimuli and motor responses. We conclude with a review of the changes engendered by long-term practice.

Implicit Sequence Learning

Most of the work examining implicit sequence learning has used the serial response time task (SRTT) developed by Nissen and Bullemer (1987). On each trial a stimulus appears in one of four positions and the subject must push one of four response keys as quickly as possible, whereupon the stimulus is extinguished and a new stimulus appears. In the implicit version of this task, subjects are not told that the stimuli appear in a repeating sequence (usually 10 or 12 units long). Although subjects often remain unaware that some stimuli are sequenced, they nevertheless learn the sequence, as revealed by their response times (RTs), which decrease with continued practice. RTs increase if a new sequence or random stimuli are introduced, indicating that the RT decrease is not due to learning factors general to the task (e.g., timing). A comparison of the RTs between sequenced and random stimuli is usually taken as a relatively pure measure of implicit sequence knowledge (figure 5.1).

The SRTT has been administered in at least 10 brain imaging studies, and there is fair consistency in the pattern of results of learning-related changes. The supplementary motor area (SMA; medial BA 6) and posterior parietal cortex (BA 7 and 40) are consistently implicated in implicit sequence learning, and anterior cingulate activation is also typically observed (Bischoff-Grethe et al., 2004; Doyon et al., 1996; Doyon et al., 2002; Grafton et al., 1998; Rauch, Savage, et al., 1997). Posterior parietal cortex may represent the sequence locations in an abstract spatial code. One study varied the motor response requirements, and observed changes in the activation of secondary motor cortices, but consistency in parietal activation (Grafton et al., 1998). The SMA may represent the sequence in a motor code; single-cell recording studies of nonhuman primates have implicated this area in motor sequencing (Lee

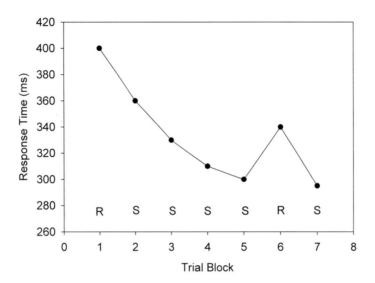

Figure 5.1
Idealized graph of RT data from the SRTT. Sequenced blocks (S) include eight repetitions of the
sequence; random blocks (R) present 96 random stimuli. RTs decrease with sequence practice, and
increase when random stimuli are reintroduced. The difference in RTs to random and sequenced stimuli
is taken as an implicit measure of learning.

& Quessy, 2003; Tanji, 2001). Cingulate activity may be related to motor preparation
associated with predicting part of the sequence. Other experiments have shown that
cingulate cortex is active when a previously repeating pattern is violated (Huettel
et al., 2002). It is possible that prediction is part of sequence learning; in explicit
sequencing tasks, cingulate activity declines once a motor sequence is well learned
(Jenkins et al., 1994; Jueptner, Frith, et al., 1997), perhaps because predictions are
infrequently violated once the sequence has been learned.

Most studies do not report striatal activity, which may be surprising, given its
anatomic relationship with the SMA and the data indicating that sequencing is
impaired in patients with striatal abnormalities (Jackson et al., 1995; Willingham &
Koroshetz, 1993). Although robust striatal activity is not always observed, two
studies that focused on the striatum (Peigneux et al., 2000; Rauch, Whalen, et al.,
1997) did observe such activity.

Activation in primary motor cortex (M1) has been observed in about half of
existing studies of implicit motor sequence learning (Bischoff-Grethe et al., 2002;
Grafton et al., 1995; Grafton et al., 1998, 2002; Hazeltine et al., 1997). This inconsistency may be due to differences in analytic methods. Activity associated with
sequence learning may be assessed by subtracting activations associated with
sequenced stimuli and with random stimuli or by applying a linear contrast to

performance on sequenced trials. Activity in M1 has not been observed when the former technique is used, but is observed with the latter.

The role of the cerebellum in implicit sequence learning also remains unclear. Neuropsychological studies consistently report profound deficits in the face of cerebellar abnormality (Gomez-Beldarrain et al., 1998; Molinari et al., 1997) but data from imaging studies are less clear, with some studies reporting activation (Doyon et al., 1996; Rauch, Whalen, et al., 1997), whereas others report none (Rauch et al., 1995; Willingham et al., 2002) and still others report an early increase, followed by a rapid decrease (Doyon et al., 2002). Seidler et al. (2002) argued that the cerebellum contributes not to the learning of implicit sequences but to the expression of sequence knowledge. Learning and expression are usually confounded in the SRTT. To dissociate them, the researchers trained subjects in the SRTT, but with a concurrent secondary task (monitoring color patches for a target color). Behaviorally, subjects showed no sequence-related improvement during training, but when transferred to the SRTT alone, they showed robust sequence knowledge, indicating that the secondary task did not inhibit learning, but prevented the expression of learning. The researchers examined images obtained during training for increasing and decreasing activations that predicted the learning that was later observed at transfer. Areas implicated in sequence learning included those typically observed—primary and secondary motor cortices, posterior parietal and prefrontal cortices—but not cerebellum. At transfer, however, there was robust bilateral activation in cerebellar lobule VI; thus the cerebellum was associated not with learning but with expressing learning (figure 5.2, plate 7).

Tracking tasks are venerable measures of motor skill and might be considered implicit sequencing tasks because they entail a set of simple movements made repeatedly. For example, in the pursuit rotor task, the subject uses a hand-held stylus to track a small target on a rotating platter. The brain areas implicated match those involved in the SRTT: the SMA and posterior parietal cortex (Grafton et al., 1992; Grafton et al., 2001; Grafton et al., 1994). Basal ganglia activation has not been observed, but it may require a focused investigation, as was necessary with SRTT learning.

Explicit Sequence Learning

Explicit sequence learning has been the subject of a number of studies, some of them using button presses as in the SRTT, and some of them employing opposing movements of the fingers and thumb. In either case, subjects are given a brief sequence—typically 6 units—to learn explicitly by trial and error, sometimes outside the scanner and sometimes during the scanning session.

As with implicit learning, the activations associated with explicit sequence learning are fairly, but not perfectly, consistent. The premotor cortex (PMC; lateral BA

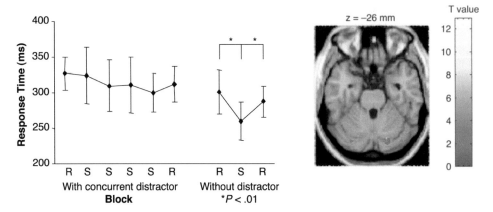

Figure 5.2
Behavioral and neuroimaging results adapted from from Seidler et al. (2002). Behavioral results (left) show that during training with a concurrent distractor task, subjects show no evidence of sequence learning. However, once the secondary task is removed, they show robust sequence knowledge. Cerebellar activity was associated only with the expression of learning at transfer (right), but not with learning. See plate 7 for color version.

6), posterior parietal (BA 7 and 40), and prefrontal cortices (BA 45 and 46) are most often implicated in explicit sequence learning (De Weerd et al., 2003; Eliassen et al., 2001; Muller et al., 2002; Toni et al., 1998). This pattern appears to be consonant with the roles of posterior parietal and prefrontal cortices in spatial working memory (Wager & Smith, 2003).

As with implicit motor sequence learning, the cerebellum's contribution is unclear. About half of extant studies report cerebellar activation (Doyon et al., 1996; Eliassen et al., 2001; Muller et al., 2002; Toni et al., 1998; Willingham et al., 2002). Perhaps more surprising is the lack of activation in the medial temporal lobe, which is known to be vital for explicit memory (Squire, 1992). Many of the early studies used PET, with which the medial temporal lobe is notoriously difficult to image. One fMRI study (Schendan et al., 2003) targeted the medial temporal lobe as a region of interest and showed reliable learning-related activation of hippocampus for an explicit version of the SRTT.

Perceptual-Motor Relationships
Some skills do not require learning sequences of motor acts, but rather require learning new relationships between perceptual stimuli and motor behaviors. Sometimes the relationship between stimulus and response is arbitrary, as when one learns to depress the brake pedal in response to a red traffic light. In other situations, there is an orderly but unfamiliar relationship between the visual stimuli that one

uses to set a goal and the movements which will accomplish that goal. For example, the goal of where to move a computer cursor is determined by the configuration of stimuli on the screen, but the movements necessary to position the cursor are not made in the plane of the screen, but in the plane of the desktop as one maneuvers a mouse. A novice computer user must learn the translation between them. Arbitrary perceptual motor relationships (such as the traffic light) and systematic ones (such as the mouse) appear to be learned by different neural circuits.

Learning a systematic mapping (often called *adaptation*) has been studied using prism spectacles, which displace the visual world some degrees to the right or left, and in paradigms where subjects manipulate a cursor with a joystick, but the joystick-cursor relationship is rotated. Movements are initially quite inaccurate, but practice with visual feedback leads to rapid improvement. Adaptation studies show substantial activation in posterior parietal cortex (BA 7) (Clower et al., 1996; Flament et al., 1996). This result is consistent with in vivo recordings in nonhuman primates, which indicate that this area may support the translation of retinotopic spatial information to other spatial frames (Andersen et al., 1997).

More controversial is the role of the cerebellum in adaptation. Patients with cerebellar abnormalities are impaired in adapting to prism spectacles (Sanes et al., 1990; Weiner et al., 1974). The lack of cerebellar activation in imaging studies is therefore somewhat surprising. Some researchers (e.g., Fiez et al., 1992; Wang et al., 1987) have suggested that the cerebellum is important in processing movement error, which naturally abounds early in adaptation learning. Flament et al. (1996) noted that their subjects' cerebellar activation was highest when the relationship between joystick and cursor was random, so that learning was not possible but error was high. Clower et al. (1996) observed no cerebellar activation associated with learning, possibly because their control condition (the activation of which was subtracted from learning) included the target jumping 7 cm during the reach, thus ensuring the detection of error in the control. Imamizu et al. (2000) offered a different account of the role of the cerebellum in adaptation. They argued that part of the cerebellum is indeed devoted to processing error signals, but a smaller region is also the site of plasticity for adaptation learning. They had subjects track a moving target for 11 sessions with a mouse rotated 120 degrees. The baseline condition included no rotation, but used a faster target speed to equate performance. Although error was the same in both conditions, cerebellar activation was greater in the adaptation condition, which the authors interpreted as reflecting an internal model of the rotation.

Shadmehr and Holcomb (1997, 1999) used a different adaptation task. Subjects used a manipulandum to direct a computer cursor to targets. Torque motors applied forces to the manipulandum so that the subject moved in a force field—the motors produced a force perpendicular to the actual direction of the hand. Subjects adapted to this new dynamic environment with practice, and made accurate movements (figure 5.3). Brain imaging studies show learning-associated activity in prefrontal cortex (BA 46), with smaller activations in striatum and thalamus. The different pattern of activation in this task compared with other adaptation tasks is notable. Other tasks use a spatial transformation and rely strongly on parietal cortex, which does not contribute to this force learning task.

Learning arbitrary relationships between stimuli and appropriate motor actions has been studied extensively in nonhuman primates using single-cell and ablation techniques. The underlying neural network has largely been identified (Wise & Murray, 2000), and includes ventral prefrontal cortex (inferior frontal sulcus) posterior parietal cortex (BA 7 and 40), PMC (lateral BA 6), and parts of the basal ganglia and medial temporal lobe. Brain imaging data are in accord with investigations using these other techniques. For example, Toni et al. (2001) had subjects learn to make finger movements to each of four abstract visual patterns. Across scans taken at four points in learning, significant activation was observed in the lingual gyrus, parahippocampal cortex, caudate nucleus and inferior frontal sulcus. The extent to which some of these structures are best characterized as dedicated to learning arbitrary visuomotor mappings is not clear—at least some (e.g., medial temporal lobe) are more general mnemonic structures.

The foregoing data can be summarized as follows. Different types of motor skills appear to be supported by different neural circuits. Implicit sequence learning is supported by posterior parietal cortex, the SMA, anterior cingulate, and striatum.

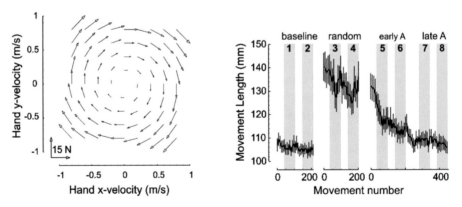

Figure 5.3
Example of perceptual-motor adaptation (adapted from Shadmehr & Holcomb, 1997). Subjects used a manipulandum to move a cursor to a target. Continuous feedback was provided, and the dependent measure was distance traveled. In the baseline condition, no forces perturbed the movement, and movements were short because they went directly to the target. In the random condition, movement was perturbed by a field of random forces; movements were circuitous, and subjects don't improve. They do improve with practice on Field A, however, which is depicted on the right.

Explicit sequence learning is supported by posterior parietal and dorsolateral prefrontal cortices, and the PMC. Adaptation is supported by the posterior parietal cortex and perhaps the cerebellum. Arbitrary visuomotor mappings are supported by ventral prefrontal, medial temporal, and posterior parietal cortices, as well as the PMC.

A couple of points should be borne in mind. First, there is some overlap in the structures that support these different types of skill, but not a great deal. The most notable area of overlap is the posterior parietal cortex, which likely supports spatial representations relevant to the skill. This consistency in PPC activation may be observed because space is integral to almost all of the tasks tested to date; the spatial organization of movements is what is to be learned in the skill. The sole exception is the force-field task, and indeed, learning-related activation in the PPC was not observed in that task. Another important point to keep in mind is that all of the studies cited used rather brief training regimens—typically a single session of an hour or less. Thus, the data described may not represent motor skill learning in general, but rather the early stages of motor skill learning. One of the hallmarks of skill is that behavioral changes accrue slowly, and high levels of practice are necessary for movements to become smooth and for the demands of attention to decrease. We turn now to studies that have examined changes in brain activation with practice.

Practice Effects

A number of studies have sought to examine the changes in learning-related brain activations as subjects practice and attain greater levels of skill. One might expect a qualitative change in the anatomy underlying skill because most subjects report that early practice is associated with conscious direction of movements, whereas late practice is associated with automaticity (Fitts & Posner, 1967).

It is difficult to generalize across studies because different research groups have used somewhat different tasks, although most have used some variant of a sequencing task. More important, different studies have employed quite different amounts of practice. Some studies used fewer than 50 training trials (Eliassen et al., 2001; Muller et al., 2002; Sakai et al., 1998), whereas others used hundreds (Penhune & Doyon, 2002; Petersen et al., 1998). In all cases researchers categorized activations as associated with "early" or "late" training, but it is clear that the "late" training for one study would correspond to the "early" training of another.

Despite these complications to interpretation, there are some points of agreement. Most studies of sequence learning report PMC activation early in training and SMA activation later in training (Doyon et al., 2002; Eliassen et al., 2001; Petersen et al., 1998; Toni et al., 1998), with the exception of Grafton et al. (1994), who used a pursuit tracking task. Also, striatal activation is more often associated with advanced training (Doyon et al., 2002; Grafton et al., 1994; Penhune & Doyon, 2002). These generalizations are consistent with the idea that sequence learning is supported by explicit processes early in training, but implicit processes come to play a greater role with increased practice. When cerebellar activation is reported, it is consistently observed early in training (Doyon et al., 2002; Eliassen et al., 2001; Grafton et al., 1994; Petersen et al., 1998; Toni et al., 1998). As noted, there is still controversy as to whether such activation is due to error detection and correction, or to learning processes per se.

There are also points of disagreement in this literature. Several studies using a short training regimen suggest that M1 contributes to learning early in training (Eliassen et al., 2001; Grafton et al., 1994; Toni et al., 1998), but other studies suggest that it has an effect late in training (Petersen et al., 1998) or both early and late (De Weerd et al., 2003). It is of course possible that activation profiles could be nonlinear. Results from Karni et al. (1995) are consistent with this hypothesis. They had subjects practice a finger sequence 1–20 min each day over the course of 4 to 6 weeks. They reported an initial decrease in the extent of M1 activation, followed by a later increase after sustained training.

The role of prefrontal cortex across practice is also unclear. Given the role of PFC in supporting spatial working memory, one might expect strong activation as the sequence was learned and practiced, but a diminution once the behavior became automatic. Jueptner, Stephan, et al. (1997) provided an interesting test of that hypothesis (figure 5.4). They showed that PFC is more active when learning a new sequence than when performing a well-learned sequence, but PFC is reactivated when subjects are instructed to perform the well-learned sequence while paying attention to what they were doing (i.e., planning each movement).

This result is consistent with other brain-imaging work on motor control that indicates a role for PFC in the conscious planning of movement (Frith et al., 1991; Pochon et al., 2001; Seitz et al., 2000). As logical as this interpretation appears, the

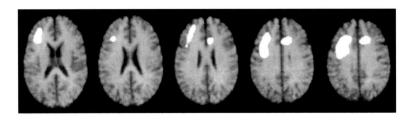

Figure 5.4
Activity related to attention during motor sequence learning (adapted from Jueptner et al., 1997). Significant increases of rCBF when subjects are asked to attend to the movements of a well-learned sequence are compared with when they are not asked to attend. Activations correspond to left prefrontal cortex (BA 46 and 9) and right anterior cingulate (BA 32, 34).

data do not line up neatly to fit it. Although activation is often reported in dorsal PFC (BA 8, 9, 45, and 46) in explicit sequencing studies (Grafton et al., 1995; Jueptner, Stephan, et al., 1997; Muller et al., 2002; Sakai et al., 1998; Toni et al., 1998; Willingham et al., 2002), those studies comparing early and late activation seldom report activity in this region, and when they do, it is neither consistently early nor consistently late. This uncertainty is likely due to differences in analysis techniques and in the behavioral tasks: some had subjects learn the sequence before scanning, others during scanning by instruction, and still others during scanning by trial and error.

Imaging of Perceptual Skill Learning

Perceptual skill learning encompasses tasks in which the subject learns to process novel perceptual stimuli, to make increasingly fine distinctions among familiar stimuli, or to process perceptually transformed versions of familiar stimuli. The term "perceptual learning" is often used within the psychophysics literature to refer to learning of psychophysical discriminations; as used here, the term "perceptual skill learning" encompasses those tasks but also includes higher-level tasks that may have conceptual components.

Mirror Reading

In the mirror-reading task, subjects are presented with geometrically transformed text and asked either to read the text aloud or to make decisions about the text (e.g., lexical decision). With training, subjects can come to identify novel words written in the transformed typeface more rapidly. The nature of learning in the mirror-reading task remains a point of debate; whereas some researchers have argued that learning on the task occurs primarily at the level of letters or letter clusters (Masson, 1986), other work suggests that learning may also be occurring at higher levels of organization (e.g., Horton, 1989). In addition, an important aspect of learning on the task may relate to the direction of attention to the right side of the word (for mirror-reversed English words). Neuropsychology has demonstrated that amnesic patients are normal at learning the mirror-reading skill (N. J. Cohen & Squire, 1980; Martone et al., 1984), whereas patients with HD are at least mildly impaired (Martone et al., 1984).

Several studies have examined activation during mirror-reading prior to extensive training on the task; unlike motor skill learning tasks, where learning often occurs relatively quickly, learning on the mirror-reading task evolves over the course of many hours. Compared with reading of normally oriented text, mirror-reading has been associated with activation in both ventral and dorsal visual streams, including occipital, inferior temporal, and superior parietal cortices (Dong et al., 2000; Goebel et al., 1998; Kassubek et al., 2001; Poldrack et al., 1998; Poldrack & Gabrieli, 2001). Connectivity analyses by Goebel et al. (1998) showed that inferior occipitotemporal cortex and intraparietal sulcus were correlated in their activity, suggesting that they act as a common network. Activity has also been observed in the caudate nucleus in English (Poldrack & Gabrieli, 2001) and Japanese kana (Dong et al., 2000) mirror-reading, consistent with the finding of impairments of mirror-reading in patients with Huntington's disease (Martone et al., 1984). The finding of these effects with Japanese kana by Dong et al. (2000) is important because it suggests that caudate activation is not related to the oculomotor effects of mirror-reversal, since kana are read vertically and mirror-reversal thus does not interfere with the direction of reading, as it does in English.

A smaller set of studies has examined learning-related changes in activation related to training on the mirror-reading task. In two of these studies (Poldrack et al., 1998; Poldrack & Gabrieli, 2001), subjects were trained for several hours and scanned before and after training. In both studies, increased activity was observed in the inferior temporal cortex (BA 37) after training, and in each case the region of increase was within about a centimeter of the "visual word-form area" that is preferentially responsive to visual words (e.g., L. Cohen & Dehaene, 2004). In the Poldrack et al. (1998) study, response times did not differ between the pretraining and posttraining scans, suggesting that learning-related changes were not due to changes in time on task.

Two findings suggest that these increases do not reflect a specific representation of mirror-reversed letters. First, Poldrack & Gabrieli (2001) examined the selectivity of the learning-related increase by presenting subjects with a practiced transformation (mirror-reversal) as well as two other unpracticed transformations (inverted-reversed and spelled-backward). The learning-related increase in inferior temporal cortex was found to occur similarly for both practiced and unpracticed transformations, suggesting that it most likely reflects some general aspect of reading transformed text rather than a specific representation of mirror-reversed letters, as initially proposed by Poldrack et al. (1998). Second, Kassubek et al. (2001) examined the learning of vertically transformed text (which is read from left to right), and failed to find any significant learning-related increases; however, an unspecified portion of inferior temporal cortex was not imaged in this study, so it is unclear whether it was possible to find such changes, if they existed. One likely possibility is that the increased activity seen in some studies reflects top-down attentional modulation related to the direction of attention to the right side of the stimulus (cf. Poldrack & Gabrieli, 2001).

Learning-related increases have also been observed in the body of the caudate nucleus (Poldrack & Gabrieli, 2001); it is unclear whether this reflects visual association learning or strategic aspects of learning on the task. Learning-related decreases have been consistently observed in the superior parietal cortex (Kassubek et al., 2001; Poldrack et al., 1998); Poldrack & Gabrieli (2001) failed to find decreases in superior parietal cortex, but this region was not fully covered due to missing data for some subjects in the most superior slices.

Skilled Object Recognition

It is well known that a region in the fusiform gyrus (known as the "fusiform face area," or FFA) in humans is selectively responsive to faces in comparison with other classes of objects (e.g., Kanwisher et al., 1997; Puce et al., 1995). Whereas some researchers have taken this to reflect specialization for faces per se, others have suggested that it may reflect a more general specialization of the FFA for expert subordinate-level individuation of stimuli, faces or otherwise. Skill learning with novel nonface objects was assessed by Gauthier et al. (1999), using a set of synthetic stimuli known as "Greebles." Subjects were taught to classify and individuate a large number of exemplars, and were scanned before and after training using fMRI (only occipital/temporal regions were imaged in this study). Learning-related increases in activity were observed in the fusiform gyri bilaterally; of particular interest was the fact that regions initially responsive to human faces but not Greebles became responsive to both stimulus classes after training. These results suggest that the FFA is sensitive to objects other than faces after training, but a caveat on these results is that the Greebles have facelike features, and thus may be engaging face-specific processes.

In addition to training effects, the nature of expertise in visual object recognition has been investigated in groups of subjects who are expert in particular visual domains. Gauthier et al. (2000) examined regions involved in the perception of faces as well as of cars and birds in two groups of subjects, one of which was expert with cars and the other of which was expert with birds. The results showed that activation in the fusiform gyrus was greater for the category of stimuli in which the subject was expert, in addition to being sensitive to faces in both groups. The primary goal of this study was to investigate whether the FFA was equally sensitive to faces and expert recognition of nonface objects. Its claims in this regard have been questioned by Kanwisher (2000) and Rhodes et al. (2004), who pointed out that the definition of the FFA used in this study was not standard. Regardless of the relation to face processing, the results of Gauthier et al. (2000) do show an interaction between expertise and object type for cars versus birds, suggesting that some aspects of object recognition skill may rely upon the fusiform gyrus.

A study by Rhodes et al. (2004) examined expert object recognition for faces and butterflies in both novices and experts. Comparison of butterfly experts and novices showed that the experts had greater activation in the fusiform gyrus for butterflies than did novices, consistent with the Gauthier et al. (2000) results. However, they also showed that the experts had greater activation for faces than did the novices, suggesting that the differences between these groups are not specific to expertise with this visual class (figure 5.5). In addition, the majority of voxels activated for butterflies were outside of the FFA (defined in a standard manner).

Finally, Grill-Spector et al. (2004) found that whereas behavioral performance on face perception was predicted by activity in the fusiform gyrus, performance of car experts on car perception was not predicted by activity in this area, suggesting that the fusiform gyrus may play a more central role in face perception than in perception of other expert object classes. It is clear from these studies that expert object perception relies in a general sense on representations in the occipitotemporal cortex, though the degree to which these representations overlap with those involved in face perception seems to be in doubt.

Orientation Discrimination

The neural basis of perceptual learning has been investigated using an orientation discrimination task, in which subjects judge the orientation of a noisy grating (Schiltz et al., 1999; Schiltz et al., 2001). The advantage of this task is that training on one orientation (e.g., +45 degrees) transfers only minimally to the oblique orientation (e.g., –45 degrees). In both studies, learning on this task was associated with decreased activity in striate (BA 17) and extrastriate (BA 18/19) cortices that is specific to the trained compared with the untrained orientation. These changes are consistent with the changes in cortical receptive fields observed in single-unit studies using the same task (Schoups et al., 2001); however, decreases in visual cortices could also reflect repetition priming or habituation for the trained stimulus. In one study (Schiltz et al., 2001), learning was also associated with increased activity in the caudate nucleus. Thus, there is some reason to believe that the striatum may be involved very generally in the acquisition of perceptual skills.

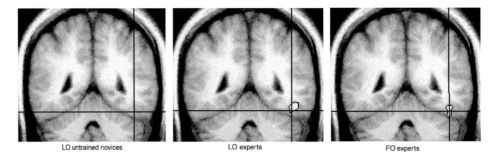

LO untrained novices   LO experts   FO experts

Figure 5.5
Results from Rhodes et al. (2004). Coronal slices through the fusiform gyrus are presented, showing activation for LO (butterflies) versus objects in novice butterfly viewers (*left*) and butterfly experts (*middle*), and activation for faces versus objects in butterfly experts (*right*).

References

Aguirre, G. K., & D'Esposito, M. (1999). Experimental design for fMRI. In C. T. W. Moonen & P. A. Bandettini (Eds.), *Functional MRI*, 369–380. Berlin: Springer-Verlag.

Aguirre, G. K., Zarahn, E., & D'Esposito, M. (1998). The variability of human, BOLD hemodynamic responses. *NeuroImage* 8, 360–369.

Bandettini, P. A., & Cox, R. W. (2000). Event-related fMRI contrast when using constant interstimulus interval: Theory and experiment. *Magnetic Resonance in Medicine* 43, 540–548.

Basser, P. J., Pajevic, S., Pierpaoli, C., Duda, J., & Aldroubi, A. (2000). In vivo fiber tractography using DT-MRI data. *Magnetic Resonance in Medicine* 44, 625–632.

Beauchamp, M. S., Cox, R. W., & DeYoe, E. A. (1997). Graded effects of spatial and featural attention on human area MT and associated motion processing areas. *Journal of Neurophysiology* 78, 516–520.

Beauchamp, M. S., Petit, L., Ellmore, T. M., Ingeholm, J., & Haxby, J. V. (2000). A parametric fMRI study of overt and covert shifts of visuospatial attention. *Society for Neuroscience Abstracts* 26, 1586.

Birn, R. M., Bandettini, P. A., Cox, R. W., & Shaker, R. (1999). Event-related fMRI of tasks involving brief motion. *Human Brain Mapping* 7, 106–114.

Biswal, B. B., & Ulmer, J. L. (1999). Blind source separation of multiple signal sources of fMRI data sets using independent component analysis. *Journal of Computational Assisted Tomography* 23, 265–271.

Blakemore, S. J., Winston, J., & Frith, U. (2004). Social cognitive neuroscience: Where are we heading? *Trends in Cognitive Sciences* 8, 216–222.

Blamire, A. M., Ogawa, S., Ugurbil, K., Rothman, D., McCarthy, G., Ellermann, J. M., et al. (1992). Dynamic mapping of the human visual cortex by high-speed magnetic resonance imaging. *Proceedings of the National Academy of Sciences USA* 89, 11069–11073.

Boynton, G. M., & Finney, E. M. (2003). Orientation-specific adaptation in human visual cortex. *Journal of Neuroscience* 23, 8781–8787.

Brewer, J. B., Zhao, Z., Desmond, J. E., Glover, G. H., & Gabrieli, J. D. E. (1998). Making memories: Brain activity that predicts how well visual experience will be remembered. *Science* 281, 1185–1187.

Buckner, R. L., Bandettini, P. A., O'Craven, K. M., Savoy, R. L., Petersen, S. E., Raichle, M. E., & Rosen, B. R. (1996). Detection of cortical activation during averaged single trials of a cognitive task using functional magnetic resonance imaging. *Proceedings of the National Academy of Sciences USA* 93, 14878–14883.

Buckner, R. L., & Braver, T. S. (1999). Event-related functional MRI. In C. T. W. Moonen & P. A. Bandettini (Eds.), *Functional MRI*, 441–452. Berlin: Springer-Verlag.

Buckner, R. L., & Logan, J. M. (2001). Functional neuroimaging methods: PET and fMRI. In R. Cabeza & A. Kingstone (Eds.), *Handbook of Functional Neuroimaging of Cognition*, 27–48. Cambridge, MA: MIT Press.

Chao, L. L., & Martin, A. (2000). Representation of manipulable man-made objects in the dorsal stream. *NeuroImage* 12, 478–484.

Chein, J. M., & Schneider, W. (2003). Designing effective fMRI experiments. In J. Grafman & I. Robertson (Eds.), *Handbook of Neuropsychology*. Amsterdam: Elsevier Science.

Colby, C. L., Duhamel, J.-R., & Goldberg, M. E. (1996). Visual, presaccadic, and cognitive activation of single neurons in monkey lateral intraparietal area. *Journal of Neurophysiology* 76, 2841–2851.

Corbetta, M., Akbudak, E., Conturo, T. E., Snyder, A. Z., Ollinger, J. M., Drury, H. A., et al. (1998). A common network of functional areas for attention and eye movements. *Neuron* 21, 761–773.

Crick, F., & Jones, E. (1993). Backwardness of human neuroanatomy. *Nature* 361, 109–110.

Culham, J., He, S., Dukelow, S., & Verstraten, F. A. (2001). Visual motion and the human brain: What has neuroimaging told us? *Acta Psychologica* (Amsterdam) 107, 69–94.

Culham, J. C. (2003). Human brain imaging reveals a parietal area specialized for grasping. In N. Kanwisher & J. Duncan (Eds.), *Attention and Performance XX: Functional Brain Imaging of Human Cognition*. Oxford: Oxford University Press.

For example, in the commonly used "weather prediction task" (Knowlton et al., 1994), subjects learn to predict one of two outcomes (rain or sunshine), depending upon the presence of four features (cards with geometric shapes), each of which is probabilistically associated with one of those outcomes. Particular interest has focused on the role of the basal ganglia in PCL, since it is known to be impaired in patients with basal ganglia disorders (Knowlton et al., 1996a; Knowlton et al., 1996b). All reported studies of classification learning in normal subjects have found activity in the basal ganglia (Aron et al., 2004; Moody et al., 2004; Poldrack et al., 2001; Poldrack et al., 1999), as well as a broad network of prefrontal, parietal, and occipitotemporal cortical regions. Poldrack et al. (2001) compared the standard version of the weather prediction task, in which subjects learn on the basis of feedback, with an "observational learning" version of the task in which subjects learn on the basis of category labels without making a categorization response. Activity in the caudate nucleus and midbrain (SN/VTA) was decreased in the observational version compared with the feedback-based version, suggesting that the role of basal ganglia may be in the processing of response-contingent feedback. Consistent with this result, patients with Parkinson's disease were unimpaired at learning an observational version of the weather prediction task, whereas they were impaired at learning the same classification in a feedback-based task (Shohamy et al., 2004).

Rapid event-related fMRI was used by Aron et al. (2004) to separately estimate the hemodynamic response to stimulus, delay, and feedback in the weather prediction task. In order to estimate these trial components separately, intervals of randomly varying length were placed between the stimulus and feedback presentation. This analysis showed that the striatum was active during both the stimulus presentation/motor response phase and the feedback phase, though there was more activity during stimulus/response than during feedback. A comparison of trials on which positive versus negative feedback was presented (i.e., the feedback stated that the subject was correct or incorrect, respectively) showed greater activity in the midbrain (SN/VTA) and orbitofrontal cortex for negative feedback (figure 5.7, plate 8); other analyses (Poldrack, unpublished) using a different basis set also showed greater activity for negative feedback in the ventral striatum. These results are consistent with the role of the basal ganglia in error correction (cf. Lawrence, 2000), but they seem on their face inconsistent with the results of Schultz and colleagues (e.g., Schultz et al., 2000), who have shown, using single-unit recordings, that the absence of an expected reward leads to decreased firing of dopaminergic (DA) cells in the midbrain. The results can be reconciled by noting that fMRI is primarily a measure of afferent synaptic inputs rather than of local spiking (e.g., Lauritzen, 2001). Thus, the afferent signals (primarily from striatum) that result in decreased DA neuron firing in the midbrain may result in increased fMRI signal. Alternatively,

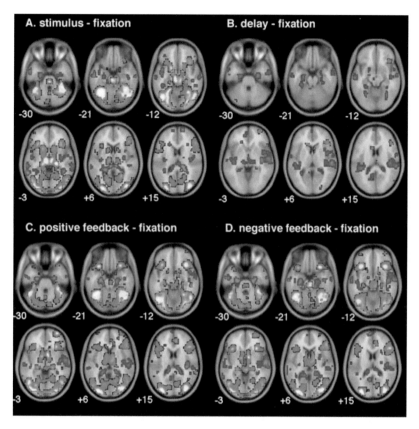

Figure 5.7
Results from Aron et al. (2004), depicting activation during each trial component of a probabilistic classification task. See plate 8 for color version.

the response of DA neurons may differ across either tasks or species in ways that lead to differences in activity across these studies.

Another consistent finding in studies of PCL has been a decrease in signal in the MTL versus baseline (Poldrack et al., 1999; Poldrack et al., 2001; Aron et al., 2004; Moody et al., 2004). This deactivation is greater under feedback-based learning compared with observational learning (Poldrack et al., 2001), but decomposition using event-related fMRI has shown that the deactivation occurs to both the stimulus and the feedback, and is not modulated by feedback valence. Using functional connectivity analysis, Poldrack et al. (2001) found that activity in the MTL is negatively correlated with activity in the caudate nucleus (i.e., greater striatal activation is associated with greater MTL deactivation) across subjects; furthermore, these regions also showed reciprocal changes in their evoked response over time during the early part of learning. These results were interpreted to reflect a competitive interaction between the basal ganglia and MTL; see "Current Issues," below, for additional discussion of this issue.

A study by Moody et al. (2004) used fMRI to compare the neural basis of classification learning in PD patients and controls. The patients, who were in the early stages of PD, were not impaired at learning on the task. However, their pattern of neural activity during task performance differed from controls. Whereas controls exhibited activation in the striatum and deactivation of the MTL, the PD patients exhibited activation in the MTL but no activation in the striatum. These results are consistent with those from several other studies (e.g., Dagher et al., 2001; Rauch, Savage, Alpert, et al., 1997), showing that disorders of the basal ganglia result in an altered balance of activity between the striatum and the MTL.

To summarize, the pattern of striatal activation and MTL deactivation has been strikingly consistent across studies of PCL. The role of the striatum appears to be modulated by the need to process feedback, but striatal activity is not limited to the feedback component of the task.

Artificial Grammar Learning
The learning of novel artificial grammars has been extensively investigated in cognitive psychology, with a particular focus on the degree to which subjects may abstract knowledge about the underlying rules of the grammar without conscious awareness of those rules. What is learned, and the degree to which this knowledge is available to awareness, remain a topic of substantial controversy (e.g., Dulany et al., 1984; Knowlton & Squire, 1994). A number of neuroimaging studies have investigated the neural basis of learning on this task. Early studies used blocked designs to compare grammatical judgments with baseline tasks (Fletcher et al., 1999; Seger et al., 2000). These studies found activity in a network including bilateral occipital cortex and bilateral ventrolateral and dorsolateral frontal cortex. Two subsequent studies have used event-related designs to examine differences between grammatical and nongrammatical items during classification. Skosnik et al. (2002) found differences between grammatical and ungrammatical items in posterior visual regions, including superior occipital (BA 19) and fusiform gyrus (BA 37). Lieberman et al. (2004) separately manipulated grammaticality and the similarity of bigram and trigram "chunks" between grammatical and ungrammatical items, based on previous behavioral work suggesting that knowledge of grammatical rules and superficial similarity of letter strings exert separate influences on grammar judgment (Chang & Knowlton, 2004; Knowlton & Squire, 1996).

The comparison of grammatical and ungrammatical items with low chunk strength (which are presumably classified on the basis of rules) showed differential activation in the caudate nucleus and occipital cortex, consistent with the notion that the striatum is involved in the acquisition of rulelike regularities. Comparison of items with high versus low chunk strength (i.e., fragment familiarity) showed that the hippocampus is modulated by chunk strength, regardless of grammatical status of the item. These results converge with previous behavioral results to suggest that grammar learning and fragment knowledge rely upon separate neural systems.

The finding of activity in the medial temporal lobe during artificial grammar learning is unexpected, since amnesic patients exhibit normal learning on artificial grammar tasks (Knowlton et al., 1992; Knowlton & Squire, 1994). It appears that the medial temporal lobe may be engaged in the course of grammar learning in normal individuals even though it is not necessary for learning to occur. A similar finding has been observed in the classical conditioning literature, wherein delay eyeblink conditioning (where the conditioned and unconditioned stimuli overlap in time) results in activation of the hippocampus even though the hippocampus is not necessary for this form of learning (Blaxton et al., 1996). These results are consistent with the fact that neuroimaging cannot demonstrate the necessity of a region for any particular cognitive process (cf. Poldrack, 2000), and highlight the importance of converging results across imaging and neuropsychological patient studies (e.g., Shohamy et al., 2004).

Visual Prototype Learning

The learning of visual categories has been examined using tasks where subjects are exposed to exemplars derived (by distortion) from a prototype, and are then asked to classify novel distortions. Using dot patterns as stimuli, Posner and Keele (1968) found that subjects were able to classify new distortions after training with an original set of distortions; furthermore, the prototype was classified with high accuracy even though it had never been presented. Several studies by Reber and colleagues have used fMRI to examine learning on this task. Subjects are first trained with dot patterns in an incidental learning paradigm, followed by scanning while they classify distortion from either the trained prototype or a novel prototype. These studies have found consistently that activity in the occipital cortex (BA 17/18) is decreased for distortions of the trained prototype compared with distortions of the novel prototype (P. J. Reber et al., 2003; P. J. Reber et al., 1998a, 1998b). The location of these decreases was quite consistent across the studies by Reber and colleagues. This effect has been conceptualized as a "category fluency" effect, similar to the priming-related decreases that are often observed with other stimuli (e.g., Wiggs & Martin, 1998). Aizenstein et al. (2000) found a similar decrease for category versus noncategory stimuli in an incidental discriminative learning paradigm in which subjects were exposed to prototype distortions along with random dot patterns, though the region of the decrease was quite superior to the medial occipital region found in the studies by Reber and colleagues.

There is conflicting evidence regarding the neural basis of explicit prototype learning. P. J. Reber et al. (2003) examined whether the category-specific decrease was specific to incidental learning. One group of subjects received incidental learning instructions, whereas a second group was alerted to the presence of a category and told to try to determine how the patterns were categorized. The incidental learning group exhibited decreased activity in the occipital cortex for distortions of the trained compared with the novel category. The intentional learning group showed a very different pattern, with a number of regions exhibiting greater activity for novel distortions of the trained prototype versus distortions of the novel prototype, including right anterior PFC (BA 10), left inferior occipital/temporal cortex (BA 37), posterior cingulate (BA 31), and right dorsolateral PFC (BA 9).

Region-of-interest analyses showed that there was a small but nonsignificant decrease in occipital cortex for distortions of the trained prototype in the intentional learning group, but this effect was significantly greater in the incidental group. There was also a significant difference in activity in anterior hippocampus for the intentional compared with the incidental group, consistent with the notion that these subjects were using declarative memory to perform the task. Aizenstein et al. (2000) examined explicit prototype learning following implicit learning of a different prototype by the same subjects. In contrast with the previously described findings, this study found greater activity in the medial temporal lobe for noncategory versus category distortions; however, this effect was observed in the posterior MTL, whereas the opposite effect in the Reber et al. (2003) study was found in the anterior hippocampus. Given previous suggestions of functional dissociations between anterior and posterior hippocampal regions (e.g., Gabrieli et al., 1997), this may not be surprising, but a full understanding of the neural basis of explicit prototype learning will require additional work.

Whereas most studies of dot pattern learning have used observational learning (i.e., subjects encounter only distortions of a single prototype during training), Seger et al. (2000) examined prototype learning based on feedback, using a checkboard pattern task initially presented by Fried and Holyoak (1984) in which subjects learn to classify patterns into one of two categories. Compared with a baseline task, classification resulted in activation of bilateral inferior PFC (BA 45/47), right dorsolateral PFC (BA 9/46), bilateral inferior parietal (BA 7), bilateral occipital (BA 18), and anterior cingulate (BA 32) cortex. It is of interest that basal ganglia activity was not observed, given the findings of Poldrack et al. (2001); however, this may reflect the limited power of imaging deep structures at 1.5T that is often noted. Learning was associated with increasing activity in the bilateral occipital and left parietal cortex. This suggests that the substrates of learning in this task are likely to differ from those in dot pattern learning, but it is not clear whether this relates to differences in stimuli or differences in the training paradigm.

Perceptual Categorization

A substantial literature has examined how subjects learn classifications based on decision boundaries within a multidimensional stimulus space. Ashby and colleagues (1998) have proposed that learning of classifications based on a verbalizable rule relies upon a verbal system involving the prefrontal cortex, anterior cingulate, and head of the caudate, whereas learning of more complex problems (termed "information integration") relies upon an implicit system involving the tail of the caudate nucleus and dopaminergic midbrain systems. This question was examined by Seger and Cincotta (2002), who compared categorization based on a verbal rule (i.e., whether the height of the stimulus was greater than its width) with information integration classification based on either linear or quadratic decision bounds (which have no easily verbalizable definitions). Subjects were scanned while learning with feedback in a blocked design. Activation of the anterior cingulate and bilateral striatum occurred in all conditions, whereas left occipital cortex (BA 18/19/37) was activated in the decision bound problems but not in the verbal condition.

These results are somewhat inconsistent with the predictions of the COVIS (Competition between Verbal and Implicit Systems) theory (Ashby et al., 1998), which argues that the verbal task should engage the head of the caudate, whereas the implicit task should engage the tail of caudate. However, Ashby and colleagues (1998) argue that the two systems are in competition during learning, which could explain activity throughout the striatum in both tasks. The results are consistent with the notion that the striatum is involved in the processing of feedback during category learning (Poldrack et al., 2001).

Issues

The Neural Basis of Skill Learning: A General Framework

The range of tasks in which skill learning is examined and the range of cognitive and neural processes engaged by these tasks make it extraordinarily difficult to formulate a theory that can explain all of the data reviewed here. However, at an abstract level the data can be accounted for mostly by a relatively old concept that was introduced above in the section on motor skill learning: namely, the idea that skill learning involves changes in the processors that are directly involved in performing the task. An early version of this idea was proposed by Hirst (1974), who argued that hippocampal-independent learning occurred "on the perfomance line," that is, in the processors that are directly engaged in the task. This concept is also central in the procedural/declarative distinction (N. J. Cohen & Squire, 1980; N. J. Cohen, 1984):

This implicitly represented procedural knowledge is tied to and expressible only through activation of the particular processing structures and procedures engaged by the learning tasks; it is acquired and retained by virtue of the plasticity inherent in these processing structures or procedures. (Cohen, 1984, 96)

Motivation for this view also came from the work of Kolers (e.g., 1975, 1978), who performed extensive studies of subjects learning to read geometrically transformed text (e.g., mirror-reading). Kolers argued that learning on this task was tied to changes in the pattern-analyzing procedures involved in reading, without explicit access to this knowledge (see also Kolers & Roediger, 1984). One attractive feature of this procedural view of skill acquisition is that it provides a direct point of contact between neuroimaging work on skills and neurophysiological work examining synaptic plasticity in cortical and subcortical regions (e.g., Buonomano & Merzenich, 1998); this point is developed extensively by N. J. Cohen and Eichenbaum (1993).

With regard to the results reviewed above, there is substantial evidence in favor of a procedural view of skill learning. For motor skill learning, changes have been observed in a set of regions involved in motor control and execution, including SMA, PMC, cerebellum, striatum, and M1. For perceptual skill learning, changes have been consistently observed in the occipitotemporal regions involved in visual perception; the particular locus has varied depending upon the task, with changes for simple visual tasks occurring in posterior occipital cortices and changes for higher-level object recognition tasks occurring in inferior temporal cortices. For classification learning, there is at least some evidence of such a pattern as well, particularly for visual prototype learning, which is associated with changes in early visual cortices.

There are, of course, exceptions to this rule. In particular, changes have often been observed in regions of the prefrontal cortex that are not directly involved in motor control, such as dorsolateral prefrontal cortex and the anterior cingulate. There are at least two possible explanations for the involvement of these regions. First, a primary role of the prefrontal cortex is thought to be in the control and modulation of processes subserved by more posterior cortices (e.g., Miller & Cohen, 2001). To the degree that learning involves a decrease in the need for executive control (i.e., as the behavior becomes more automatic), it is likely that the prefrontal cortex will become less necessary to guide behavior toward the intended goal. In this way, the prefrontal cortex can provide the "scaffolding" (Petersen et al., 1998) for learning to occur. A second possible explanation is that these regions are involved not in executive control but in the monitoring of behavior. For example, the anterior cingulate cortex (ACC) is thought to respond to the presence of response conflict, leading to subsequent exertion of executive control by other regions, including the dorsolateral prefrontal cortex (e.g., Kerns et al., 2004). As learning progresses, performance is likely to result in reduced conflict between the intended response and its competitors, leading to decreased responses in the ACC. Further work is needed to directly test these hypotheses in the context of skill learning.

What Role(s) Do the Basal Ganglia Play in Skill Learning?

The basal ganglia seem to play a central role in many forms of skill learning, consistent with a number of earlier proposals based on neuropsychological data (e.g., Mishkin et al., 1984; Saint-Cyr & Taylor, 1992). Although not particularly surprising for motor skills, given the importance of the basal ganglia for motor control, the role of the basal ganglia in perceptual and cognitive skill learning was rather surprising, and understanding the basal ganglia's role in skill learning is a current issue of great interest. A number of theories posit different roles for the basal ganglia in the acquisition of skills. It is important to keep in mind that the basal ganglia are a complex and heterogeneous set of structures (including the striatum, pallidum, subthalamic nucleus, and substantia nigra), and that different substructures may play very different roles in learning. Furthermore, the basal ganglia do not perform their functions in isolation, but are part of large-scale "loops" from the cortex to the striatum and then back to the cortex via the pallidum and thalamus (Alexander et al., 1986).

Habit Learning

One of the longest-standing claims regarding the striatum is that it is involved in the acquisition of "habits," referring to stimulus-response associations (e.g., Mishkin et al., 1984). Consistent with this claim are lesion results demonstrating that the tail of the caudate nucleus is necessary for the gradual learning of response associations to complex visual stimuli (Fernandez-Ruiz et al., 2001; Teng et al., 2000), and results from brain imaging studies showing caudate activation associated with learning arbitrary visuomotor associations (Toni & Passingham, 1999). It is the tail of the caudate nucleus that is most strongly connected to higher-order visual cortices in primates, suggesting that it may serve to connect visual representations with particular actions. There is also evidence of neural plasticity (long-term potentiation/depression) at corticostriatal synapses, which could serve as the basis for habit learning. This plasticity in the striatum is modulated by dopamine release from the SN/VTA (e.g., Wickens & Kotter, 1995), suggesting that reinforcement may be important for the development of habits. However, an important aspect of habit learning is that, once established, habits do not require reinforcement for their continued expression. This has been demonstrated, for example, by showing that overtrained performance on a win-stay maze task (which is known to rely upon the striatum;

Packard et al., 1989) is not affected by devaluation of the unconditioned stimulus (US) (e.g., through taste aversion), whereas early performance on the same task is affected by US devaluation (Sage & Knowlton, 2000).

Action Sequences

Graybiel and her colleagues (Graybiel, 1998; Jog et al., 1999) have proposed that the basal ganglia are critical for the development and expression of particular sequences of actions (or "action repertoires"). First, striatal lesions result in deficits in the expression of established action sequences. For example, Berridge and Whishaw (1992) found that lesions to the striatum resulted in lasting deficits in the execution of stereotyped grooming sequences in rats, whereas cortical and cerebellar lesions did not. Studies of patients with basal ganglia abnormalities, such as Huntington's and Parkinson's disease also show that they have difficulty with movement sequencing (e.g., Benecke et al., 1987; Serrien et al., 2001). Second, work using multiunit neurophysiology has shown changes in striatal response related to the acquisition of novel motor sequences. Using chronic tetrode recordings in a T-maze task in rats, Jog et al. (1999) found that striatal responses changed with learning. Whereas early in training there was a large population of neurons that responded to the turn at the end of the runway, training was associated with the development of responses at the beginning and end of the maze, consistent with the notion that the striatum was representing the initial execution of the overlearned sequence as well as its conclusion.

Reinforcement Learning

The basal ganglia are thought to play an important role in modulating behavior on the basis of environmental feedback, such as rewards. This has been formalized in the application of reinforcement learning models, such as actor/critic models, to understanding basal ganglia function (e.g., Houk et al., 1995). The actor-critic model comprises an "actor" that is responsible for selecting actions in order to maximize reinforcement, and a "critic" that provides a signal reflecting predictions of reinforcement. In the Houk et al. model, the role of the basal ganglia is to integrate information about reinforcement into the selection of actions, with the striatal matrix performing action selection and striosomal modules (involving striatal patch neurons, subthalamic nucleus, and dopamine cells in the midbrain) providing an error prediction signal. Neuroimaging studies have provided recent evidence in favor of the notion that the basal ganglia (particularly the ventral striatum) codes for prediction errors in a way consistent with actor-critic models (e.g., McClure et al., 2003; O'Doherty et al., 2003). Evidence consistent with the role of reinforcement learning in skill acquisition includes the finding that patients with basal ganglia disorders are impaired at learning probabilistic classifications using feedback, but can learn the same information when it is provided under conditions that do not require the processing of behaviorally contingent feedback (Shohamy et al., 2004). It is less clear whether this idea is relevant to tasks such as the SRTT, where the nature of the reinforcement is not apparent.

Set Switching

The basal ganglia are thought to be involved generally in the process of switching between task sets. For example, patients with PD are impaired at switching dimensions in an analogue to the Wisconsin Card Sorting Task (Owen et al., 1993), and are impaired at switching between task sets and motor sequences (Hayes et al., 1998). The relevance of set switching to skill acquisition arises from proposals that learning may involve a transition between different methods of performing a task (e.g., Logan, 1988). Although there are currently some data to support this idea, the relevant experiments remain to be performed. In particular, the corticostriatal loops involving the caudate nucleus and dorsolateral prefrontal cortex may be particularly important for this function, as may the dopaminergic projections from the midbrain.

Evaluation

Evaluation of these theories suggests that there will not be a grand unified theory of the role of the basal ganglia in skill learning. Rather, it is more likely that different skill learning domains may tap into different aspects of basal ganglia function. For example, motor skill learning may engage the basal ganglia structures involved in the representation of action sequences, whereas classification learning may rely upon the structures responsible for reinforcement learning. To the degree that this divergence is not currently understood, it may reflect a limitation on the anatomical resolution of many imaging studies. Future imaging studies that provide a more reliable anatomical subdivision of the basal ganglia may help address this issue.

The Role of Awareness in Learning

The role of awareness in learning has been a topic of great controversy over the last several decades (cf. Shanks & St. John, 1994). A number of researchers have claimed to find evidence for learning in the absence of awareness, but such claims are routinely challenged on the basis of an incomplete assessment of the contents of awareness. Functional imaging does not obviate the need for assessments of awareness. However, once awareness has been properly assessed, it does allow the examination of differences in brain function based on the results of those assessments.

If, as is often claimed by critics, learning with awareness and learning without awareness are really reflections of the same underlying learning mechanism, then qualitative differences should not be evident in the comparison of subjects who learn with and without awareness. The foregoing review makes clear that learning with awareness and learning without awareness are clearly associated with the engagement of different neural systems. Most impressive are findings that the neural systems involved in the expression of learning differ depending upon how the task was acquired, even though the task at test is exactly the same (e.g., P. J. Reber et al., 2003). These results pose a direct challenge to the psychologists who have argued against separate systems underlying different forms of learning in favor of a single system (e.g., Kinder & Shanks, 2003): Regardless of the theoretical possibility that dissociations could be produced by a single system, these data provide strong evidence that different forms of memory reflect different underlying brain systems.

At the same time, neuroimaging results have pointed to a degree of complexity in the architecture of implicit learning that was not evident from cognitive or neuropsychological studies. For example, implicit learning researchers have claimed that artificial grammar learning occurs without awareness of the underlying rules or features that determine grammaticality (but see Dulany et al., 1984; A. S. Reber, 1993). Consistent with this claim, Knowlton and colleagues (B. J. Knowlton et al., 1992; B. J. Knowlton & Squire, 1994) found that amnesic patients were not impaired at artificial grammar learning, suggesting that explicit memory is not necessary for this form of learning. However, neuroimaging of grammar learning in normal subjects has shown that the hippocampus is active during grammaticality judgments, particularly for items with high chunk strength (Lieberman et al., 2004).

The role of the striatum in grammar learning is also a point of conflict between neuropsychological and imaging results. Patients with Parkinson's disease and patients with Huntington's disease exhibit normal artificial grammar learning (Knowlton et al., 1996b; P. J. Reber & Squire, 1999; Smith et al., 2001; Witt et al., 2002), suggesting that the striatum is not necessary for this task. However, Lieberman et al. (2004) found that the caudate nucleus was active in relation to grammatical knowledge in normal subjects. A more or less parallel set of results may be observed in implicit sequence learning in the SRTT. Researchers have claimed that sequence learning may be implicit (e.g., Willingham et al., 1989), and amnesic patients learn the task normally (e.g., Nissen et al., 1989; P. J. Reber & Squire, 1994, 1998), indicating that explicit memory is unnecessary, although one study argued for a subtle deficit in amnesics' learning of complex sequences (Curran, 1997). Neuroimaging studies of neurologically intact subjects typically do not show learning-related activity in the medial temporal lobe, but a recent study using a region-of-interest analysis and complex sequences did report hippocampal activation (Schendan et al., 2003). These results highlight the importance of converging methods and the limitations of neuropsychological studies: the lack of necessity of a particular neural structure in patients does not imply that normal subjects will not employ the structure in performing a task.

Memory Systems: Independent or Interactive?

The existence of dissociations between memory systems has long been taken to suggest that those systems are independent, meaning that they are based on separate brain systems and operate by separate mechanisms that do not influence each other. However, a substantial amount of evidence suggests that memory systems, although dissociable by lesion methods, may interact with each other during behavior in normal individuals. The initial impetus for this notion came from lesion studies in animals showing that under some conditions, lesions to the hippocampus actually result in better learning on basal ganglia-dependent tasks than in control animals (e.g, Packard et al., 1989), and from pharmacological studies showing that the engagement of either system is related to the balance of activity between hippocampus and basal ganglia (e.g., Packard, 1999). These results have been interpreted to reflect a competition between the medial temporal lobe and basal ganglia memory systems, likely owing to the fact that these systems are optimized for learning different aspects of the environment (Packard, 1999; Poldrack & Rodriguez, 2004).

Functional neuroimaging has subsequently provided evidence for memory system interactions in humans as well (cf. Poldrack & Packard, 2003). This was first suggested on the basis of deactivation of the MTL during classification learning (Poldrack et al., 1999). Analyses of functional connectivity in two studies (Poldrack et al., 2001; Lieberman et al., 2004) have since shown negative correlation (across subjects) between the engagement of the basal ganglia and MTL during learning. Other evidence for interaction comes from imaging studies with patient groups, including Parkinson's disease (Moody et al., 2004) and obsessive-compulsive disorder (Rauch, Savage, et al., 1997). In each of these studies, decreased basal ganglia activity in the patient group during learning was associated with increased activity in the MTL, which allowed the patients to perform at a normal level, albeit using different mechanisms. For anatomical reasons it is unlikely that the basal ganglia and MTL exert a direct negative influence on one another; rather, this interaction may be mediated by the prefrontal cortex at the level of response selection (White & McDonald, 2002), or through the effects of neuromodulatory systems (particularly dopamine). Recent analyses using effective connectivity modeling of classification learning data are consistent with prefrontal mediation of the interaction (Poldrack & Rodriguez, 2004).

It is of course possible that some memory systems do *not* interact, and indeed there is evidence to that effect, even for systems that learn identical tasks. Willingham and Goedert-Eschmann (1999) trained subjects on the SRTT to learn the sequence either implicitly or explicitly. All subjects then performed a version of the task in which they thought the stimuli appeared randomly; in fact, the sequence from the training phase was occasionally slipped in among the random stimuli. The comparison of RTs with the sequenced and random stimuli was a measure of implicit learning. The results showed equivalent implicit knowledge regardless of whether training had been implicit or explicit. The authors interpreted these data as showing parallel development of implicit and explicit knowledge without any interaction between the two systems. A brain-imaging study supported this conjecture, showing learning-related activity in structures putatively supporting implicit learning even during explicit task training in the SRTT (Willingham et al., 2002).

The data from classification learning studies (indicating system interaction), and those from motor sequence learning studies (indicating system independence) need not be viewed as inconsistent, since the task demands in these different domains may determine the nature of the memory system interaction. Implicit and explicit versions of classification tasks have conflicting cognitive demands—explicit versions demand attention to exemplars, whereas implicit versions demand that one ignore exemplars and abstract central tendencies. Motor sequencing does not have this property, since what is learned in the implicit and explicit versions of the task does not conflict. Hence, system interactions or lack thereof may be determined by task demands.

Acknowledgments

The authors would like to thank James Ashe and Barbara Knowlton for comments on a draft of this chapter. This work was supported by the National Science Foundation (BCS-0223843), Whitehall Foundation, and the National Institutes of Health (NS40106–01; MH065598–01A1).

References

Aizenstein, H. J., MacDonald, A. W., Stenger, V. A., Nebes, R. D., Larson, J. K., Ursu, S., et al. (2000). Complementary category learning systems identified using event-related functional MRI. *Journal of Cognitive Neuroscience* 12(6), 977–987.

Alexander, G. E., DeLong, M. R., & Strick, P. L. (1986). Parallel organization of functionally segregated circuits linking basal ganglia and cortex. *Annual Review of Neuroscience* 9, 357–381.

Andersen, R. A., Snyder, L. H., Bradley, D. C., & Xing, J. (1997). Multimodal representation of space in posterior parietal cortex and its use in planning movements. *Annual Review of Neuroscience* 20, 303–330.

Aron, A. R., Shohamy, D., Clark, J., Myers, C., Gluck, M. A., & Poldrack, R. A. (2004). Human midbrain sensitivity to cognitive feedback and uncertainty during classification learning. *Journal of Neurophysiology* 92, 1144–1152.

Ashby, F. G., Alfonso-Reese, L. A., Turken, A. U., & Waldron, E. M. (1998). A neuropsychological theory of multiple systems in category learning. *Psychology Review* 105(3), 442–481.

Benecke, R., Rothwell, J. C., Dick, J. P., Day, B. L., & Marsden, C. D. (1987). Simple and complex movements off and on treatment in patients with Parkinson's disease. *Journal of Neurology, Neurosurgery & Psychiatry* 50(3), 296–303.

Berns, G. S., Song, A. W., & Mao, H. (1999). Continuous functional magnetic resonance imaging reveals dynamic nonlinearities of "dose-response" curves for finger opposition. *Journal of Neuroscience* 19(14), RC17.

Berridge, K. C., & Whishaw, I. Q. (1992). Cortex, striatum and cerebellum: Control of serial order in a grooming sequence. *Experimental Brain Research* 90(2), 275–290.

Bischoff-Grethe, A., Goedert, K. M., Willingham, D. T., & Grafton, S. T. (2004). Neural substrates of response-based sequence learning using fMRI. *Journal of Cognitive Neuroscience* 16(1), 127–138.

Bischoff-Grethe, A., Ivry, R. B., & Grafton, S. T. (2002). Cerebellar involvement in response reassignment rather than attention. *Journal of Neuroscience* 22(2), 546–553.

Blaxton, T. A., Zeffiro, T. A., Gabrieli, J. D. E., Bookheimer, S. Y., Carrillo, M. C., Theodore, W. H., et al. (1996). Functional mapping of human learning: A positron emission tomography activation study of eyeblink conditioning. *Journal of Neuroscience* 16, 4032–4040.

Buonomano, D. V., & Merzenich, M. M. (1998). Cortical plasticity: From synapses to maps. *Annual Review of Neuroscience*, 21, 149–186.

Chang, G. Y., & Knowlton, B. J. (2004). Visual feature learning in artificial grammar classification. *Journal of Experimental Psychology: Learning, Memory, and Cognition* 30(3), 714–722.

Clower, D. M., Hoffman, J. M., Votaw, J. R., Faber, T. L., Woods, R. P., & Alexander, G. E. (1996). Role of posterior parietal cortex in the recalibration of visually guided reaching. *Nature* 383(6601), 618–621.

Cohen, L., & Dehaene, S. (2004). Specialization within the ventral stream: The case for the visual word form area. *NeuroImage* 22(1), 466–476.

Cohen, N. J. (1984). Preserved learning capacity in amnesia: Evidence for multiple memory systems. In L. R. Squire & N. Butters (Eds.), *Neuropsychology of memory* (pp. 83–103). New York: Guilford.

Cohen, N. J., & Eichenbaum, H. (1993). *Memory, Amnesia, and the Hippocampal System.* Cambridge, MA: MIT Press.

Cohen, N. J., Eichenbaum, H., Deacedo, B. S., & Corkin, S. (1985). Different memory systems underlying acquisition of procedural and declarative knowledge. *Annals of the New York Academy of Sciences*, 444, 54–71.

Cohen, N. J., & Squire, L. R. (1980). Preserved learning and retention of pattern-analyzing skill in amnesia: Dissociation of knowing how and knowing that. *Science* 210(4466), 207–210.

Corkin, S. (1968). Acquisition of motor skill after bilateral medial temporal-lobe excision. *Neuropsychologia* 6, 255–265.

Curran, T. (1997). Higher-order associative learning in amnesia: Evidence from the serial reaction time task. *Journal of Cognitive Neuroscience* 9(4), 522–533.

Dagher, A., Owen, A. M., Boecker, H., & Brooks, D. J. (2001). The role of the striatum and hippocampus in planning: A PET activation study in Parkinson's disease. *Brain* 124(5), 1020–1032.

De Weerd, P., Reinke, K., Ryan, L., McIsaac, T., Perschler, P., Schnyer, D., et al. (2003). Cortical mechanisms for acquisition and performance of bimanual motor sequences. *NeuroImage* 19(4), 1405–1416.

Dong, Y., Fukuyama, H., Honda, M., Okada, T., Hanakawa, T., Nakamura, K., et al. (2000). Essential role of the right superior parietal cortex in Japanese kana mirror reading: An fMRI study. *Brain* 123(4), 790–799.

Doyon, J., Owen, A. M., Petrides, M., Sziklas, V., & Evans, A. C. (1996). Functional anatomy of visuomotor skill learning in human subjects examined with positron emission tomography. *European Journal of Neuroscience* 8(4), 637–648.

Doyon, J., Song, A. W., Karni, A., Lalonde, F., Adams, M. M., & Ungerleider, L. G. (2002). Experience-dependent changes in cerebellar contributions to motor sequence learning. *Proceedings of the National Academy of Sciences USA* 99(2), 1017–1022.

Dulany, D. E., Carlson, R. A., & Dewey, G. I. (1984). A case of syntactical learning and judgment—how conscious and how abstract? *Journal of Experimental Psychology: General* 113(4), 541–555.

Eliassen, J. C., Souza, T., & Sanes, J. N. (2001). Human brain activation accompanying explicitly directed movement sequence learning. *Experimental Brain Research* 141(3), 269–280.

Fernandez-Ruiz, J., Wang, J., Aigner, T. G., & Mishkin, M. (2001). Visual habit formation in monkeys with neurotoxic lesions of the ventrocaudal neostriatum. *Proceedings of the National Academy of Sciences USA* 98(7), 4196–4201.

Fiez, J. A., Petersen, S. E., Cheney, M. K., & Raichle, M. E. (1992). Impaired non-motor learning and error detection associated with cerebellar damage. A single case study. *Brain* 115, 155–178.

Fitts, P. M., & Posner, M. I. (1967). *Human Performance.* Belmont, CA: Brooks-Cole.

Flament, D., Ellerman, J. M., Kim, S. G., Ugurbil, K., & Ebner, T. J. (1996). Functional magnetic resonance imaging of cerebellar activation during the learning of a visuomotor dissociation task. *Human Brain Mapping* 4, 210–226.

Fletcher, P., Buchel, C., Josephs, O., Friston, K., & Dolan, R. (1999). Learning-related neuronal responses in prefrontal cortex studied with functional neuroimaging. *Cerebral Cortex* 9(2), 168–178.

Fried, L. S., & Holyoak, K. J. (1984). Induction of category distributions: A framework for classification learning. *Journal of Experimental Psychology: Learning, Memory, and Cognition* 10(2), 234–257.

Frith, C. D., Friston, K., Liddle, P. F., & Frackowiak, R. S. (1991). Willed action and the prefrontal cortex in man: A study with PET. *Proceedings of the Royal Society of London* B244(1311), 241–246.

Gabrieli, J. D. E. (1998). Cognitive neuroscience of human memory. *Annual Review of Psychology* 49, 87–115.

Gabrieli, J. D. E., Brewer, J. B., Desmond, J. E., & Glover, G. H. (1997). Separate neural bases of two fundamental memory processes in the human medial temporal lobe. *Science* 276(5310), 264–266.

Gauthier, I., Skudlarski, P., Gore, J. C., & Anderson, A. W. (2000). Expertise for cars and birds recruits brain areas involved in face recognition. *Nature Neuroscience* 3(2), 191–197.

Gauthier, I., Tarr, M. J., Anderson, A. W., Skudlarski, P., & Gore, J. C. (1999). Activation of the middle fusiform "face area" increases with expertise in recognizing novel objects. *Nature Neuroscience* 2(6), 568–573.

Goebel, R., Linden, D. E., Lanfermann, H., Zanella, F. E., & Singer, W. (1998). Functional imaging of mirror and inverse reading reveals separate coactivated networks for oculomotion and spatial transformations. *NeuroReport* 9(4), 713–719.

Gomez-Beldarrain, M., Garcia-Monco, J. C., Rubio, B., & Pascual-Leone, A. (1998). Effect of focal cerebellar lesions on procedural learning in the serial reaction time task. *Experimental Brain Research* 120(1), 25–30.

Grafton, S. T., Hazeltine, E., & Ivry, R. (1995). Functional mapping of sequencing learning in normal humans. *Journal of Cognitive Neuroscience* 7(4), 497–510.

Grafton, S. T., Hazeltine, E., & Ivry, R. B. (1998). Abstract and effector-specific representations of motor sequences identified with PET. *Journal of Neuroscience* 18(22), 9420–9428.

Grafton, S. T., Hazeltine, E., & Ivry, R. B. (2002). Motor sequence learning with the nondominant left hand. A PET functional imaging study. *Experimental Brain Research* 146(3), 369–378.

Grafton, S. T., Mazziotta, J. C., Presty, S., Friston, K. J., Frackowiak, R. S., & Phelps, M. E. (1992). Functional anatomy of human procedural learning determined with regional cerebral blood flow and PET. *Journal of Neuroscience* 12(7), 2542–2548.

Grafton, S. T., Salidis, J., & Willingham, D. B. (2001). Motor learning of compatible and incompatible visuomotor maps. *Journal of Cognitive Neuroscience* 13(2), 217–231.

Grafton, S. T., Woods, R. P., & Tyszka, M. (1994). Functional imaging of procedural motor learning: Relating cerebral blood flow with individual subject performance. *Human Brain Mapping* 1, 221–234.

Graybiel, A. M. (1998). The basal ganglia and chunking of action repertoires. *Neurobiology of Learning and Memory* 70(1–2), 119–136.

Grill-Spector, K., Knouf, N., & Kanwisher, N. (2004). The fusiform face area subserves face perception, not generic within-category identification. *Nature Neuroscience* 7(5), 555–562.

Hayes, A. E., Davidson, M. C., Keele, S. W., & Rafal, R. D. (1998). Toward a functional analysis of the basal ganglia. *Journal of Cognitive Neuroscience* 10(2), 178–198.

Hazeltine, E., Grafton, S. T., & Ivry, R. (1997). Attention and stimulus characteristics determine the locus of motor-sequence encoding. A PET study. *Brain* 120(1), 123–140.

Heindel, W. C., Salmon, D. P., Shults, C. W., Wallicke, P. A., & Butters, N. (1989). Neuropsychological evidence for multiple implicit memory systems: A comparison of Alzheimer's, Huntington's and Parkinson's disease patients. *Journal of Neuroscience* 9, 582–587.

Hirst, R. (1974). The hippocampus and contextual retrieval from memory: A theory. *Behavioral Biology* 12, 421–444.

Horton, K. D. (1989). The processing of spatially transformed text. *Memory and Cognition* 17(3), 283–291.

Houk, J. C., Adams, J. L., & Barto, A. G. (1995). A model of how the basal ganglia generate and use neural signals that predict reinforcement. In J. C. Houk, J. L. Davis, & D. G. Beiser (Eds.), *Models of Information Processing in the Basal Ganglia*, 249–270. Cambridge, MA: MIT Press.

Huettel, S. A., Mack, P. B., & McCarthy, G. (2002). Perceiving patterns in random series: Dynamic processing of sequence in prefrontal cortex. *Nature Neuroscience* 5, 485–490.

Imamizu, H., Miyauchi, S., Tamada, T., Sasaki, Y., Takino, R., Putz, B., et al. (2000). Human cerebellar activity reflecting an acquired internal model of a new tool. *Nature* 403(6766), 192–195. (See comment.)

Jackson, G. M., Jackson, S. R., Harrison, J., Henderson, L., & Kennard, C. (1995). Serial reaction time learning and Parkinson's disease: Evidence for a procedural learning deficit. *Neuropsychologia* 33(5), 577–593.

Jenkins, I. H., Brooks, D. J., Nixon, P. D., Frackowiak, R. S., & Passingham, R. E. (1994). Motor sequence learning: A study with positron emission tomography. *Journal of Neuroscience* 14(6), 3775–3790.

Jog, M. S., Kubota, Y., Connolly, C. I., Hillegaart, V., & Graybiel, A. M. (1999). Building neural representations of habits. *Science* 286(5445), 1745–1749.

Jueptner, M., Frith, C. D., Brooks, D. J., Frackowiak, R. S., & Passingham, R. E. (1997). Anatomy of motor learning. II. Subcortical structures and learning by trial and error. *Journal of Neurophysiology* 77(3), 1325–1337.

Jueptner, M., Stephan, K. M., Frith, C. D., Brooks, D. J., Frackowiak, R. S., & Passingham, R. E. (1997). Anatomy of motor learning. I. Frontal cortex and attention to action. *Journal of Neurophysiology* 77(3), 1313–1324.

Kanwisher, N. (2000). Domain specificity in face perception. *Nature Neuroscience* 3(8), 759–763.

Kanwisher, N., McDermott, J., & Chun, M. M. (1997). The fusiform face area: A module in human extrastriate cortex specialized for face perception. *Journal of Neuroscience* 17(11), 4302–4311.

Karni, A., Meyer, G., Jezzard, P., Adams, M. M., Turner, R., & Ungerleider, L. G. (1995). Functional MRI evidence for adult motor cortex plasticity during motor skill learning. *Nature* 377(6545), 155–158.

Kassubek, J., Schmidtke, K., Kimmig, H., Lucking, C. H., & Greenlee, M. W. (2001). Changes in cortical activation during mirror reading before and after training: An fMRI study of procedural learning. *Cognitive Brain Research* 10(3), 207–217.

Kerns, J. G., Cohen, J. D., MacDonald, A. W. III, Cho, R. Y., Stenger, V. A., & Carter, C. S. (2004). Anterior cingulate conflict monitoring and adjustments in control. *Science* 303(5660), 1023–1026.

Kinder, A., & Shanks, D. R. (2003). Neuropsychological dissociations between priming and recognition: A single-system connectionist account. *Psychology Review* 110(4), 728–744.

Knowlton, B. J., Squire, L. R., & Gluck, M. A. (1994). Probabilistic classification in amnesia. *Learning and Memory* 1, 106–120.

Knowlton, B. J., Mangels, J. A., & Squire, L. R. (1996a). A neostriatal habit learning system in humans. *Science* 273, 1399–1402.

Knowlton, B. J., Ramus, S. J., & Squire, L. R. (1992). Intact artificial grammar learning in amnesia: Dissociation of classification learning and explicit memory for specific instances. *Psychological Science* 3(3), 172–179.

Knowlton, B. J., & Squire, L. R. (1994). The information acquired during artificial grammar learning. *Journal of Experimental Psychology: Learning Memory and Cognition* 20, 79–91.

Knowlton, B. J., & Squire, L. R. (1996). Artificial grammar learning depends on implicit acquisition of both abstract and exemplar-specific information. *Journal of Experimental Psychology: Learning, Memory, and Cognition* 22(1), 169–181.

Knowlton, B. J., Squire, L. R., Paulsen, J. S., Swerdlow, N. R., Swenson, M., & Butters, N. (1996b). Dissociations within nondeclarative memory in Huntington's disease. *Neuropsychology* 10, 538–548.

Kolers, P. A. (1975). Specificity of operations in sentence recognition. *Cognitive Psychology* 7(3), 289–306.

Kolers, P. A., & Magee, L. E. (1978). Specificity of pattern-analyzing skills in reading. *Canadian Journal of Psychology* 32(1), 43–51.

Kolers, P. A., & Roediger, H. L. (1984). Procedures of mind. *Journal of Verbal Learning and Verbal Behavior* 23(4), 425–449.

Lauritzen, M. (2001). Relationship of spikes, synaptic activity, and local changes of cerebral blood flow. *Journal of Cerebral Blood Flow and Metabolism* 21(12), 1367–1383.

Lawrence, A. D. (2000). Error correction and the basal ganglia: Similar computations for action, cognition and emotion? *Trends in Cognitive Sciences* 4(10), 365–367.

Lee, D., & Quessy, S. (2003). Activity in supplementary motor area related to learning and performance during a sequential visuomotor task. *Journal of Neurophysiology* 89(2), 1039–1056.

Lieberman, M. D., Chang, G. Y., Chiao, J., Bookheimer, S. Y., & Knowlton, B. J. (2004). An event-related fMRI study of artificial grammar learning in a balanced chunk strength design. *Journal of Cognitive Neuroscience* 16(3), 427–438.

Logan, G. D. (1988). Toward an instance theory of automatization. *Psychological Review* 95(4), 492–527.

Martone, M., Butters, N., Payne, M., Becker, J. T., & Sax, D. (1984). Dissociations between skill learning and verbal recognition in amnesia and dementia. *Archives of Neurology* 41(9), 965–970.

Masson, M. E. (1986). Identification of typographically transformed words: Instance-based skill acquisition. *Journal of Experimental Psychology: Learning, Memory, and Cognition* 12(4), 479–488.

McClure, S. M., Berns, G. S., & Montague, P. R. (2003). Temporal prediction errors in a passive learning task activate human striatum. *Neuron* 38(2), 339–346.

Miller, E. K., & Cohen, J. D. (2001). An integrative theory of prefrontal cortex function. *Annual Review of Neuroscience* 24, 167–202.

Milner, B., Corkin, S., & Teuber, H. L. (1968). Further analysis of the hippocampal amnesia syndrome. *Neuropsychologia* 6, 215–234.

Mishkin, M., Malamut, B., & Bachevalier, J. (1984). Memory and habits: Some implications for the analysis of learning and retention. In L. R. Squire & N. Butters (Eds.), *Neuropsychology of Memory,* 287–296. New York: Guilford.

Molinari, M., Leggio, M. G., Solida, A., Ciorra, R., Misciagna, S., Silveri, M. C., et al. (1997). Cerebellum and procedural learning: Evidence from focal cerebellar lesions. *Brain* 120(10), 1753–1762.

Moody, T. D., Bookheimer, S. Y., Vanek, Z., & Knowlton, B. J. (2004). An implicit learning task activates medial temporal lobe in patients with Parkinson's disease. *Behavioral Neuroscience* 118(2), 438–442.

Muller, R. A., Kleinhans, N., Pierce, K., Kemmotsu, N., & Courchesne, E. (2002). Functional MRI of motor sequence acquisition: Effects of learning stage and performance. *Cognitive Brain Research* 14(2), 277–293.

Nissen, M. J., & Bullemer, P. (1987). Attentional requirements of learning: Evidence from performance measures. *Cognitive Psychology* 19(1), 1–32.

Nissen, M. J., Willingham, D., & Hartman, M. (1989). Explicit and implicit remembering: When is learning preserved in amnesia? *Neuropsychologia* 27(3), 341–352.

O'Doherty, J. P., Dayan, P., Friston, K., Critchley, H., & Dolan, R. J. (2003). Temporal difference models and reward-related learning in the human brain. *Neuron* 38(2), 329–337.

Owen, A. M., Roberts, A. C., Hodges, J. R., Summers, B. A., Polkey, C. E., & Robbins, T. W. (1993). Contrasting mechanisms of impaired attentional set-shifting in patients with frontal lobe damage or Parkinson's disease. *Brain* 116(5), 1159–1175.

Packard, M. G. (1999). Glutamate infused posttraining into the hippocampus or caudate-putamen differentially strengthens place and response learning. *Proceedings of the National Academy of Sciences USA* 96(22), 12881–12886.

Packard, M. G., Hirsh, R., & White, N. M. (1989). Differential effects of fornix and caudate nucleus lesions on two radial maze tasks: Evidence for multiple memory systems. *Journal of Neuroscience* 9(5), 1465–1472.

Packard, M. G., & Knowlton, B. J. (2002). Learning and memory functions of the basal ganglia. *Annual Review of Neuroscience* 25, 563–593.

Peigneux, P., Maquet, P., Meulemans, T., Destrebecqz, A., Laureys, S., Degueldre, C., et al. (2000). Striatum forever, despite sequence learning variability: A random effect analysis of PET data. *Human Brain Mapping* 10(4), 179–194.

Penhune, V. B., & Doyon, J. (2002). Dynamic cortical and subcortical networks in learning and delayed recall of timed motor sequences. *Journal of Neuroscience* 22(4), 1397–1406.

Petersen, S. E., van Mier, H., Fiez, J. A., & Raichle, M. E. (1998). The effects of practice on the functional anatomy of task performance. *Proceedings of the National Academy of Sciences USA* 95(3), 853–860.

Pochon, J. B., Levy, R., Poline, J. B., Crozier, S., Lehericy, S., Pillon, B., et al. (2001). The role of dorsolateral prefrontal cortex in the preparation of forthcoming actions: An fMRI study. *Cerebral Cortex* 11(3), 260–266.

Poldrack, R. A. (2000). Imaging brain plasticity: Conceptual and methodological issues—a theoretical review. *NeuroImage* 12(1), 1–13.

Poldrack, R. A., Clark, J., Paré-Blagoev, J., Shohamy, D., Creso Moyano, J., Myers, C., et al. (2001). Interactive memory systems in the human brain. *Nature* 414, 546–550.

Poldrack, R. A., Desmond, J. E., Glover, G. H., & Gabrieli, J. D. E. (1998). The neural basis of visual skill learning: An fMRI study of mirror-reading. *Cerebral Cortex* 8, 1–10.

Poldrack, R. A., & Gabrieli, J. D. (2001). Characterizing the neural mechanisms of skill learning and repetition priming: Evidence from mirror reading. *Brain* 124(1), 67–82.

Poldrack, R. A., & Packard, M. G. (2003). Competition among multiple memory systems: Converging evidence from animal and human brain studies. *Neuropsychologia* 41(3), 245–251.

Poldrack, R. A., Prabakharan, V., Seger, C., & Gabrieli, J. D. E. (1999). Striatal activation during cognitive skill learning. *Neuropsychology* 13, 564–574.

Poldrack, R. A., & Rodriguez, P. (2004). How do memory systems interact? Evidence from human classification learning. *Neurobiology of Learning and Memory* 82(3), 324–332.

Posner, M. I., and Keele, S. W. (1968). On the genesis of abstract ideas. *Journal of Experimental Psychology* 77, 353–363.

Puce, A., Allison, T., Gore, J. C., & McCarthy, G. (1995). Face-sensitive regions in human extrastriate cortex studied by functional MRI. *Journal of Neurophysiology* 74(3), 1192–1199.

Rauch, S. L., Savage, C. R., Alpert, N. M., Dougherty, D., Kendrick, A., Curran, T., et al. (1997). Probing striatal function in obsessive-compulsive disorder: A PET study of implicit sequence learning. *Journal of Neuropsychiatry and Clinical Neuroscience* 9(4), 568–573.

Rauch, S. L., Savage, C. R., Cary, R., Brown, H. D., Curran, T., Alpert, N. M., et al. (1995). A PET investigation of implicit and explicit sequence learning. *Human Brain Mapping* 3(4), 271–286.

Rauch, S. L., Whalen, P. J., Savage, C. R., Curran, T., Kendrick, A., Brown, H. D., et al. (1997). Striatal recruitment during an implicit sequence learning task as measured by functional magnetic resonance imaging. *Human Brain Mapping* 5(2), 124–132.

Reber, A. S. (1993). *Implicit Learning and Tacit Knowledge*. New York: Oxford University Press.

Reber, P. J., Gitelman, D. R., Parrish, T. B., & Mesulam, M. M. (2003). Dissociating explicit and implicit category knowledge with fMRI. *Journal of Cognitive Neuroscience* 15(4), 574–583.

Reber, P. J., & Squire, L. R. (1994). Parallel brain systems for learning with and without awareness. *Learning & Memory* 1(4), 217–229.

Reber, P. J., & Squire, L. R. (1998). Encapsulation of implicit and explicit memory in sequence learning. *Journal of Cognitive Neuroscience* 10(2), 248–263.

Reber, P. J., & Squire, L. R. (1999). Intact learning of artificial grammars and intact category learning by patients with Parkinson's disease. *Behavioral Neuroscience* 113(2), 235–242.

Reber, P. J., Stark, C. E., & Squire, L. R. (1998a). Contrasting cortical activity associated with category memory and recognition memory. *Learning & Memory* 5(6), 420–428.

Reber, P. J., Stark, C. E., & Squire, L. R. (1998b). Cortical areas supporting category learning identified using functional MRI. *Proceedings of the National Academy of Sciences USA* 95(2), 747–750.

Rhodes, G., Byatt, G., Michie, P. T., & Puce, A. (2004). Is the fusiform face area specialized for faces, individuation, or expert individuation? *Journal of Cognitive Neuroscience* 16(2), 189–203.

Sage, J. R., & Knowlton, B. J. (2000). Effects of US devaluation on win-stay and win-shift radial maze performance in rats. *Behavioral Neuroscience* 114(2), 295–306.

Saint-Cyr, J. A., & Taylor, A. E. (1992). The mobilization of procedural learning: The "key signature" of the basal ganglia. In L. R. Squire & N. Butters (Eds.), *Neuropsychology of Memory*, 2nd ed., 188–202. New York: Guilford.

Sakai, K., Hikosaka, O., Miyauchi, S., Takino, R., Sasaki, Y., & Putz, B. (1998). Transition of brain activation from frontal to parietal areas in visuomotor sequence learning. *Journal of Neuroscience* 18(5), 1827–1840.

Sanes, J. N., Dimitrov, B., & Hallett, M. (1990). Motor learning in patients with cerebellar dysfunction. *Brain* 113, 103–120.

Schendan, H. E., Searl, M. M., Melrose, R. J., & Stern, C. E. (2003). An fMRI study of the role of the medial temporal lobe in implicit and explicit sequence learning. *Neuron* 37, 1013–1025.

Schiltz, C., Bodart, J. M., Dubois, S., Dejardin, S., Michel, C., Roucoux, A., et al. (1999). Neuronal mechanisms of perceptual learning: Changes in human brain activity with training in orientation discrimination. *NeuroImage* 9(1), 46–62.

Schiltz, C., Bodart, J. M., Michel, C., & Crommelinck, M. (2001). A PET study of human skill learning: Changes in brain activity related to learning an orientation discrimination task. *Cortex* 37(2), 243–265.

Schoups, A., Vogels, R., Qian, N., & Orban, G. (2001). Practising orientation identification improves orientation coding in V1 neurons. *Nature* 412(6846), 549–553.

Schultz, W., Tremblay, L., & Hollerman, J. R. (2000). Reward processing in primate orbitofrontal cortex and basal ganglia. *Cerebral Cortex* 10(3), 272–284.

Seger, C. A., & Cincotta, C. M. (2002). Striatal activity in concept learning. *Cognitive, Affective, and Behavioral Neuroscience* 2(2), 149–161.

Seger, C. A., Poldrack, R. A., Prabhakaran, V., Zhao, M., Glover, G. H., & Gabrieli, J. D. (2000). Hemispheric asymmetries and individual differences in visual concept learning as measured by functional MRI. *Neuropsychologia* 38(9), 1316–1324.

Seidler, R. D., Purushotham, A., Kim, S. G., Ugurbil, K., Willingham, D., & Ashe, J. (2002). Cerebellum activation associated with performance change but not motor learning. *Science* 296(5575), 2043–2046.

Seitz, R. J., Stephan, K. M., & Binkofski, F. (2000). Control of action as mediated by the human frontal lobe. *Experimental Brain Research* 133(1), 71–80.

Serrien, D. J., Burgunder, J. M., & Wiesendanger, M. (2001). Grip force scaling and sequencing of events during a manipulative task in Huntington's disease. *Neuropsychologia* 39(7), 734–741.

Shadmehr, R., & Holcomb, H. H. (1997). Neural correlates of motor memory consolidation. *Science* 277(5327), 821–825.

Shadmehr, R., & Holcomb, H. H. (1999). Inhibitory control of competing motor memories. *Experimental Brain Research* 126(2), 235–251.

Shanks, D. R., & St. John, M. F. (1994). Characteristics of dissociable human learning systems. *Behavioral and Brain Sciences* 17, 367–447.

Shohamy, D., Myers, C. E., Grossman, S., Sage, J., Gluck, M. A., & Poldrack, R. A. (2004). Cortico-striatal contributions to feedback-based learning: Converging data from neuroimaging and neuropsychology. *Brain* 127(4), 851–859.

Skosnik, P. D., Mirza, F., Gitelman, D. R., Parrish, T. B., Mesulam, M. M., & Reber, P. J. (2002). Neural correlates of artificial grammar learning. *NeuroImage* 17(3), 1306–1314.

Smith, J., Siegert, R. J., McDowall, J., & Abernethy, D. (2001). Preserved implicit learning on both the serial reaction time task and artificial grammar in patients with Parkinson's disease. *Brain and Cognition* 45(3), 378–391.

Squire, L. R. (1992). Memory and the hippocampus: A synthesis from findings with rats, monkeys, and humans. *Psychological Review* 99(2), 195–231.

Tanji, J. (2001). Sequential organization of multiple movements: Involvement of cortical motor areas. *Annual Review of Neuroscience* 24, 631–651.

Teng, E., Stefanacci, L., Squire, L. R., & Zola, S. M. (2000). Contrasting effects on discrimination learning after hippocampal lesions and conjoint hippocampal-caudate lesions in monkeys. *Journal of Neuroscience* 20(10), 3853–3863.

Toni, I., Krams, M., Turner, R., & Passingham, R. E. (1998). The time course of changes during motor sequence learning: A whole-brain fMRI study. *NeuroImage* 8(1), 50–61.

Toni, I., & Passingham, R. E. (1999). Prefrontal-basal ganglia pathways are involved in the learning of arbitrary visuomotor associations: A PET study. *Experimental Brain Research* 127(1), 19–32.

Toni, I., Ramnani, N., Josephs, O., Ashburner, J., & Passingham, R. E. (2001). Learning arbitrary visuomotor associations: Temporal dynamic of brain activity. *NeuroImage* 14(5), 1048–1057.

Wager, T. D., & Smith, E. E. (2003). Neuroimaging studies of working memory: A meta-analysis. *Cognitive, Affective & Behavioral Neuroscience* 3(4), 255–274.

Wang, J. J., Kim, J. H., & Ebner, T. J. (1987). Climbing afferent modulation during a visually guided, multi-joint arm movement in the monkey. *Brain Research* 410(2), 323–329.

Weiner, M. J., Hallett, M., & Funkenstein, H. H. (1974). Adaptation to lateral displacement of vision in patients with lesions of the central nervous system. *Neurology* 33(6), 766–772.

White, N. M., & McDonald, R. J. (2002). Multiple parallel memory systems in the brain of the rat. *Neurobiology of Learning and Memory* 77(2), 125–184.

Wickens, J. R., & Kotter, R. (1995). Cellular models of reinforcement. In J. C. Houk, J. L. Davis & D. G. Beiser (Eds.), *Models of Information Processing in the Basal Ganglia*, 187–214. Cambridge, MA: MIT Press.

Wiggs, C. L., & Martin, A. (1998). Properties and mechanisms of perceptual priming. *Current Opinion in Neurobiology* 8(2), 227–233.

Willingham, D. B. (1992). Systems of motor skill. In L. R. Squire & N. Butters (Eds.), *Neuropsychology of Memory*, 2nd ed., 166–178. New York: Guilford.

Willingham, D. B., & Goedert-Eschmann, K. (1999). The relation between implicit and explicit learning: Evidence for parallel development. *Psychological Science* 10, 531–534.

Willingham, D. B., & Koroshetz, W. J. (1993). Evidence for neurally dissociable motor skill systems in Huntington's disease patients. *Psychobiology* 21, 173–182.

Willingham, D. B., Nissen, M. J., & Bullemer, P. (1989). On the development of procedural knowledge. *Journal of Experimental Psychology: Learning, Memory, & Cognition* 15(6), 1047–1060.

Willingham, D. B., Salidis, J., & Gabrieli, J. D. (2002). Direct comparison of neural systems mediating conscious and unconscious skill learning. *Journal of Neurophysiology* 88(3), 1451–1460.

Wise, S. P., & Murray, E. A. (2000). Arbitrary associations between antecedents and actions. *Trends in Neuroscience* 23(6), 271–276.

Witt, K., Nuhsman, A., & Deuschl, G. (2002). Intact artificial grammar learning in patients with cerebellar degeneration and advanced Parkinson's disease. *Neuropsychologia* 40(9), 1534–1540.

6 Functional Neuroimaging of Semantic Memory

Sharon L. Thompson-Schill, Irene P. Kan, and Robyn T. Oliver

> *Five senses; an incurably abstract intellect; a haphazardly selective memory; a set of preconceptions and assumptions so numerous that I can never examine more than a minority of them—never become even conscious of them all. How much of total reality can such an apparatus let through?*
> —C. S. Lewis

> *Nothing, at first view, may seem more unbounded than the thought of man.*
> —David Hume

Centuries of philosophers, psychologists, and, most recently, neuroscientists have become fascinated with questions of what we know and how we know it, and their attempts to find answers have taken many forms. This chapter approaches these questions using the new tools, and hopefully new insights, of the first generations of cognitive neuroscientists, who have searched for knowledge about knowledge in images of the brain.

Introduction

Linguists use the term "semantics" to refer to the meaning of a word or phrase. Thus, Endel Tulving borrowed the word "semantic" to refer to a memory system for "words and other verbal symbols, their meaning and referents, about relations among them, and about rules, formulas, and algorithms" for manipulating them (Tulving, 1972, 386). Today, most psychologists conceive of a broader meaning than "meaning" when they use the term "semantic memory." In the previous edition of this *Handbook*, Alex Martin defined semantic memory as "a broad domain of cognition composed of knowledge acquired about the world, including facts, concepts, and beliefs" (2001, 153). Following in this tradition, we use the term "semantic memory" to refer to *world* knowledge, not just *word* knowledge.

The study of world knowledge has its origins in philosophy, although the terminology has changed across the years: Where Locke wrote of "ideas," psychologists today would substitute the word "concepts" to refer to "those expressed by the words 'whiteness, hardness, sweetness, thinking, motion, man, elephant, army, drunkenness,' and others." And while the British empiricists asked about "human understanding," cognitive neuroscientists today speak of "semantic memory" to refer to our shared knowledge of the world. Despite the new vocabulary, many of the central themes remain. Consider the question of the relation between knowledge and experience: Locke argued "Whence comes [the mind] by that vast store, which the busy and boundless fancy of man has painted on it with an almost endless variety? . . . To this I answer, in one word, From experience." Three centuries later, the British psychologist Alan Allport, continuing in the tradition of his empiricist compatriots, argued that the sensorimotor systems used to experience the world are also used to represent meaning: "The essential idea is that the *same* neural elements that are involved in coding the sensory attributes of a (possibly unknown) object presented to eye or hand or ear also make up the elements of the auto-associated activity-patterns that represent familiar object-concepts in 'semantic memory'" (1985, 53). Allport's theory, which is reminiscent of a description of concepts offered by Freud in his 1891 monograph on aphasia, was derived from a consideration of patterns of impairments to semantic memory following brain damage. In this chapter, we examine evidence from neuroimaging studies for an isomorphism between the architecture of semantic memory and the architecture of our sensorimotor systems. These neuroimaging studies provide new insights about the relation between knowledge and experience, using methods that Locke may never have imagined possible.

We have organized the review into three main divisions that reflect parallel (but interacting) lines of inquiry into the neural bases of semantic memory.

Semantic Memory—Episodic Memory Distinction

Is semantic memory a distinct memory system from episodic memory? If so, what neural systems are involved in learning and retrieval of semantic memory? The putative division between knowledge of the world and memories of personal events emerged in philosophical writings of Broad and Furlong in the first half of the twentieth century, although it was not introduced into the language of cognitive psychology until 1972 (Tulving, 1972). Today, the extent to which the distinction between semantic memory and episodic memory is realized in neural systems is the subject of ongoing debate. Much of the evidence brought to bear on this question has come from studies of selective impairments of either semantic memory or episodic memory. In this section, we highlight some of the complementary neuroimaging findings that have addressed this distinction.

Organization of Semantic Memory

What psychological distinctions are realized in the neural systems that support semantic memory? Does the neural architecture of semantic memory obey categorical subdivisions among concepts? Is conceptual knowledge distributed among distinct sensorimotor systems? How is abstract knowledge represented? Distributed theories of semantic memory, such as those of Freud and Allport described above, emphasize the relation between concepts and their sensorimotor features. In contrast, many psychological investigations of concepts have focused on the hierarchical relations among them (see Margolis & Laurence, 1999). Discussion of the neural instantiation of these relations has been fueled by reports of selective degradation of branches of this putative hierarchy (e.g., animals). We begin by reviewing historical and recent evidence that bears on the question of how taxonomic category relations may be represented. Then, following a more in-depth discussion of sensorimotor theories, we reconsider the interpretation of some of these startlingly specific impairments, drawing on new insights from neuroimaging studies of the sensorimotor organization of semantic memory. We end with a brief discussion of the representation of abstract semantic knowledge—brief, because investigations of the representations of physical attributes and categorical relationships have, by and large, excluded consideration of abstract concepts and features. In particular, we discuss the proposal that distributed sources of information are united in a neural "convergence zone" that represents abstract relations.

Semantic Memory Retrieval

During retrieval of semantic memory, do different input modalities have preferential access to certain representations? How do executive control mechanisms guide the retrieval process? Our review of sensorimotor theories of object knowledge naturally relates to debates about the representation of visual knowledge—Is it propositional, is it imagistic, or are there multiple representations? We present evidence that the input modality affects the way in which knowledge is retrieved (rather than the format in which it is stored). Finally, once semantic memory has been taken apart, we are left with the problem of how to put Humpty together again. One consequence of distributed concept representations is the likely occurrence of representational conflict when partial, incompatible representations are activated. At the end of this section, we argue for the important role that prefrontal cortex (PFC) plays in guiding the selection of representations when there are conflicting sources of information.

Throughout this tour of neuroimaging studies of semantic memory, we occasionally make reference to contributions from other methodologies; however, in keeping with the goals of this volume, our focus will remain on the recent advances that have been made in our understanding of semantic memory by examining regional hemodynamic changes in normal volunteers who are busy thinking about the world.

Functional Neuroimaging of Semantic Memory

Semantic Memory—Episodic Memory Distinction

Tulving's proposal for a distinction between episodic and semantic memory went beyond the mere difference in the *content* of the memories (i.e., about a personal episode vs. about the world). He argued for two functionally distinct memory systems on the basis of a dozen sources of evidence, ranging from "armchair speculation" to stochastic independence (1984). Since Tulving's treatise on the organization of memory, the cognitive psychology and cognitive neuroscience communities have continued to debate the relation between semantic and episodic memory and the extent to which this distinction should be viewed as anything more than a useful heuristic (e.g., Graham et al., 2000).

Studies of patients with medial temporal lobe amnesia, which were so instrumental in separating episodic and procedural memory, generally have reported impairments in both episodic and semantic memory (Gabrieli et al., 1988; Stefanacci et al., 2000). However, the study of children with early hippocampal damage (i.e., "developmental amnesia") has revealed grossly impaired episodic memory but seemingly normal semantic memory (Vargha-Khadem et al., 2001). These data argue against hypotheses that semantic memory is an abstraction of accumulated episodic memories. On the flip side, numerous patients have been described who show a progressive and profound deterioration in the knowledge of facts, object concepts, and vocabulary, despite otherwise normal language, memory, and perception (Hodges et al., 1994). Patients with *semantic dementia*, as this syndrome is commonly called, typically have a temporal variant of frontotemporal dementia, with extensive but asymmetric (left more than right) polar and inferolateral temporal atrophy (Galton et al., 2001).

The description of these neuropsychological impairments, now coupled with increasingly sophisticated methods for quantitatively describing the location and extent of lesions, has increased attention to the relation between semantic and episodic memory systems (e.g., Graham et al., 2000). Neuroimaging studies provide a complementary source of evidence for the divide between medial and lateral temporal cortical contributions to these systems. Direct comparisons of semantic and episodic memory have revealed activation specific to semantic memory in lateral temporal and parietal cortex, lateral and medial PFC, and the dorsomedial nucleus of the thalamus (e.g., Maguire & Frith, 2004). The content of the memory (whether episodic or semantic) can affect the patterns of activation, as studies of concrete words (Dalla Barba et al., 1998), musical tunes (Platel et al., 2003), and spatial information (Mayes et al., 2004) have illustrated. Some of the previously reported differences between episodic and semantic retrieval may reflect confounded differences in content (e.g., semantic retrieval of spatial information activates the hippocampus; Mayes et al., 2004).

One of the more controversial hypotheses about the neural substrates of episodic and semantic memory to emerge from the neuroimaging literature is referred to by the acronym HERA (Hemispheric Encoding-Retrieval Asymmetry). The HERA model describes the relative specialization of left and right PFC for episodic encoding and retrieval, respectively (Tulving et al., 1994). Although formulated as an explanation of differences during encoding and retrieval of *episodic* memory, many of the studies cited as investigations of episodic encoding could just as easily be characterized as studies of semantic retrieval (but see Lee, Robbins et al., 2002 for an example of an attempt to dissociate episodic encoding and semantic retrieval). Thus, the bulk of the data speak to a Hemispheric Episodic Semantic Asymmetry (though we hesitate to introduce the acronym HESA in any way other than jest!) that is relevant for the current discussion. While the HERA model focuses on differences in PFC activation patterns, commonalities across semantic and episodic retrieval tasks have been reported in a number of studies (Buckner et al., 1995; Dalla Barba et al., 1998; Nyberg et al., 2003; Wiggs et al., 1999). In particular, both semantic and episodic retrieval activate regions in the anterior cingulate and left PFC; we discuss a possible domain-general role for PFC that may be relevant to these observations near the end of the chapter.

One problem with the attempt to form generalizations about the neural bases of semantic memory based on a list of studies such as those briefly reviewed here is that the devil lies in the details. Each new way of manipulating or measuring semantic retrieval is likely to affect the component processes, of which there are almost certainly many, that are involved in each task. The operations involved in monitoring a list of words for animals (Dalla Barba et al., 1998) will not be identical to those involved in completing a word stem (Buckner et al., 1995). Differences in the results across studies may be noise, or they may reflect the systematic (but perhaps as yet unidentified) manipulation of processes beyond semantic retrieval per se. For example, at the end of the chapter we present one such hypothesis for the role of left PFC in (some) semantic retrieval tasks. As we argue, the extent to which PFC is engaged by a semantic memory task depends on factors that are not, strictly speaking, semantic.

That said, neuroimaging studies comparing episodic and semantic memory can be roughly summarized thusly: semantic memory and episodic memory systems rely in part on common neural circuitry, activation of which might be understood in terms of variables orthogonal to the episodic/semantic distinction, such as content (e.g., spatial, verbal) or cognitive control processes. Nonetheless, semantic memory retrieval does have a distinct neural signature, which includes regions of temporal and frontal cortex. In the remaining sections of this chapter, we will begin to tease apart the unique contributions that these regions make to semantic memory processes.

Organization of Semantic Memory

Categories of Semantic Memory

Throughout the twentieth century, clinical neurologists began to notice strikingly selective language impairments: anecdotal case studies described patients who were unable to understand or produce the names of colors (A. R. Damasio et al., 1979), body parts (Dennis, 1976), people (McKenna & Warrington, 1980), actions (Goodglass et al., 1966), concrete entities (Warrington, 1975), inanimate objects (Nielsen, 1936), small, manipulable objects (Konorski, 1967), and indoor objects (Yamadori & Albert, 1973). However, it was not until the systematic, experimental investigations of Elizabeth Warrington and her colleagues that these so-called category-specific deficits began to change the way cognitive psychologists thought about the organization of semantic memory.

In 1983, Warrington and McCarthy described a patient with a specific impairment of understanding object names. The next year, Warrington and Shallice (1984) described four patients who showed the reverse dissociation, a selective impairment in visual identification and verbal comprehension of living things and foods. Thus began, in the words of two of its leaders, "the modern era of the study of the representation of object concepts in the human brain" (Martin & Caramazza, 2003, 195). It is a question for historians of science why these two papers captivated the field in a way that those which came before had not. But the outcome is clear: not only did these studies alter the course of investigations of semantic memory, but they also provided a foundational example of the critical role that neuropsychology could play in cognitive science (Shallice, 1988).

There are several excellent reviews of the growing literature reporting category-specific deficits (e.g., Capitani et al., 2003; Saffran & Schwartz, 1994). Here, we highlight just a few of the important points to emerge from these investigations, emphasizing those which have relevance in subsequent sections of this chapter.

First, in most cases, category-specific impairments are observed across multiple testing modalities (e.g., pictorial and verbal stimuli). However, deficits have been described that are restricted to a single modality (e.g., Hart et al., 1985), and within-modality item consistency can exceed between-modality consistency (Warrington

& Shallice, 1984). These observations have been interpreted by some as evidence for multiple formats of semantic memory.

Second, selective impairments in knowledge of both living things (something described as "animate" or "biological kinds") and nonliving things (sometimes described as "inanimate" or "artifacts") have been reported, but the frequency of these two deficits is not equal. In a 2003 review, Martin and Caramazza identified reports of over 100 patients with a living things deficit in contrast to about 25 patients with a nonliving things deficit. Although artifactual accounts of living things deficits (e.g., complexity, familiarity) have been ruled out in some cases (Basso et al., 1988; Farah et al., 1991), it is possible that confounding variables have created part of the discrepancy in the incidence of these two types of category-specific deficits. However, the disparity could also reflect important differences in the way living and nonliving things are represented that affect the susceptibility of semantic knowledge.

Third, the neuroanatomical correlates of category-specific disorders are hardly precise, given the extent of damage present in many cases, but a few generalities have been proposed: patients with a living things deficit most commonly have lesions that include anterior, inferior, and medial temporal cortex, bilaterally (but left more than right). In contrast, patients with a nonliving things deficit typically have large, left frontoparietal lesions. However, exceptions to these patterns have been noted in both cases (Caramazza & Shelton, 1998; Tippett et al., 1996).

Fourth, finer-grained examinations of category-specific deficits have been both informative and controversial. In some cases these analyses revealed impairments that are broader than "living things": patients with impaired knowledge of animals, fruits, and vegetables have been reported to have concurrent deficits identifying gemstones (Warrington & Shallice, 1984), liquids and materials (Borgo & Shallice, 2001), and musical instruments (Silveri & Gainotti, 1988). In other cases, these analyses have revealed strikingly narrow category-specific impairments of knowledge of only fruits and vegetables (Crutch & Warrington, 2003) or only animals (Caramazza & Shelton, 1998). These exceptions to the broad living/nonliving distinction continue to inform theories of the organization of semantic memory.

The dozens of neuropsychological studies reporting category-specific impairments are now complemented by dozens of investigations of category-specificity in neurologically intact subjects using functional neuroimaging. One rich source of data about category-specificity comes from studies of visual responses to highly specific object categories, such as faces (Kanwisher et al., 1997), places (Epstein & Kanwisher, 1998), and body parts (Downing et al., 2001). These studies, and the controversy that surrounds them (Haxby et al., 2001; Tarr & Gauthier, 2000), are discussed in detail in Kanwisher (2003). The neuroimaging studies of category-specificity reviewed in this chapter are confined to those in which the subject was required to retrieve some unpictured information about an object (e.g., its name, color, size, etc.). We have excluded studies in which subjects had to passively view or briefly remember an object; the difficulty in determining where to draw this line highlights the continuity between these two areas of inquiry.

Initial reports of category-specific activation during semantic processing came from studies of word retrieval. For example, a comparison of PET activation during verbal fluency (generation of examplars of living and nonliving things) revealed differences in left anteromedial temporal cortex (increased for living things) and left posterior temporal cortex (increased for nonliving things; Mummery et al., 1996). Martin and colleagues (1996) found increased PET activation in left medial occipital cortex during animal-naming and in left premotor and middle temporal cortex during tool-naming. Both animal-naming and tool-naming activated common regions of ventral temporal cortex bilaterally and left PFC; however, in a subsequent fMRI study (with better spatial resolution), this group observed multiple, small category-specific sites (for animals, tools, faces, and houses) in ventral temporal cortex (Chao et al., 1999). Spitzer and colleagues (Spitzer et al., 1998; Spitzer et al., 1995) also reported small regions of category-specific activity in frontal and tempo-roparietal cortex during covert naming of living and nonliving things. Although there were no consistent areas of category-specific activation across subjects, consistent activation was observed in one subject on two scanning dates. These findings were taken as evidence for category-specific semantic representations that are highly variable across subjects as a result of different life histories. Damasio and colleagues (H. Damasio et al., 1996; Grabowski et al., 1998) reported category-specific PET activation in the left hemisphere during naming of people (temporal pole), animals (middle portion of inferior temporal gyrus and medial occipital cortex), and tools (posterior portion of inferior temporal gyrus and premotor cortex). A similar category-specific organization was observed in patients with lesions to these regions (H. Damasio et al., 1996); however, these patients had anomia (i.e., word retrieval deficits) rather than semantic knowledge deficits. Thus, the evidence for category-specific representations in studies of verbal fluency and picture naming may reflect principles of lexical organization rather than semantic organization.

The few studies that have examined category-specific differences with nonverbal tasks have reported mixed results. Perani and colleagues (1995, 1999) compared PET activation during same-different judgments about animals and tools. In one study they reported that tool judgments activated left frontal cortex (although not the same premotor region reported elsewhere), but animal judgments were associated with no consistent locus of activation (Perani et al., 1995). In a subsequent study, they identified common regions of activation for both pictures and words: across modalities, tool judgments were associated with middle temporal activation, whereas animal judgments were associated with left fusiform gyrus activation (Perani et al., 1999). Although this study might be seen as an improvement over strictly verbal studies, the extent to which semantic knowledge was required for these tasks is not clear (e.g., their word task required matching two stimuli presented in different fonts, which is arguably non-semantic).

Tyler and colleagues have conducted a series of experiments that have failed to find reliable category-specific activity during word comprehension: across three experiments, they observed activity during lexical decision and category judgments in a network of areas including the left inferior frontal lobe, left posterior temporal cortex, and the anterior temporal poles bilaterally (Devlin et al., 2002). While they did find category differences in some of the same regions as previous studies (i.e., the left anterior-medial temporal pole activated specifically for animals and the left posterior middle temporal gyrus specifically for tools), these effects were present only at lowered statistical thresholds. Utilizing the same category judgment task (i.e., Is the fourth item in a list of words from the same semantic category as the first three items?), Pilgrim et al. (2002) found no significant differences between artifact and natural kind concepts in an event-related fMRI study. The only significant activation difference between the two categories emerged in a region of interest analysis in the fusiform gyrus (artifacts greater than natural kinds—oddly, the reverse of other studies). Finally, in a third fMRI study, they repeated the experiment but restricted the object types to tools and animals (Tyler et al., 2003). Again, they failed to find category-specific effects at either a statistically corrected threshold or a lowered one.

In summary, attempts to find category-specific activation patterns using neuroimaging methods have had mixed success. In principle, the failure to find category-specific responses could result from neural category-specificity at a spatial resolution higher than that of our neuroimaging methods. However, in light of the relatively remote lesion sites that have been implicated in category-specific deficits, this is an unsatisfying explanation. More likely is the possibility that activation has been observed in areas which are not necessary for the performance of a task. Category judgments about animals, for example, might activate a widely distributed neural network, all of which represents information about animals, but only portions of which are necessary to perform the task. Clearly, additional work is necessary to discern what specializations exist within this rather extensive collection of regions that are recruited during semantic processing. In the next section, we consider one candidate organizing principle of a distributed semantic network.

Attribute Domains of Semantic Memory

At the outset of this chapter, we briefly introduced a model of semantic memory that describes object concepts as distributed mental representations implemented in functionally and physically distinct attribute domains (Allport, 1985). These attribute domains correspond to different sensory or motor domains of which they are also a part. In fact, according to Allport, these modules are the very same areas of the brain that are dedicated to processing sensorimotor information. Among the ideas discussed in this seminal paper, Allport suggested that (1) the class of attribute domains that pertain to any given object concept, and thus that serve to represent that concept, will vary across objects; (2) object concepts are less vulnerable to brain damage, by virtue of their widely distributed representation, than linguistic representations (e.g., word forms); (3) those object concepts which are defined over few attribute domains will be more vulnerable to brain damage than those which are defined over many attribute domains. We will revisit some of these claims, and implications of this model for understanding category-specificity, later in the chapter. For now, we turn to investigations of attribute domains—namely, what are they, and where are they?

The distinction between *visual* and *functional* attributes is the most common and perhaps also the coarsest division among attribute domains in the semantic memory literature. Research in several diverse areas, from language acquisition (e.g., Gentner, 1978; Nelson, 1974) to language dysfunction (e.g., Warrington & Shallice, 1984), from word reading (e.g., Schreuder et al., 1984) to object categorization (e.g., Rosch et al., 1976), indicates that semantic knowledge may be divided into visual and functional attributes. Now adding to these sources of evidence, a number of functional neuroimaging studies have reported neuroanatomical dissociations between visual and functional attributes (Cappa et al., 1998; Mummery et al., 1998; Thompson-Schill, Aguirre et al., 1999), or between abstract and concrete words, which, by definition, differ with regard to visual knowledge (Beauregard et al., 1997; D'Esposito et al., 1997; but see Kiehl et al., 1999). For example, retrieving the color of an object activates ventral temporal cortex bilaterally, while retrieving an associated action activates left middle temporal and prefrontal cortex (Martin et al., 1995). Note that the operationalization of "function" knowledge has varied widely across these studies (e.g., actions, uses, etc), so, to be more accurate, we organize the next two sections of the chapter around the principal neuroimaging findings relating to visual and *nonvisual* semantic knowledge.

Visual Attribute Domains   One interpretation of the studies reviewed above is that knowledge about visual attributes of an object is represented differently from knowledge of nonvisual attributes. This conjecture is related to a central debate in cognitive science about the extent to which any type of conceptual knowledge relies on perceptual representations (for a review, see Barsalou, 1999). This controversy has perhaps been played out most thoroughly in the investigation of mental imagery. On one side of the imagery debate are those who maintain that mental images are propositional or symbolic, such as language, and therefore do not share representations with perception (e.g., Pylyshyn, 1981). On the other side of the debate are those who believe that mental images have a spatial format and share representations with those used during perception (e.g., Kosslyn, 1980). There is mounting support for the hypothesis that visual imagery and visual perception share common processes, including evidence from brain-damaged patients (Farah, 2000); transcranial magnetic stimulation (Kosslyn et al., 1999), ERP recordings (Farah, Peronnet et al., 1988); and now neuroimaging.

Numerous neuroimaging studies have found activation in visual cortex during mental imagery (e.g., Charlot et al., 1992; D'Esposito et al., 1997; Goldenberg et al., 1991; Goldenberg et al., 1987; Roland & Friberg, 1985), in extrastriate and occasionally striate cortex. Furthermore, images of different sizes produce different patterns of activation, consistent with what is known about the retinotopic mapping of visual cortex (Kosslyn et al., 1993). Across neuroimaging studies of mental imagery, there is some disagreement about whether the activation is confined to higher-order visual association cortex or whether it includes primary visual cortex. Despite this controversy, there is near agreement that visual imagery activates some retinotopically organized cortical regions, which supports the hypothesis that imagery and perception have common representations.

We have taken a slightly different approach recently (Kan et al., 2003), in which we examined activation in visual association cortex during a property verification task (e.g., Does a camel have a hump?). With no explicit imagery instructions, we observed activation in visual association cortex (i.e., fusiform gyrus) only under conditions in which conceptual knowledge was required (i.e., not when word association strength would suffice to make a correct response); this pattern indicates a specific reliance of conceptual knowledge on perceptual representations.

If one believes that knowledge of visual attributes depends on visual representations, then one might logically ask whether divisions that have been observed in visual perception exist in our representations of visual knowledge. For example, it is well known that regions of cortex are specialized for color perception, motion perception, and form perception. Recently, investigators have used functional neuroimaging to probe for similar distinctions within semantic knowledge.

Color   Knowledge of color—and its relation to perception of color—has been investigated in more neuroimaging studies than any other visual attribute domain. Across a wide variety of tasks—including reporting the color of a pictured line drawing (Chao & Martin, 1999; Martin et al., 1995; Wiggs & Martin, 1998), verifying the color of a visually or auditorily named object (Kellenbach et al., 2001; Noppeney & Price, 2003), and making similarity judgments across a triad of object names (Mummery et al., 1998)—activation is typically observed in left or bilateral ventral temporal cortex, with a high degree of consistency across studies. Chao and Martin (1999) directly compared activation during color perception and color knowledge retrieval, and found activation during color naming just anterior to the areas responsible for processing color information. A similar finding was reported in a comparison of color perception and color imagery (Howard et al., 1998).

Unlike other regions that are active during a broad range of semantic retrieval tasks (e.g., PFC), ventral temporal cortex may be active *specifically* during color retrieval (e.g., in contrast to retrieval of object size knowledge (Kellenbach et al., 2001). However, contrary to this claim, Noppeney and Price (2003) reported *less*, not more, activation in left ventral temporal cortex during a color retrieval task ("Red?") for fruits compared with an "origin" retrieval task ("Tropical?"). Whether this anomalous finding is specific to the origin task remains to be determined.

Motion   Several early neuroimaging studies of semantic memory reported that retrieval of action knowledge activates, among other areas (discussed more below), the left middle temporal gyrus (Martin et al., 1995; Warburton et al., 1996; Wise et al., 1991), anterior to the region associated with motion perception (MT/MST; e.g., Watson et al., 1993; Zeki et al., 1991). Similarly, Decety and colleagues reported activation in lateral temporal cortex while imagining actions or observing semantically meaningful actions (Decety et al., 1997; Ruby & Decety, 2001). Kable and colleagues (2002) observed increased activity in (or just anterior to) functionally defined MT/MST while subjects made semantic judgments about actions (relative to objects). Because of the coincidence of these locations, lateral temporal activation during retrieval of action attributes has been attributed to retrieval of motion knowledge (Martin et al., 2000).

In addition to object motion, the lateral temporal lobe has also been implicated in biological motion. Specifically, the superior temporal sulcus, which is slightly anterior and dorsal to MT, has been shown to be involved when subjects observe face and leg motion, mouth movements (e.g., Buccino et al., 2001; Buccino et al., 2004; Calvert et al., 1997; Calvert & Campbell, 2003; Campbell et al., 2001; Wheaton et al., 2004), eye movements (e.g., Pelphrey et al., 2003; Puce et al., 1998), and body movements (e.g., Bonda et al., 1996; Grezes et al., 2001; E. Grossman et al., 2000; Howard et al., 1996). Given the spatial separation and the consistency of the localization of these two types of motions, Martin and colleagues (Martin et al., 2000) proposed a dorsal-ventral divide in the representations of biological and nonbiological motion. Consistent with this hypothesis, Beauchamp et al. (2002, 2003) reported more activity during viewing of human movement (either videos or point-light displays) compared to tool movement in the superior temporal sulcus, and the reverse pattern in the middle temporal gyrus. To date, this putative distinction has not been tested during semantic retrieval tasks.

Size   The findings of the few studies that specifically examined retrieval of size knowledge have been a bit more mixed than those which have looked at color or motion: when compared with other semantic retrieval tasks, retrieval of size knowledge has resulted in either no areas of selective activation (Vandenberghe et al., 1996), activation of medial parietal cortex (Kellenbach et al., 2001), or activation of lateral parietal cortex (Oliver & Thompson-Schill, 2003). Selective activation of medial parietal cortex during size retrieval (relative to color retrieval) was attributed to activation of spatial representations that encode relative size (Kellenbach et al., 2001). However, in our study, parietal activation (albeit lateral, not medial) was greater during retrieval of size, but also shape, relative to retrieval of color knowledge (Oliver & Thompson-Schill, 2003). We discuss the role of the dorsal visual processing stream in representing physical properties of objects, including size and shape, below.

Form   Most of the studies that have probed the representation of form information have focused on the recognition of objects from pictures to explore the question of category differences in representation of form information in occipitotemporal cortex (Chao et al., 1999; Ishai et al., 2000; Ishai et al., 1999). Likewise, activation has been reported in ventral occipitotemporal cortex during mental imagery of object shape (e.g., De Volder et al., 2001; Ganis et al., 2004) or during semantic decisions based on object form (Cappa et al., 1998). Even in blind subjects, retrieval of shape knowledge activates occipitotemporal cortex, to the same extent as in sighted subjects (Noppeney et al., 2003; Pietrini et al., 2004). While results from blind subjects have been used to argue that ventral occipitotemporal representations of form are abstract and supramodal, this pattern may reflect reorganization of function in blind individuals (e.g., what may serve as a visual processing area in sighted individuals may operate as a spatial or tactile processing region in blind individuals).

Our investigations of shape retrieval highlighted the potential role of the *dorsal* visual processing stream in the representation of object concepts (Oliver & Thompson-Schill, 2003). When we compared shape retrieval to color retrieval, the most prominent selective activation was found in parietal cortex, in regions also activated (although less so) during size retrieval. The hypothesized involvement of parietal cortex in shape recognition is not without precedent (Murata et al., 2000; Peuskens et al., 2004), although the precise role of this region during semantic retrieval has not yet been determined. However, the field of visual perception suggests some avenues to explore in further research.

Extrastriate visual areas can be divided into a ventral stream running from occipital cortex through temporal cortex and a dorsal stream extending from occipital cortex through the parietal lobe (Ungerleider & Mishkin, 1982). It has been proposed that the ventral stream processes the identity of objects during perception, while the dorsal stream has been ascribed different roles, including spatial processing (Ungerleider & Mishkin, 1982) and processing performed during visually mediated actions (Goodale & Milner, 1992). By analogy, the dorsal stream may also be involved in *retrieval* of aspects of attributes that are acquired through spatial processing or through visually mediated actions. In other words, spatiomotor processing may provide another source of information about the shape and size of objects, at least for some categories of objects. In particular, objects that have a strong relationship between their form and their manner of manipulation (i.e., a strong affordance for action; Gibson, 1979) would be more likely to have motor representations that also carry information about their form. Below, we consider implications of this additional source of information when discussing vulnerability of semantic memory to brain damage.

Nonvisual Attribute Domains   The term "functional knowledge," typically used to contrast with visual knowledge when talking about types of semantic memory, has been rendered almost meaningless through its abundance of uses. For example, the term has been used by some to denote any abstract property that is not physically defined (e.g., Schreuder et al., 1984), and by others to denote an attribute that is physically defined, but by motor properties rather than sensory properties (e.g., Farah & McClelland, 1991; Warrington & McCarthy, 1987). Abandoning this terminology completely, we focus here on action knowledge and how that knowledge may be further subdivided into function ("what for") knowledge and manipulation ("how") knowledge. Then, we briefly review investigations of other nonvisual (but sensory) attributes—sound, smell, and taste.

Action   Dozens of neuroimaging studies have investigated the neural bases of action knowledge retrieval (e.g., Binkofski, Buccino, Posse, et al., 1999; Binkofski, Buccino, Stephan, et al., 1999; Buccino et al., 2001; Gerlach, Law, Gade, et al., 2002; Gerlach, Law, & Paulson, 2002; Grabowski et al., 1998; Grafton et al., 1996; Grafton et al., 1997; Kable et al., 2002; Kellenbach et al., 2003; Martin et al., 1995; Martin et al., 1996; Perani et al., 1999; Warburton et al., 1996; Wheaton et al., 2004). Across a variety of explicit retrieval tasks (e.g., verb generation, similarity judgments) and implicit retrieval tasks (e.g., tool identification, pleasantness ratings), a distributed network of brain regions including left ventral prefrontal, posterior temporal, and parietal areas has consistently been identified. In a recent meta-analysis of 24 neuroimaging studies of action knowledge retrieval, Grezes and Decety (2001) identified considerable overlap in the neural bases of action execution, simulation, observation, and verbalization.

In particular, the relation between action knowledge in premotor cortex has received considerable attention, fueled in part by parallel findings that neurons in monkey premotor cortex are involved in the recognition of motor actions (Rizzolatti et al., 1996). Differences within premotor cortex have been observed, depending on the body part involved in the retrieved action (e.g., Pulvermuller et al., 2001). An area of left ventrolateral premotor cortex that is activated by imagined grasping and other hand movements with the right hand (Decety, 1996; Decety et al., 1994; Stephan et al., 1995) is almost identical to the area activated during tool naming (Martin et al., 1996). Based on these results, Martin and colleagues have argued that knowledge of tool use is stored in this region (see also Chao & Martin, 2000; Grabowski et al., 1998; Grafton et al., 1997, for similar findings and interpretations).

There are two distinct meanings of tool use, and of action knowledge more generally: knowledge of the function of an object (e.g., a key opens a door) and knowledge of the manner of manipulation (e.g., using a key involves twisting and turning of the hand) have been doubly dissociated in neuropsychological investigations (e.g., Buxbaum & Saffran, 1998; Buxbaum et al., 2000; Sirigu et al., 1991). Kellenbach and colleagues (2003) reported that PET activation in frontal, middle temporal, and parietal cortex is linked to manipulation knowledge, not function knowledge. Similarly, Boronat and colleagues (2005) reported selective fMRI activation of the inferior parietal cortex during retrieval of manipulation information. Neither of these studies found reliable activation associated with retrieval of function knowledge; information about the function of an object (i.e., what it is used for) may depend on more abstract representations, which we will consider shortly.

Other Sensory Domains   The few neuroimaging studies that have investigated retrieval of auditory knowledge (e.g., animal sounds) have found selective activity in the superior aspect of the temporal pole (Noppeney & Price, 2002), temporoparietal cortex near auditory association areas (Kellenbach et al., 2001), and the superior temporal gyrus (Adams & Janata, 2002; Wheeler et al., 2000). Overall, it appears that the temporal lobe, and in particular auditory association areas in the superior temporal lobe, may be selectively involved in the retrieval of auditory semantic information.

Several recent neuroimaging studies have examined selective activation during retrieval of information about smell and taste of objects; however, there are methodological issues (e.g., fMRI signal dropout in orbital regions) that make research in these areas difficult. Failures to find taste-specific activation (e.g., Noppeney & Price, 2003) may reflect these challenges. That said, at least one study has reported that taste imagery and taste perception activate common regions within frontal cortex (Levy et al., 1999). Research on odor knowledge has found that, in large part, the regions associated with olfactory perception, including orbitofrontal, pyriform, and insular cortex, are involved in identification of odors (Cerf-Ducastel & Murphy, 2003; Dade et al., 1998; Karaken et al., 2003). The tasks used in these studies are the olfactory equivalent of a picture-naming task (i.e., subjects must retrieve a name, given modality-specific input). To date, there have been no studies of olfactory retrieval that are not potentially confounded with effects of olfactory perception. Also, olfactory semantic studies that utilized an odor perception baseline task failed to find involvement of one or more of these regions (Karaken et al., 2003; Qureshy et al., 2000; Royet et al., 1999).

Abstract Semantic Representations

Thus far, our discussion of the representation of semantic memory has been confined to physical properties of concrete objects. When Allport articulated his theory of the representation of meanings, he limited himself, "for simplicity," to the domain of object concepts. Of course, any complete theory of semantic memory has a bit more work to do: there are abstract concepts (e.g., peace), abstract features of object concepts (e.g., "alive" as a feature of a plant), and abstract relations between concepts (e.g., the ways in which a "bat" is more similar to a "bear" than to a "bird").

There is ample neuropsychological evidence for a dissociation between the representation of abstract and concrete concepts (e.g., Breedin et al., 1994) that may reflect any number of qualitative differences in their acquisition and representational format. Neuroimaging comparisons of abstract and concrete words have identified an inconsistent array of regions associated with abstract concepts in the left superior temporal gyrus (Wise et al., 2000), right anterior temporal pole (Kiehl et al., 1999), and left posterior middle temporal gyrus (M. Grossman et al., 2002). Noppeney and Price (2004) compared fMRI activation while subjects made similarity judgments about triads of visual words, sound words, action words, and abstract words that were matched for difficulty. Relative to the three other conditions, retrieval of abstract concepts activated the left inferior frontal gyrus, middle temporal gyrus, superior temporal sulcus, and anterior temporal pole. The authors suggest that these differences reflect activation of areas involved in sentence comprehension, although this is clearly an area in need of more investigation.

There is, to date, even less work addressing abstract features. One particular problem with using functional neuroimaging to compare abstract and concrete features is that abstract semantic decisions typically take longer to resolve. The left inferior PFC has been implicated in extended or controlled semantic processing on the basis of studies that might confound effort with abstractness (Roskies et al., 2001); for example, PFC activity increased when subjects decided that "candle" and "halo" were similar, compared to deciding that "candle" and "flame" were similar

(Wagner et al., 2001), arguably a comparison that confounds effort with abstraction. To unconfound these processes, Goldberg and colleagues (2004) compared the effects of increasing semantic abstractness and increasing difficulty on activity in PFC while subjects verified perceptual or abstract facts about animals. fMRI activation in left PFC (BA 47) was specifically associated with an increased reliance on abstract properties but not increased semantic difficulty. This finding is consistent with recent evidence showing that neurons in a primate analogue of this region represent abstract rules (Wallis et al., 2001).

Many cognitive models of semantic memory have described hierarchical networks that reflect abstract relations between concepts (e.g., a tree is a plant and a plant is a living thing). This description is quite different from the distributed representation we have been describing thus far. However, Rogers and colleagues have articulated a formal model of semantic memory that includes units which integrate information across all of the attribute domains (including verbal descriptions and object names; McClelland & Rogers, 2003). As a consequence, "abstract semantic representations emerge as a product of statistical learning mechanisms in a region of cortex suited to performing cross-modal mappings by virtue of its many interconnections with different perceptual-motor areas" (Rogers et al., 2004, 206). The interaction between content-bearing perceptual representations and verbal labels produces a similarity space that is not captured in any single attribute domain; rather, they argue, it reflects abstract similarity (cf. Caramazza et al., 1990; A. R. Damasio, 1989; Plaut, 2002; Tyler et al., 2000). The cortical region they offer as a candidate for these abstract representations is the temporal pole, based both on the anatomical connectivity of this region and the degeneration of this region in semantic dementia.

The notion that interactions between perceptual and verbal representations lead to the emergence of new, abstract representations may be relevant for a puzzle that has emerged in neuroimaging tests of Allport's (1985) sensorimotor model of semantic memory: that there is a consistent trend for retrieval of a given physical attribute to be associated with activation of cortical areas 2–3 cm anterior to regions associated with perception of that attribute (Martin et al., 1995; Thompson-Schill, 2003). This pattern, which has been interpreted as coactivation of the "same areas" involved in sensorimotor processing, as Allport hypothesized, could alternatively be used as grounds to reject the Allport model. What does this anterior shift reflect? We believe the answer may lie in the ideas developed by Rogers and colleagues (2004). The process of abstracting away from modality-specific representations may occur gradually across a number of cortical regions (perhaps converging on the temporal pole). As a result, a gradient of abstraction may emerge in the representations throughout a given region of cortex (e.g., the ventral extrastriate visual pathway), and the anterior shift may reflect activation of a more abstract representation (Kosslyn & Thompson, 2000). The tasks that have been used to study conceptual retrieval of visual attributes have not consistently required the subject to retrieve perceptual information. For example, in order to recall that a banana is "yellow," activation of color representations that are more abstract than those necessary for perception could suffice. The conceptual similarity space in more anterior regions may depart a bit from the similarity space in the environment, perhaps moving in the direction of abstract relations. More work is needed to uncover the nature of the representations—and how the similarity space may gradually change across different cortical regions.

Categories of Semantic Memory—Redux

Thus far, we have presented two potentially orthogonal views about the organization of semantic memory. We initially considered the hypothesis that representations of specific categories of semantic knowledge are instantiated in spatially distinct neural regions. As we saw, there is ample support for this hypothesis from the neuropsychological literature, but only partial support from neuroimaging studies. Then, we reviewed neuroimaging studies that support models of distributed representations of semantic memory, where different attribute domains of object knowledge are represented in distinct sensorimotor systems. As the reader having even a passing familiarity with these literatures will know, these two hypotheses about the organization of semantic memory are intertwined, by virtue of the fact that the taxonomic category of an object and its associated attribute domains are not at all orthogonal. The confound between these two putative organizing principles has made it challenging to uncover the neural architecture of semantic memory.

Warrington and McCarthy (1983) first called attention to implications of this relation for the interpretation of category-specific deficits: whereas sensory attributes are important for discriminating between members of the category of living things, functional attributes are more important for discriminating between members of the category of nonliving things. Thus, category-specific deficits could result from the degradation of an attribute domain of semantic memory. Since the mid-1980s, this *sensory-functional theory* has persisted in a variety of accounts of category-specific deficits, all of which hold that semantic knowledge is stored in sensorimotor channels, and that the relative importance of information contained in these channels varies across items in different categories (e.g., Farah & McClelland, 1991; Martin et al., 2000; Saffran & Schwartz, 1994; Simmons & Barsalou, 2003).

Accordingly, one explanation of category-specific activation in neuroimaging studies is that these differences reflect the differential weighting of visual and functional knowledge across categories (e.g., Martin et al., 1996). In order to test this account, Patterson and colleagues have reported two PET studies that have unconfounded object category and attribute domain. In the first, subjects made similarity judgments about living or nonliving things on the basis of either visual or nonvisual information. With this fully crossed design, the authors compared the magnitude of category-specific effects and attribute-specific effects directly, and concluded that the latter were more prominent neurally (Mummery et al., 1998). In a second study, subjects generated visual or nonvisual features in response to an object name (Lee, Graham, et al., 2002). Although they found no category-specific effects, they did find an effect of attribute type: visual retrieval activated left posterior inferior temporal cortex, and nonvisual retrieval activated left middle temporal cortex and right fusiform cortex.

The relationship between visual processing demands and object category was elegantly demonstrated in a PET study by Rogers and colleagues (2005). Subjects categorized photographs of animals and vehicles at one of three levels of specificity (e.g., animal, bird, or robin; vehicle, boat, or ferry). Posterior fusiform activation was greater for animals than for vehicles *only* when subjects were categorizing pictures at an intermediate level (e.g., bird). The authors argued that the fusiform gyrus responds to the discrimination of items with similar visual representations, and that at the intermediate level of description only, animals have more overlapping visual properties than do vehicles. In addition, the modulation of the category effect by task demands provides a plausible explanation for the inconsistent pattern of category-specific effects described earlier.

The sensory-functional theory has been debated and refined as new observations have challenged the ability of this theory to parsimoniously account for the relevant neuropsychological data. Caramazza and colleagues have frequently called attention to some of the more problematic findings for the sensory-functional theory. An early objection was based on the observation that patients with living-things deficits have impairments across multiple attribute domains (Caramazza & Shelton, 1998). The sensory-functional theory, which presumes that living-things deficits result from loss of visual knowledge, would seem to predict normal nonvisual knowledge of living things. This objection was initially answered by Farah and McClelland (1991), who used a computational model to demonstrate the emergence of category-specific effects (across attributes) following damage to an interactive, attribute-specific systems. Key to the behavior of this model was the assumption that retrieval of a weakly represented attribute of a concept would depend on the activation of more strongly represented attributes, thus exhibiting a critical-mass effect. Thompson-Schill and colleagues (1999) sought physiological evidence for this assumption: for living things, retrieval of visual or nonvisual information should require activation of visual representations, because of the disproportionate weighting of visual information in the representations of living things. For nonliving things, no such dependence on visual knowledge should occur. As predicted, areas involved in visual knowledge retrieval were active during judgments about visual *and* nonvisual attributes of living things but only during judgments about visual attributes of non-living things. These results lend credence to claims that category-specific activations actually reflect attribute-specific representations. (For a different interpretation of these data, see Caramazza, 2000).

A second criticism of Caramazza and colleagues' has proven more difficult to answer: the sensory-functional theory would seem to predict that patients with a degradation of the visual attribute domain would have impaired visual knowledge of all concepts, not just of living things. However, at least some patients with a living-things deficit have normal visual knowledge of nonliving things (Caramazza & Shelton, 1998). Here, we suggest a possible way to answer this objection, on the basis of some of the ideas that have emerged from the neuroimaging studies reviewed above. As we argued earlier, visual knowledge is most probably not a *single* attribute domain. Under this revised description of visual knowledge, in which visual knowl-edge itself is a distributed representation, a different set of predictions emerges: objects with multiple sources of knowledge about their appearance (e.g., vision, touch, actions) will be less susceptible to loss of any single source of visual knowl-edge (cf. Crutch & Warrington, 2003). We tend to have more sources of knowledge of the appearance of nonliving things, or at least of certain nonliving things. Thus, damage to ventral visual processing regions, which represent only one source of information, will not necessarily cause an impairment to other representations of appearance for these things. This idea was present in Allport's (1985) description of attribute domains (he used the example "cloud"), but it was not included in many sensory-functional theories that, in effect, collapsed across all types of visual knowledge. We argue here that the consideration of multiple sources of visual knowledge—and the way those sources vary across categories—may be crucial to our ability to explain category-specific phenomena.

There are some provocative data that lend credence to this conjecture: Borgo and Shallice (2001) described a patient with a living-things deficit who was also unable to identify nonliving things without a solid form (e.g., liquids). They argued that the affected attribute domains were purely visual qualities, such as color and texture, which are unrelated to object use. However, his knowledge—including visual knowl-edge—of artifacts presumed to have strong form-action links (i.e., affordances) was preserved (cf. De Renzi & Lucchelli, 1994; Tyler & Moss, 1997). Wolk and colleagues (2005) more directly examined the role of affordances in a patient with an apparent living-things deficit. They noted that this patient was impaired at recognizing not only animals but also artifacts that minimally afforded a particular action. In con-trast, for artifacts that strongly afforded an action (e.g., piano), the patient could identify a line drawing of the object. The patient's ability to recognize shape, in the absence of a functional occipitotemporal representation of form, may have been mediated by action representations (for objects where the form affords the action). Subsequently, we demonstrated that this patient's knowledge of the *color* of objects was impaired (in contrast to his normal knowledge of both shape and size; Oliver et al., 2004).

In summary, the relationship between taxonomic categories and attribute domains, and the implications of that relationship for our understanding of phenomena such as category-specific deficits and activation patterns, is continuing to be informed by new neuroimaging studies of semantic memory. It is likely that at least some of the category-specific phenomena will be better understood as the result of processing within a distributed semantic system organized around a broad collection of senso-rimotor attributes. However, refinements to the sensory-functional theory—perhaps beginning by abandoning the term "functional"—are clearly warranted by both the neuropsychological and the neuroimaging literature (figure 6.1). Finally, it is worth noting that evidence for attribute-specific representations does not necessarily refute the hypothesis that there are category-specific representations (and vice versa); it is possible that the organization of semantic representations has more than one governing principle. Several investigators have proposed the emergence of category representations as an intermediary between sensorimotor knowledge and language (e.g., Coltheart et al., 1998). The relationship of semantic memory to language, and the extent to which category-specific representations exist in either or both, should be the subject of future research.

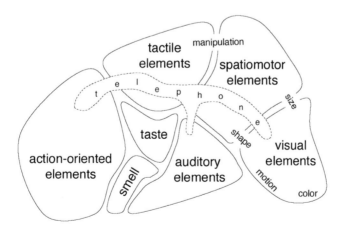

Figure 6.1
A revised version of Allport's (1985) influential model of distributed sensorimotor semantic representations, incorporating attribute domains that have been the subject of recent neuroimaging investigations.

Semantic Memory Retrieval

In the preceding section, we argued that semantic memory comprises, at least in part, a distributed set of representations that are tied to sensorimotor channels. Now we turn to the question of how these distributed representations are retrieved when one accesses semantic memory. In particular, we focus on two questions: First, we consider the relationship between the input modality and the process of semantic retrieval. Second, we discuss evidence that regions of PFC, in certain contexts, function to bias activity across distributed representations in semantic memory.

Accessing Semantic Memory from Words and Pictures

In neuropsychological investigations of semantic memory impairments, striking dissociations have been noted between visual and verbal input modalities. For example, patients with optic aphasia are unable to name visually presented objects, despite relatively spared perception of stimulus surface structure (Beauvois, 1982; Riddoch & Humphreys, 1987), and other patients perform significantly better with pictures than with words (e.g., Bub et al., 1988; Lambon Ralph & Howard, 2000; Saffran et al., 2003). These dissociations have led researchers to examine whether information from different input modalities may have differential access to different content within the conceptual system (see also Paivio, 1971; Shallice, 1988).

Many of the neuroimaging studies examining modality differences have reported regions of common activation and regions of modality-specific activations. For example, Vandenberghe and colleagues (1996) reported that semantic judgments of both words and pictures activated common regions in inferior temporal and frontal cortex, but also that a few areas were uniquely activated only by pictures (left posterior inferior temporal sulcus) or only by words (left anterior middle temporal gyrus and left inferior frontal sulcus). Similarly, Postler and colleagues (2003) observed common areas of activation across verbal and visual modalities (left inferior frontal gyrus and middle temporal gyrus) along with modality-specific areas (see also Bright et al., 2004 for a meta-analysis and report of similar findings).

Across various neuroimaging studies, a few regions have emerged as candidate regions for an amodal semantic system: left inferior frontal gyrus, middle temporal areas, and ventral temporal lobe, centered on the fusiform gyrus (see also Bookheimer et al., 1995; Moore & Price, 1999; Perani et al., 1999). Since activity in these common regions is invariant to input modality, these data seem to provide support for a unitary semantic system, such as that described by Caramazza and colleagues (1990). However, one must be cautious in interpreting "common activation" as "common representations." Given the limited spatial resolution of fMRI and PET, it is difficult to determine whether commonly activated brain regions indicate involvement of the same network of neurons or involvement of different networks of neurons existing in the same regions. One possible way to sidestep this limitation is discussed in "Issues" (below).

Neuroimaging evidence for input modality-specific activations proves equally problematic to interpret. One possibility is that these patterns reflect the existence of separate visual and verbal semantic systems (cf. Warrington & Shallice, 1984). Under this account, there is a redundant representation of semantic information in two different formats. A second possibility is that modality-specific activation patterns reflect differences in presemantic processing (Bright et al., 2004). This account might explain why the locations of putative modality-specific regions have been inconsistent across studies. We favor a third explanation: different input modalities may be preferentially associated with (or have preferential access to) different attribute domains in the distributed semantic system. By this logic, modality-specific effects do not reveal differences in the format of the representations accessed by different modalities, nor do they indicate redundant representations of the same semantic information. Rather, under this account, modality-specific effects reflect relations across attribute domains. For example, consider the relationship between form and manipulation knowledge (described in the Form section): Pictorial stimuli, which contain form information, may have preferential access to manipulation knowledge compared with word stimuli. Consistent with this claim, Chainay and Humphreys (2002) reported that normal subjects were faster at making action decision (e.g., pour or twist?) about picture stimuli than word stimuli. Also, using a free association task, Saffran et al. (2003) observed that subjects generated more action words (i.e., verbs) in response to pictures of objects than to written names of objects. Thus, activation patterns that appear specific to pictures could instead be pointing to areas specialized to represent action information. These three accounts of modality-specific activations have yet to be distinguished within the neuroimaging literature.

Selection of Semantic Representations

Consider the task of deciding whether a cherry is more similar to a rose or to a banana: On the one hand, cherries and bananas are both the fruits of a tree, both are edible, and both taste sweet. On the other hand, cherries and roses (at least the canonical ones) are red and approximately (in the case of the rose) spherical. If the attribute domains representing these three items were "polled" to assess similarity, conflict would occur. In order to answer the question, presuming you were not content simply to choose randomly, you might try to pay attention to some sources of information more than others. The process of resolving this sort of conflict is the subject of this section of the chapter.

In any model in which information is represented as a distributed pattern across multiple units, there exists the possibility for the partial activation of multiple, incompatible representations. The process of resolving this conflict and arriving at a stable representation can be referred to by the term *selection*: In any step along an information-processing stream, an appropriate representation must be selected for further processing. In some cases, selection of a representation may proceed successfully based entirely on local constraints (e.g., bottom-up inputs to a system). However, in other cases, conflict among competing representations may require top-down modulation of the selection process. We suggest that this intervention comes in the form of a modulatory signal from PFC that aids in the selection of an appropriate representation (cf. Fletcher et al., 2000; Miller & Cohen, 2001).

One example of variation in selection demands can be seen in the verb generation task: In response to the probe "cat," the activation of many weakly associated actions (e.g., "scratch," "purr") and/or of a strongly associated non-action (e.g., dog) might fail to produce sufficient activation to select any action representation. Both of these situations (underdetermined representations and prepotent representations) can induce conflict among active representations in working memory that requires top-down intervention (Botvinick et al., 2001). In contrast, in response to the probe "scissors," the strongly associated action "cut" might be activated from the input without additional demands for conflict resolution. The process of generating a verb related to "cat" and "scissors" thus differs in the selection demands.

Systematic manipulation of selection demands during semantic processing effectively modulates the fMRI response in the posterior left inferior frontal gyrus (pLIFG; Thompson-Schill et al., 1997). Subsequent studies have shown that this effect is specific to PFC (Thompson-Schill, D'Esposito, et al., 1999); is not limited to production tasks or to certain stimulus types, such as verbs (Thompson-Schill et al., 1997); is not an effect of response conflict (which has been linked to the anterior cingulate; Barch et al., 2000); and is not simply a reflection of task difficulty (Thompson-Schill, D'Esposito, et al., 1999). Rather, it appears that activity in the pLIFG is modulated by increasing demands to select a representation among competing sources of information (for a more detailed review, see Thompson-Schill, 2003). This conclusion is bolstered by evidence that patients with lesions to the pLIFG have impairments in word retrieval under high selection demands that are proportional to the extent of their lesion in the left frontal operculum (Thompson-Schill et al., 1998).

There are, naturally, other hypotheses about the role of ventrolateral PFC in semantic retrieval. Early observations of pLIFG activation during semantic retrieval led to consideration of the specific role this area may play in semantic memory (Petersen et al., 1988; Tulving et al., 1994) because the one region that is most consistently activated during semantic retrieval, across categories, attributes, and modalities, is the pLIFG. Our hypothesis that pLIFG is necessary for the selection of semantic information from competing alternatives, and not semantic retrieval per se, was motivated in part by the observation that naming pictures and making semantic comparisons do not consistently lead to pLIFG activation, despite the prima facie involvement of semantic knowledge in these tasks (e.g., Wise et al., 1991), and in part by the absence of converging evidence from lesion studies of the necessity of pLIFG for semantic retrieval. For example, Price and colleagues (1999) described a patient with pLIFG damage who was able to make semantic similarity judgments; PET activation in this patient revealed temporal, not frontal, activation associated with semantic processing.

Another, more specific, hypothesis about the role of pLIFG in semantic processing came from reports of increased activation in this region during semantic tasks involving tools. As was discussed above, knowledge about tool use has been hypothesized to depend on regions at or near ventral premotor cortex (adjacent to hand representations in motor cortex), typically including the region of pLIFG described above but extending more posteriorly into premotor cortex. To examine whether the left frontal response to tools can be further dissociated, we systematically manipulated object category (animals vs. tools) and selection demands (based on name agreement measures, cf. Kan & Thompson-Schill, 2004) in a picture-naming task. We identified two distinct neural components that jointly contribute to the previously reported tool-specific response: a posterior region, centered in left ventrolateral premotor cortex, that responds to motor knowledge retrieval, and an anterior region, centered in the left frontal operculum, that responds to selection among competing alternatives (Kan et al., 2006).

Other accounts of the role of the ventrolateral PFC in semantic retrieval draw a clear distinction between areas that represent semantic memory and areas that serve to maintain or manipulate those representations. One such proposal is that PFC is involved in temporary maintenance of semantic attributes in working memory (Gabrieli et al., 1998). Another alternative proposal is that activity in PFC reflects "controlled semantic retrieval" (Wagner et al., 2001). One key difference between these hypotheses and our own (see also Barch et al., 2000; Fletcher et al., 2000) is that we have described a potentially general-purpose mechanism that is not specific to semantic processing, whereas proposals of semantic working memory or controlled semantic retrieval are clearly specific to semantic retrieval. A mechanism that guides selection among competing representations may be necessary not only for some semantic retrieval tasks, but also for the successful performance of many tasks, including the ability to identify a color type instead of reading a word (i.e., the Stroop task; Milham, 2001; Perret, 1974), to reduce interference during working memory, or to maintain fixation instead of making a saccade to a target (i.e., the anti-saccade task; Guitton et al., 1985). For example, we have discussed the relation between the putative selection mechanism and working memory (Thompson-Schill et al., 2002), language processing (Novick et al., 2005; Thompson-Schill, in press) and visual selective attention (Kan & Thompson-Schill, 2004).

One reason to favor a more general account is that numerous lines of evidence suggest that PFC is not organized by stimulus content or domain but rather by processing type (for a review, see D'Esposito et al., 1998; Owen, 1997). Although many of these studies have compared visual and spatial forms of working memory, we have reported a similar lack of material specificity in pLIFG in a comparison of semantic and phonological working memory (Barde & Thompson-Schill, 2002). At least one other study also has failed to find differences between phonological and semantic processing (Gold & Buckner, 2002). However, these two studies exist alongside many reports of increased pLIFG activation during phonological processing (relative to semantic processing; e.g., Poldrack et al., 1999). What accounts for this discrepancy? We believe that the so-called phonological activation may actually reflect increased selection demands in response to representational conflict during the phonological tasks. These tasks typically require subjects to make judgments about the syllable structure or vowel sounds of words, as in the cherry-rose-banana example above. Such a comparison will likely involve ignoring other forms of similarity (e.g., similarity in various semantic attribute domains) in order to focus solely on phonological similarity. It is noteworthy that the two studies which have failed to find differences between phonological and semantic tasks in pLIFG (Barde & Thompson-Schill, 2002; Gold & Buckner, 2002) are the only two reported comparisons of semantic processing of words to phonological processing of *non-words* (where conflicting semantic similarity would not be a problem).

Summary

In this review of neuroimaging studies of semantic memory, we have presented evidence for a semantic memory system in which concept representations are distributed across sensorimotor domains. Expanding on previous descriptions of these sensorimotor representations, the model we have depicted in figure 6.1 includes putative subdivisions that are emerging from neuropsychological and neuroimaging studies of perception, action, and semantic retrieval. For example, we argue for multiple representations of visual knowledge attributes that parallel distinctions made in visual neuroscience. We also propose a subdivision of action knowledge across motor domains and abstract domains of knowledge. These modifications provide a more complete description of the many sources of information that we have about concepts, and may prove useful in understanding selective breakdowns in semantic memory. We have argued that activation of information represented across these various sensorimotor domains will depend on the nature of the specific concept being retrieved (i.e., what is known about it), the input modality (i.e., what part of the distributed pattern is determined by the input), and biasing mechanisms that guide competitive interactions between representations. Consideration of these factors can be crucial for the interpretation of neuroimaging patterns across the wide variety of tasks and stimuli that we have described here. Finally, we have described how interactions between different domains (e.g., linguistic and perceptual) may alter sensorimotor representations and allow for the emergence of abstract semantic representations.

Issues

Tulving titled his 1986 response to the commentaries on his précis on the organization of memory "Episodic and semantic memory: Where should we go from here?" We might ask the same question today. And more precisely, for this volume, we ask, "Where should neuroimaging studies go from here?" Throughout this chapter, we have tried to highlight areas of inquiry that are still in need of clarification. Here, we outline a few new directions in which we believe the field is (or should be) moving. These are our predictions for three general questions about semantic memory that will be covered in the third edition of this volume.

Adapting to Change

One way to characterize the kind of information that is represented by a population of neurons is with a description of the similarity space of neural responses. Just as one can discern the function of an individual neuron by determining what stimulus variations affect its firing rate and what variations do not, so the description of a population of neurons can be informed by an understanding of the factors that determine overlap in firing patterns. In a distributed representation of some aspect of semantic memory, the similarity of two patterns will reflect the similarity between two concepts along some dimension: If you can figure out the organizing principles behind the similarity space, you will understand what properties the area represents.

Until recently, attempts to determine the population code of a region using functional neuroimaging methods seemed well beyond any hoped-for resolution of these methods. However, several investigators have made arguments about representational similarity using a technique that is referred to as "fMRI adaptation" (Grill-Spector & Malach, 2001). The logic of the approach depends on the assumption that the integrated fMRI response to a sequentially presented pair of stimuli that are representationally similar will be less than to a pair of stimuli that are representationally distinct, because in the former case, the repeated activation of the same set of neurons will produce a reduced (i.e., adapted) response (Muller et al., 1999).

This logic has been applied to studies of object and space representations in occipital and temporal cortex (Epstein et al., 2003; Grill-Spector et al., 1999; Kourtzi & Kanwisher, 2001).

There are a number questions that could be addressed using this technique. An obvious place to begin would be to characterize the similarity space of regions hypothesized to function as attribute domains in semantic memory. For example, as illustrated in figure 6.2, a region that represents color knowledge should show weaker (i.e., adapted) responses during retrieval of concepts that are the same color than it does for concepts that vary in color (but are similar in other ways). Likewise, the technique could also be used to investigate the similarity space of anterior temporal cortex, which has been described as the repository of more abstract representations. Finally, fMRI adaptation could be used to understand the phenomenon that we have referred to as the "anterior shift" in semantic representations. If this shift represents the gradual transformation from sensorimotor to abstract representa-

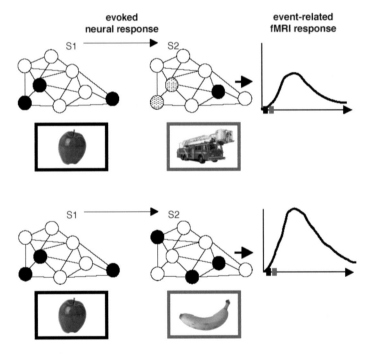

Figure 6.2
A hypothetical example of the application of fMRI adaptation to the study of semantic memory representations. In the example shown here, the fMRI response in an area that represents color knowledge (e.g., V4) should be less to a pair of stimuli with similar colors than to a pair with different colors, regardless of other similarities and differences. In contrast, the reverse pattern should be expected in an area that represents more abstract properties of objects. Figure courtesy of Russell Epstein.

Imaging of Classification Learning

Several of the tasks used most widely to study implicit learning involve the learning of novel stimulus classifications (figure 5.6). Some of these tasks are clearly similar to the perceptual skill-learning tasks described above; we have grouped them together here to emphasize the commonality in task procedures, rather than to suggest that they must share common underlying neural mechanisms.

Probabilistic Classification Learning

Probabilistic classification learning (PCL) is a paradigm in which subjects learn to classify stimuli into novel categories based on imperfect (probabilistic) feedback.

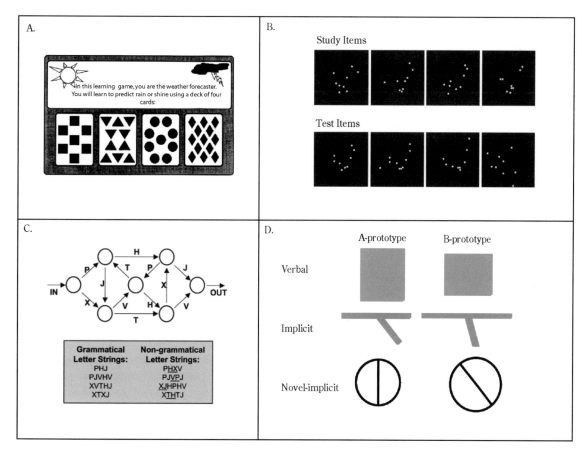

Figure 5.6
Examples of tasks used to study classification learning. (*A*) Probabilistic classification learning (from Knowlton et al., 1994). (*B*) Dot-pattern classification (from Reber et al., 1998). (*C*) Artificial grammar learning (from Skosnik et al., 2002). (*D*) Perceptual categorization (from Seger & Cincotta, 2002).

Embracing Differences

Psychologists can be divided into those who treat subject variability as noise and those who treat it as data. In the short history of functional neuroimaging, subject variability has been treated almost exclusively as noise. We hate it. We try to get rid of it. Anything to get those random-effects t-values higher!

Of course, as the "other half" could tell us, variability is noise only if you can't explain it. And, as cognitive neuroscientists have started making attempts to explain subject variability in activation patterns, they are discovering that, in many cases, it can be explained. We are now witnessing the gradual emergence of a cognitive neuroscience of individual differences: variation in V1 activation is related to contrast discrimination thresholds (Boynton et al., 1999); variation in parahippocampal cortex activation is related to navigational competence (Epstein et al., 2005); variation in amygdala activation is related to baseline mood (Schaefer et al., 2002) and personality variables (Canli et al., 2002); and variation in PFC activation is related to fluid intelligence (Gray et al., 2003). Closer to the topic of this chapter, Farah and Peronnet (1989) observed that ERP patterns evoked during mental imagery varied as a function of self-reported skill in imagery, and Kosslyn and colleagues (1996) reported PET activation in V1 that correlated with response time on a visualization task. But, by and large, investigators using neuroimaging to study semantic memory have not yet jumped on the "individual differences" bandwagon. Perhaps this is because many define semantic memory as *shared* knowledge, to distinguish it from the individual experiences that form our episodic memory. But semantic memories are shared only to the extent that our experiences are shared.

There have been occasional attempts to explain variation in behavioral category-specific effects (in normal subjects and brain-damaged patients) in terms of individual experience (Laws, 2000). For example, Wilson and colleagues (1995) described the living-things deficit of a professional musician (Patient C) who, unlike many patients with living-things deficits, displayed preserved knowledge of musical instruments; one explanation of the variation in this pattern is that a musician has more sources of information (e.g., tactile, motor) about instruments than others do, leaving the category of musical instruments less susceptible to degradation following focal damage. There are also reports of the effects of *extreme* variation in experience on neuroimaging patterns, such as that observed in comparisons of blind and sighted individuals (e.g., Burton et al., 2003; Roder et al., 2002). For example, Noppeney and colleagues (2003) compared activation during semantic retrieval in sighted and early-blind subjects. Interestingly (relevant to the point about networks above), they found similar profiles of activation but different patterns of functional connectivity within those networks that the authors attribute to an abnormal pruning process.

We observed variation during semantic retrieval that may result from slightly *less* extreme variations in experience: left- and right-handed tool use. We found that naming photographs of manipulable objects was, as expected, associated with increased activity in left inferior frontal cortex, extending from the frontal operculum to ventrolateral premotor cortex (Kan et al., 2006). Crucial to the interpretation of the premotor response, individual variation in motor experience with these objects was highly correlated with the magnitude of the response in ventrolateral premotor cortex, but not in the frontal operculum. These results provide the first demonstration of a domain-specific response in premotor cortex during retrieval of stored knowledge that is both linked to motor experience and distinguishable from domain-general cognitive control functions of prefrontal cortex.

A complete theory of the neural bases of semantic memory not only will describe the "average" semantic network but also will be able to predict individual variation around that average. It is easy to talk about the role of sensorimotor experience in the formation of a semantic network, but it is another matter to measure it, to manipulate it, and to quantify its effects. We anticipate seeing efforts to do just that in the neuroimaging of semantic memory, such as What factors predict the developmental progression to mature semantic activation patterns? How does motor experience affect object representations in dorsal and ventral visual areas? How are activation patterns during semantic retrieval related to other visuomotor competencies?

Returning to *An Essay Concerning Human Understanding*, Locke argued that individuals "come to be furnished with fewer or more simple ideas from without, according as the objects they converse with afford greater or less variety; and from the operations of their minds within, according as they more or less reflect on them" (p. 61). Variations both in our experiences with the world and in the way in which those experiences are represented should have profound, and perhaps predictable, effects on the organization and retrieval of semantic memory. A complete understanding of the representation of "shared knowledge" may depend on our ability to describe aspects of these representations that aren't shared, to characterize variations in the neural bases of semantic memory.

Acknowledgments

We would like to thank the individuals who have contributed in various ways to the ideas we have discussed in this chapter. We've talked about all of these ideas in some form or another with members of the Thompson-Schill lab, including Laura Barde, Marina Bedny, Rob Goldberg, Dawn Morales, Stacey Schaefer, Tatiana Schnur, Geeta Shivde, and numerous undergraduate research assistants. We are continually appreciative of frequent discussions and active collaborations with our colleagues at Penn, including Geoff Aguirre, David Brainard, Anjan Chatterjee, Andy Connolly, Branch Coslett, Marc Egeth, Russell Epstein, Martha Farah, Lila Gleitman, Amishi Jha, Joe Kable, Jared Novick, Marianna Stark, and John Trueswell. From farther away, we acknowledge the contributions of our collaborators, including Larry Barsalou, Laurel Buxbaum, Mark D'Esposito, John Jonides, Bob Knight, Myrna Schwartz, Ed Smith, Diane Swick, and Lynette Tippett. Finally, we are grateful to the National Institutes of Health, the Searle Scholars Program, and the University of Pennsylvania Research Foundation for the generous support of our research program.

References

Adams, R. B., & Janata, P. (2002). A comparison of neural circuits underlying auditory and visual object categorization. *NeuroImage* 16(2), 361–377.

Allport, D. A. (1985). Distributed memory, modular subsystems and dysphasia. In S. K. Newman & R. Epstein (Eds.), *Current Perspectives in Dysphasia*, 32–60. Edinburgh: Churchill Livingstone.

Barabási, A. (2002). *Linked: How Everything Is Connected to Everything Else and What It Means for Business, Science, and Everyday Life.* New York: Plume.

Barch, D. M., Braver, T. S., Sabb, F. W., & Noll, D. C. (2000). Anterior cingulate and the monitoring of response conflict: Evidence from an fMRI study of overt verb generation. *Journal of Cognitive Neuroscience* 12(2), 298–309.

Barde, L. H., & Thompson-Schill, S. L. (2002). Models of functional organization of the lateral prefrontal cortex in verbal working memory: Evidence in favor of the process model. *Journal of Cognitive Neuroscience* 14(7), 1054–1063.

Barsalou, L. W. (1999). Perceptual symbol systems. *Behavioral Brain Science* 22, 577–660.

Basso, A., Capitani, E., & Laiacona, M. (1988). Progressive language impairment without dementia: A case with isolated category specific semantic defect. *Journal of Neurology, Neurosurgery & Psychiatry* 51(9), 1201–1207.

Beauchamp, M. S., Lee, K. E., Haxby, J. V., & Martin, A. (2002). Parallel visual motion processing streams for manipulable objects and human movements. *Neuron* 34(1), 149–159. (See comment.)

Beauchamp, M. S., Lee, K. E., Haxby, J. V., & Martin, A. (2003). FMRI responses to video and point-light displays of moving humans and manipulable objects. *Journal of Cognitive Neuroscience* 15(7), 991–1001.

Beauregard, M., Chertkow, H., Bub, D., Murtha, S., Dixon, R., & Evans, A. (1997). The neural substrate for concrete, abstract, and emotional word lexica: A positron emission tomography study. *Journal of Cognitive Neuroscience* 9, 441–461.

Beauvois, M. F. (1982). Optic aphasia: A process of interaction between vision and language. *Philosophical Transactions of the Royal Society of London*, B298, 35–47.

Binkofski, F., Buccino, G., Posse, S., Seitz, R. J., Rizzolatti, G., & Freund, H. (1999). A fronto-parietal circuit for object manipulation in man: Evidence from an fMRI-study. *European Journal of Neuroscience* 11(9), 3276–3286.

Binkofski, F., Buccino, G., Stephan, K. M., Rizzolatti, G., Seitz, R. J., & Freund, H. J. (1999). A parieto-premotor network for object manipulation: Evidence from neuroimaging. *Experimental Brain Research* 128(1–2), 210–213.

Bokde, A. L., Tagamets, M. A., Friedman, R. B., & Horwitz, B. (2001). Functional interactions of the inferior frontal cortex during the processing of words and word-like stimuli. *Neuron* 30(2), 609–617.

Bonda, E., Petrides, M., Ostry, D., & Evans, A. (1996). Specific involvement of human parietal systems and the amygdala in the perception of biological motion. *Journal of Neuroscience* 16(11), 3737–3744.

Bookheimer, S. Y., Zeffiro, T. A., Blaxton, T., Gaillard, W., & Theodore, W. (1995). Regional cerebral blood flow during object naming and word reading. *Human Brain Mapping* 3, 93–106.

Borgo, F., & Shallice, T. (2001). When living things and other "sensory quality" categories behave in the same fashion: A novel category specificity effect. *Neurocase* 7, 201–220.

Boronat, C. B., Buxbaum, L. J., Coslett, H. B., Tang, K., Saffran, E. M., Kimberg, D. Y., & Detre, J. A. (2005). Distinctions between manipulation and function knowledge of objects: Evidence from functional magnetic resonance imaging. *Cognitive Brain Research* 23, 361–373.

Botvinick, M. M., Braver, T. S., Barch, D. M., Carter, C. S., & Cohen, J. D. (2001). Conflict monitoring and cognitive control. *Psychological Review* 108(3), 624–652.

Boynton, G. M., Demb, J. B., Glover, G. H., & Heeger, D. J. (1999). Neuronal basis of contrast discrimination. *Vision Research* 39(2), 257–269.

Breedin, S. D., Saffran, E. M., & Coslett, H. B. (1994). Reversal of the concreteness effect in a patient with semantic dementia. *Cognitive Neuropsychology* 11, 617–660.

Bright, P., Moss, H., & Tyler, L. K. (2004). Unitary vs multiple semantics: PET studies of word and picture processing. *Brain and Language* 89, 417–432.

Bub, D., Black, S., Hampson, E., & Kertesz, A. (1988). Semantic encoding of pictures and words: Some neuropsychological observations. *Cognitive Neuropsychology* 5(1), 27–66.

Buccino, G., Binkofski, F., Fink, G. R., Fadiga, L., Fogassi, L., Gallese, V., et al. (2001). Action observation activates premotor and parietal areas in a somatotopic manner: An fMRI study. *European Journal of Neuroscience* 13(2), 400–404.

Buccino, G., Lui, F., Canessa, N., Patteri, I., Lagravinese, G., Benuzzi, F., et al. (2004). Neural circuits involved in the recognition of actions performed by nonconspecifics: An fMRI study. *Journal of Cognitive Neuroscience* 16(1), 114–126.

Buckner, R. L., Petersen, S. E., Ojemann, J. G., Miezin, F. M., Squire, L. R., & Raichle, M. E. (1995). Functional anatomical studies of explicit and implicit memory retrieval tasks. *Journal of Neuroscience* 15(1), 12–29.

Burton, H., Diamond, J. B., & McDermott, K. B. (2003). Dissociating cortical regions activated by semantic and phonological tasks: A fMRI study in blind and sighted people. *Journal of Neurophysiology* 90(3), 1965–1982.

Buxbaum, L. J., & Saffran, E. M. (1998). Knowing "how" vs. "what for": A new dissociation. *Brain and Language* 65, 73–86.

Buxbaum, L. J., Veramonti, T., & Schwartz, M. F. (2000). Function and manipulation tool knowledge in apraxia: Knowing "what for" but not "how." *Neurocase* 6, 83–97.

Calvert, G. A., Bullmore, E. T., Brammer, M. J., Campbell, R., Williams, S. C., McGuire, P. K., et al. (1997). Activation of auditory cortex during silent lipreading. *Science* 276(5312), 593–596.

Calvert, G. A., & Campbell, R. (2003). Reading speech from still and moving faces: The neural substrates of visible speech. *Journal of Cognitive Neuroscience* 15(1), 57–70.

Campbell, R., MacSweeney, M., Surguladze, S., Calvert, G., McGuire, P., Suckling, J., et al. (2001). Cortical substrates for the perception of face actions: An fMRI study of the specificity of activation for seen speech and for meaningless lower-face acts (gurning). *Cognitive Brain Research* 12(2), 233–243.

Canli, T., Sivers, H., Whitfield, S. L., Gotlib, I. H., & Gabrieli, J. D. (2002). Amygdala response to happy faces as a function of extraversion. *Science* 296(5576), 2191.

Capitani, E., Laiacona, M., Mahon, B., & Caramazza, A. (2003). What are the facts of semantic category-specific deficits? A critical review of the evidence. *Cognitive Neuropsychology* 20, 213–261.

Cappa, S. F., Perani, D., Schnur, T., Tettamanti, M., & Fazio, F. (1998). The effects of semantic category and knowledge type on lexical-semantic access: A PET study. *NeuroImage* 8(4), 350–359.

Caramazza, A. (2000). Minding the facts: A comment on Thompson-Schill et al.'s "A neural basis for category and modality specificity of semantic knowledge." *Neuropsychologia* 38(7), 944–949. (comment.)

Caramazza, A., Hillis, A. E., Rapp, B. C., & Romani, C. (1990). The multiple semantics hypothesis: Multiple confusions? *Cognitive Neuropsychology* 7, 161–189.

Caramazza, A., & Shelton, J. R. (1998). Domain-specific knowledge systems in the brain: The animate-inanimate distinction. *Journal of Cognitive Neuroscience* 10(1), 1–34.

Cerf-Ducastel, B., & Murphy, C. (2003). fMRI brain activation in response to odors is reduced in primary olfactory areas of elderly subjects. *Brain Research* 986(1–2), 39–53.

Chainay, H., & Humphreys, G. W. (2002). Privileged access to action for objects relative to words. *Psychonomic Bulletin & Review* 9(2), 348–355.

Chao, L., Haxby, J. V., & Martin, A. (1999). Attribute-based neural substrates in temporal cortex for perceiving and knowing about objects. *Nature Neuroscience* 2, 913–919.

Chao, L., & Martin, A. (1999). Cortical regions associated with perceiving, naming, and knowing about colors. *Journal of Cognitive Neuroscience* 11(1), 25–35.

Chao, L., & Martin, A. (2000). Representation of manipulable man-made objects in the dorsal stream. *NeuroImage* 12, 478–484.

Charlot, V., Tzourio, N., Zilbovicius, M., Mazoyer, B., & Denis, M. (1992). Different mental imagery abilities result in different regional cerebral blood flow activation patterns during cognitive tasks. *Neuropsychologia* 30, 565–580.

Coltheart, M., Inglis, L., Cupples, L., Michie, P., Bates, A., & Budd, B. (1998). A semantic subsystem of visual attributes. *Neurocase* 4, 353–370.

Crutch, S. J., & Warrington, E. K. (2003). The selective impairment of fruit and vegetable knowledge: A multiple processing channels account of fine-grain category specificity. *Cognitive Neuropsychology* 20, 355–372.

D'Esposito, M., Aguirre, G. K., Zarahn, E., Ballard, D., Shin, R. K., & Lease, J. (1998). Functional MRI studies of spatial and nonspatial working memory. *Cognitive Brain Research* 7(1), 1–13.

D'Esposito, M., Detre, J. A., Aguirre, G. K., Stallcup, M., Alsop, D. C., Tippet, L. J., et al. (1997). A functional MRI study of mental image generation. *Neuropsychologia* 35(5), 725–730.

Dade, L. A., Jones-Gotman, M., Zatorre, R. J., & Evans, A. C. (1998). Human brain function during odor encoding and recognition. A PET activation study. *Annals of the New York Academy of Sciences* 855, 572–574.

Dalla Barba, G., Parlato, V., Jobert, A., Samson, Y., & Pappata, S. (1998). Cortical networks implicated in semantic and episodic memory: Common or unique? *Cortex* 34(4), 547–561.

Damasio, A. R. (1989). The brain binds entities and events by multiregional activation from convergence zones. *Neural Computation* 1, 123–132.

Damasio, A. R., McKee, J., & Damasio, H. (1979). Determinants of performance in color anomia. *Brain & Language* 7(1), 74–85.

Damasio, H., Grabowski, T. J., Tranel, D., Hichwa, R. D., & Damasio, A. R. (1996). A neural basis for lexical retrieval. *Nature* 380(6574), 499–505. (See comments.) Published erratum appears in *Nature* 381(6595) (1996), 810.

De Renzi, E., & Lucchelli, F. (1994). Are semantic systems separately represented in the brain? The case of living category impairment. *Cortex* 30, 3–25.

De Volder, A. G., Toyama, H., Kimura, Y., Kiyosawa, M., Nakano, H., Vanlierde, A., et al. (2001). Auditory triggered mental imagery of shape involves visual association areas in early blind humans. *NeuroImage* 14(11), 129–139.

Decety, J. (1996). Do imagined and executed actions share the same neural substrate? *Cognitive Brain Research* 3(2), 87–93.

Decety, J., Grezes, J., Costes, N., Perani, D., Jeannerod, M., Procyk, E., et al. (1997). Brain activity during observation of actions: Influence of action content and subject's strategy. *Brain* 120(10), 1763–1777.

Decety, J., Perani, D., Jeannerod, M., Bettinardi, V., Tadary, B., Woods, R., et al. (1994). Mapping motor representations with positron emission tomography. *Nature* 371, 600–602.

Dennis, M. (1976). Dissociated naming and locating of body parts after left anterior temporal lobe resection: An experimental case study. *Brain and Language* 3, 147–163.

Devlin, J. T., Russell, R. P., Davis, M. H., Price, C. J., Moss, H. E., Fadili, M. J., et al. (2002). Is there an anatomical basis for category-specificity? Semantic memory studies in PET and fMRI. *Neuropsychologia* 40(1), 54–75.

Downing, P. E., Jiang, Y., Shuman, M., & Kanwisher, N. (2001). A cortical area selective for visual processing of the human body. *Science* 293(5539), 2470–2473. (See comment.)

Epstein, R., Graham, K. S., & Downing, P. E. (2003). Viewpoint-specific scene representations in human parahippocampal cortex. *Neuron* 37(5), 865–876.

Epstein, R., Higgins, J. S., & Thompson-Schill, S. L. (2005). Learning places from views: Variation in scene processing as a function of experience and navigational ability. *Journal of Cognitive Neuroscience* 17, 73–83.

Epstein, R., & Kanwisher, N. (1998). A cortical representation of the local visual environment. *Nature* 392(6676), 598–601.

Farah, M. J. (2000). *The Cognitive Neuroscience of Vision.* Malden, MA: Blackwell.

Farah, M. J., & McClelland, J. L. (1991). A computational model of semantic memory impairment: Modality specificity and emergent category specificity. *Journal of Experimental Psychology: General* 120(4), 339–357.

Farah, M. J., McMullen, P. A., & Meyer, M. M. (1991). Can recognition of living things be selectively impaired? *Neuropsychologia* 29, 185–193.

Farah, M. J., & Peronnet, F. (1989). Event-related potentials in the study of mental imagery. *Journal of Psychophysiology* 3, 99–109.

Farah, M. J., Peronnet, F., Gonon, M. A., & Giard, M. H. (1988). Electrophysiological evidence for a shared representational medium for visual images and visual percepts. *Journal of Experimental Psychology: General* 117(3), 248–257.

Fletcher, P. C., Shallice, T., & Dolan, R. J. (2000). "Sculpting the response space"—an account of left prefrontal activation at encoding. *NeuroImage* 12(4), 404–417.

Gabrieli, J. D., Cohen, N. J., & Corkin, S. (1988). The impaired learning of semantic knowledge following bilateral medial temporal-lobe resection. *Brain and Cognition* 7(2), 157–177.

Gabrieli, J. D., Poldrack, R. A., & Desmond, J. E. (1998). The role of left prefrontal cortex in language and memory. *Proceedings of the National Academy of Sciences USA* 95(3), 906–913.

Galton, C. J., Patterson, K., Graham, K., Lambon-Ralph, M. A., Williams, G., Antoun, N., et al. (2001). Differing patterns of temporal atrophy in Alzheimer's disease and semantic dementia. *Neurology* 57(2), 216–225.

Ganis, G., Thompson, W. L., & Kosslyn, S. M. (2004). Brain areas underlying visual mental imagery and visual perception: An fMRI study. *Cognitive Brain Research* 20, 226–241.

Gentner, D. (1978). On relational meaning: The acquisition of verb meaning. *Child Development* 49(4), 988–998.

Gerlach, C., Law, I., Gade, A., & Paulson, O. B. (2002). The role of action knowledge in the comprehension of artefacts—a PET study. *NeuroImage* 15(1), 143–152.

Gerlach, C., Law, I., & Paulson, O. B. (2002). When action turns into words: Activation of motor-based knowledge during categorization of manipulable objects. *Journal of Cognitive Neuroscience* 14(8), 1230–1239.

Gibson, J. J. (1979). *The Ecological Approach to Visual Perception.* Boston: Houghton Mifflin.

Gold, B. T., & Buckner, R. L. (2002). Common prefrontal regions coactivate with dissociable posterior regions during controlled semantic and phonological tasks. *Neuron* 35(4), 803–812.

Goldberg, R. F., Perfetti, C. A., & Schneider, W. (2004). *The role of left inferior prefrontal cortex in semantic processing.* Paper presented at the Eleventh Annual Meeting of the Cognitive Neuroscience Society, San Francisco.

Goldenberg, G., Podreka, I., Steiner, M., Franzen, P., & Deecke, L. (1991). Contributions of occipital and temporal brain regions to visual and acoustic imagery—a spect study. *Neuropsychologia* 29(7), 695–702.

Goldenberg, G., Podreka, I., Steiner, M., & Willmes, K. (1987). Patterns of regional cerebral blood flow related to memorizing of high and low imagery words: An emission computer tomography study. *Neuropsychologia* 25(3), 473–485.

Goodale, M. A., & Milner, A. D. (1992). Separate visual pathways for perception and action. *Trends in Neurosciences* 15, 20–25.

Goodglass, H., Klein, B., Carey, P., & Jones, K. J. (1966). Specific semantic word categories in aphasia. *Cortex* 2, 74–89.

Grabowski, T. J., Damasio, H., & Damasio, A. R. (1998). Premotor and prefrontal correlates of category-related lexical retrieval. *NeuroImage* 7, 232–243.

Grafton, S. T., Arbib, M. A., Fadiga, L., & Rizzolatti, G. (1996). Localization of grasp representations in humans by positron emission tomography. 2. Observation compared with imagination. *Experimental Brain Research* 112(1), 103–111.

Grafton, S. T., Fadiga, L., Arbib, M. A., & Rizzolatti, G. (1997). Premotor cortex activation during observation and naming of familiar tools. *NeuroImage* 6, 231–236.

Graham, K. S., Simons, J. S., Pratt, K. H., Patterson, K., & Hodges, J. R. (2000). Insights from semantic dementia on the relationship between episodic and semantic memory. *Neuropsychologia* 38(3), 313–324.

Gray, J. R., Chabris, C. F., & Braver, T. S. (2003). Neural mechanisms of general fluid intelligence. *Nature Neuroscience* 6(3), 316–322. (See comment.)

Grèzes, J., & Decety, J. (2001). Functional anatomy of execution, mental simulation, observation, and verb generation of actions: A meta-analysis. *Human Brain Mapping* 12(1), 1–19.

Grèzes, J., Fonlupt, P., Bertenthal, B., Delon-Martin, C., Segebarth, C., & Decety, J. (2001). Does perception of biological motion rely on specific brain regions? *NeuroImage* 13(5), 775–785.

Grill-Spector, K., Kushnir, T., Edelman, S., Avidan, G., Itzchak, Y., & Malach, R. (1999). Differential processing of objects under various viewing conditions in the human lateral occipital complex. *Neuron* 24(1), 187–203.

Grill-Spector, K., & Malach, R. (2001). fMR-adaptation: A tool for studying the functional properties of human cortical neurons. *Acta Psychologica* (Amsterdam), 107(1–3), 293–321.

Grossman, E., Donnelly, M., Price, R., Pickens, D., Morgan, V., Neighbor, G., et al. (2000). Brain areas involved in perception of biological motion. *Journal of Cognitive Neuroscience* 12(5), 711–720.

Grossman, M., Koenig, P., DeVita, C., Glosser, G., Alsop, D., Detre, J., et al. (2002). The neural basis for category-specific knowledge: An fMRI study. *NeuroImage* 15(4), 936–948.

Guitton, D., Buchtel, H. A., & Douglas, R. M. (1985). Frontal lobe lesions in man cause difficulties in suppressing reflexive glances and in generating goal-directed saccades. *Experimental Brain Research* 58, 455–472.

Hart, J., Berndt, R. S., & Caramazza, A. (1985). Category-specific naming deficit following cerebral infarction. *Nature* 316, 439–440.

Haxby, J. V., Gobbini, M. I., Furey, M. L., Ishai, A., Schouten, J. L., & Pietrini, P. (2001). Distributed and overlapping representations of faces and objects in ventral temporal cortex. *Science* 293(5539), 2425–2430. (See comment.)

Hodges, J. R., Patterson, K., & Tyler, L. K. (1994). Loss of semantic memory: Implications for the modularity of mind. *Cognitive Neuropsychology* 11(5), 505–542.

Howard, R. J., Brammer, M., Wright, I., Woodruff, P. W., Bullmore, E. T., & Zeki, S. (1996). A direct demonstration of functional specialization within motion-related visual and auditory cortex of the human brain. *Current Biology* 6(8), 1015–1019.

Howard, R. J., ffytche, D. H., Barnes, J., McKeefry, D., Ha, Y., Woodruff, P. W., et al. (1998). The functional anatomy of imagining and perceiving colour. *NeuroReport* 9, 1019–1023.

Ishai, A., Ungerleider, L. G., Martin, A., & Haxby, J. V. (2000). The representation of objects in the human occipital and temporal cortex. *Journal of Cognitive Neuroscience* 12(supp. 2), 35–51.

Ishai, A., Ungerleider, L. G., Martin, A., Schouten, J. L., & Haxby, J. V. (1999). Distributed representation of objects in the human ventral visual pathway. *Proceedings of the National Academy of Sciences USA* 96(16), 9379–9384.

Kable, J. W., Lease-Spellmeyer, J., & Chatterjee, A. (2002). Neural substrates of action event knowledge. *Journal of Cognitive Neuroscience* 14(5), 795–805.

Kan, I. P., Barsalou, L. W., Solomon, K. O., Minor, J. K., & Thompson-Schill, S. L. (2003). Role of mental imagery in a property verification task: fMRI evidence for perceptual representations of conceptual knowledge. *Cognitive Neuropsychology* 20, 525–540.

Kan, I. P., Kable, J. W., Van Scoyoc, A., Chatterjee, A., & Thompson-Schill, S. L. (2006). Fractionating left frontal response to tools: Dissociable effects of selection and action. *Journal of Cognitive Neuroscience* 18.

Kan, I. P., & Thompson-Schill, S. L. (2004). Effect of name agreement on prefrontal activity during overt and covert picture naming. *Cognitive, Affective, & Behavioral Neuroscience* 4, 43–57.

Kan, I. P., & Thompson-Schill, S. L. (2004). Selection from perceptual and conceptual representations. *Cognitive, Affective, & Behavioral Neuroscience* 4, 466–482.

Kanwisher, N., & Duncan, J. (Eds.). (2003). *Attention and Performance XX: Functional Neuroimaging of Visual Cognition.* Oxford: Oxford University Press.

Kanwisher, N., McDermott, J., & Chun, M. M. (1997). The fusiform face area: A module in human extrastriate cortex specialized for face perception. *Journal of Neuroscience* 17(11), 4302–4311.

Karaken, D. A., Mosnik, D. M. M., Doty, R. L., Dzemidzic, M., & Hutchins, G. D. (2003). Functional anatomy of human odor sensation, discrimination, and identification in health and aging. *Neuropsychology* 17(3), 482–495.

Kellenbach, M. L., Brett, M., & Patterson, K. (2001). Large, colorful or noisy? Attribute- and modality-specific activations during retrieval of perceptual attribute knowledge. *Cognitive, Affective, & Behavioral Neuroscience* 1(3), 207–221.

Kellenbach, M. L., Brett, M., & Patterson, K. (2003). Actions speak louder than functions: The importance of manipulability and action in tool representation. *Journal of Cognitive Neuroscience* 15(1), 30–46.

Kiehl, K. A., Liddle, P. F., Smith, A. M., Mendrek, A., Forster, B. B., & Hare, R. D. (1999). Neural pathways involved in the processing of concrete and abstract words. *Human Brain Mapping* 7(4), 225–233.

Konorski, J. (1967). *Integrative Activity of the Brain.* Chicago: University of Chicago Press.

Kosslyn, S. M. (1980). *Image and Mind.* Cambridge, MA: Harvard University Press.

Kosslyn, S. M., Alpert, N. M., Thompson, W. L., Maljkovic, V., Weise, S., Chabris, C. F., et al. (1993). Visual mental imagery activates topographically organized visual cortex: PET investigations. *Cognition* 5, 139–181.

Kosslyn, S. M., Pascual-Leone, A., Felician, O., Camposano, S., Keenan, J. P., Thompson, W. L., et al. (1999). The role of area 17 in visual imagery: Convergent evidence from PET and rTMS. [erratum appears in Science 1999 May 7;284(5416):197]. *Science* 284(5411), 167–170. (See comment.) Erratum appears in *Science* 284(5416) (1999), 197.

Kosslyn, S. M., & Thompson, W. L. (2000). Shared mechanisms in visual imagery and visual perception: Insights from cognitive neuroscience. In M. S. Gazzaniga (Ed.), *The New Cognitive Neurosciences*, 2nd ed., 975–985. Cambridge, MA: MIT Press.

Kosslyn, S. M., Thompson, W. L., Kim, I. J., Rauch, S. L., & Alpert, N. M. (1996). Individual differences in cerebral blood flow in area 17 predict the time to evaluate visualized letters. *Journal of Cognitive Neuroscience* 8, 78–82.

Kourtzi, Z., & Kanwisher, N. (2001). Representation of perceived object shape by the human lateral occipital complex. *Science* 293(5534), 1506–1509.

Lambon-Ralph, M. A., & Howard, D. (2000). Gogi aphasia or semantic dementia? Simulating and accessing poor verbal comprehension in a case of progressive fluent aphasia. *Cognitive Neuropsychology* 17, 437–465.

Laws, K. R. (2000). Category-specific naming errors in normal subjects: The influence of evolution and experience. *Brain & Language* 75(1), 123–133.

Lee, A. C., Graham, K. S., Simons, J. S., Hodges, J. R., Owen, A. M., & Patterson, K. (2002). Regional brain activations differ for semantic features but not categories. *NeuroReport* 13(12), 1497–1501.

Lee, A. C., Robbins, T. W., Graham, K. S., & Owen, A. M. (2002). "Pray or Prey?" Dissociation of semantic memory retrieval from episodic memory processes using positron emission tomography and a novel homophone task. *NeuroImage* 16(3, pt 1), 724–735.

Levy, L. M., Henkin, R. I., Lin, C. S., Finley, A., & Schellinger, D. (1999). Taste memory induces brain activation as revealed by functional MRI. *Journal of Computer Assisted Tomography* 23(4), 499–505.

Lewis, C. S. (1989). *A Grief Observed*. New York: HarperCollins.

Locke, J. (1690/1995). *An Essay Concerning Human Understanding*. New York: Prometheus Books.

Maguire, E. A., & Frith, C. D. (2004). The brain network associated with acquiring semantic knowledge. *NeuroImage* 22(1), 171–178.

Margolis, E., & Laurence, S. (Eds.). (1999). *Concepts: Core Readings*. Cambridge, MA: MIT Press.

Martin, A. (2001). Functional neuroimaging of semantic memory. In R. Cabeza & A. Kingstone (Eds.), *Handbook of Functional Neuroimaging of Cognition*, 153–186. Cambridge, MA: MIT Press.

Martin, A., & Caramazza, A. (2003). Neuropsychological and neuroimaging perspectives on conceptual knowledge: An introduction. *Cognitive Neuropsychology* 20, 195–212.

Martin, A., Haxby, J. V., Lalonde, F. M., Wiggs, C. L., & Ungerleider, L. G. (1995). Discrete cortical regions associated with knowledge of color and knowledge of action. *Science* 270(5233), 102–105.

Martin, A., Ungerleider, L. G., & Haxby, J. V. (2000). Category-specificity and the brain: The sensory-motor model of semantic representations of objects. In M. S. Gazzaniga (Ed.), *The Cognitive Neurosciences*, 2nd ed. Cambridge MA: MIT Press.

Martin, A., Wiggs, C. L., Ungerleider, L. G., & Haxby, J. V. (1996). Neural correlates of category-specific knowledge. *Nature* 379, 649–652.

Mayes, A. R., Montaldi, D., Spencer, T. J., & Roberts, N. (2004). Recalling spatial information as a component of recently and remotely acquired episodic or semantic memories: An fMRI study. *Neuropsychology* 18(3), 426–441.

McClelland, J. L., & Rogers, T. T. (2003). The parallel distributed processing approach to semantic cognition. *Nature Reviews Neuroscience* 4(4), 310–322.

McKenna, P., & Warrington, E. K. (1980). Testing for nominal dysphasia. *Journal of Neurology, Neurosurgery & Psychiatry* 43(9), 781–788.

Milham, M. P., Banich, M. T., Webb, A., Barad, V., Cohen, N. J., Wszalek, T., & Kramer, A. F. (2001). The relative involvement of anterior cingulate and prefrontal cortex in attentional control depends on nature of conflict. *Cognitive Brain Research* 12, 467–473.

Miller, E. K., & Cohen, J. D. (2001). An integrative theory of prefrontal cortex function. *Annual Review of Neuroscience* 24, 167–202.

Moore, C. J., & Price, C. (1999). Three distinct ventral occipitotemporal regions for reading and object naming. *NeuroImage* 10, 181–192.

Muller, J. R., Metha, A. B., Krauskopf, J., & Lennie, P. (1999). Rapid adaptation in visual cortex to the structure of images. *Science* 285(5432), 1405–1408.

Mummery, C. J., Patterson, K., Hodges, J. R., & Price, C. J. (1998). Functional neuroanatomy of the semantic system: Divisible by what? *Journal of Cognitive Neuroscience* 10(6), 766–777.

Mummery, C. J., Patterson, K., Hodges, J. R., & Wise, R. J. (1996). Generating "tiger" as an animal name or a word beginning with T: Differences in brain activation. *Proceedings of the Royal Society of London* B263(1373), 989–995. Erratum published in *Proceedings of the Royal Society of London* B263(1377) (1996), 1755–1756.

Murata, A., Gallese, V., Luppino, G., Kaseda, M., & Sakata, H. (2000). Selectivity for the shape, size, and orientation of objects for grasping in neurons of monkey parietal area AIP. *Journal of Neurophysiology* 83(5), 2580–2601.

Nelson, K. (1974). Concept, word, and sentence: Interrelations in acquisition and development. *Psychological Review* 81(4), 267–285.

Nielsen, J. M. (1936). *Agnosia, Apraxia, and Aphasia: Their Value in Cerebral Localization.* New York: Paul Hoeber.

Noppeney, U., Friston, K. J., & Price, C. J. (2003). Effects of visual deprivation on the organization of the semantic system. *Brain* 126(7), 1620–1627.

Noppeney, U., & Price, C. J. (2002). Retrieval of visual, auditory, and abstract semantics. *NeuroImage* 15(4), 917–926.

Noppeney, U., & Price, C. J. (2003). Functional imaging of the semantic system: Retrieval of sensory-experienced and verbally learned knowledge. *Brain & Language* 84(1), 120–133.

Noppeney, U., & Price, C. J. (2004). Retrieval of abstract semantics. *NeuroImage* 22(1), 164–170.

Novick, J. M., Trueswell, J. C., & Thompson-Schill, S. L. (2005). Toward the neural basis of parsing: Prefrontal cortex and the role of selectional processes in language. *Cognitive, Affective, & Behavioral Neuroscience* 5, 263–281.

Nyberg, L., Marklund, P., Persson, J., Cabeza, R., Forkstam, C., Petersson, K. M., et al. (2003). Common prefrontal activations during working memory, episodic memory, and semantic memory. *Neuropsychologia* 41(3), 371–377.

Olesen, P. J., Nagy, Z., Westerberg, H., & Klingberg, T. (2003). Combined analysis of DTI and fMRI data reveals a joint maturation of white and grey matter in a fronto-parietal network. *Cognitive Brain Research* 18(1), 48–57.

Oliver, R. T., Coslett, H. B., Wolk, D., Geiger, E. J., & Thompson-Schill, S. L. (2004). *What does the parietal lobe know about objects?* Paper presented at the Annual Meeting of the Cognitive Neuroscience Society, San Francisco.

Oliver, R. T., & Thompson-Schill, S. L. (2003). Dorsal stream activation during retrieval of object size and shape. *Cognitive, Affective & Behavioral Neuroscience* 3(4), 309–322.

Owen, A. (1997). The functional organization of working memory processes within human lateral frontal cortex: The contribution of functional neuroimaging. *European Journal of Neuroscience* 9, 1329–1339.

Paivio, A. (1971). *Imagery and Verbal Processes.* New York: Holt, Rinehart, and Winston.

Pelphrey, K. A., Singerman, J. D., Allison, T., & McCarthy, G. (2003). Brain activation evoked by perception of gaze shifts: The influence of context. *Neuropsychologia*, 41(2), 156–170. Erratum appears in *Neuropsychologia* 41(11) (2003), 1561–1562.

Perani, D., Cappa, S. F., Bettinardi, V., Bressi, S., Gorno-Tempini, M., Matarrese, M., et al. (1995). Different neural systems for the recognition of animals and man-made tools. *NeuroReport* 6(12), 1637–1641.

Perani, D., Schnur, T., Tettamanti, M., Gorno-Tempini, M., Cappa, S. F., & Fazio, F. (1999). Word and picture matching: A PET study of semantic category effects. *Neuropsychologia* 37, 293–306.

Perret, E. (1974). The left frontal lobe of man and the suppression of habitual responses in verbal categorical behavior. *Neuropsychologia* 12, 323–330.

Petersen, S. E., Fox, P. T., Posner, M. I., Mintun, M., & Raichle, M. E. (1988). Positron emission tomographic studies of the cortical anatomy of single-word processing. *Nature* 331(6157), 585–589.

Petrides, M., & Pandya, D. N. (2002). Comparative cytoarchitectonic analysis of the human and the macaque ventrolateral prefrontal cortex and corticocortical connection patterns in the monkey. *European Journal of Neuroscience* 16(2), 291–310.

Peuskens, H., Claeys, K. G., Todd, J. T., Norman, J. F., Van Hecke, P., & Orban, G. A. (2004). Attention to 3-D shape, 3-D motion, and texture in 3-D structure from motion displays. *Journal of Cognitive Neuroscience* 16(4), 665–682.

Pietrini, P., Furey, M. L., Ricciardi, E., Gobbini, M. I., Wu, W. H., Cohen, L., et al. (2004). Beyond sensory images: Object-based representation in the human ventral pathway. *Proceedings of the National Academy of Sciences USA* 101(15), 5658–5663.

Pilgrim, L. K., Fadili, J., Fletcher, P., & Tyler, L. K. (2002). Overcoming confounds of stimulus blocking: An event-related fMRI design of semantic processing. *NeuroImage* 16(3, pt 1), 713–723.

Platel, H., Baron, J. C., Desgranges, B., Bernard, F., & Eustache, F. (2003). Semantic and episodic memory of music are subserved by distinct neural networks. *NeuroImage* 20(1), 244–256.

Plaut, D. C. (2002). Graded modality-specific specialization in semantics: A computational account of optic aphasia. *Cognitive Neuropsychology* 19, 603–639.

Poldrack, R. A., Wagner, A. D., Prull, M. W., Desmond, J. E., Glover, G. H., & Gabrieli, J. D. E. (1999). Functional specialization for semantic and phonological processing in the left inferior prefrontal cortex. *NeuroImage* 10(1), 15–35.

Postler, J., De Bleser, R., Cholewa, J., Glauche, V., Hamzei, F., & Weiller, C. (2003). Neuroimaging of the semantic system(s). *Aphasiology* 17(9), 799–814.

Price, C. J., Mummery, C. J., Moore, C. J., Frakowiak, R. S., & Friston, K. J. (1999). Delineating necessary and sufficient neural systems with functional imaging studies of neuropsychological patients. *Journal of Cognitive Neuroscience* 11(4), 371–382.

Puce, A., Allison, T., Bentin, S., Gore, J. C., & McCarthy, G. (1998). Temporal cortex activation in humans viewing eye and mouth movements. *Journal of Neuroscience* 18(6), 2188–2199.

Pulvermuller, F., Harle, M., & Hummel, F. (2001). Walking or talking? Behavioral and neurophysiological correlates of action verb processing. *Brain & Language* 78(2), 143–168.

Pylyshyn, Z. W. (1981). The imagery debate: Analogue media versus tacit knowledge. *Psychological Review* 88, 16–45.

Qureshy, A., Kawashima, R., Imran, M. B., Sugiura, M., Goto, R., Okada, K., et al. (2000). Functional mapping of human brain in olfactory processing: A PET study. *Journal of Neurophysiology* 84(3), 1656–1666.

Riddoch, M. J., & Humphreys, G. W. (1987). A case of integrative visual agnosia. *Brain* 110, 1431–1462.

Rizzolatti, G., Fadiga, L., Gallese, V., & Fogassi, L. (1996). Premotor cortex and the recognition of motor actions. *Cognitive Brain Research* 3(2), 131–141.

Roder, B., Stock, O., Bien, S., Neville, H., & Rosler, F. (2002). Speech processing activates visual cortex in congenitally blind humans. *European Journal of Neuroscience* 16(5), 930–936.

Rogers, T. T., Hocking, J., Mechelli, A., Patterson, K., & Price, C. (2005). Fusiform activation to animals is driven by the process, not the stimulus. *Journal of Cognitive Neuroscience* 17, 434–445.

Rogers, T. T., Lambon-Ralph, M. A., Garrard, P., Bozeat, S., McClelland, J. L., Hodges, J. R., et al. (2004). Structure and deterioration of semantic memory: A neuropsychological and computational investigation. *Psychological Review* 111(1), 205–235.

Roland, P. E., & Friberg, L. (1985). Localization of cortical areas activated by thinking. *Journal of Neurophysiology* 53, 1219–1243.

Rosch, E., Mervis, C. B., Gray, W., Johnson, D., & Boyes-Braem, P. (1976). Basic objects in natural categories. *Cognitive Psychology* 8, 382–439.

Roskies, A. L., Fiez, J. A., Balota, D. A., Raichle, M. E., & Petersen, S. E. (2001). Task-dependent modulation of regions in the left inferior frontal cortex during semantic processing. *Journal of Cognitive Neuroscience* 13(6), 829–843.

Royet, J. P., Koenig, O., Gregoire, M. C., Cinotti, L., Lavenne, F., Le Bars, D., et al. (1999). Functional anatomy of perceptual and semantic processing for odors. *Journal of Cognitive Neuroscience* 11(1), 94–109.

Ruby, P., & Decety, J. (2001). Effect of subjective perspective taking during simulation of action: A PET investigation of agency. *Nature Neuroscience* 4(5), 546–550.

Saffran, E. M., Coslett, H. B., & Keener, M. T. (2003). Differences in word associations to pictures and words. *Neuropsychologia* 41, 1541–1546.

Saffran, E. M., & Schwartz, M. F. (1994). Of cabbages and things: Semantic memory from a neuropsychological perspective—A tutorial review. In C. M. M. Umiltà (Ed.), *Attention and Performance XV: Conscious and Nonconscious Information Processing*, 507–536. Cambridge, MA: MIT Press.

Schaefer, S. M., Jackson, D. C., Davidson, R. J., Aguirre, G. K., Kimberg, D. Y., & Thompson-Schill, S. L. (2002). Modulation of amygdalar activity by the conscious regulation of negative emotion. *Journal of Cognitive Neuroscience* 14(6), 913–921.

Schreuder, R., Flores D'Arcais, G. B., & Glazenborg, G. (1984). Effects of perceptual and conceptual similarity in semantic priming. *Psychological Research* 45, 339–354.

Shallice, T. (1988). *From Neuropsychology to Mental Structure.* New York: Cambridge University Press.

Silveri, M. C., & Gainotti, G. (1988). Interaction between vision and language in category-specific semantic impairment. *Cognitive Neuropsychology* 5, 677–709.

Simmons, W. K., & Barsalou, L. W. (2003). The similarity-in-topography principle: Reconciling theories of conceptual deficits. *Cognitive Neuropsychology* 20, 451–486.

Sirigu, A., Duhamel, J. R., & Poncet, M. (1991). The role of sensorimotor experience in object recognition. A case of multimodal agnosia. *Brain* 114(6), 2555–2573. Erratum appears in *Brain* 115(2) (1992), 645.

Spitzer, M., Kischka, U., Guckel, F., Bellemann, M. E., Kammer, T., Seyyedi, S., et al. (1998). Functional magnetic resonance imaging of category-specific cortical activation: Evidence for semantic maps. *Cognitive Brain Research* 6(4), 309–319.

Spitzer, M., Kwong, K. K., Kennedy, W., Rosen, B. R., & Belliveau, J. W. (1995). Category-specific brain activation in fMRI during picture naming. *NeuroReport* 6, 2109–2112.

Stefanacci, L., Buffalo, E. A., Schmolck, H., & Squire, L. R. (2000). Profound amnesia after damage to the medial temporal lobe: A neuroanatomical and neuropsychological profile of patient E. P. *Journal of Neuroscience* 20(18), 7024–7036.

Stephan, K. M., Fink, G. R., Passingham, R. E., Silbersweig, D., Ceballos-Baumann, A. O., Frith, C. D., et al. (1995). Functional anatomy of the mental representation of upper extremity movements in healthy subjects. *Journal of Neurophysiology* 73, 373–386.

Tarr, M. J., & Gauthier, I. (2000). FFA: A flexible fusiform area for subordinate-level visual processing automatized by expertise. *Nature Neuroscience* 3(8), 764–769.

Thompson-Schill, S. L. (2003). Neuroimaging studies of semantic memory: Inferring "how" from "where." *Neuropsychologia* 41(3), 280–292.

Thompson-Schill, S. L. (in press). Dissecting the language organ: A new look at the role of Broca's area in language processing. In A. Cutler (Ed.), *Twenty-first Century Psycholinguistics: Four Cornerstones.* Hillsdale, NJ: Erlbaum.

Thompson-Schill, S. L., Aguirre, G. K., D'Esposito, M., & Farah, M. J. (1999). A neural basis for category and modality specificity of semantic knowledge. *Neuropsychologia* 37(6), 671–676.

Thompson-Schill, S. L., D'Esposito, M., Aguirre, G. K., & Farah, M. J. (1997). Role of left inferior prefrontal cortex in retrieval of semantic knowledge: A reevaluation. *Proceedings of the National Academy of Sciences USA* 94(26), 14792–14797.

Thompson-Schill, S. L., D'Esposito, M., & Kan, I. P. (1999). Effects of repetition and competition on activity in left prefrontal cortex during word generation. *Neuron* 23(3), 513–522.

Thompson-Schill, S. L., Jonides, J., Marshuetz, C., Smith, E. E., D'Esposito, M., Kan, I. P., et al. (2002). Effects of frontal lobe damage on interference effects in working memory. *Cognitive, Affective, and Behavioral Neuroscience* 2(2), 109–120.

Thompson-Schill, S. L., Swick, D., Farah, M. J., D'Esposito, M., Kan, I. P., & Knight, R. T. (1998). Verb generation in patients with focal frontal lesions: A neuropsychological test of neuroimaging findings. *Proceedings of the National Academy of Sciences USA* 95, 15855–15860.

Tippett, L. J., Glosser, G., & Farah, M. J. (1996). A category-specific naming deficit after temporal lobectomy. *Neuropsychologia* 34, 139–146.

Tulving, E. (1972). Episodic and semantic memory. In E. Tulving & W. Donaldson (Eds.), *Organization of Memory.* New York: Academic Press.

Tulving, E. (1984). Précis of *Elements of episodic memory. Behavioral and Brain Sciences* 7, 223–268.

Tulving, E. (1986). Episodic and semantic memory: Where should we go from here? *Behavioral & Brain Sciences* 9, 573–577.

Tulving, E., Kapur, S., Craik, F. I. M., Moscovitch, M., & Houle, S. (1994). Hemispheric encoding/retrieval asymmetry in episodic memory: Positron emission tomography findings. *Proceedings of the National Academy of Sciences USA* 91(6), 2016–2020.

Tyler, L. K., & Moss, H. E. (1997). Functional properties of concepts: Studies of normal and brain-damaged patients. *Cognitive Neuropsychology* 14, 511–545.

Tyler, L. K., Moss, H. E., Durrant-Peatfield, M. R., & Levy, J. P. (2000). Conceptual structure and the structure of concepts: A distributed account of category-specific deficits. *Brain & Language* 75(2), 195–231.

Tyler, L. K., Stamatakis, E. A., Dick, E., Bright, P., Fletcher, P., & Moss, H. (2003). Objects and their actions: Evidence for a neurally distributed semantic system. *NeuroImage* 18(2), 542–557.

Ungerleider, L. G., & Mishkin, M. (1982). Two cortical visual systems. In D. J. Ingle, M. A. Goodale, & R. J. W. Mansfield (Eds.), *Analysis of Visual Behavior*, 549–586. Cambridge, MA: MIT Press.

Vandenberghe, R., Price, C., Wise, R., Josephs, O., & Frackowiak, R. S. J. (1996). Functional anatomy of a common semantic system for words and pictures. *Nature* 383(6597), 254–256.

Vargha-Khadem, F., Gadian, D. G., & Mishkin, M. (2001). Dissociations in cognitive memory: The syndrome of developmental amnesia. *Philosophical Transactions of the Royal Society of London*, B356(1413), 1435–1440.

Wagner, A. D., Pare-Blagoev, E. J., Clark, J., & Poldrack, R. A. (2001). Recovering meaning: Left prefrontal cortex guides controlled semantic retrieval. *Neuron* 31(2), 329–338.

Wallis, J. D., Anderson, K. C., & Miller, E. K. (2001). Single neurons in prefrontal cortex encode abstract rules. *Nature* 411(6840), 953–956.

Warburton, E., Wise, R. J., Price, C. J., Weiller, C., Hadar, U., Ramsay, S., et al. (1996). Noun and verb retrieval by normal subjects. Studies with PET. *Brain* 119(1), 159–179.

Warrington, E. K. (1975). The selective impairment of semantic memory. *Quarterly Journal of Experimental Psychology* 27, 635–657.

Warrington, E. K., & McCarthy, R. (1983). Category specific access dysphasia. *Brain* 106, 859–878.

Warrington, E. K., & McCarthy, R. A. (1987). Categories of knowledge: Further fractionations and an attempted integration. *Brain* 110(5), 1273–1296.

Warrington, E. K., & Shallice, T. (1984). Category specific semantic impairments. *Brain* 107, 829–854.

Watson, J. D. G., Myers, R., Frackowiak, R. S. J., Hajnal, J. V., Woods, R. P., Mazziotta, J. C., et al. (1993). Area V5 of the human brain: Evidence from a combined study using positron emission tomography and magnetic resonance imaging. *Cerebral Cortex* 3(2), 79–94.

Wheaton, K. J., Thompson, J. C., Syngeniotis, A., Abbott, D. F., & Puce, A. (2004). Viewing the motion of human body parts activates different regions of premotor, temporal, and parietal cortex. *NeuroImage* 22(1), 277–288.

Wheeler, M. E., Petersen, S. E., & Buckner, R. L. (2000). Memory's echo: Vivid remembering reactivates sensory-specific cortex. *Proceedings of the National Academy of Sciences USA* 97(20), 11125–11129. Erratum appears in *Proceedings* 101(14) (2004), 5181.

Wiggs, C. L., & Martin, A. (1998). Properties and mechanisms of perceptual priming. *Current Opinion in Neurobiology* 8(2), 227–233.

Wiggs, C. L., Weisberg, J., & Martin, A. (1999). Neural correlates of semantic and episodic memory retreival. *Neuropsychologia* 37(1), 103–118.

Wilson, B. A., Baddeley, A. D., & Kapur, N. (1995). Dense amnesia in a professional musician following herpes simplex virus encephalitis. *Journal of Clinical & Experimental Neuropsychology* 17(5), 668–681.

Wise, R. J., Chollet, F., Hadar, U., Friston, K., Hoffner, E., & Frackowiak, R. (1991). Distribution of cortical neural networks involved in word comprehension and word retrieval. *Brain* 114(4), 1803–1817.

Wise, R. J., Howard, D., Mummery, C. J., Fletcher, P., Leff, A., Buchel, C., et al. (2000). Noun imageability and the temporal lobes. *Neuropsychologia* 38(7), 985–994.

Wolk, D. A., Coslett, H. B., & Glosser, G. (2005). The role of sensory-motor information in object recognition: Evidence from category-specific visual agnosia. *Brain and Language* 94, 131–146.

Yamadori, A., & Albert, M. L. (1973). Word category aphasia. *Cortex* 9, 112–125.

Zeki, S., Watson, J. D., Lueck, C. J., Friston, K. J., Kennard, C., & Frackowiak, R. S. (1991). A direct demonstration of functional specialization in human visual cortex. *Journal of Neuroscience* 11(3), 641–649.

7   Functional Neuroimaging of Language

Richard J. S. Wise and Cathy J. Price

Introduction

For the most part, the study of speech and language function can be based only on human data. The study of birdsong offers interesting parallels with a human infant's acquisition of language (Doupe & Kuhl, 1999). Further, the use of anatomical tracer studies (Romanski et al., 1999), single cell recordings (Tian et al., 2001), and metabolic brain studies (Poremba et al., 2004) in the monkey is directing attention to auditory processing streams (Kaas & Hackett, 2000; Rauschecker & Tian, 2000). As a result, inferences are being made from nonhuman primate research that can be profitably applied to research into human speech perception and comprehension (Scott & Johnsrude, 2003) and production (Wise et al., 2001). Nevertheless, because human communication is so complex and versatile, there are strict limits to what zebra finches and macaques can teach us about everyday human discourse.

The introduction of functional neuroimaging has given us the potential to view the functional anatomy of the normal human brain as it perceives, comprehends, and produces language. However, we had better state at the outset what this chapter will not do. It will not provide a detailed overview of all functional imaging studies of human communication. This is for two reasons. First, since functional imaging is used predominantly as an anatomical tool, attributing a particular brain function to a particular cortical or subcortical region, a conscientious "overview" may end up reading a little like a modern-day phrenology text, of the kind "here lies phoneme perception and there lies theory of mind." Second, the literature is now vast and encompasses papers of real excellence as well as ones that are less memorable. We will confine our review to results that we consider have raised issues of interest in the study of the functional anatomy of language, issues that, in many instances, are still the subject of lively debate.

The Imaging of Communication

Although we will mainly discuss studies that used positron emission tomography (PET) and functional magnetic resonance imaging (fMRI), we will refer to an electroencepaholographic (EEG) or magnetoencephalographic (MEG) study when it helps to make a point. The great advantage of EEG and MEG techniques, which directly record electrical activity in the brain, is that they have a temporal resolution of a few milliseconds. This compares with the seconds of fMRI and the parts of a minute of PET, techniques that rely on the much more slowly evolving changes in regional blood flow that accompany increased synaptic activity in cerebral gray matter. Although PET and fMRI have much greater spatial resolution than surface EEG recordings, newer analysis techniques have considerably improved the spatial resolution of MEG over the cortical surface (Dale & Halgren, 2001). However, MEG does not "see" many areas of the brain well, such as midline and subcortical gray matter, and so MEG complements PET and fMRI but is not imminently about to replace them.

The signal from PET and fMRI studies depends on a change in local blood flow, which is related to the local field potential (Logothetis et al., 2001). Thus, the signal predominantly reflects the input of encoded information to a region and its local processing, and not the output from that region to other brain areas. When functional neuroimaging has been used to study the human language system, the purpose has usually been to identify the functional anatomy and physiological responsiveness associated with one or more of the traditional subsystems of language. Thus, there are studies that have investigated issues in phonetics (the articulatory and perceptual characteristics of speech sounds), phonology (language-specific rules by which speech sounds are represented and manipulated) and orthography (language-specific rules by which words are represented in alphabetic or ideographic scripts). Some have also investigated whole word forms (a lexicon each for familiar spoken and written words), although only some models of language specify their existence as distinct mental representations. There have also been many studies investigating the neural organization of semantic memory and the manner in which words map onto long-term representations of meaning. Finally, there have been different approaches attempting to identify distinct neural substrates for the rules that govern the combining of words into sentences (syntax).

It should not be forgotten that each of these areas had been studied intensively long before functional imaging came on the scene. Language scientists, in their many guises, have come late into the field of brain imaging and its attendant demand for a working knowledge of neuroanatomy. However, most psychological models of language processing owe little, if anything, to the physical organization of the brain. Thus, the boxes and arrows that constitute an information-processing model of

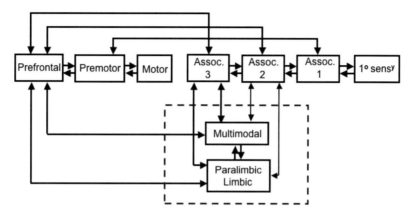

Figure 7.1
A general map of anatomical connectivity in the primate brain, redrawn from Gloor (1997). It demonstrates the connections among three ascending levels of unimodal association (Assoc) cortex, polysensory (multimodal) and paralimbic/limbic cortex, and prefrontal and premotor cortex. The hatched line around multimodal and paralimbic cortex indicates that these are the main sites for the "transmodal areas" of Mesulam (1998), and are probably the location of the "convergence zones" of Damasio (1989).

language do not necessarily map readily onto a general wiring diagram of the cortical connections of the primate brain (mostly, for ethical reasons, worked out in nonhuman primates) (figure 7.1). Although some are making progress in reconciling them, sometimes the interpretation attached to a particular focal activation on an image is anatomically naïve. This is a two-way learning experience, as neurologists and neuroanatomists are learning why, for example, the past tense of regular and irregular verbs so excites some language psychologists (Pinker, 1999)—described memorably by one worker in the field as the *Drosophila* of linguistics, analogous to the impact that the fruit fly has had on research in genetics.

The Relative Merits and Demerits of PET and fMRI

The majority of studies have investigated the perception, recognition, and comprehension of language; with the notable exceptions of cued word retrieval and single word repetition, only a few have looked at language production. This is for a methodological reason: most workers have access to fMRI, and the blood-oxygen-level-dependent (BOLD) signal with this technique becomes very noisy as the result of movements of the articulators and the movement of air in the nasal passages. Therefore, continuous speech cannot be studied with the most commonly used fMRI method, although alternative methods are being investigated (Kemeny et al., 2004). Even with single word production, experimenters have frequently resorted to investigating "covert" speech (the subjects have been asked to think of the word but not articulate it). An alternative has been to measure the relatively prolonged hemody-namic response function, which peaks only after a few seconds and is prolonged for ~10–12 sec, after articulation has been completed. This technique (Hall et al., 1999) has more often been used to present auditory stimuli in silence, before the subject experiences the noise of MRI data acquisition. By contrast, PET has the major advantage that it can be used to investigate continuous overt speech without articulation-related artifact. It is also a relatively silent technique.

Both authors have a strong regard for the use of PET in language studies that go beyond its value in the study of speech production and its relative silence in opera-tion. Its other main advantage is that it is equally sensitive to signal throughout the brain. fMRI with gradient-echo (GE), echo-planar imaging (EPI), the most widely used technique, has problems in regions where air-bone-tissue interfaces disturb the homogeneity of the magnetic field, reducing the signal-to-noise ratio (for one of the few direct comparisons of PET and fMRI in a language-related study, see Devlin, Russell et al., 2000). This susceptibility artifact occurs particularly in the basal regions (the undersurfaces) of the temporal and frontal lobes. EPI results in geometric distortion, which means the signal acquired with EPI does not coregister accurately onto the subject's structural image. PET is also nowhere nearly as claustrophobic an environment as fMRI, and we have rarely had a subject climb out of the PET scanner in protest at the lack of space. Patients, in particular those who are elderly and somewhat stiff, dislike the long, narrow bore of a scanning magnet, and are sometimes reluctant to come back for a second session in a serial fMRI study.

However, fMRI has two major advantages. The first is that the blood flow mea-surement with PET is prolonged over many tens of seconds, and event-related measurements are possible only with fMRI. Thus, as an example, if one wishes to know whether a difference in hemodynamic response distinguishes words in a list that are subsequently remembered in a recognition memory test from those that are not (Wagner et al., 1998), the recording of a hemodynamic response to each stimulus offers a sensitivity that is greater than averaging recognition memory success over a block of stimuli.

The second relates to the number of scans (observations) that can be acquired in any one subject. PET relies on the quantitative localization of a tracer amount of water labeled with positron-emitting ^{15}oxygen to index regional cerebral blood flow. The number of observations (individual scans) that can be made on single subjects with PET is limited for two reasons. First, each dose of radiolabeled water has to be allowed to decay before the next observation can be made following a fresh bolus of radiolabeled water. Second, the subject is exposed to a dose of radiation. In these risk-averse times, there is a widely held view that any radiation is bad for you, although there is no good evidence of linearity of risk (and people do not take cold baths on the principle that because a bath of boiling water is universally fatal, a warm bath must carry a finite risk of morbidity and mortality). Popular prejudice means that permitted radiation dosimetry is a fine balance between adequate data collection, regulation by government advisory bodies, and ease of subject recruitment after informed consent. The practical outcome is that any single-subject PET ^{15}O water study is limited to 12–16 scans, which usually does not give sufficient statistical power. Therefore, group studies are required. Speed of data acquisition and the absence of ionizing radiation often allow fMRI data to be analyzed as a single-subject series, which emphasizes the differences between individuals in the distribution of activated tissue relative to sulcal and gyral anatomy, such as in Broca's area (Amunts et al., 1999; Amunts et al., 2004).

Anatomical resolution is less in grouped data. Variations of anatomy and inhomogeneities in the relationship between structure and function in a population are only partially overcome by anatomical normalization; an averaged focal activation in a group analysis is a composite of distributed individual foci. Obviously, the more anatomically constant a functional brain region is across subjects, the better the spatial resolution and the less noisy the signal. Noise is further reduced by smoothing the signal, which enlarges the apparent extent of activation but does not shift the position of the peak. This is why many functional imaging studies publish tables of the coordinates of peaks, which, although as dull as a railway timetable to the nonspecialist, are the unit of trade when comparing "my study" with "your study."

Spatial resolution is also affected by other factors that differ in PET and fMRI. The theoretical limit of spatial resolution is no better than 2–4 mm with PET, and "in the field" spatial resolution (after small head movements, etc.) is of the order of 5–7 mm. By contrast, the spatial resolution of fMRI depends primarily on magnet strength and the scanning technique employed. The BOLD response at 1.5–3 Tesla has a spatial resolution of perhaps 3–5 mm. This functional spatial resolution is considerably worse than anatomical resolution, and arises from the predominant source of signal, which is not the tissue compartment in which neural activity takes place but blood in draining venules a few millimeters away (Ugurbil et al., 2003). Obtaining the majority of the signal from capillaries close to the neural tissue will allow much improved (submillimeter) spatial resolution, but this will depend on more powerful magnets (e.g., Yacoub et al., 2005).

Parallel Processes

Depending on the study design, functional imaging potentially "sees" other systems engaged during the performance of language-related tasks—those related to episodic encodement of verbal information, attention, and the maintenance and manipulation of the stimuli over a short time span—before arriving at a task-specific decision to make a response. Thus, at first it may seem a little confusing that word lists are used by some to study the processes up to and including lexical semantics, while others use essentially identical word lists to investigate episodic memory encodement and retrieval. The two forms of long-term declarative memory, semantic and episodic, are inextricably related, and saying *pink elephant* to a subject lying in a scanner will automatically result in the retrieval of specific semantic knowledge and episodic encodement of that verbal event. To which aspect of memory the experimenter then attributes the activation associated with that stimulus may be a matter of preference. Not infrequently, the only way around this dilemma is to use converging evidence from clinical studies on the effects of focal lesions on language, memory, and other cognitive functions to arrive at a plausible interpretation of one's data.

Therefore, compelling though functional imaging is in the study of brain-function relationships, it complements but does not replace the hard slog of careful behavioral observations on patients. As an example, theories about the role of paracingulate cortex in "theory of mind," that aspect of social cognition which allows us to infer the beliefs and intentions of another, have arisen from a number of studies using functional neuroimaging (Frith & Frith, 1999). Nevertheless, the clinical study of one patient with anterior frontal infarction (Bird et al., 2004), which obliterated her paracingulate cortex, showed her to be nearly flawless on tasks designed to reveal impaired "theory of mind." Therefore, the observations with functional imaging had not predicted the behavioral impairment consequent upon destruction of this region (at least in one well-documented case). One of us in particular, CJP, has championed the need to combine functional imaging studies on normal subjects with clinical studies on patients to achieve the most reliable interpretations of one's data (Price et al., 1999). That said, functional imaging has some major advantages compared with clinical studies, and these will be discussed in the next section.

The Advantages of Functional Imaging over the "Lesion Deficit" Method

The time-honored method of inferring the normal organization of brain function has been to observe *abnormal* speech and language processing after a focal lesion. However, human cerebral lesions (the "experiments" of nature) are rarely subtle. Nevertheless, there is a natural tendency to attribute lost function to the location of the cortical lesion observed on an anatomical X-ray, CT, or MR image. Some workers have deliberately sought to relate the loss of a white matter tract to the observed deficit, or to the disconnection of cortical areas otherwise unaffected by the lesion (for example, Alexander et al., 1989; Naeser et al., 1989), but this is relatively rare. A notable exception is the syndrome of "conduction" aphasia, most often attributed to the disconnection of the area of Wernicke, centered on the left posterior temporal lobe, from the area of Broca, in the left inferior frontal gyrus, by a lesion of the arcuate fasciculus. However, the distribution of vascular or other destructive pathological lesions of the human brain will mean that any aphasic syndrome will be a mixture of cortical and conduction deficits.

In an attempt to study the effects of cortical pathology alone, detailed neuropsychological assessments have been performed on patients with focal neurodegenerative conditions presenting as primary progressive aphasia. The difficulty here is that the distribution of degenerate cortex is not governed by functional boundaries; and further, the degree of atrophy in any one region may not correlate linearly with the behavior under study. Thus, in patients with the temporal variant of frontotemporal dementia, it has been demonstrated that the degree of anomia correlates well with left anterior temporal lobe atrophy, but impairment on more direct tests of semantic knowledge is dependent on the presence of bilateral temporal polar atrophy (Lambon-Ralph et al., 2001). However, the appearance of right temporal atrophy will, in all probability, be accompanied by progressing anterior-posterior atrophy in the left temporal lobe. Those who believe that knowledge of word meaning is entirely a function of the left cerebral hemisphere can argue that the right temporal lobe atrophy is simply a marker of advancing atrophy in an entirely left-lateralized semantic system.

This significance of white matter tract damage after stroke must also relate to the connections of the posterior and anterior temporal lobe to prefrontal cortex. These initially pursue separate routes in the superior longitudinal fasciculus (which includes the arcuate fasciculus) and the uncinate fasciculus, respectively. However, both converge in white matter underlying the inferior frontal operculum and gyrus, close to the location of the cortical area of Broca. Mohr and colleagues (1978) attributed at least some of the behavioral differences between patients with a "small" and a "large" Broca's lesion to underlying white matter damage. Thus, the consequences of a typical Broca's lesion may be as much about disruption of distributed fronto-temporal connections as about damage to Brodmann's areas 44 and 45. Similar arguments apply to lesions in and around Wernicke's area.

Nevertheless, the sometimes surprisingly specific effects on human behavior following strokes, tumors, bullet wounds, blows, and degenerative diseases can be very informative. Furthermore, one does not have to care about relating function to structure. Models of language processing can be constructed entirely from the reaction times and errors of normal subjects while they make forced-choice decisions on language stimuli or produce speech under normal or experimental conditions (e.g., Levelt, 1989). However, if one is interested in the branch of systems neuroscience that relates function to structure, the advent of functional neuroimaging would seem, at the very least, to complement the lesion-deficit method.

Functional Neuroimaging of Language

The Mapping of Speech onto Meaning

The perception of speech activates the length of both superior temporal gyri (Binder et al., 1997). Since speech contains many nonverbal cues, activity will include the perception of prosodic cues, and the affect and identity of the speaker. Thus, activity relates to more than the phonetic cues and features that allow mapping of the speech signal onto both long-term representations of word meaning and syntax and the sensorimotor systems responsible for speech production.

Much of the functional imaging work on speech perception over the past few years has been influenced by studies of the auditory cortex of the nonhuman primate (Scott & Johnsrude, 2003). There are good reasons for thinking that "primate vocal behavior represents an excellent model system for studying the substrates of speech perception" (Ghafanzar & Hauser, 1999). Initially, at least in the nonhuman primate (anatomical tracer studies and single cell recordings are never and rarely, respectively, possible in vivo in man), there is a hierarchy of processing in primary auditory (core) and adjacent periauditory cortex (belt and parabelt) (Kaas et al., 1999). Subsequent projections pass in anterior and posterior directions (Romanski et al., 1999) and to memory-related polysensory medial temporal lobe cortex (Lavenex et al., 2002), with the entire length of the superior temporal gyrus connected reciprocally to prefrontal cortex via the superior longitudinal fasciculus (posteriorly), external capsule, and uncinate fasciculus (anteriorly) (Pandya & Yeterian, 1985). The length of the dorsal bank of the superior temporal sulcus is activated by the human voice (Belin et al., 2000), a region, as in the nonhuman primate (Poremba et al., 2003), likely to be polysensory cortex. A study that combined the perception of visual objects and the sounds that those objects make, supports the suggestion that the human superior temporal polysensory area does indeed lie within the superior temporal sulcus (Beauchamp et al., 2004).

Cortical analysis of the acoustic features that result in word recognition relies on analysis of both temporal and spectral features. Details of the many studies that have studied the response to manipulation of sublexical auditory stimuli have been reviewed by Scott and Johnsrude (2003). An area of particular interest has been the culture-specific sounds of spoken language, and the brain responses to speech sounds or consonant-vowel combinations in native and nonnative speakers of a particular language (e.g., Näätänen et al., 1997; Jacquemot et al., 2003). This is of considerable relevance to the shaping of auditory cortex to the particular phonetic and phonological features of the native language that occurs in the first year of life. There has also been debate about hemispheric specialization for particular acoustic features and the contribution of functional imaging to this debate. Some claim that there is good evidence for a left hemisphere specialization for temporal features and a right hemisphere specialization for pitch (Zatorre & Belin, 2001; Zatorre et al., 2002), but others disagree (Scott & Wise, 2004). In this debate, attention to detail is of particular importance, such as the functional distinction between resolving differences in pitch and resolving differences in spectral features.

There is, however, disagreement about the anatomical route by which speech maps onto meaning. One model proposes that the route to lexical semantics is via the temporo-parieto-occipital junction (Hickok & Poeppel, 2000) or posterior middle and inferior temporal gyri (Hickok & Poeppel, 2004), a model that accords with the literature on loss of comprehension following stroke. A second model proposes that the mapping of speech onto meaning proceeds from the superior temporal gyrus in a ventral direction toward the superior temporal sulcus, and then to the middle and inferior temporal gyri, the site, it is proposed, of long-term representations of meaning (Binder et al., 2000). The third alternative is that mapping of speech onto meaning occurs in an auditory processing stream that passes forward in the temporal lobe toward the anterior superior temporal sulcus and to temporal polar cortex (Scott et al., 2000; Crinion et al., 2003; Davis & Johnsrude, 2003). The notion that meaning is associated with the anterior reaches of the temporal lobe accords with the views of those who study loss of semantic knowledge in patients with the temporal variant of frontotemporal dementia (semantic dementia) (see, e.g., Gorno-Tempini et al., 2004).

A number of review articles and papers have presented the evidence, both clinical and functional imaging, that the temporo-parieto-occipital junction/angular gyrus and inferolateral temporal cortex provide supramodal access to meaning (Grabowski & Damasio, 2000; Hickok & Poeppel, 2000, 2004; Binder & Price, 2001; Binder, 2002). However, as discussed by Marinkovic and colleagues (2003), fMRI studies are relatively insensitive to signal in the temporal pole due to susceptibility artifact (Devlin et al., 2000). Figure 7.2 demonstrates the strong temporal polar signal associated with a contrast of hearing intelligible speech with hearing unintelligible speech when the study is carried out with PET. A number of functional imaging studies have suggested that the anterior temporal signal is predominantly associated with syntactic rather than lexical semantic comprehension. However, since others have clearly related activation of the anterior superior temporal sulcus and temporal pole to explicit access to single word meaning (Marinkovic et al., 2003; Scott et al., 2003; Sharp et al., 2004a) it seems that a "syntax-only" explanation for the anterior "stream" of language processing is unlikely. It also accords with the loss of single-word semantic knowledge with preserved syntactic knowledge observed in semantic dementia (e.g., Gorno-Tempini et al., 2004).

There is less controversy that the anterior part of the fusiform gyrus, part of the "basal language area" (Burnstine et al., 1990) of the temporal lobe, is involved in

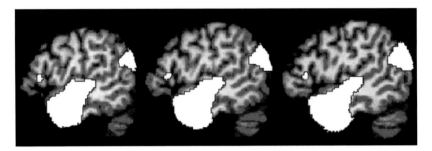

Figure 7.2
Listening to narratives versus listening to unintelligible but acoustically equivalent (i.e., spectrally rotated) versions (Scott et al., 2000) of the same narratives in 11 subjects, with the result displayed on three sagittal slices taken from the left cerebral hemisphere (single-subject MR template) spaced 4 mm apart, lateral-medial. The greatest distribution of activity was in the anterior temporal pole, with a second region of activation in the left temporo-parieto-occipital junction and a small region in the left inferior gyrus. PET is better at revealing temporal polar cortical activity than conventional fMRI. The Broca's Area activity is seen to be centered anterior to the ascending ramus of the lateral fissure, and thus may be located (with some uncertainty; see Amunts et al. 1999) in Brodmann's Area 45. Statistical threshold P < 0.00001, uncorrected, fixed-effects statistical model.

mapping language onto meaning. It and the closely related perirhinal cortex respond across language modalities (Buchel et al., 1998; Wise et al., 2000). This is perhaps surprising, for the anterior fusiform gyrus consists of high-order visual cortex (Insausti et al., 1998). However, it clearly responds to speech during both automatic and controlled access to meaning (Crinion et al., 2003; Sharp et al., 2004a). Activity in this region is reduced when the perception of speech is impaired, either by distortion of the speech signal (in normal subjects) or by the presence of left superior temporal lobe damage (in stroke patients) (Sharp et al., 2004b). Therefore, despite its location in unimodal visual association cortex, this region behaves, in the manner described by Mesulam (1998), as a "transmodal area" where unimodal processing of heard and written speech converges prior to amodal cognitive processing.

The Organization of Semantic Memory

The neural organization of semantic memory is currently the subject of three main theories. These attempt to explain category-specific deficits described in the clinical neuropsychological literature, the most common distinction being that between living kinds and nonliving kinds. An attempt to bring them together, using the concept of convergence zones (Damasio, 1989), is presented in a paper by Simmons and Barsalou (2003). In clinical practice, category-specific deficits are rare, and in semantic dementia, they are excessively rare (Lambon-Ralph et al., 2003). The sensory-functional theory has dominated functional imaging studies. This proposes that knowledge of a specific category is located near the sensory or motor areas that process experiences of that item (hence object-based vision for animals and motion-based vision and motor execution for tools). Although there have been many striking studies that seem to support this theory (see Martin et al., 1995; Hauk et al., 2004), a recent series of analyses, reanalyses, and meta-analyses has begun to question interpretations of the observed regional activations. The current thinking is that they may not indicate long-term sensorimotor representations of semantic knowledge, but a transient interaction between bottom-up and top-down neural activity that is as much dependent on the brain's response to a particular stimulus within the context of a particular task as to the neural organization of semantic memories (Joseph, 2001; Devlin, Moore, et al., 2002; Devlin, Moore, et al., 2002; Mechelli et al., 2003; Mechelli et al., 2004). It would seem that improved methods of study design and data analysis—and dynamic causal modeling of effective connectivity is being proposed as a promising approach (Penny et al., 2004)—may modify some of the interpretations that have arisen from functional imaging studies of object knowledge since the mid-1990s.

The Mapping of Speech onto Articulation

Binder and colleagues (1996) demonstrated that the planum temporale, lying on the supratemporal plane behind primary auditory cortex in Heschl's gyrus and long considered "speech cortex," responds as strongly to acoustically simple nonspeech sounds as to speech. New theories are now being proposed about functions of the planum temporale unrelated to speech processing (Griffiths & Warren, 2002). Nevertheless, functional imaging studies have demonstrated a role for subregions of auditory cortex posterior to Heschl's gyrus. Within or close to the left planum temporale, subregions hold a sequence of speech in short-term memory and provide a sensorimotor interface by which heard speech can be mapped onto articulatory gestures (Hickok et al., 2000; Wise et al., 2001; Hickok et al., 2003). This is an important route for the acquisition of language (Kuhl, 2004). The hypothesis that matching an acoustic representation (either short- or long-term) to an articulatory gesture occurs via reciprocal projections through a posterior auditory pathway to dorsal prefrontal/premotor regions is in keeping with the original ideas of Wernicke about the function of the arcuate fasciculus. To strengthen the evidence that the auditory and articulatory features of speech strongly interact at the neural level, it has been demonstrated that the perception of speech activates the motor output to articulatory muscles (Fadiga et al., 2002; Wilson et al., 2004).

Controlled Retrieval of Meaning—The Role of the Left Inferior Frontal Gyrus

Whatever the neural organization of semantic knowledge, it is generally accepted that the representations principally lie within posterior cortex. During the automatic retrieval of meaning during the "passive" comprehension of single words and syntactically simple sentences and narratives, little activity is observed in the left inferior frontal gyrus (Mummery et al., 1999; Scott et al., 2000; Crinion et al., 2003) (see also figure 7.2). However, in the context of the controlled retrieval of single-word information, in which a decision and a response are required, the left inferior frontal gyrus and adjacent premotor cortex become strongly activated. One hypothesis proposes a domain-specific organization, in which the anterior inferior frontal gyrus (Brodmann's areas 45/47) is specialized for the controlled processing of semantic information, whereas its posterior part (Brodmann's area 44, extending into BA 6) processes only phonological information (Poldrack et al., 1999; Wagner et al., 2001). Alternatively, a process-specific organization has been proposed, in which neural activity is associated with the maintenance and the retrieval or selection of verbal information, irrespective of the type of information (Barde & Thompson-Schill, 2002; Gold & Buckner, 2002).

Evidence in favor of a domain-specific organization includes the observations that the anterior left inferior frontal gyrus is recruited during the processing of semantic information (Poldrack et al., 1999) and that the signal is modulated by the extent of semantic processing (Wagner et al., 2001). By contrast, activation of the posterior left inferior frontal gyrus has been observed during tasks that depend upon processing the sound structure of words held in working memory, such as during word-stem completion (Buckner et al., 1995; Poldrack et al., 1999). A domain-specific organization for the inferior frontal gyrus predicts that tasks which involve the controlled processing of nonsemantic information should not activate the anterior part. However, activation of this region has been observed during phonological processing (Devlin et al., 2003), and similar levels of activation have been seen within this region when phonological and semantic processing have been directly compared (Barde & Thompson-Schill, 2002; Gold & Buckner, 2002). These results suggest that the anterior left inferior frontal gyrus does not exclusively process semantic information, and provide evidence in favor of a process-specific organization. What is not clear at present is how these observations on metalinguistic task performance relate to the role of Broca's area in the comprehension of complex syntax and the production of connected speech, which are the topics of the next two sections.

Syntax

Despite the agrammatic production of speech in Broca's aphasia, it seemed that many such patients have relatively intact speech comprehension, including comprehension of grammatically simple sentences (Goodglass, 1993). However, it became apparent that certain sentence types, such as those that contain a center-embedded object relative clause or have a reversible passive structure, cause problems for patients with the behavioral syndrome of Broca's aphasia (Caramazza and Zurif, 1976; Schwartz et al., 1980). By contrast, studies have suggested that Wernicke's aphasics not only produce grammatically correct, although semantically "empty," speech but also make use of syntactic information in comprehension (Swinney, 1996). This double dissociation led to the belief that a lesion of the left inferior frontal gyrus resulted in an impaired ability to process syntax during both comprehension and production. However agrammatic aphasia may be a deficit of syntactic processing rather than syntactic knowledge, and thus Broca's area need not be the region of cortex where syntactic knowledge is stored (Kolk & Friederici, 1985; Swaab et al., 1998). More recently, it has been proposed that the loss of Broca's area results in only a very specific impairment of grammatical processing (for example, Grodzinsky, 2000), although the methods by which patients were included for analysis and by which their performance on sentence comprehension were statistically analyzed by Grodzinsky and colleagues have come under critical scrutiny (Caramazza et al., 2001).

However, these behavioral studies often provided little or no neuroimaging evidence of the lesion sites (some were performed before X-ray CT scanning became available). Because classical aphasic syndromes predict lesion site rather poorly (Basso et al., 1985), these studies do not tell us anything reliable about the location of something akin to a "grammar module" in the brain for sentence comprehension. Further, patients with the syndrome of Broca's aphasia who perform poorly on comprehension tasks that depend on syntax may be accurate when making decisions about whether sentences are grammatically correct or not. Therefore, grammatical knowledge can remain intact in patients unable to use this knowledge to arrive at sentence-level meaning (Linebarger et al., 1983).

By contrast, a study of 22 unselected patients with a mix of aphasic syndromes has shown both that aphasic patients are commonly impaired at grammaticality judgement and that their deficits are not restricted to particular sentence types (Wilson & Saygin, 2004). Their relative performance on "easy" and "difficult" sentences was not different, which contrasts with performance on tasks of sentence comprehension. The authors suggest that sentence comprehension is assisted by cues such as canonical word order but fail with noncanonical sentence structures, since interpretation is then heavily dependent on morphological cues, which may be particularly vulnerable in aphasia. By contrast, grammaticality judgment tasks depend on a correct assessment of all elements of a sentence to arrive at a correct decision, which makes "easy" sentences as hard to analyze as "difficult" sentences in a task-dependent manner. A strong feature of this study is the descriptions of lesion distribution, using voxel-based lesion-symptom mapping (VLSM) (Bates et al., 2003). Lesion location did not predict severity, and a Wernicke's area lesion most reliably predicted poor performance at grammaticality judgments.

This accords with other studies, which have suggested that a neural system distributed along left (and possible right) perisylvian cortex is responsible for syntactic comprehension (Caplan et al., 1996; Dick et al., 2001). In another study using VLSM to investigate sentence comprehension (Dronkers et al., 2004), which used a range of sentence types in a large group of chronic aphasic patients, impaired comprehension correlated with damage to left prefrontal, temporal, and inferior parietal loci, but not with damage to "classic" Broca's (Brodmann's areas 44 and 45) and Wernicke's (posterior Brodmann's area 22) areas. Impaired comprehension of certain sentence subtypes correlated better with damage to particular regions, and damage to the left middle temporal gyrus in particular affected single-word comprehension, to an extent that its contribution to sentence-level processing was less certain. In the light of earlier comments about the potential effects of white matter damage on cortical processing, this study emphasized a correlation between impaired comprehension and temporal lobe white matter damage.

In addition to the stroke literature, observations on patients with neurodegenerative disorders presenting as progressive aphasia are informative about the localization of word and sentence comprehension. Patients with the temporal variant of frontotemporal dementia, so-called semantic dementia, have prominent anterior temporal lobe atrophy associated with anomia, progressive loss of single-word comprehension but intact production of syntax, and, within the limits imposed by their level of loss of single-word comprehension, intact comprehension of syntax. In a recent study (Gorno-Tempini et al., 2004) that contrasted three variants of progressive aphasia—nonfluent progressive aphasia, semantic dementia, and so-called logopenic progressive aphasia (the last perhaps being an atypical presentation of Alzheimer's disease), the logopenic variant was associated with the most marked loss of sentence comprehension. The focal atrophy in these patients was most evident in the left temporoparietal region. Nonfluent progressive aphasia resulted in loss of comprehension only of more complex sentence types, and the anterior temporal atrophy of semantic dementia was associated with almost flawless sentence comprehension.

Therefore, contrary to an earlier belief that Broca's area is the "seat of syntax," the lateral temporal and inferior parietal cortex have emerged as important sites in sentence comprehension in the recent studies of stroke and focal neurodegeneration that have used sophisticated analyses of structural brain images. After a review of the functional neuroimaging literature on studies of grammaticality judgment and sentence comprehension (Kaan & Swaab, 2002), Kaan and Swaab come to a similar conclusion: that sentence comprehension depends on a widely distributed neural system, possibly involving both hemispheres.

A number of studies have attempted to isolate syntactic processing. When contrasting syntactically complex sentences with simple sentences, Broca's area has been consistently activated (for example, Caplan et al., 1998; Caplan et al., 1999; Stowe et al., 1998; Dapretto and Bookheimer, 1999). However, sentence complexity increases the load not only on syntactic operations but also on short-term memory, because various components of the sentence have to be "kept in mind" before final integration of the whole sentence structure. The role of working memory in sentence comprehension has been much debated in the psychological literature (Just & Carpenter, 1992; Waters & Caplan, 1996; Caplan & Waters, 1999; MacDonald & Christiansen, 2002). Evidence for an increasing memory or processing load for Broca's area has been demonstrated in a number of ways. They include the use of sentences containing ambiguous words (Stowe et al., 1998), sentences constructed with a noncanonical word order containing low-frequency words (Keller et al., 2001), and sentences in which words need to be retained prior to syntactic and semantic integration (Cooke et al., 2002; Waters et al., 2003; Fiebach, Schlesewsky, et al., 2004; Fiebach, Vos, et al., 2004).

One difficulty with a contrast between complex and simple sentences is that it may mask activations associated with shared syntactic operations. Comparing sentences with lists of unrelated words is an alternative (Stowe et al., 1999; Friederici et al., 2000; Kuperberg et al., 2000). These studies have not emphasized Broca's area; instead, activity for sentences has been observed in temporal cortex, including the temporal pole, often bilaterally. Anterior temporal activation has also been found when sentences were compared with a rest condition or a nonword control (Mazoyer et al., 1993; Perani et al., 1996; Stowe et al., 1999; Humphries et al., 2001). However, a baseline that does not control for the acoustic complexity of the sentence activation condition creates many potential confounds when interpreting the data. Further, and as discussed previously, anterior temporal lobe activity cannot be specific to the processing of syntax, because it is also observed during both the automatic and the controlled lexical semantic processing of single-content words. Other study designs have used "Jabberwocky" or "syntactic prose," in which semantic processing is reduced by substituting pseudo words for content words (e.g., Friederici et al., 2000), and yet other studies have employed syntactic and semantic violations of the kind used in ERP studies (Embick et al., 2000; Meyer et al., 2000; Ni et al., 2000; Indefrey et al., 2001; Moro et al., 2001). Overall, these studies have been associated with widely distributed syntax-related activations throughout the temporal and fontal lobes.

In summary, despite considerable efforts and ingenuity in study design, a consistent "grammar module" has not been identified. It would appear that these studies, along with the recent lesion-deficit studies, are far from consistent with the idea that grammar localizes to Broca's area. Ullman (2001) has proposed that "the mental lexicon depends on declarative memory and is rooted in the temporal lobe, whereas the mental grammar involves procedural memory and is rooted in the frontal cortex and basal ganglia." Most would agree with his localization of the mental lexicon, but the present evidence indicates that mental grammar is more widely distributed than he suggests. However, teaching adults the grammar of foreign languages, with rules that obey the universal principles of grammar, was associated with increased activity in the left inferior frontal gyrus (Musso et al., 2003). The same activity was not observed when the subjects learned "unreal" grammar that violated the universal principles of grammar. This intriguing study does indicate a central role for prefrontal cortex in the left inferior frontal gyrus in human linguistic competence.

Speech Production

At one level, the production of speech can be described in terms of a source-filter system. Energy comes from controlled expiration; quasi-periodic vibration of the vocal folds provides the noise source; and the filter is formed by sequential movements of the articulators (jaw, soft palate, tongue, and lips; Fitch, 2000). Studying speech production at this level means examining premotor and motor systems and feedback loops through auditory and somatosensory cortex, monitoring and matching the intended to the actual acoustic product, and the shaping of the articulators that produced that sound. At an entirely different level, normal speech production concerns concept formation (itself dependent on retrieval of episodic and semantic memories), the selection of words (with appropriate affixes and suffixes), and their ordering in a sentence structure, prior to phonological encoding and the formulation of a transient phonetic code (Levelt, 1989) (see figure 7.1). Imaging these processes compared with nonspeech or nonpropositional speech baselines, and irrespective of whether the motor output is through the mouth or hands (sign language), it is not surprising that activations distributed throughout frontal, temporal, and parietal lobes are observed (Braun et al., 2001; Blank et al., 2002; Blank et al., 2003).

Although Broca's area (Brodmann's areas 44 and 45) is active during propositional speech, adjacent regions have very different response profiles to different forms of speech (e.g., counting aloud as opposed to conversational speech; figure 7.3, plate 9). Further, the extent of prefrontal activation is considerably less than in cued word retrieval tasks (Blank et al., 2002), another instance when metalinguistic tasks show systems that are not engaged during normal communication. A more complete understanding of the function of these regions has hardly begun. It will depend on converging evidence from lesion-deficit analyses and functional imaging designs that may not at first seem to address communication. An example is the very prominent activity observed in the superior frontal gyrus during both propositional speech and speech comprehension (Binder et al., 1997; Binder et al., 2003). Infarction of this region may result in the syndrome of transcortical motor aphasia, characterized by a preserved ability to repeat but impaired initiation of speech

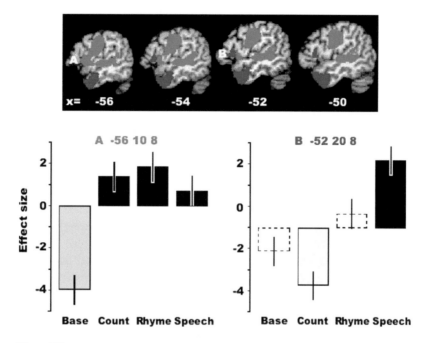

Figure 7.3
Results from a PET study of speech production on 12 subjects (Blank et al., 2002; 2003). Two contrasts are displayed: in red, the contrast of all speech conditions—propositional speech, the recitation of over-learned nursery rhymes, and counting—with a baseline condition of low-level auditory attention; and in blue, the contrast of propositional speech with counting. The results are displayed on sagittal single-subject MR slices. The peak in pars opercularis (A) for the first contrast (−56 10 8) lies only 12 mm away from the peak in pars triangularis (B) in the second contrast (−52 20 8). See plate 9 for color version.

production. A number of functional imaging studies are attempting to describe activity in this region in relation to the cognitive control of seemingly unrelated tasks (Goel et al., 1997; Zysset et al., 2002; Scott et al., 2003; Sharp et al., 2004a). It will be fascinating to see whether a unifying hypothesis about the role of anterior and medial prefrontal cortex in normal human communication emerges.

Issues

Advances in the reliable statistical testing of PET and fMRI data, and the method-ologies being used to extend the scope of imaging techniques and extracting the most information from the data obtained (particularly for fMRI data), have become truly daunting. We will confine ourselves to some general issues that affect study design and data interpretation. Then, ideally, the final paper describing one's func-tional imaging study should survive the test that is recommended for reading clinical research reports (Montori et al., 2004). The dispassionate reader should scrutinize only the methods and results sections in the first instance, and draw his or her own conclusions about what hypothesis is being proposed and whether it has been proved or disproved. Only then should the introduction and discussion sections be read. In this manner, one-sided interpretation of the data will be more apparent.

Problems with the "Passive" Condition

The generation of local field potentials accompanies the continuous mental activity present in the conscious human brain, whether or not the subject is exposed to external stimuli or task demands. Thus, one pervasive reason why some functional imaging studies are found wanting is in the choice of baseline condition, because there is no universal baseline state of cognitive "neutrality" with which to compare all activation conditions.

Certain regions are consistently more active in a "rest" or "passive" baseline state, and the studies that have examined this issue, and the possible explanations underlying the activity within these regions, have been reviewed (Gusnard and Raichle, 2001). One compelling explanation is that a "rest" state permits the subject to "ruminate" or "daydream"—in other words, to have stimulus-independent thoughts (Binder et al., 1999). Even if the subject is exposed to stimuli during scanning, the "passive" perception of the stimuli, or the intervals when a response has been made and the next stimulus is awaited in an "active" condition with stimuli presented at a fixed rate, may be accompanied by periods of stimulus-independent thoughts.

The brain regions most strongly associated with the "rest" or "passive" states are midline cortex, anterior and posterior, and bilateral posterior parietal cortex. Therefore, any activity in these regions associated with an activation condition will be "subtracted" when the baseline condition is a "rest" or "passive" condition. The posterior regions have recently been associated in the functional imaging literature with episodic memory retrieval (Gilboa et al., 2004; Shannon & Buckner, 2004); and, of course, one cannot have thoughts without retrieving memories. These regions show the earliest metabolic changes in Alzheimer's disease, which usually presents initially as impairment of memory retrieval (Reiman et al., 1996). The role of posterior midline cortex in memory has also been observed in clinical neuropsychological studies (e.g., Rudge & Warrington, 1991).

Subtracting processes to do with episodic memory in a study of language processing might be desirable, but there is a strong possibility that other cognitive processes accompanying the awake thinking brain may also be involved in "seeing beneath" the surface meaning of what one has heard or read, or in selecting how best to respond to a question. Losing these activations in a contrast may be a disadvantage if one is interested in conceptual or inferential processes associated with communication. It has been proposed that one possible solution is to use a simple, unmemorable, but demanding task as a baseline condition, such as an odd/even decision on random presentation of single digits. This approach, when put to the test, improved the signal observed within medial temporal lobe structures in studies on the encoding and retrieval of episodic memories (Stark & Squire, 2001). An example, using both "passive" and "active" baseline conditions in a language study, is shown in figure 7.4.

Activity in orbitofrontal cortex is also commonly observed in "passive" relative to "active" conditions (figure 7.4). The first author, who is a veteran of a number of PET and fMRI studies, can attest to the bodily discomforts that accompany lying, confined and still, for prolonged periods in a scanner. These sensations are temporarily alleviated by paying attention to the performance of a task, only to return during "passive" conditions. The rich sensory, somatosensory and visceral connections of orbitofrontal cortex, and its role in emotional responsiveness to internal as well as external sensations (Öngür & Price, 2000) suggest one reason why the contemplation of one's present discomforts during "passive" conditions increases activity in orbitofrontal cortex.

The signal from unimodal primary and association sensory cortex is confounded less by cognitive processes that accompany the "rest" or "passive" state. However, adequately controlling for potential confounds across stimulus sets is not straightforward. Thus, for example, the stimulus to "subtract" the sublexical processing of such a complex but overfamiliar acoustic signal as speech has varied widely across studies, and none are entirely satisfactory (Scott & Wise, 2004). If the sublexical component of sensory processing is not matched across conditions, or the rate of presentation of the stimuli is not the same (Price et al., 1992; Dhankar et al., 1997), then cognitive subtractions purporting to demonstrate lexical or syntactic processes are difficult to interpret, especially because early sensory processing is associated with a particularly strong signal (Norris & Wise, 2000). An example demonstrating the effects of both the sensory complexity of verbal and nonverbal stimuli and their rate of presentation is shown in figure 7.5 (plate 10). One solution is to use a variety of stimuli and a factorial design. For example, it was possible to show that speech signal from which fine temporal and spectral detail had been removed, while preserving intelligibility, activated part of the left anterior temporal lobe more strongly than speech signal that had been rendered unintelligible without loss of any of the acoustic detail present in normal speech (Scott et al., 2000). Therefore, this study separated responses to speech intelligibility from responses to acoustic complexity (figure 7.6, plate 11).

Finally, there is the effect of attention, which may strongly modulate the observed signal. For example, modality-dependent selective attention modulates the blood flow observed in auditory and visual cortex (Woodruff et al., 1996). Within

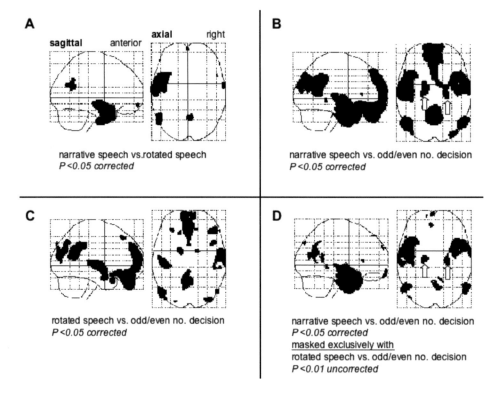

A

sagittal   anterior   **axial**   right

narrative speech vs.rotated speech
P<0.05 corrected

B

narrative speech vs. odd/even no. decision
P<0.05 corrected

C

rotated speech vs. odd/even no. decision
P<0.05 corrected

D

narrative speech vs. odd/even no. decision
P<0.05 corrected
<u>masked exclusively with</u>
rotated speech vs. odd/even no. decision
P<0.01 uncorrected

Figure 7.4
This PET study illustrates the effects of using "passive" presentation of stimuli, and how the use of different baseline conditions in cognitive "subtractions" from a single activation condition results in major differences in the visualization of cortical activity. Eleven subjects heard narratives without an explicit task demand; that is, they were simply asked to listen to the passages. A second condition was "passive" listening to the same passages after the speech signal had been rendered unintelligible by spectral rotation (Scott et al., 2000). The third condition was a repetitive "active" task on numbers, one originally proposed by Stark and Squire (2001) to reveal activity related to episodic memory encodement in the medial temporal lobes. The results are displayed as statistical parametric maps in sagittal and axial views (Wellcome Department of Cognitive Neurology, Institute of Neurology, London, UK; www.fil.ion.ucl. ac.uk/spm/).

(*A*)"Passive" listening to narrative speech contrasted with "passive" listening to unintelligible rotated speech showed a prominent activation in the left anterior temporal lobe. There were smaller volumes of activation in the right anterior temporal lobe, the left temporo-parietal-occipital junction, and two midline regions: anterior prefrontal cortex and anterior precuneus.

(*B*) By contrast, "passive" listening to narrative speech contrasted with the odd/even number decision showed extensive midline and posterior parietal activity. There was activity in both medial temporal lobes (arrows) and in posterior regions, which probably indicates memory processing of the content of the narratives.

(*C*) "Passive" listening contrasted with the odd/even number decision also demonstrated activity in anterior and posterior cortex, and at least some of this distributed activity may be attributed to the retrieval of memories and knowledge during stimulus independent thoughts.

(*D*) When those voxels in (*C*) were excluded from (*B*), regions that were related to the "passive" state were excluded. Although this excludes processes that may be common both to the comprehension and the interpretation of concepts contained within intelligible narratives and to the initiation and pursuit of lines of coherent thoughts that intrude while "passively" listening to unintelligible rotated speech, it reveals that the automatic processing of intelligible narratives is associated with extensive activity in both anterior temporal lobes.

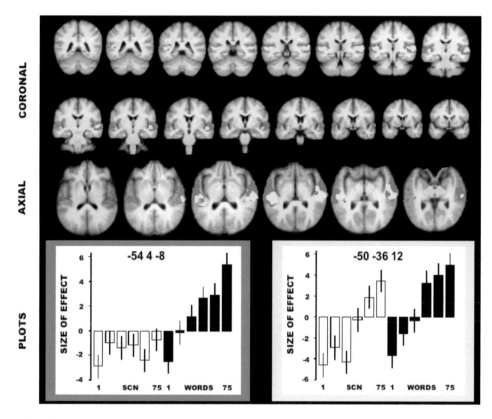

Figure 7.5
This PET study (Mummery et al., 1999) investigated the brain responses to listening to increasing rates of single, unrelated, bisyllabic nouns (range 1–75 words/min) and signal-correlated noise (SCN) at the same rates (SCN comprises the time-amplitude envelopes of the words with all spectrotemporal detail removed by filling the envelopes with white noise). Voxels in which there was a linear increase in activity to both SCN and words were identified separately from voxels where the response was to words and not to SCN. These were coregistered, in yellow and red, respectively, onto an averaged T1-weighted MRI template. The slices are 4 mm apart, displayed posterior-anterior for the coronal slices and dorsal-ventral for the axial slices. The "speech-specific" (at least specific relative to SCN) extended forward along both left and right superior temporal gyri. Two plots of activity (arbitrary units centered around zero) for SCN and words at the different rates of presentation are shown, one taken from a voxel in the left anterior superior temporal gyrus (stereotactic coordinates –54 4 –8) and the other from the left planum temporale (–50 –36 12). In the latter region, the responses to SCN and words were indistinguishable. See plate 10 for color version.

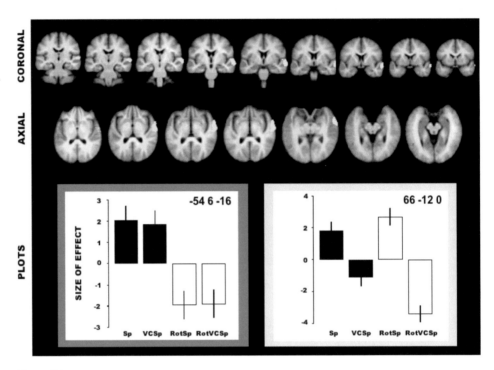

Figure 7.6
This result is taken from the PET study of Scott and colleagues (2000). The subjects "passively" heard normal speech (Sp), degraded but intelligible speech (VCSp), spectrally rotated normal speech (RotSp; unintelligible, but closely matched the acoustic complexity of normal speech) and spectrally rotated degraded speech (RotVCSp). The response (displayed on successive posterior-anterior coronal and dorsal-ventral axial MR templates, spaced 4 mm apart) in the left anterior superior temporal sulcus (−54 6 −16, in red) corresponded to the intelligibility of the stimulus, whereas the signal in the right superior temporal gyrus (66 −12 0, in yellow) corresponded to acoustic complexity. See plate 11 for color version.

modality-specific sensory cortex, there may be regions that respond to unattended stimuli, whereas activity in adjacent regions may be strongly modulated by attention (Petkov et al., 2004). When listening to two speakers but attending only to one, the magnitude of activity in regions within the listener's auditory cortex indicated an attention-independent response to both speech inputs (Scott et al., 2004). With overt speech conditions, it remains unclear how much of the recorded temporal lobe activity is due to the retrieval of lexical forms prior to utterance and how much to the sound of the speaker's own voice. The attention one pays to one's own speech production after rather than before articulation may depend much on the context (Levelt, 1989). Electroencephalographic (EEG) recordings of event-related potentials (ERPs) or magnetoencephalographic (MEG) recordings could give the millisecond timing to answer this question, but the muscle activity associated with continuous speech production is a major confound, although recordings can be made using very brief utterances (Gunji et al., 2001). Blood flow studies have shown that the activity recorded in superior temporal cortex in response to the subject's own voice is different from that recorded when the subject listens to another voice, at least during single-word repetition (Wise et al., 1999). Studies of the effects of delayed auditory feedback of one's own voice suggest one method of further investigating automatic and explicit self-monitoring of speech output (Hashimoto & Sakai, 2003).

Problems with the "Active" Condition

Most commonly, studies use "active" tasks to isolate components of the language system. One reason for this is obvious: many workers have arrived in functional imaging from a research background in which reaction times and error rates were the only measures. You carry on doing what you are used to doing. The advantages are that task accuracy and error rate ensure that the subjects are paying attention to the stimuli and processing them in the way intended; for example, deciding that *tiger* is a dangerous animal, but *antelope* is not, must probe controlled access to associative knowledge. Alternatively, requiring the subjects to make an explicit decision on a nonlinguistic feature present in verbal stimuli allows one to investigate obligatory parallel automatic linguistic processing while ensuring that the subjects pay attention to each stimulus (Price et al., 1996). Further, performance measures are often very useful measures with which to correlate the relative magnitude of regional cerebral activity.

A real problem, however, is that it may not be at all obvious how the nature of the task may be influencing the observed signal. Listening to or reading a linguistic stimulus; making a decision based on sublexical, lexical, semantic or syntactic criteria; and indicating this decision to the experimenter, usually through a button box, is very different from simply listening to speech or reading for meaning, which proceed largely automatically. A particular example is a task that requires the mental segmentation of a heard word or nonword to identify the presence or otherwise of a particular phoneme. To do this task, the subject must make use of the same neural systems required for the perception and recognition of heard words. However, the subject must also use additional resources that depend on awareness of the alphabet; illiterate subjects, who have no problem perceiving and understanding speech, are incapable of deciding, for example, whether a *t* sound is present in *bitten* (Read et al., 1986).

There is usually an attempt to control for task-dependent processes that are not under investigation, such as working memory and decision-making, by incorporating an equivalent task in the baseline condition to subtract the signal from these processes. However, the precise equivalence of these processes between the activation and the baseline conditions is usually assumed rather than determined from direct experimental evidence. Thus, categorizing the pitch of a tone as the same or different relative to one or more exemplars is not the same as making a decision on the semantic associations of a word. Such a contrast will undoubtedly result in the demonstration of prefrontal activity (Binder et al., 1997), but the relation of this activity to normal language comprehension may not be readily apparent. However, such task-related activity may itself be worthy of investigation and interpretation (Scott et al., 2003; Sharp et al., 2004a).

In addition to prefrontal activity that may be task-specific rather than language-specific, there may be uncertainty about the effects of task-specific, top-down modulation altering activity in posterior cortex. Physiologists and anatomists have long recognized that forward neural pathways are almost invariably accompanied by feedback pathways. In the visual system, neurons relatively early in the visual pathway respond to simple features, such as color or line orientation, but in anterior visual association cortex the more broadly tuned neurons respond to complex conjunctions of features (Tanaka, 1996; Lerner et al., 2004). Research in nonhuman primates has shown, after appropriate behavioral training, that a population of single neurons in the anterior part of the ventral visual pathway respond to one complex, arbitrary visual shape and not another. Further, training can result in these neurons responding to another shape with which the sample shape is arbitrarily paired. This acquired knowledge depends on neural interactions between "pair-encoding" neurons far forward in high-order visual association cortex and adjacent polysensory perirhinal cortex (Naya et al., 2003). To speculate that cross-modal, visual-auditory, pair-encoding neurons develop in the human polysensory perirhinal cortex as an infant learns to match an object with its heard word is compelling, with increasing experience resulting in greater specificity of the tuning of these neurons—learning, for example, that a *Pekingese* is a particular, if rather unusual-looking, dog.

These and similar observations and speculations have motivated studies which have shown, for example, that retrieving the name of an object will increase activity in perirhinal cortex, but only if the basic name is generated (*it's a monkey* rather than *it's a living thing*) (Tyler et al., 2004). However, it has been observed in a number of studies that various word- and picture-related tasks contrasting animals and tools have demonstrated activity early in the ventral visual stream. This result has not been interpreted as a demonstration that detailed associative knowledge about animals is represented in occipital cortex; rather, it is proposed that our knowledge about animals is dependent more on their visual features than is our knowledge about tools. Thus, the animal-related occipital activity is viewed as the result of category-specific feedback from higher-order to lower-order unimodal visual association cortex (for references and discussion, see Martin & Chao, 2001). Ultimately, access to knowledge about any object or word will depend on activity in both forward and feedback pathways, with the general rule that the earlier the activity is in the processing "stream," the simpler are the associative features that are represented. The relative weight of activity in reciprocal pathways will depend on the context within which that knowledge is being retrieved.

Related phenomena may occur in linguistic processing. In particular, there is the likelihood of frontotemporal interactions in the controlled processing of language stimuli. To illustrate this possibility, we take the example of the interpretation of studies of syntactic processing. A number of groups have published data suggesting that syntactic processing occurs in the anterior superior temporal gyrus (left and/or right)—in other words, in unimodal auditory association cortex, even as close to primary auditory cortex as the planum polare (for example, Friederici et al., 2000; Kuperberg et al., 2000). These studies used auditory presentation of the stimuli. Studies on syntactical processing that have used written stimuli have not demonstrated activity in the same region of the superior temporal gyrus. Figure 7.7 (see plate 12) illustrates one of our recent studies, using the "passive" perception of written narratives contrasted with "passive" perception of an unintelligible visual baseline. It is evident, as far as this simple contrast goes, that the processing of the visually perceived narratives, both semantic and syntactic, activates the length of the left superior temporal sulcus, but this activity does not spread into the superior temporal gyrus or superior temporal plane.

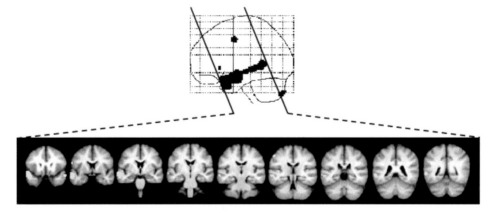

Figure 7.7
This result from an unpublished PET study included reading narratives contrasted with reading illegible textlike arrays of pseudo script. The contrast showed activity along the length of the left superior temporal sulcus. Activity displayed on the sagittal statistical parametric map has also been displayed on coronal MR slices, in the same manner as in figures 7.5 and 7.6. See plate 12 for color version.

If the result from this study is combined with the results of the auditory language studies depicted in figures 7.5 and 7.6, it would seem that spoken and written language converge on the superior temporal sulcus, a region in the primate known to be an important neocortical polysensory area, and forwards to the temporal pole. This is a strikingly similar result to the MEG study of the "active" semantic processing of both spoken and written single words (Marinkovic et al., 2003). This raises a number of issues. First, anterior temporal activation is not synonymous with the processing of syntax alone; it is observed in both "passive" and "active" single-word conditions (see also Scott et al., 2003; Sharp et al., 2004a). Second, if unimodal auditory association cortex in the superior temporal gyrus is indeed involved in syntactic processing (and there is no a priori reason why neural networks for the acoustic processing of the speech signal and syntax are not colocalized in overlapping but separate neural networks), the implication is that syntactic processing must be, at least in part, modality-specific. Finally, and this is the rub, activity in the anterior superior temporal gyrus in association with syntactic tasks on heard stimuli may be a task-specific modulation of activity relatively early in the speech-processing "stream."

Therefore, although the "passive" presentation of stimuli is open to the criticism "You don't know what the subjects were doing," metalinguistic tasks may produce a physiological signal that does not map in a simple manner onto the psychological process under study. Rather, it is the sum of forward and feedback neural activity associated with linguistic and task-specific processing on perceptually odd stimuli, such as pseudo words, Jabberwocky sentences, syntactic prose, and so on. (Friston et al., 1996). There is a potential way around this problem: the combination of millisecond resolution of MEG with techniques to give better spatial resolution of this technique (Dale and Halgren, 2001) offers the potential to separate forward processes from later feedback modulation of activity. Even then, this may not be an entirely straightforward exercise when investigating syntactic comprehension, for studies using scalp electroencephalography to measure event-related potentials indicate that there are early (automatic) and late (controlled) phases in the normal comprehension of syntax (Friederici, 2002; Friederici for Kotz, 2003). An alternative is to model fMRI data to examine task-specific and context-specific effective connectivity. Such an approach no longer displays the data as a set of functionally specialized regions, but as functionally integrated units (Penny et al., 2004). The strength of the connections between regions may then reveal the differences in bottom-up and top-down modulations, modulations that are very likely to vary with the type of stimulus and the context of the task (Mechelli et al., 2003; Mechelli et al., 2004).

The Problem of the Null Result

This is a problem with any branch of science, and perhaps more so with functional imaging. If, across different studies purporting to investigate the same mental process or representation, the individual populations studied are small and the statistical power is marginal, then lack of agreement ensues. To counter this, several centers are constructing large databases to which individual institutions can send their raw data for subsequent reanalysis or inclusion in a meta-analysis by any contributor to the scheme.

We have already alluded to uncertainties that may accompany the choice of activation and baseline conditions. A further example concerns theories about the representation of nouns and verbs. Although a number of clinical neuropsychological studies have suggested that verbs and nouns are differentially sensitive to focal brain damage (Goodglass et al., 1966; Damasio & Tranel, 1993), and some imaging studies support the hypothesis of regional neural differentiation within the semantic system (e.g., (Perani et al., 1999), others do not (Tyler et al., 2001). In the face of a previously published positive result, Tyler and colleagues had to argue two points. The first was that their design was less susceptible to confounds than the earlier study. The second was that their null result was not a consequence of inadequate statistical power. Since it is less easy to publish an absence of an effect, especially if a presence of an effect has been "established" by a prior publication, this leads to both a bias in the literature and a certain reluctance for workers to expend effort (and money) seeing if an earlier result is reproducible. Therefore, strong claims based on the results of a single study should be treated with circumspection unless there is strong converging evidence from another discipline, such as clinical neuropsychology. As with any branch of the behavioral sciences, the devil is in the details with functional imaging studies, and a small change in stimulus type or in task demand *may* be accompanied by a large difference in outcome.

The Problems of Scale, Modularity, and Regional Selectivity

We will illustrate these points by referring to the current lively debate about the so-called visual word-form area (VWFA). Although originally a neuropsychological concept, the VWFA became anatomically localized to part of the left basal occipitotemporal cortex after analysis of structural images of patients with pure alexia (see, e.g., Binder & Mohr, 1992). Subsequently, a large body of work, from one group in particular, has been interpreted as a demonstration of the regional specialization of part of the left fusiform gyrus for the recognition of written words (Cohen et al., 2000; McCandliss et al., 2003; Cohen & Dehaene, 2004). The arguments are compelling to those neurologists who take an interest in acquired alexia, since patients with pure alexia may exhibit striking dissociations: a patient who can only laboriously read *hundred* aloud may quickly produce the response *one million, six hundred and seventy-three thousand, and four* when presented with *1,673,004*. However, the claim for regional word-form specialization has been challenged by Price and Devlin (2003, 2004). Modularity of the VWFA, in the Fodorian sense (Fodor, 1983), implies both domain specificity (the response is to words and not other visual objects) and mandatory processing (whatever the written word-related task, that region will always be engaged, regardless of what other neural systems are involved) (Cerullo et al., 2004). In particular, the domain specificity of the proposed VWFA is being questioned (for recent examples, see (Kao et al., 2004; Vandenbulcke et al., 2004).

An important part of the debate centers on resolution. One possibility, as discussed by Cohen and Dehaene (2004), is that domain specificity may occur at the level of cortical columns (Tsunoda et al., 2001). If this is so, it will require high-field fMRI scanning with spin-echo data acquisition and resulting submillimeter resolution. Thus, an important consideration at the beginning of a study is to ask whether one's hypothesis includes the expectation that the function under study is served by a regionally specialized patch of cortex that is at least several millimeters in size. Such hypotheses may best be applied to input rather than central systems (as originally proposed by Fodor, 1983). A series of single case studies will give the best anatomical resolution. Using a range of different stimuli in the experimental design will help to confirm domain specificity and mandatory processing. If one has a more distributed system in mind, with involvement of a number of local neural systems and their connections, then spatial resolution is less of a concern, and MEG studies with fine temporal resolution may be the answer (Tarkiainen et al., 1999; Marinkovic et al., 2003). An alternative is a more sophisticated analysis of the fMRI data to reveal effective connectivity—in other words, a statistical measure of the strength of functional connections, as indexed by regionally correlated changes in blood flow between different brain regions in response to a particular experimental context.

Concluding Remarks

We have covered a lot in this chapter, and missed out much more. We have not covered, as a few examples, studies of recovery after aphasic stroke, the abnormal control of speech during stuttering, culture-specific brain activity related to different kinds of script, or bilingualism. However, there have been about 1,000 papers directly or indirectly exploring the functional imaging of human communication published since the first edition of this chapter. Lines, usually around personal preferences, were drawn. We hope that we have achieved two ends: to introduce the wide diversity of activity in the study of human communication with functional imaging, and to highlight the fact that performing a meaningful functional imaging study requires more than taking a snapshot of the brain "in action."

We will end with a general point. The recent debate about the visual word-form area has highlighted what it means to define a brain module in terms of a change in local blood flow. In earlier days one "knew" where to look and simply drew a "region of interest," followed up by a t-test. These have gone except for a small handful of specialized studies. Viewing the brain as an array of specialized functional units has a long tradition, and is the general concept that has supported a host of functional imaging studies since the mid-1980s. Now we are entering the era, long predicted and awaiting practical and validated methodological solutions, of interpreting activations in terms of transient interactions between specialized regions, with the strength of local signal governed as much by the stimulus and task as is the process (lexical semantics, syntax, etc.) under investigation. We return to the MEG study of Marinkovic and colleagues (2003, 105). If you give a subject a task (*is a larger or smaller than 1 foot [one-third of a meter] in length*), and then flash *tiger* on a screen, activity spreads from the occipital to the frontal pole in <500 ms. In passing, all the brain regions depicted in figure 7.1 become involved (if recording had been continued up to the time of a motor response to the decision, activity in premotor and motor cortex would have been observed). Forward and feedback projections between unimodal association, polysensory, paralimbic and limbic, and prefrontal cortex are universal. Although observations on regional specialization will continue, additional information from studies of "effective connectivity" will add depth to our understanding of language processing in the normal brain, and perhaps even more to neural compensation after a focal brain injury.

References

Alexander, M. P., Hiltbrunner, B., & Fischer, R. S. (1989). Distributed anatomy of transcortical sensory aphasia. *Archives of Neurology* 46, 885–892.

Amunts, K., Schleicher, A., Burgel, U., Mohlberg, H., Uylings, H. B., & Zilles, K. (1999). Broca's region revisited: Cytoarchitecture and intersubject variability. *Journal of Comparative Neurology* 412, 319–341.

Amunts, K., Weiss, P. H., Mohlberg, H., Pieperhoff, P., Eickhoff, S., Gurd, J. M., Marshall, J. C., Shah, N. J., Fink, G. R., & Zilles, K. (2004). Analysis of neural mechanisms underlying verbal fluency in cytoarchitectonically defined stereotaxic space—the roles of Brodmann areas 44 and 45. *NeuroImage* 22, 42–56.

Barde, L. H., & Thompson-Schill, S. L. (2002). Models of functional organization of the lateral prefrontal cortex in verbal working memory: Evidence in favor of the process model. *Journal of Cognitive Neuroscience* 14, 1054–1063.

Basso, A., Lecours, A. R., Moraschini, S., & Vanier, M. (1985). Anatomoclinical correlations of the aphasias as defined through computerized tomography: Exceptions. *Brain and Language* 26, 201–229.

Bates, E., Wilson, S. M., Saygin, A. P., Dick, F., Sereno, M. I., Knight, R. T., & Dronkers, N. F. (2003). Voxel-based lesion-symptom mapping. *Nature Neuroscience* 6, 448–450.

Beauchamp, M. S., Lee, K. E., Argall, B. A., & Martin, A. (2004). Integration of auditory and visual information about objects in superior temporal sulcus. *Neuron* 41, 809–823.

Belin, P., Zatorre, R. J., Lafaille, P., Ahad, P., & Pike, B. (2000). Voice-selective areas in human auditory cortex. *Nature* 403, 309–312.

Binder, J. R. (2002). Wernicke aphasia: A disorder of central language processing. In M. E. D'Esposito (Ed.), *Neurological Foundations of Cognitive Neuroscience*, 175–238. Cambridge, MA: MIT Press.

Binder, J. R., Frost, J. A., Hammeke, T. A., Bellgowan, P. S. F., Rao, S. M., & Cox, R. W. (1999). Conceptual processing during the conscious resting state: A functional MRI study. *Journal of Cognitive Neuroscience* 11, 80–93.

Binder, J. R., Frost, J. A., Hammeke, T. A., Bellgowan, P. S., Springer, J. A., Kaufman, J. N., & Possing, E. T. (2000). Human temporal lobe activation by speech and nonspeech sounds. *Cerebral Cortex* 10, 512–528.

Binder, J. R., Frost, J. A., Hammeke, T. A., Cox, R. W., Rao, S. M., & Prieto, T. (1997). Human brain language areas identified by functional magnetic resonance imaging. *Journal of Neuroscience* 17, 353–362.

Binder, J. R., Frost, J. A., Hammeke, T. A., Rao, S. M., & Cox, R. W. (1996). Function of the left planum temporale in auditory and linguistic processing. *Brain* 119, 1239–1247.

Binder, J. R., McKiernan, K. A., Parsons, M. E., Westbury, C. F., Possing, E. T., Kaufman, J. N., & Buchanan, L. (2003). Neural correlates of lexical access during visual word recognition. *Journal of Cognitive Neuroscience* 15, 372–393.

Binder, J. R., & Mohr, J. P. (1992). The topography of callosal reading pathways. A case-control analysis. *Brain* 115, 1807–1826.

Binder, J. R., & Price, C. P. (2001). Functional imaging of language. In R. Cabeza & A. Kingstone (Eds.), *Handbook of Functional Neuroimaging of Cognition*, 187–251. Cambridge, MA: MIT Press.

Bird, C. M., Castelli, F., Malik, O., Frith, U., & Husain, M. (2004). The impact of extensive medial frontal lobe damage on "theory of mind" and cognition. *Brain* 127, 914–928.

Blank, S. C., Bird, H., Turkheimer, F., & Wise, R. J. (2003). Speech production after stroke: The role of the right pars opercularis. *Annals of Neurology* 54, 310–320.

Blank, S. C., Scott, S. K., Murphy, K., Warburton, E., & Wise, R. J. (2002). Speech production: Wernicke, Broca and beyond. *Brain* 125, 1829–1838.

Braun, A. R., Guillemin, A., Hosey, L., & Varga, M. (2001). The neural organization of discourse: An $H_2^{15}O$-PET study of narrative production in English and American sign language. *Brain* 124, 2028–2044.

Büchel, C., Price, C., & Friston, K. (1998). A multimodal language region in the ventral visual pathway. *Nature* 394, 274–277.

Buckner, R. L., Raichle, M. E., & Petersen, S. E. (1995). Dissociation of human prefrontal cortical areas across different speech production tasks and gender groups. *Journal of Neurophysiology* 74, 2163–2173.

Burnstine, T. H., Lesser, R. P., Hart, J., Jr., Uematsu, S., Zinreich, S. J., Krauss, G. L., Fisher, R. S., Vining, E. P., & Gordon, B. (1990). Characterization of the basal temporal language area in patients with left temporal lobe epilepsy. *Neurology* 40, 966–970.

Caplan, D., Alpert, N., & Waters, G. (1998). Effects of syntactic structure and propositional number on patterns of regional cerebral blood flow. *Journal of Cognitive Neuroscience* 10, 541–552.

Caplan, D., Alpert, N., & Waters, G. (1999). PET studies of syntactic processing with auditory sentence presentation. *NeuroImage* 9, 343–351.

Caplan, D., Hildebrandt, N., & Makris, N. (1996). Location of lesions in stroke patients with deficits in syntactic processing in sentence comprehension. *Brain* 119, 933–949.

Caplan, D., & Waters, G. S. (1999). Verbal working memory and sentence comprehension. *Behavioral and Brain Sciences* 22, 77–94.

Caramazza, A., Capitani, E., Rey, A., & Berndt, R. S. (2001). Agrammatic Broca's aphasia is not associated with a single pattern of comprehension performance. *Brain and Language* 76, 158–184.

Caramazza, A., & Zurif, E. B. (1976). Dissociation of algorithmic and heuristic processes in language comprehension: Evidence from aphasia. *Brain and Language* 3, 572–582.

Cerullo, M. A., Mier, C. R., & Joseph, J. E. (2004). Testing the modularity of cognitive domains with functional magnetic resonance imaging. Abstract Viewer & Itinerary Planner. Washington DC: Society for Neuroscience, 2004. Online.

Cohen, L., & Dehaene, S. (2004). Specialization within the ventral stream: The case for the visual word form area. *NeuroImage* 22, 466–476.

Cohen, L., and Dehaene, S., Naccache, L., Lehéricy, S., Dehaene-Lambertz, G., Hénaff, M., & Michel, F. (2000). The visual word form area: Spatial and temporal characterization of an initial stage of reading in normal subjects and posterior split-brain patients. *Brain* 123, 291–307.

Cooke, A., Zurif, E. B., DeVita, C., Alsop, D., Koenig, P., Detre, J., Gee, J., Pinango, M., Balogh, J., & Grossman, M. (2002). Neural basis for sentence comprehension: Grammatical and short-term memory components. *Human Brain Mapping* 15, 80–94.

Crinion, J. T., Lambon-Ralph, M. A., Warburton, E. A., Howard, D., & Wise, R. J. (2003). Temporal lobe regions engaged during normal speech comprehension. *Brain* 126, 1193–1201.

Dale, A. M., & Halgren, E. (2001). Spatiotemporal mapping of brain activity by integration of multiple imaging modalities. *Current Opinion in Neurobiology* 11, 202–208.

Damasio, A. R. (1989). Time-locked multiregional retroactivation: A systems-level proposal for the neural substrates of recall and recognition. *Cognition* 33, 25–62.

Damasio, A. R., & Tranel, D. (1993). Nouns and verbs are retrieved with differently distributed neural systems. *Proceedings of the National Academy of Sciences USA* 90, 4957–4960.

Dapretto, M., & Bookheimer, S. Y. (1999). Form and content: Dissociating syntax and semantics in sentence comprehension. *Neuron* 24, 427–432.

Davis, M. H., & Johnsrude, I. S. (2003). Hierarchical processing in spoken language comprehension. *Journal of Neuroscience* 23, 3423–3431.

Devlin, J. T., Matthews, P. M., & Rushworth, M. F. (2003). Semantic processing in the left inferior prefrontal cortex: A combined functional magnetic resonance imaging and transcranial magnetic stimulation study. *Journal of Cognitive Neuroscience* 15, 71–84.

Devlin, J. T., Moore, C. J., Mummery, C. J., Gorno-Tempini, M. L., Phillips, J. A., Noppeney, U., Frackowiak, R. S., Friston, K. J., & Price, C. J. (2002). Anatomic constraints on cognitive theories of category specificity. *NeuroImage* 15, 675–685.

Devlin, J. T., Russell, R. P., Davis, M. H., Price, C. J., Moss, H. E., Fadili, M. J., & Tyler, L. K. (2002). Is there an anatomical basis for category-specificity? Semantic memory studies in PET and fMRI. *Neuropsychologia* 40, 54–75.

Devlin, J. T., Russell, R. P., Davis, M. H., Price, C. J., Wilson, J., Moss, H. E., Matthews, P. M., & Tyler, L. K. (2000). Susceptibility-induced loss of signal: Comparing PET and fMRI on a semantic task. *NeuroImage* 11, 589–600.

Dhankhar, A., Wexler, B. E., Fulbright, R. K., Halwes, T., Blamire, A. M., & Shulman, R. G. (1997). Functional magnetic resonance imaging assessment of the human brain auditory cortex response to increasing word presentation rates. *Journal of Neurophysiology* 77, 476–483.

Dick, F., Bates, E., Wulfeck, B., Utman, J. A., Dronkers, N., & Gernsbacher, M. A. (2001). Language deficits, localization, and grammar: Evidence for a distributive model of language breakdown in aphasic patients and neurologically intact individuals. *Psychological Review* 108, 759–788.

Doupe, A. J., & Kuhl, P. K. (1999). Birdsong and human speech: Common themes and mechanisms. *Annual Review of Neuroscience* 22, 567–631.

Dronkers, N. F., Wilkins, D. P., Van Valin, R. D., Jr., Redfern, B. B., & Jaeger, J. J. (2004). Lesion analysis of the brain areas involved in language comprehension. *Cognition* 92, 145–177.

Embick, D., Marantz, A., Miyashita, Y., O'Neil, W., & Sakai, K. L. (2000). A syntactic specialization in Broca's area. *Proceedings of the National Academy of Sciences USA* 97, 6150–6154.

Fadiga, L., Craighero, L., Buccino, G., & Rizzolatti, G. (2002). Speech listening specifically modulates the excitability of tongue muscles: A TMS study. *European Journal of Neuroscience* 15, 399–402.

Fiebach, C. J., Schlesewsky, M., Lohmann, G., von Cramon, D. Y., & Friederici, A. D. (2004). Revisiting the role of Broca's area in sentence processing: Syntactic integration versus syntactic working memory. *Human Brain Mapping* 24, 79–91.

Fiebach, C. J., Vos, S. H., & Friederici, A. D. (2004). Neural correlates of syntactic ambiguity in sentence comprehension for high and low span readers. *Journal of Cognitive Neuroscience* 16, 1562–1575.

Fitch, W. T. (2000). The evolution of speech: A comparative review. *Trends in Cognitive Sciences* 4, 258–267.

Fodor, J. (1983). *The Modularity of Mind*. Cambridge, MA: MIT Press.

Friederici, A. D. (2002). Towards a neural basis of auditory sentence processing. *Trends in Cognitive Sciences* 6, 78–84.

Friederici, A. D., & Kotz, S. A. (2003). The brain basis of syntactic processes: Functional imaging and lesion studies. *NeuroImage* 20(supp. 1), S8–S17.

Friederici, A. D., Meyer, M., & von Cramon, D. Y. (2000). Auditory language comprehension: An event-related fMRI study on the processing of syntactic and lexical information. *Brain and Language* 74, 289–300.

Friston, K. J., Price, C. J., Fletcher, P., Moore, C., Frackowiak, R. S. J., & Dolan, R. J. (1996). The trouble with cognitive subtraction. *NeuroImage* 4, 97–104.

Frith, C. D., & Frith, U. (1999). Interacting minds—a biological basis. *Science* 286, 1692–1695.

Ghafanzar, A. A., & Hauser, M. D. (1999). The neuroethology of primate vocal communication: Substrates for the evolution of speech. *Trends in Cognitive Sciences* 3, 377–384.

Gilboa, A., Winocur, G., Grady, C. L., Hevenor, S. J., & Moscovitch, M. (2004). Remembering our past: Functional neuroanatomy of recollection of recent and very remote personal events. *Cerebral Cortex* 14, 1214–1225.

Gloor, P. (1997). *The Temporal Lobe and Limbic System*. New York: Oxford University Press.

Goel, V., Gold, B., Kapur, S., & Houle, S. (1997). The seats of reason? An imaging study of deductive and inductive reasoning. *NeuroReport* 8, 1305–1310.

Gold, B. T., & Buckner, R. L. (2002). Common prefrontal regions coactivate with dissociable posterior regions during controlled semantic and phonological tasks. *Neuron* 35, 803–812.

Goodglass, H. (1993). *Understanding Aphasia*. San Diego: Academic Press.

Goodglass, H., Klein, B., Carey, P., & Jones, K. J. (1966). Specific semantic word categories in aphasia. *Cortex* 2, 74–89.

Gorno-Tempini, M. L., Dronkers, N. F., Rankin, K. P., Ogar, J. M., Phengrasamy, L., Rosen, H. J., Johnson, J. K., Weiner, M. W., & Miller, B. L. (2004). Cognition and anatomy in three variants of primary progressive aphasia. *Annals of Neurology* 55, 335–346.

Grabowski, T. J., & Damasio, A. R. (2000). Investigating language with functional neuroimaging. In A. W. Toga & J. C. Mazziotta (Eds.), *Brain Mapping: The Systems*, 425–461. San Diego: Academic Press.

Griffiths, T. D., & Warren, J. D. (2002). The planum temporale as a computational hub. *Trends in Neurosciences* 25, 348–353.

Grodzinsky, Y. (2000). The neurology of syntax: Language use without Broca's area. *Behavioral and Brain Sciences* 23, 1–21.

Gunji, A., Hoshiyama, M., & Kakigi, R. (2001). Auditory response following vocalization: A magnetoencephalographic study. *Clinical Neurophysiology* 112, 514–520.

Gusnard, D. A., & Raichle, M. E. (2001). Searching for a baseline: Functional imaging and the resting human brain. *Nature Neuroscience Review* 2, 685–694.

Hall, D. A., Haggard, M. O., Akeroyd, M. A., Palmer, A. R., Summerfield, A. O., Elliott, M. R., Gurney, E. M., & Bowtell, R. W. (1999). "Sparse" temporal sampling in auditory fMRI. *Human Brain Mapping* 7, 213–223.

Hashimoto, Y., & Sakai, K. L. (2003). Brain activations during conscious self-monitoring of speech production with delayed auditory feedback: An fMRI study. *Human Brain Mapping* 20, 22–28.

Hauk, O., Johnsrude, I., & Pulvermuller, F. (2004). Somatotopic representation of action words in human motor and premotor cortex. *Neuron* 22(41), 301–307.

Hickok, G., Buchsbaum, B., Humphries, C., & Muftuler, T. (2003). Auditory-motor interaction revealed by fMRI: Speech, music, and working memory in area Spt. *Journal of Cognitive Neuroscience* 15, 673–682.

Hickok, G., Erhard, P., Kassubek, J., Helms-Tillery, A. K., Naeve-Velguth, S., Strupp, J. P., Strick, P. L., & Ugurbil, K. (2000). A functional magnetic resonance imaging study of the role of left posterior superior temporal gyrus in speech production: Implications for the explanation of conduction aphasia. *Neuroscience Letters* 287, 156–160.

Hickok, G., & Poeppel, D. (2000). Towards a functional neuroanatomy of speech perception. *Trends in Cognitive Sciences* 4, 131–138.

Hickok, G., & Poeppel, D. (2004). Dorsal and ventral streams: A framework for understanding aspects of the functional anatomy of language. *Cognition* 92, 67–99.

Humphries, C., Willard, K., Buchsbaum, B., & Hickok, G. (2001). Role of anterior temporal cortex in auditory sentence comprehension: An fMRI study. *NeuroReport* 12, 1749–1752.

Indefrey, P., Hagoort, P., Herzog, H., Seitz, R. J., & Brown, C. M. (2001). Syntactic processing in left pre-frontal cortex is independent of lexical meaning. *NeuroImage* 14, 546–555.

Insausti, R., Juottonen, K., Soininen, H., Insausti, A. M., Partanen, K., Vainio, P., Laakso, M. P., & Pitkanen, A. (1998). MR volumetric analysis of the human entorhinal, perirhinal, and temporopolar cortices. *American Journal of Neuroradiology* 19, 659–671.

Jacquemot, C., Pallier, C., LeBihan, D., Dehaene, S., & Dupoux, E. (2003). Phonological grammar shapes the auditory cortex: A functional magnetic resonance imaging study. *Journal of Neuroscience* 23, 9541–9546.

Joseph, J. E. (2001). Functional neuroimaging studies of category specificity in object recognition: A critical review and meta-analysis. *Cognitive, Affective, and Behavioral Neuroscience* 1, 119–136.

Just, M. A., & Carpenter, P. A. (1992). A capacity theory of comprehension: Individual differences in working memory. *Psychological Review* 98, 122–149.

Just, M. A., Carpenter, P. A., Keller, T. A., Eddy, W. F., & Thulborn, K. R. (1996). Brain activation modulated by sentence comprehension. *Science* 274, 114–116.

Kaan, E., & Swaab, T. Y. (2002). The brain circuitry of syntactic comprehension. *Trends in Cognitive Sciences* 6, 350–356.

Kaas, J. H., & Hackett, T. A. (2000). Subdivisions of auditory cortex and processing streams in primates. *Proceedings of the National Academy of Sciences USA* 97, 11793–11799.

Kaas, J. H., Hackett, T. A., & Tramo, M. J. (1999). Auditory processing in primate cerebral cortex. *Current Opinion in Neurobiology* 9, 164–170.

Kao, C., Hue, C., Chen, C., Chen, D., Liang, K., & Chen, J. (2004). The role of the left fusiform gyrus in the processing of Chinese characters. Abstract Viewer and Itinerary Planner, Washington DC: Society for Neuroscience, 2004. Online.

Keller, T., Carpenter, M. A., & Just, M. A. (2001). The neural basis of sentence comprehension: An fMRI examination of syntactic and lexical processing. *Cerebral Cortex* 11, 223–237.

Kemeny, S., Ye, F. Q., Birn, R., & Braun, A. R. (2004). Comparison of continuous overt speech fMRI using BOLD and arterial spin labeling. *Human Brain Mapping* 24, 173–183.

Kolk, H. H., & Friederici, A. D. (1985). Strategy and impairment in sentence understanding by Broca's and Wernicke's aphasics. *Cortex* 21, 47–67.

Kuhl, P. K. (2004). Early language acquisition: Cracking the speech code. *Nature Reviews Neuroscience* 5, 831–843.

Kuperberg, G. R., McGuire, P. K., Bullmore, E. T., Brammer, M. J., Rabe-Hesketh, S., Wright, I. C., Lythgoe, D. J., Williams, S. C., & David, A. S. (2000). Common and distinct neural substrates for pragmatic, semantic and syntactic processing of spoken word sentences: An fMRI study. *Journal of Cognitive Neuroscience* 12, 321–341.

Lambon-Ralph, M. A., McClelland, J. L., Paterson, K., Galton, C. J., & Hodges, J. R. (2001). No right to speak? The relationship between object naming and semantic impairment: Neuropsychological evidence and a computational model. *Journal of Cognitive Neuroscience* 13, 341–356.

Lambon-Ralph, M. A., Patterson, K., Garrard, P., & Hodges, J. R. (2003). Semantic dementia with category-specificity: A comparative case-series study. *Cognitive Neuropsychology* 20, 307–326.

Lavenex, P., Suzuki, W. A., & Amaral, D. G. (2002). Perirhinal and parahippocampal cortices of the macaque monkey: Projections to the neocortex. *Journal of Comparative Neurology* 447, 394–420.

Lerner, Y., Hendler, T., Ben-Bashat, D., Harel, M., & Malach, R. (2004). A hierarchical axis of object processing stages in the human visual cortex. *Cerebral Cortex* 11, 287–297.

Levelt, W. J. M. (1989). *Speaking: From Intention to Articulation.* Cambridge, MA: MIT Press.

Linebarger, M. C., Schwartz, M. F., & Saffran, E. M. (1983). Sensitivity to grammatical structure in so-called agrammatic aphasics. *Cognition* 13, 361–392.

Logothetis, N. K., Pauls, J., Augath, M., Trinath, T., & Oeltermann, A. (2001). Neurophysiological investigation of the basis of the fMRI signal. *Nature* 412, 150–157.

MacDonald, M. C., & Christiansen, M. H. (2002). Reassessing working memory: Comment on Just and Carpenter (1992) and Waters and Caplan (1996). *Psychological Review* 109, 35–54.

Marinkovic, K., Dhond, R. P., Dale, A. M., Glessner, M., Carr, V., & Halgren, E. (2003). Spatiotemporal dynamics of modality-specific and supramodal word processing. *Neuron* 38, 487–497.

Martin, A., & Chao, M. L. (2001). Semantic memory and the brain: structure and processes. *Current Opinion in Neurobiology* 11, 194–201.

Martin, A., Haxby, J. V., Lalonde, F. M., Wiggs, C. L., & Ungerleider, L. G. (1995). Discrete cortical regions associated with knowledge of color and knowledge of action. *Science* 270, 102–105.

Mazoyer, B. M., Tzourio, N., Frak, V., Syrota, A., Murayama, N., Levrier, O., Salamon, G., Dehaene, S., Cohen, L., & Mehler, J. (1993). The cortical representation of speech. *Journal of Cognitive Neuroscience* 5, 467–479.

McCandliss, B. D., Cohen, L., & Dehaene, S. (2003). The visual word form area: Expertise for reading in the fusiform gyrus. *Trends in Cognitive Sciences* 7, 293–299.

Mechelli, A., Price, C. J., Friston, K. J., & Ishai, A. (2004). Where bottom-up meets top-down: Neuronal interactions during perception and imagery. *Cerebral Cortex* 14, 1256–1265.

Mechelli, A., Price, C. J., Noppeney, U., & Friston, K. J. (2003). A dynamic causal modeling study on category effects: Bottom-up or top-down mediation? *Journal of Cognitive Neuroscience* 15, 925–934.

Mesulam, M. M. (1998). From sensation to cognition. *Brain* 121, 1013–1052.

Meyer, M., Friederici, A. D., & von Cramon, D. Y. (2000). Neurocognition of auditory sentence comprehension: Event-related fMRI reveals sensitivity to syntactic violations and task demands. *Cognitive Brain Research* 9, 19–33.

Mohr, J. P., Pessin, M. S., Finkelstein, S., Funkenstein, H. H., Duncan, G. W., & Davis, K. R. (1978). Broca aphasia: Pathologic and clinical. *Neurology* 28, 311–324.

Montori, V. M., Jaeschke, R., Schünemann, H. J., Bhandari, M., Brozek, J. L., Devereaux, P. J., & Guyatt, G. H. (2004). Users' guide to detecting misleading claims in clinical research reports. *British Medical Journal* 329, 1093–1096.

Moro, A., Tettamanti, M., Perani, D., Donati, C., Cappa, S. F., & Fazio, F. (2001). Syntax and the brain: Disentangling grammar by selective anomalies. *NeuroImage* 13, 110–118.

Mummery, C. J., Ashburner, J., Scott, S. K., & Wise, R. J. (1999). Functional neuroimaging of speech perception in six normal and two aphasic subjects. *Journal of the Acoustical Society of America* 106, 449–457.

Musso, M., Moro, A., Glauche, V., Rijntjes, M., Reichenbach, J., Buchel, C., & Weiller, C. (2003). Broca's area and the language instinct. *Nature Neuroscience* 6, 774–781.

Näätänen, R., Lehtokoski, A., Lennes, M., Cheour, M., Huotilainen, M., Iivonen, A., Vainio, M., Alku, P., Ilmoniemi, R. J., Luuk, A., Allik, J., Sinkkonen, J., & Alho, K. (1997). Language-specific phoneme representations revealed by electric and magnetic brain responses. *Nature* 385, 432–434.

Naeser, M. A., Palumbo, C. L., Helm-Estabrooks, N., Stiassny-Eder, D., & Albert, M. L. (1989). Severe nonfluency in aphasia: Role of the medial subcallosal fasciculus and other white matter pathways in recovery of spontaneous speech. *Brain* 112, 1–38.

Naya, Y., Yoshida, M., & Miyashita, Y. (2003). Forward processing of long-term associative memory in monkey inferotemporal cortex. *Journal of Neuroscience* 23, 2860–2871.

Ni, W., Constable, R. T., Menci, W. E., Pugh, K. R., Fulbright, R. K., Shaywitz, S. E., Shaywitz, B. A., Gore, J. C., & Shankweiler, D. (2000). An event-related neuroimaging study distinguishing form and content in sentence processing. *Journal of Cognitive Neuroscience* 12, 120–133.

Norris, D., & Wise, R. (2000). The study of prelexical and lexical processes in comprehension: Psycholinguistics and functional neuroimaging. In M. S. Gazzaniga (Ed.), *The New Cognitive Neurosciences*, 867–880. Cambridge, MA: MIT Press.

Öngür, D., & Price, J. L. (2000). The organization of networks within the orbital and medial prefrontal cortex of rats, monkeys and humans. *Cerebral Cortex* 10, 206–219.

Pandya, D. N., & Yeterian, E. H. (1985). Architecture and connections of cortical association areas. In A. Peters & E. F. Jones (Eds.), *Cerebral Cortex*, vol 4, *Association and Auditory Cortices*, 3–61. New York: Plenum Press.

Penny, W. D., Stephan, K. E., Mechelli, A., & Friston, K. J. (2004). Modelling functional integration: A comparison of structural equation and dynamic causal models. *NeuroImage* 23(supp. 1), S264–S274.

Perani, D., Cappa, S. F., Schnur, T., Tettamanti, M., Collinia, S., & Rosa, M. (1999). The neural correlates of verb and noun processing: A PET study. *Brain* 122, 2337–2344.

Perani, D., Dehaene, S., Grassi, F., Cohen, L., Cappa, S. F., Dupoux, E., Fazio, F., & Mehler, J. (1996). Brain processing of native and foreign languages. *NeuroReport* 7, 2439–2444.

Petkov, C. I., Kang, X., Alho, K., Bertrand, O., Yund, E. W., & Woods, D. L. (2004). Attentional modulation of human auditory cortex. *Nature Neuroscience* 6, 658–663.

Petrides, M., & Pandya, D. N. (2002). Comparative cytoarchitectonic analysis of the human and the macaque ventrolateral prefrontal cortex and corticocortical connection patterns in the monkey. *European Journal of Neuroscience* 16, 291–310.

Pinker, S. (1999). *Words and Rules: The Ingredients of Language.* London: Weidenfield and Nicholson.

Poldrack, R. A., Wagner, A. D., Prull, M. W., Desmond, J. E., Glover, G. H., & Gabrieli, J. D. E. (1999). Functional specialization for semantic and phonological processing in the left inferior prefrontal cortex. *NeuroImage* 10, 15–35.

Poremba, A., Malloy, M., Saunders, R. C., Carson, R. E., Herscovitch, P., & Mishkin, M. (2004). Species-specific calls evoke asymmetric activity in the monkey's temporal poles. *Nature* 427, 448–451.

Poremba, A., Saunders, R. C., Crane, A. M., Cook, M., Sokoloff, L., & Mishkin, M. (2003). Functional mapping of the primate auditory system. *Science* 299, 568–572.

Price, C., Wise, R., Ramsay, S., Friston, K., Howard, D., Patterson, K., & Frackowiak, R. (1992). Regional response differences within the human auditory cortex when listening to words. *Neuroscience Letters* 146, 179–182.

Price, C. J., & Devlin, J. T. (2003). The myth of the visual word form area. *NeuroImage* 19, 473–481.

Price, C. J., & Devlin, J. T. (2004). The pros and cons of labelling a left occipitotemporal region: "The visual word form area." *NeuroImage* 22, 477–479.

Price, C. J., Mummery, C. J., Moore, C. J., Frackowiak, R. S., & Friston, K. J. (1999). Delineating necessary and sufficient neural systems with functional imaging studies of neuropsychological patients. *Journal of Cognitive Neuroscience* 11, 371–382.

Price, C. J., Wise, R. J. S., & Frackowiak, R. S. J (1996). Demonstrating the implicit processing of visually presented words and pseudowords. *Cerebral Cortex* 6, 62–70.

Rauschecker, J. P., & Tian, B. (2000). Mechanisms and streams for processing of "what" and "where" in auditory cortex. *Proceedings of the National Academy of Sciences USA* 97, 11800–11806.

Read, C. A., Zhang, Y., Nie, H., & Ding, B. (1986). The ability to manipulate speech sounds depends on knowing alphabetic reading. *Cognition* 24, 31–44.

Reiman, E. M., Caselli, R. J., Yun, L. S., Chen, K., Bandy, D., Minoshima, S., Thibodeau, S. N., & Osborne, D. (1996). Preclinical evidence of Alzheimer's disease in persons homozygous for the ε4 allele for apolipoprotein E. *New England Journal of Medicine* 334, 752–758.

Romanski, L. M., Tian, B., Fritz, J., Mishkin, M., Goldman-Rakic, P. S., & Rauschecker, J. P. (1999). Dual streams of auditory afferents target multiple domains in the primate prefrontal cortex. *Nature Neuroscience* 2, 1131–1136.

Rudge, P., & Warrington, E. K. (1991). Selective impairment of memory and visual perception in splenial tumours. *Brain* 114, 349–360.

Schwartz, M. F., Saffran, E. M., & Marin, O. S. (1980). The word order problem in agrammatism: I. Comprehension. *Brain and Language* 10, 249–262.

Scott, S. K., Blank, S. C., Rosen, S., & Wise, R. J. S. (2000). Identification of a pathway for intelligible speech in the left temporal lobe. *Brain* 123, 2400–2406.

Scott, S. K., & Johnsrude, I. S. (2003). The neuroanatomical and functional organization of speech perception. *Trends in Neurosciences* 26, 100–107.

Scott, S. K., Leff, A., & Wise, R. J. S. (2003). Going beyond the information given: A neural system supporting semantic interpretation. *NeuroImage* 19, 870–876.

Scott, S. K., Rosen, S., Wickham, L., & Wise, R. J. (2004). A positron emission tomography study of the neural basis of informational and energetic masking effects in speech perception. *Journal of the Acoustical Society of America* 115, 813–821.

Scott, S. K., & Wise, R. J. S. (2004). The functional neuroanatomy of prelexical processing in speech perception. *Cognition* 92, 13–45.

Shannon, B. J., & Buckner, R. L. (2004). Functional-anatomic correlates of memory retrieval that suggest nontraditional processing roles for multiple distinct regions within posterior parietal cortex. *Journal of Neuroscience* 24, 10084–10092.

Sharp, D. J., Scott, S. K., & Wise, R. J. S. (2004a). Monitoring and the controlled processing of meaning: Distinct prefrontal systems. *Cerebral Cortex* 14, 1–10.

Sharp, D. J., Scott, S. K., & Wise, R. J. (2004b). Retrieving meaning after temporal lobe infarction: The role of the basal language area. *Annals of Neurology* 56, 836–846.

Simmons, W. K., & Barsalou, L. W. (2003). The similarity-in-topography principle: Reconciling theories of conceptual deficits. *Cognitive Neuropsychology* 20, 451–486.

Stark, C. E. L., & Squire, L. R. (2001). When zero is not zero: The problem of ambiguous baseline conditions in fMRI. *Proceedings of the National Academy of Sciences USA* 98, 12760–12766.

Stowe, L. A., Broere, C. A., Paans, A. M., Wijers, A. A., Mulder, G., Vaalburg, W., & Zwarts, F. (1998). Localizing components of a complex task: Sentence processing and working memory. *NeuroReport* 9, 1995–1999.

Stowe, L. A., Paans, A. M., Wijers, A. A., Zwarts, F., Mulder, G., & Vaalburg, W. (1999). Sentence comprehension and word repetition: A positron emission tomography investigation. *Psychophysiology* 36, 786–801.

Swaab, T. Y., Brown, C., & Hagoort, P. (1998). Understanding ambiguous words in sentences: Electrophysiological evidence for delayed contextual selection in Broca's aphasia. *Neuropsychologia* 36, 737–761.

Swinney, D. (1996). Neurological distribution of processing resources underlying language comprehension. *Journal of Cognitive Neuroscience* 8, 174–184.

Tanaka, K. (1996). Inferotemporal cortex and object vision. *Annual Review of Neuroscience* 19, 109–140.

Tarkiainen, A., Helenius, P., Hansen, P. C., Cornelissen, P. L., & Salmelin, R. (1999). Dynamics of letter string perception in the human occipitotemporal cortex. *Brain* 122, 2119–2132.

Tian, B., Reser, D., Durham, A., Kustov, A., & Rauschecker, J. P. (2001). Functional specialization in rhesus monkey auditory cortex. *Science* 292, 290–293.

Tsunoda, K., Yamane, Y., Nishizaki, M., & Tanifuji, M. (2001). Complex objects are represented in macaque inferotemporal cortex by the combination of feature columns. *Nature Neuroscience* 4, 832–838.

Tyler, L. K., Moss, H. E., Durrant-Peatfield, M., & Levy, J. (2000). Conceptual structure and the structure of concepts: A distributed account of category-specific deficits. *Brain and Language* 75, 195–231.

Tyler, L. K., Russell, R., Fadili, J., & Moss, H. E. (2001). The neural representations of nouns and verbs: PET studies. *Brain* 124, 1619–1634.

Tyler, L. K., Stamatakis, E. A., Bright, P., Acres, K., Abdallah, S., Rodd, J. M., & Moss, H. E. (2004). Processing objects at different levels of specificity. *Journal of Cognitive Neuroscience* 16, 351–362.

Ugurbil, K., Toth, L., & Kim, D. S. (2003). How accurate is magnetic resonance imaging of brain function? *Trends in Neurosciences* 26, 108–114.

Ullman, M. T. (2001). A neurocognitive perspective on language: The declarative/procedural model. *Nature Reviews Neuroscience* 2, 717–726.

Vandenbulcke, M., Peeters, R., Vanhecke, P., & Vandenberghe, R. (2004). Activation of the visual word form area for words and pictures presented in the left or right visual field. Abstract and Itinerary Planner Washington DC: Society for Neuroscience 2004. Online.

Wagner, A. D., Pare-Blagoev, E. J., Clark, J., & Poldrack, R. A. (2001). Recovering meaning: Left prefrontal cortex guides controlled semantic retrieval. *Neuron* 31, 329–38.

Wagner, A. D., Schacter, D. L., Rotte, M., Koutstaal, W., Maril, A., Dale, A. M., Rosen, B. R., & Buckner, R. L. (1998). Building memories: Remembering and forgetting of verbal experiences as predicted by brain activity. *Science* 281, 1188–1191.

Waters, G. S., & Caplan, D. (1996). The capacity theory of sentence comprehension: Critique of Just and Carpenter (1992). *Psychological Review* 103, 761–772.

Waters, G. S., Caplan, D., Alpert, N., & Stanczak, L. (2003). Individual differences in rCBF correlates of syntactic processing in sentence comprehension: Effects of working memory and speed of processing. *NeuroImage* 19, 101–112.

Wilson, S. M., & Saygin, A. P. (2004). Grammaticality judgement in aphasia: Deficits are not specific to syntactic structures, aphasic syndromes, or lesion sites. *Journal of Cognitive Neuroscience* 16, 238–252.

Wilson, S. M., Saygin, A. P., Sereno, M. I., & Iacoboni, M. (2004). Listening to speech activates motor areas involved in speech production. *Nature Neuroscience* 7, 701–702.

Wise, R. J., Greene, J., Buchel, C., & Scott, S. K. (1999). Brain regions involved in articulation. *Lancet* 353, 1057–1061.

Wise, R. J., Howard, D., Mummery, C. J., Fletcher, P., Leff, A., Buchel, C., & Scott, S. K. (2000). Noun imageability and the temporal lobes. *Neuropsychologia* 38, 985–994.

Wise, R. J. S., Scott, S. K., Blank, S. C., Mummery, C. J., Murphy, K., & Warburton, E. A. (2001). Separate neural subsystems within "Wernicke's area." *Brain* 124, 83–95.

Woodruff, P. W., Benson, R. R., Bandettini, P. A., Kwong, K. K., Howard, R. J., Talavage, T., Belliveau, J., & Rosen, B. R. (1996). Modulation of auditory and visual cortex by selective attention is modality-dependent. *NeuroReport* 9, 1909–1913.

Yacoub, E., Van De Moortele, P. F., Shmuel, A., & Ugurbil, K. (2005). Signal and noise characteristics of Hahn SE and GE BOLD fMRI at 7T in humans. *NeuroImage* 24, 738–750.

Zatorre, R. J., & Belin, P. (2001). Spectral and temporal processing in human auditory cortex. *Cerebral Cortex* 11, 946–953.

Zatorre, R. J., Belin, P., & Penhune, V. B. (2002). Structure and function of auditory cortex: Music and speech. *Trends in Cognitive Sciences* 6, 37–46.

Zysset, S., Huber, O., Ferstl, E., & von Cramon, D. Y. (2002). The anterior frontomedian cortex and evaluative judgment: An fMRI study. *NeuroImage* 15, 983–991.

8   Functional Neuroimaging of Episodic Memory

Ian G. Dobbins and Lila Davachi

Introduction

Spelling a word, riding a bike, solving a math problem, remembering a shopping list, and finding one's car keys are all memory phenomena. However, even a cursory consideration of these various tasks suggests that they differ fundamentally with respect to key characteristics, such as the level or type of conscious awareness required and the need for contextual support during recovery. Indeed, it is now widely accepted that memory is not a unitary phenomenon, but instead depends on partially independent memory systems, each tuned to fit an environmental demand, each having different operating characteristics, and each reliant on different underlying neural architectures (Schacter & Tulving, 1994; Squire, 1992a; Tulving, 1983).

Empirical research arriving at this conclusion stems primarily from behavioral, neuropsychological, and nonhuman primate investigations; yet arguably the most powerful impetus underlying the multiple systems hypothesis has been reasoned introspection. For example, when recounting his own early thinking on the topic, Tulving (1983, 20) noted:

> Another "discovery" had to do with the relation between the learner's response and the *internal cognitive state* [emphasis added] that it represented. Identical responses could reflect different kinds of awareness. Thus for instance, making a free-association response, such as "chair," to a stimulus word, such as "table," does not mean the same thing as the same response made to a question such as, "What was the word that appeared beside the word 'table' in the list you just studied?"

The latter question specifically involves the observer's personal history, requiring recovery of information identifying an individual personal episode. Such recovery requires that the observer reflect on his or her past from a first-person perspective. In contrast, the free-association query would make sense to, and presumably would be answered similarly by, large numbers of randomly selected individuals, all with different personal histories. This represents one of the defining phenomenological differences between *episodic remembering* and *semantic knowing*, with the latter reflecting the ability to report the properties and regularities of the world that constitute the amalgam of personal experience but no one particular instance. Indeed, it is perhaps safe to say that not a single reader of the current text can recount a particular episode in which he or she learned that in a free-association context, an appropriate response to "table" is "chair"; nonetheless, most readily express this knowledge.

The introspective differences between remembering an episode and reporting semantic knowledge led Tulving (1983) to propose that they rely upon different memory systems associated with distinct types of conscious experience. If that is correct, the relative contributions of the systems could be measured simply by having subjects report their subjective experiences during recognition. This assertion led to the development of the Remember/Know procedure (Tulving 1985), whereby subjects qualify recognition by whether they retrieve a first-person experience of previously interacting with the test probe (Remember response), or whether they instead believe they have recently encountered the probe, but lack specific recollections regarding the encounter (Know response). Use of this procedure has demonstrated principled dissociations between remember and know reports across a range of encoding and retrieval manipulations (Gardiner & Java, 1993a, 1993b) consistent with the idea that they index different underlying memory systems. However, despite the fact that the pattern of Remember/Know results is compatible with a memory systems distinction, considerable controversy exists regarding whether such patterns necessitate multiple systems or can be more parsimoniously explained by a single retrieval system (Dobbins et al., 2004; W. Donaldson, 1996; Wixted & Stretch, 2004).

Although dissociations using subjective reports can be quite compelling, more objective methods also suggest dissociations between episodic and other potential memory systems. One such domain is the study of individuals with damage to medial temporal lobes (MTL) resulting in anterograde amnesia (Cohen et al., 1985; Scoville & Milner, 1957; Squire, 1992b). What has arguably been most remarkable about amnesic patients is not so much their global and prominent impairment in learning facts and remembering events, but the preservation of an immense range of memory skills (Moscovitch et al., 1994; Schacter & Graf, 1986; Tulving et al., 1988; Warrington & Weiskrantz, 1974). For example, the patient E.P., who suffers from extensive bilateral MTL damage, demonstrates a virtually complete amnesia for episodic content even when indexed by simple recognition (Hamann & Squire, 1997). Despite this, he is able to provide exquisitely detailed descriptions of the spatial layout of his boyhood hometown (Teng & Squire, 1999) indicating that his long-term semantic knowledge regarding its layout is fully intact. Despite this, he is unlikely to remember recounting this information to investigators even mere minutes later.

In addition, these patients typically demonstrate normal or near normal gains in the ability to successfully complete fragmented word probes (e.g., a_rd__rk) following study of previously intact items (e.g., aardvark), and likewise appear normal on a host of other *implicit tests* of memory, in which no overt reference to prior study episodes is made (Roediger, 1990; Warrington & Weiskrantz, 1974). Thus, although amnesic subjects are often completely unaware of the study/test relationship, performance nonetheless improves as a function of prior exposure. Findings such as these have led to the postulation of an *implicit memory* system complementing the *episodic* and *semantic systems* alluded to above.

Neuropsychological dissociations are powerful demonstrations of the relative sparing and destruction of different memory systems. However, these hypothetical systems are also dissociable experimentally in healthy subjects. For example, explicit and implicit tests have been shown to demonstrate different forgetting functions (Tulving et al., 1982).

Above we have discussed a mere fraction of the evidence for a systems approach to understanding memory behavior, and have bypassed altogether animal research also supporting similar taxonomies (Zola-Morgan & Squire, 1992). Indeed, even a nominal account of any major area (phenomenological, neuropsychological, cognitive behavioral, animal/comparative, developmental) would itself entail a very large chapter or book, and we point interested readers to several texts and reviews (Bauer, 2004; Foster & Jelicic, 1999; Mayes & Downes, 1997; Squire & Butters, 1992). However, even the cursory review offered above suggests a considerable amount of convergent evidence supporting the idea that human observers are endowed with separable memory systems that differ fundamentally in terms of their operating characteristics, conscious correlates, and behavioral affordances. In this chapter, we will focus exclusively on episodic memory.

Before turning to functional imaging studies of episodic memory, it is important to consider more carefully the behavioral techniques used to measure it and the core assumptions governing those techniques. As emphasized by Tulving's *encoding specificity principle* (Tulving, 1983), understanding episodic memory requires careful consideration of the interaction between encoding and retrieval conditions (cf. Morris et al., 1977; Roediger, 2000). More specifically, although the tendency for an event to be forgotten critically depends on the manner or circumstances in which it is encoded, consideration of the encoding conditions alone cannot determine the status of an episodic memory. For example, I may ask you whether you met anyone new at a particular event and you may emphatically state that you did not. Such a query is termed a *recall* or *cued-recall task*. Following this denial, I may then present a person to you and ask if you met him or her at that same event. During this *source recognition task*, you may indeed remember the previous meeting and perhaps recover further details about the encounter. This represents a case in which the apparent status of your memory depends heavily upon the format of the retrieval test; the reverse also holds, different conditions during the experiencing of the event critically affect whether memory will be evident on a particular type of subsequent test. Thus, although we later consider encoding and retrieval operations separately, it should be understood that the two are intimately related and, indeed, one cannot be understood without the other.

As noted above in the quote from Tulving, equivalent memory output responses can arise from fundamentally different *internal cognitive states*. This belies the fact that measures such as accuracy and response time, although vital, have inherent limitations with respect to disentangling underlying cognitive causes. In contrast to early suggestions regarding the substrates of different memory systems, researchers now have access to technology that enables the cataloging of similarities and differences across internal cognitive states (or at least their neural correlates). As we shall see below, although the functional imaging of episodic memory has laid the groundwork for characterizing episodic encoding and retrieval in terms of distributed neural systems, questions remain about the functional roles of cortical regions composing these systems, their interaction, and the compatibility of cortical activity findings with respect to the multiple memory systems framework.

Before turning to a review of the findings of functional imaging studies with respect to episodic memory, it is important to cover one more critical distinction when describing episodic memory (other than encoding versus retrieval), and that is the distinction between processes directly reflecting memory evidence versus those indicative of working with or deciding about that evidence (decision criteria) (Moscovitch & Winocur, 2002). Behaviorally, this distinction is typically formalized using statistical decision models such as signal detection theory (SDT) (Macmillan & Creelman, 1991) (figure 8.1).

During episodic recognition experiments, the primary paradigm used in functional imaging, subjects are shown a list of stimuli, such as words or pictures, during an encoding phase. These items are then re-presented during the retrieval phase, intermixed with new, unstudied items. The observer's task is to discriminate between old and new items. The SDT model assumes that memory evidence is continuous and normally distributed around two central tendencies, one for old and one for new items. Because these evidence distributions overlap, observers must select a cutoff, or criterion that reflects how much evidence is deemed sufficient to classify an item as studied. Whereas the absolute ability of observers to distinguish old and

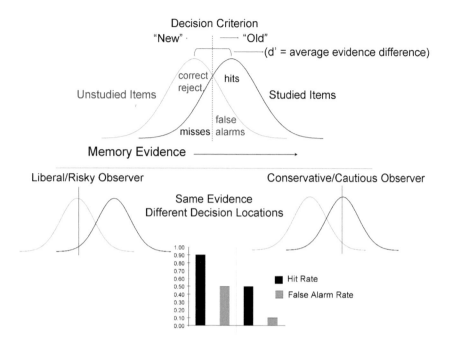

Figure 8.1

Illustration of the Signal Detection model of recognition. Top panel: The evidence underlying recognition is assumed to be continuous. Old and new items in a recognition test are assumed to be normally distributed around central values separated by a distance (d'). Because the distributions overlap, observers place a decision criterion along the evidence axis in order to parse items into "old" and "new" classifications. This yields four possible responses types (hits, false alarms, misses, and correct rejections). Bottom panel: Two observers (or the same observer on different occasions) can have identical evidence yet yield very different response patterns as a result of a shift in the decision criterion.

new items is determined by the distance between the evidence distributions (termed d'), the decision criterion determines how that evidence is overtly expressed. Hence, within SDT, overt responding is a function of both raw memory evidence (characterized as d') and decision factors regulating the placement of criterion (termed c or β). Critically, two observers with identical raw evidence may nonetheless adopt very different decision criteria. Thus, whereas Tulving (1983) emphasized that two people can express identical overt memory responses via fundamentally different internal cognitive states (see above), SDT presumes it is also possible for two people to make fundamentally different memory classifications ("old" or "new") based on *exactly* the same memory evidence. A major challenge facing the interpretation of functional imaging data is disentangling decision mechanisms that regulate valuation or monitoring of memory evidence from those which express the raw quantity or quality of that evidence.

Functional Neuroimaging of Episodic Memory

Neuroimaging techniques provide the opportunity to examine the intact, healthy functioning brain and, critically, unlike analysis of memory patterns in neuropsychological patients, allow for the study of brain activation patterns during both episodic encoding (learning phase) and retrieval. Functional imaging has provided researchers with a tool to test detailed hypotheses about how structures, such as the hippocampus and MTL cortex (whose damage leads to a global memory impairment), contribute to episodic memory. Equally important, neuroimaging has led to the discovery that brain regions, such as the prefrontal (PFC) and parietal cortices, traditionally thought to be minimally involved in simple episodic memory tasks, do indeed show correlations consistent with a role in episodic memory formation and retrieval. These insights not only have served to reveal how the brain supports episodic memory but also, and equally important, have helped to strengthen, shape, and, in some cases, challenge cognitive models of memory.

Functional Imaging of Episodic Encoding

The majority of investigations into episodic memory have focused on decision processes and evidence systems at *retrieval* because this is the time when memory strength is assessed to guide performance on memory tests. Likewise, the decision processes needed to evaluate the memory evidence arguably take place only at retrieval. On the other hand, the evidence, or the memory itself, by definition comes into existence during the study phase or the initial encounter with an item or context. Accordingly, analysis of brain activation during the encoding of information helps to reveal how episodic memories form and, perhaps, what determines the type of memory that will be recovered or experienced.

How do memories form? Surely, one can assume that we are going to remember only events that we perceive and attend to in some way. However, mere perception and global attention to a stimulus or event does not guarantee long-term memory formation for that stimulus because it is clear that we remember only a small percentage of what we perceive. Indeed, even when attention is directed toward an object, it has been shown that we do not necessarily encode, or are "blind" to, seemingly relevant aspects of the event, such as the identity of the person with whom we are conversing (D. J. Simons & Rensink, 2005; Levin et al., 2002). Therefore, in addition to attention to a stimulus, some further mechanism(s) need to be invoked to ensure the longevity of the stimulus. These further mechanisms are referred to as encoding mechanisms, processing that leads to the formation of an enduring memory trace. It is presumably these mechanisms that are lost in patients with dense amnesia, who arguably never form new episodic memories after the onset of their amnesia.

Neuroimaging has been used in a variety of ways to reveal the brain mechanisms underlying episodic memory formation. Early approaches bolstered their experimental designs on findings from the levels of processing framework which demonstrated that differential processing during encoding modulates memory formation (Craik & Lockhart, 1972). The earliest PET studies examined activation during performance of cognitive tasks that required semantic or associative processing (Fletcher et al., 1998; Montaldi et al., 1998; Rombouts et al., 1997; Shallice et al., 1994). It was reasoned that since recognition memory is known to be enhanced following semantic or associative encoding, analysis of brain activation during these forms of processing would provide clues to the neural substrates of episodic encoding. Results from these initial explorations of episodic encoding revealed that activation within left lateral PFC and the MTL was greater, on average, during semantic processing of items compared with more superficial processing (Fletcher et al., 1998; Montaldi et al., 1998; Rombouts et al., 1997; Shallice et al., 1994). Involvement of left PFC, in particular the inferior frontal gyrus, in semantic decision making has been observed consistently across many paradigms (Fiez, 1997; Poldrack et al., 1999; Thompson-Schill et al., 1997).

Other paradigms have been based on analysis of brain activation to novel versus familiar stimuli. Here, it is reasoned that encoding mechanisms are, on average, enhanced to novel stimuli compared with familiar stimuli (Tulving et al., 1994b). Using this approach, it has been demonstrated that the MTL regions show greater activation to novel compared with familiar stimuli (Dolan & Fletcher, 1997; Gabrieli et al., 1997; Stern et al., 1996), suggesting, however indirectly, that processes in these regions are related to the encoding of novel information into memory. Thus, up to this point, converging evidence had implicated a network of prefrontal and medial temporal regions under conditions of enhanced episodic encoding.

A move from PET to fMRI and from blocked to event-related designs within fMRI (see part I of this volume) enabled tighter correlations between brain activation and episodic encoding to be made. Accordingly, at present, the most powerful approach to probing episodic encoding arises from the uses of event-related fMRI (efMRI) designs. The power of efMRI is that it allows estimation of activation to a single trial or event. Thus, unlike the paradigms described above, which enabled only a contrast between different tasks or stimuli with differing experimental history, efMRI allows brain activation to events that are later remembered to be directly contrasted with those that are later forgotten. This approach, originally used in the analysis of ERP data, has been referred to as the *difference in memory* paradigm (DM) (Paller et al., 1987; Rugg, 1995; Sanquist et al., 1980; Wagner et al., 1999). This paradigm not only offers resolution of discrete events but also allows greater experimental control since one can compare events yielding successful and unsuccessful memory encoding within the *same* individual performing the *same* task.

Furthermore, encoding events can be characterized according to a variety of memory outcomes, as measured by different retrieval tests. For example, encoding activation correlated with later item recognition will likely reveal brain regions important for both encoding item familiarity and recollection because both introspective states presumably can support recognition performance. On the other hand, encoding activation that correlates with later memory specifically for source information reveals regions important for recollection of that source above and beyond item familiarity.

Initial groundbreaking studies co-opted this powerful DM paradigm and applied it to analysis of efMRI data. Wagner, Schacter, et al. (1998) recorded brain activation during a semantic decision task and found that activation in posterior parahippo-campal and left PFC regions correlated with later high-confidence recognition (figure 8.2a, plate 13). At the same time, Brewer et al. (1998) demonstrated that activation in right PFC and bilateral parahippocampal gyrus during picture viewing correlated with later subjective assessments of remembering versus knowing (figure 8.2b). These data revealed two important principles regarding episodic encoding. The first is that encoding-related activation can be process- or content-specific. It has been demonstrated that verbal semantic and phonological processing preferen-tially engages anterior and posterior portions of the left inferior frontal gyrus (Poldrack et al., 1999), while pictorial and nonnameable stimuli have been shown to preferentially engage right PFC (Kelley, 1998). Likewise, the Wagner study employed verbal stimuli and resulted in left prefrontal and parahippocampal cor-relates of memory formation, while the Brewer study utilized pictorial stimuli and resulted in right prefrontal and bilateral parahippocampal correlates of memory formation. Thus, encoding-related activation was seen in a subset of those regions initially engaged during stimulus and task processing.

The second question that arises from these data is whether there exists a special-ized system or a domain general mechanism underlying episodic memory formation. Both of these initial studies (and, more important, almost every study performed since) have found that activation within the MTL correlates with episodic memory formation. However, how the subregions within the MTL contribute to episodic encoding is under intense debate both in the animal (Meunier et al., 1993; Parkinson et al., 1988; Zola-Morgan & Squire, 1986) and in human literature (Davachi et al., 2003; Jackson & Schacter, 2004; Kirwan & Stark, 2004; Mayes et al., 2004; Squire et al., 2004; Stark & Squire, 2001, 2003). Although the precise division of labor remains to be elucidated, it is clear that the MTL plays a critical role in episodic memory encoding. Indeed, a consideration of the evidence across many disciplines suggests that the elements making up the memory trace are likely linked or constructed into a coherent unit via MTL mechanisms.

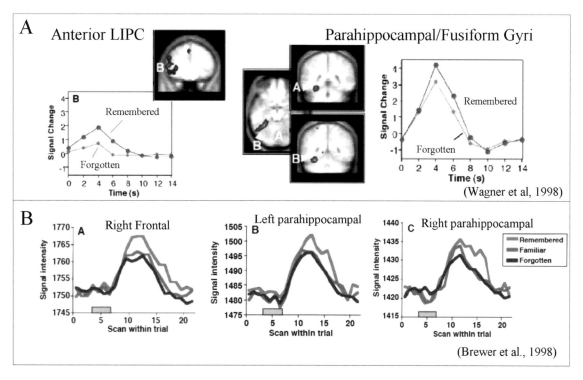

Figure 8.2

(*A*) Results of Wagner et al. (1998) showing greater activation in the anterior lateral inferior prefrontal cortex (LIPC) and left parahippocampal gyrus during encoding for items that are later recognized with high confidence compared to those later forgotten. Percent signal change is shown in line graphs, and locations from which time course data are drawn are highlighted on coronal and horizontal brain sections. (*B*) Results from Brewer et al. (1998). Displayed are three graphs depicting the MR signal intensity change over time during encoding for trials later given a "remember" response (in red), a "familiar" response (in green) and those later forgotten (in blue). Right frontal and bilateral parahippocampal regions show encoding activation that is greatest for items later "remembered," intermediate for items later "familiar," and least active for items later forgotten. See plate 13 for color version.

Encoding Specific Mechanisms Across Task and Content

Do the encoding correlates of episodic memory formation vary depending on the type of encoding task? As mentioned above, there is evidence that the specific pattern of activation in brain regions that correlates with later recognition memory varies depending on the type or form of encoding task. For example, the encoding correlates of recognition memory seem to vary depending on whether subjects perform a deep or a shallow encoding task, with those regions predicting memory being a subset of those engaged during processing (Otten & Rugg, 2001; Prince et al., 2005; Rugg et al., 2002). One such study had subjects make either animacy or syllable judgments about words followed by a recognition memory test. The results revealed that activation in the left inferior frontal gyrus, in a region known to support access to and maintenance of semantic information (Fiez, 1997; Poldrack et al., 1999; Thompson-Schill et al., 1997; Wagner et al., 2001), correlated with memory formation for items processed in the scmantic, or animacy, task. On the other hand, encoding activation in different cortical regions, including right prefrontal, bilateral parietal, and fusiform cortices, correlated with episodic memory formation for the alphabetical task (Otten & Rugg, 2001).

Thus, it appears that trial-to-trial modulations in the engagement of semantic working memory systems, as assessed by activation in anterior inferior frontal gyrus, during a semantic decision task, predict episodic memory formation for the items contained in these trials. Similarly, it has been shown that the level of activation in a network of cortical regions, including left prefrontal and parietal cortex, known to support phonological working memory (Awh et al., 1996; Chein & Fiez, 2001; Jonides et al., 1998; Paulesu et al., 1993) correlates with recognition memory for items processed in a rote rehearsal paradigm (figure 8.3) (Davachi et al., 2001). These data provide support for the guiding principle that episodic memory formation is augmented by increased activation in regions selective to task performance. This activation may represent increased attentional allocation or efforts to perform the task, trial-to-trial differences in how individual stimuli engage these processing regions, or both. In the same vein, as different stimulus classes (e.g., words, pictures) engender differential cortical processing (e.g., left vs. right hemisphere), neural correlates of successful episodic memory formation for different stimulus content have also been lateralized, usually in cortical regions (Brewer et al., 1998; Wagner, Poldrack, et al., 1998; Wagner, Schacter, et al., 1998) as well as within MTL regions (Kirchhoff et al., 2000; Stern et al., 1996), although the extent of lateralization within the MTL remains to be elucidated.

Domain General Episodic Encoding
In addition to encoding related modulation of activity in prefrontal and other cortical regions engaged during task processing, activation in other regions, particularly within the MTL, has been shown to be important in episodic memory formation *across* different tasks. The MTL is made up of highly interconnected cortical association areas (perirhinal, entorhinal and parahippocampal cortex) that project into the complex hippocampus proper (figure 8.4). Although for decades we have known that the MTL system is critical for the formation of episodic memories, the fundamental question of how each of these regions contributes to episodic memory remains unanswered. Much of the work thus far has focused on analysis of performance in animals following brain resections in addition to single-unit recordings from structures within this system. These lines of work have contributed greatly to

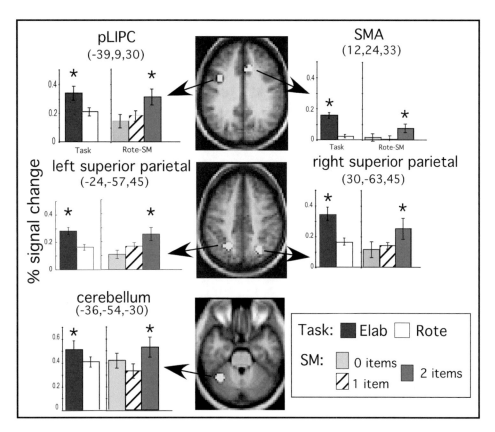

Figure 8.3
Results from Davachi et al. (2001) demonstrating the DM effect during rote rehearsal of word triplets in brain regions known to be engaged during verbal working memory. Percent signal change at the peak of the hemodynamic response is displayed in these regions (posterior LIPC, SMA, left and right superior parietal cortex and cerebellum) during both performance of the rote rehearsal task (ROTE) and the elaborative (ELAB) task, as well as during the ROTE task, dependent on how many items from a triplet were later recognized (0, 1, 2, or 3). Encoding activation is significantly greater when subjects later recognize two items from the triplet compared with when they recognize one or no items. Regions are displayed on horizontal brain sections. LIPC, lateral inferior prefrontal cortex; SMA, supplementary motor area.

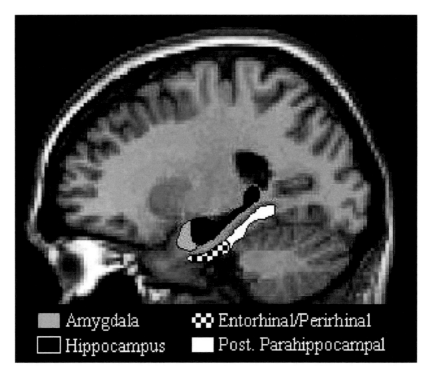

Figure 8.4
Schematic of the components of the medial temporal lobe drawn on a sagittal section of the human brain.

proposing theoretical models of MTL function in the human. Functional imaging provides a powerful method to test these models by revealing the contribution of human MTL regions to episodic memory.

Although there is general agreement that some division of labor exists between medial temporal cortex and hippocampus (figure 8.4), the precise nature of this division remains unclear and highly controversial. One influential model of MTL function posits that item and relational learning are supported by distinct, yet complementary, neural mechanisms implemented within the hippocampus and perirhinal cortex (Marr, 1971; McClelland et al., 1995; K. A. Norman & O'Reilly, 2003; O'Reilly & Rudy, 2000). Item memory refers to the memory that an item has been previously encountered, regardless of whether contextual information surrounding this past encounter is available. On the other hand, relational memory refers to the recollection of additional contextual information associated with a prior encounter. This view has sometimes been described as relating to the psychological constructs of recollection and familiarity.

Converging evidence from numerous labs has now demonstrated DM effects in the MTL (Brewer et al., 1998; Davachi & Wagner, 2002; Jackson & Schacter, 2004; Kirwan & Stark, 2004; Otten & Rugg, 2001; Ranganath et al., 2004; Sperling et al., 2003; Strange et al., 2002; Wagner, Schacter, et al., 1998; Yonelinas et al., 2001). These studies have collectively demonstrated that activation in hippocampus, and perirhinal and posterior parahippocampal gyrus correlates with later performance on different types of episodic memory tasks. In an attempt to reveal whether subregions within the MTL code for different elements of an episode, studies were then designed to distinguish the encoding contributions of these subregions. Providing evidence for a role in relational encoding, tasks that require associative or relational processing have been shown to engage the hippocampus (Davachi & Wagner, 2002; Montaldi et al., 1998; Sperling et al., 2001). On the other hand, it has been shown that attention to items instead of their relations results in differential activation of anterior rhinal cortex (Davachi & Wagner, 2002).

Although the results from these separate studies suggest differential hippocampal and anterior medial temporal cortical encoding mechanisms, only a handful of studies have selectively attempted to disentangle item encoding from relational episodic encoding (Davachi et al., 2003; Kirwan & Stark, 2004; Ranganath et al., 2004). Indeed, additional studies have analyzed encoding that correlates with later relational memory recovery versus item memory (Cansino et al., 2002; Henson et al., 1999; Jackson & Schacter, 2004; Strange et al., 2002) but only the three studies mentioned above included analysis of trials that were later forgotten, thus allowing for distinction between regions important in item memory and in relational memory. These studies all have found that encoding activation in the hippocampus and posterior parahippocampal gyrus selectively correlates with relational memory formation (figure 8.5, plate 14). Thus, hippocampal and posterior parahippocampal encoding processes seem to afford recovery of associated or related details of the episode. It is noteworthy that the tasks used in these three studies used variable stimuli (words and faces) and differed in task requirements (size and animacy judgments, spatial imagery and intentional encoding of face/name pairs), suggesting that the common involvement of hippocampal and parahippocampal regions is indicative of domain general mechanisms important in episodic memory formation.

Only a few studies have reported perirhinal engagement during encoding or retrieval. This could be due to technological difficulties or difficulties in localizing perirhinal cortex across individuals. Whatever the primary cause for the lack of reports, very little is still known about the role of the perirhinal cortex in episodic encoding compared with what has been learned regarding the roles of the hippocampus and posterior parahippocampal gyrus. That said, there are some initial reports differentiating the roles of the perirhinal cortex from that of hippocampus in episodic encoding. For example, as mentioned above, activation in anterior rhinal

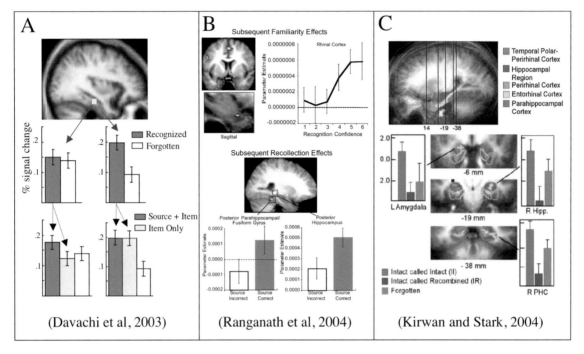

Figure 8.5

(*A*) Results from Davachi et al. (2003) showing encoding activation during scene imagery correlated with later source recollection in the hippocampus and later item recognition in the perirhinal cortex. (*B*) Results from Ranganath et al. (2004) showing increased encoding activation during size and animacy judgments in rhinal cortex correlated with later recognition confidence. Activation in hippocampus and posterior parahippocampal gyrus correlated with later source recollection (color in which word was presented). (*C*) Results from Kirwan and Stark (2004) demonstrating encoding-related activation during face-name associative encoding dependent on later associative recognition. They found that activation in both hippocampus and parahippocampal gyrus correlated with later associative recognition. Regions of interest are displayed on sagittal section as well as on coronal sections. See plate 14 for color version.

cortex, close to the perirhinal region, is more engaged during a rote rehearsal task (repeating individual words) than during a relational encoding task (making comparisons across words) (Davachi & Wagner, 2002). Furthermore, perirhinal activation during encoding has been shown to correlate specifically with later item recognition, regardless of source recollection (Davachi et al., 2003; Ranganath et al., 2004) (figure 8.5).

Importantly, as mentioned above, within these same studies, hippocampal and parahippocampal encoding activity correlated with later source recollection and not with item memory. Taken together, these data suggest a division of labor across MTL regions in their respective contributions to episodic memory formation. Although these initial distinctions between encoding mechanisms across perirhinal cortex into the hippocampus correspond to similar distinctions noted from single-cell record-ings in animals (Brown & Aggleton, 2001), whether item versus relational memory, or familiarity versus recollection fully capture the critical functional difference in the encoding operations served by these regions remains unclear. Furthermore, activation in other MTL regions, such as the posterior parahippocampal gyrus, has been shown to correlate with both item (Davachi & Wagner, 2002; Eldridge et al., 2000; Kensinger et al., 2003) and relational memory (Cansino et al., 2002; Davachi et al., 2003; Kirwan & Stark, 2004; Ranganath et al., 2004) across different paradigms. Thus, further experimentation is needed to better understand how distinct MTL regions contribute to episodic memory formation.

The diversity of experimental contexts within which MTL structures, particularly the hippocampus, have been demonstrated to correlate with episodic memory formation suggests that, unlike cortical areas, this region is important regardless of the content of the information to be remembered. Instead, what seems to be crucial is the whether later memory will contain associative or relational information. Interestingly, many studies reporting a DM effect within the hippocampus have localized this effect to the left anteriormost portion of the hippocampus (Davachi & Wagner, 2002; Jackson & Schacter, 2004; Otten et al., 2001; Sperling et al., 2003; Sperling et al., 2001). Recently, an elegant demonstration of this was reported by Prince et al. (2005). The authors demonstrated that the only brain region to predict memory formation across both shallow and deep encoding tasks was, indeed, the left anterior hippocampus. Interestingly, this same region was also correlated with successful memory retrieval at test.

In contrast to the anterior hippocampal regions, encoding related activation in the posterior portion of the hippocampus is less consistent. It has been proposed that there may exist some functional segregation along the anterior-posterior hip-pocampal axis that may explain these differences, with some authors suggesting a gradient from encoding to retrieval processes (Lepage et al., 1998; but see Schacter & Wagner, 1999); others, a gradient distinguishing different forms of novelty (Strange et al., 1999); and still others positing distinctions along stimulus type (Small et al., 2001). With further exploration and increased resolution to distinguish intrahippo-campal regions, it is clear that answers to these questions will emerge. Nonetheless, it is evident from these studies that the hippocampus, perhaps along with MTL cortex, is part of a general mechanism for episodic encoding.

Functional Imaging of Episodic Retrieval

Below we review functional imaging studies of episodic retrieval with an eye toward demonstrating the historical progression from relatively coarse comparisons across fundamentally different tasks to finer-grained comparisons suggesting process dissociations across ostensibly similar retrieval tasks. The overall picture is one of a highly flexible set of retrieval operations that are specific to different types of episodic memory demands. Owing to the structure, the review is selective, focusing primarily on PFC involvement during retrieval; therefore the interested reader is encouraged to consult other relevant reviews (Henson, 2005; Rugg et al., 2002; Rugg & Wilding, 2000; Schacter & Wagner, 1999; J. S. Simons & Spiers, 2003; Fletchen & Henson, 2001).

Coarse Memory Task Distinctions

Here we review patterns or regularities seen at the level of broad task comparisons. Such comparisons are often described as "loose" because a host of cognitive operations may be contributing to the observed activity differences across tasks (Buckner & Logan, 2001). Nevertheless, the highly reliable patterns yielded by such comparisons have provided the critical impetus for further, more selective investigations of hypothetical retrieval processes. The earliest and perhaps most widely cited regularity occurs across comparisons of encoding and retrieval tasks. Such contrasts have consistently identified asymmetric responses in PFC, with relatively greater activity in the left PFC during semantic encoding and relatively greater activity in the right PFC during episodic retrieval (usually item recognition) (Nyberg et al., 1996; Tulving, Kapur, et al., 1994). This pattern, termed HERA (hemispheric encoding-retrieval asymmetry), was quite surprising, given the paucity of neuropsychological data suggesting any critical role for PFC, particularly during simple recognition (but see Alexander et al., 2003; Schacter et al., 1996; Swick & Knight, 1999).

To further isolate the regions involved in the retrieval portion of the HERA pattern, Lepage et al. (2000) examined data across 4 PET studies and isolated 6 PFC regions that appeared to be systematically recruited during episodic recognition (compared with encoding), regardless of whether the recognition probes were predominantly new or old (Lepage et al., 2000) (figure 8.6). These regions included bilateral posterior ventrolateral areas (BA 45/47), bilateral frontopolar regions (BA 10), right dorsal PFC (BA 8/9), and a midline cingulate (BA 32) area near the supplementary motor area (SMA). As a whole these regions are frequently implicated in, though not selective to, episodic memory paradigms (Cabeza & Nyberg, 1997). Because these areas were recruited during attempted recognition (regardless of whether items were old or new), it was suggested that they contributed to *episodic retrieval mode*, a cognitive state "in which one mentally holds in the background of focal attention a segment of one's personal past, treats incoming and on-line information as 'retrieval cues' for particular events in the past, refrains from task-irrelevant processing, and becomes consciously aware of the products of successful ecphory, should it occur, as a remembered event" (Cabeza & Nyberg, 1997, 506). Because the activations were more prominent and numerous in the right compared

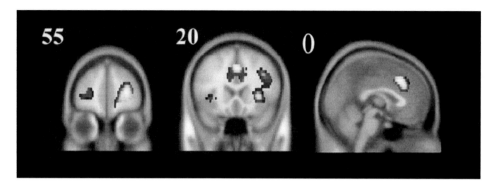

Figure 8.6
Prefrontal and midline regions linked with "retrieval mode" in Lepage et al. (2000).

with the left PFC, the authors concluded that the ubiquity of the HERA pattern was likely the result of the maintenance of retrieval mode (for electrophysiological data, see Duzel et al., 1999; Morcom & Rugg, 2002).

Although the retrieval portion of the HERA pattern is reliable, studies coarsely contrasting encoding and retrieval tasks provide little insight as to what the constituent processes involved in retrieval might be, whether they are unique to the act of episodic retrieval or instead are shared with other cognitive tasks, and similarly whether they are unique to specific types of retrieval tasks or are preserved across the broad range of explicit tests of memory (Buckner, 1996; Owen, 2003). Recent research has partially addressed this by contrasting retrieval tasks requiring different levels of contextual specificity.

Contextually Specific Memory Demands

Although it appears likely that episodic retrieval does in fact systematically recruit a subset of PFC regions, recent data also suggest finer-grained distinctions are in order. For example, the *source monitoring framework* of Johnson and colleagues (1993) stresses that not all retrieval attempts are alike. Within this framework, it is assumed that subjects monitor memory in a highly flexible fashion, weighing some types of recovered content more heavily than others, depending on specific task demands. For example, when trying to remember the location of one's car, subjects may heavily monitor for recovered visual-spatial content, whereas when trying to remember the topic of a prior conversation, one may instead try to remember prior cognitive deliberations or even emotions. To the extent that these types of information are linked with different cortical representations, the source monitoring framework predicts partially different operations during retrieval attempts emphasizing different aspects of prior experience. Within the context of interpreting neuroimaging data, these types of differences have been termed *retrieval orienta-tions* (Rugg & Wilding, 2000). Thus, whereas retrieval mode specifies a state that should not differ with respect to qualitative differences in the type of content that is to be recovered, the construct of retrieval orientation reflects the idea that target-ing different types of to-be-recovered content may require different monitoring operations.

Evidence supporting different retrieval orientations has arisen initially from elec-trophysiological research. For example, Herron and Wilding (2004) demonstrated that attempted retrieval of a probe's prior list position versus retrieval of the seman-tic operation previously performed on the probe resulted in differential activity in left PFC (subject to the restraints of ERP techniques) (see also Rugg et al., 2000; Wilding, 1999). These ERP findings are partially consistent with a highly systematic finding in fMRI studies that have contrasted contextual source tasks with item rec-ognition tasks. Whereas the former tasks require recovery of a specific aspect of prior experience—for example, remembering the type of task previously performed with an item—the latter often represent mere judgments of familiarity or novelty. Contrasts of source and item retrieval tasks have revealed a pattern strikingly different from contrasts of episodic retrieval and encoding tasks. Whereas the latter reveal the HERA pattern, implicating right PFC during retrieval, comparisons of source and item recognition have consistently implicated left PFC in contextually demanding retrieval tasks (Dobbins et al., 2002; Nolde et al., 1998; Ranganath et al., 2000; Raye et al., 2000). For example, in Dobbins et al. (2002) left frontopolar, dorsal, and ventrolateral regions all demonstrated greater activity during source recogni-tion than item recognition, with many of these regions displaying minimal if any activation during item recognition. Furthermore, there was evidence that these regions played distinct functional roles during source retrieval. Whereas dorsal and frontopolar (figure 8.7, plate 15, red regions and box plots) regions were selectively active during source recognition, anterior ventrolateral PFC was active during both source recognition and prior semantic processing performed on the items (figure 8.7, plate 16, blue region and box plots).

These findings, in conjunction with prior literature on semantic processing (Klein et al., 1997; Petersen et al., 1998; Thompson-Schill et al., 1997; Wagner et al., 2001), led to the working hypothesis that left frontopolar and dorsal regions were involved in the online monitoring of recollections, whereas the left anterior ventrolateral region is involved in semantic or conceptual elaboration of the retrieval probes. These large-scale PFC differences between source and item recognition, within the framework of Rugg and Wilding (2000), constitute fundamentally different retrieval orientations. Similarly, Nolde et al. (1998) have suggested that left PFC is engaged whenever retrieval is aimed at recovering evidence about one's prior *systematic* processing. Broadly speaking, these findings fit well with cognitive theories which

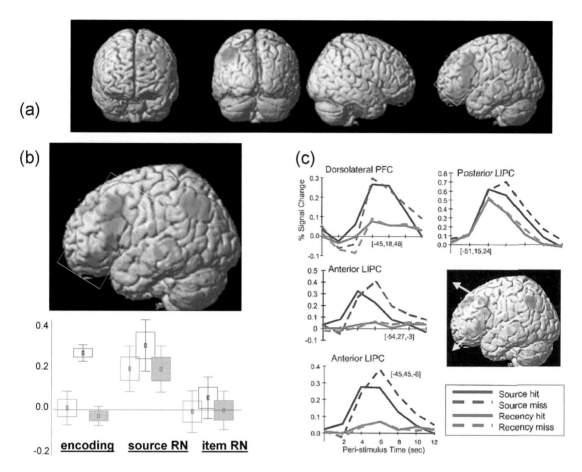

Figure 8.7
Results of Dobbins et al. (2002). (*a*) Regions demonstrating greater activity for source versus item memory on matched retrieval probes. (*b*) Regions implicated in source memory displayed different functional characteristics. Whereas dorsal and frontopolar regions (red) were selectively active during source memory, anterior ventrolateral PFC (blue) was active during both source memory and semantic processing (but not item memory). (*c*) Regions implicated in source memory were insensitive to the outcome of the source memory trial, and in fact displayed slightly higher signal during failed source retrieval attempts. See plate 15 for color version.

suggest that memory tasks dependent on the recollection of contextual information, such as source memory, require controlled search and/or evaluative processes, in contrast to familiarity/novelty-based tasks, such as item recognition (Yonelinas, 2002). This characterization also fits with discussions of controlled conceptual operations outside the domain of episodic memory (Dobbins et al., 2004; Gold & Buckner, 2002).

Given the source monitoring framework (Johnson et al., 1993) and the findings of Herron and Wilding (2004), retrieval orientations should differ not only across source and item recognition tasks, but also across source tasks that depend on monitoring fundamentally different representations. Recent fMRI evidence supports this contention. More specifically, Dobbins and Wagner (2005) considered three types of retrieval tasks performed on matched pictorial retrieval probes (figure 8.8). Conceptual source tasks required the retrieval of prior semantic operations performed on the test items. In contrast, perceptual source tasks required subjects to remember prior size information regarding the test items. Finally, item recognition merely required that subjects detect novel items, and hence made no reference to prior contextual information.

When comparing regions that were generally active during source recognition (both conceptual and perceptual) against item recognition, the ubiquitous left lateralized pattern of activity was observed, with the exception of left anterior ventrolateral PFC (BA 47) (figure 8.9, plate 16). This pattern suggests that these regions are involved in controlled aspects of retrieval, regardless of the domain of information that is to be recollected. In contrast, ventrolateral regions in the left and right hemisphere displayed qualitatively different patterns across the source retrieval questions. Whereas left anterior ventrolateral PFC demonstrated greater activity for the conceptual compared with the perceptual source task, the reverse pattern was observed in right ventrolateral areas (figure 8.9bc). Furthermore, differential activity in these ventrolateral regions correlated with different posterior regions thought to play different roles in semantic and object processing.

These findings led to the suggestion that the left and right ventrolateral regions are involved in different *attentional biasing* operations, with left anterior ventrolateral PFC involved when attention is directed toward a subset of semantic information regarding the probes, and right ventrolateral PFC more involved when attention is directed toward a subset of perceptual characteristics of the probes (in this case, size). The purpose of such biasing operations may be to increase the fidelity of memory signals by limiting the space of attended representations. Although the source tasks demonstrated differences, they also demonstrated a marked commonality compared with item recognition, in that both similarly recruited left frontopolar and dorsal PFC, suggesting a common evaluative or monitoring operation across the source tasks.

Study Phases

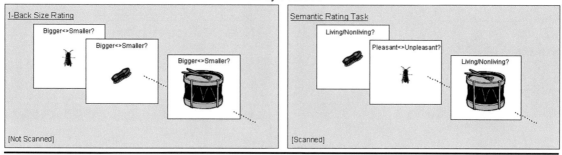

Test Phase

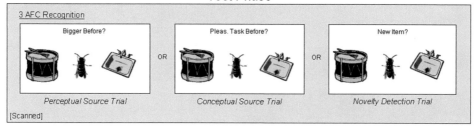

Figure 8.8

Task design Dobbins and Wagner (in press). During initial encounter, items were shown individually and subjects decided if each item occupied a bigger screen area than the immediately preceding item (1-back size rating). This manipulation was not scanned and was conducted in order to familiarize the subjects with the screen size of the objects. Immediately following, one of two semantic encoding judgments (pleasant/unpleasant or living/nonliving) was performed on pictures that maintained the same physical size as during the 1-back task. At test, three objects were shown (one novel and two studied) in an intermediate and similar size, and either novelty detection or one of two source judgments was required (source versus novelty detection). Conceptual source retrieval required selection of the item earlier rated for pleasantness, whereas the perceptual source task required selecting the one that was physically larger on the screen during previous viewings.

Temporal Profile and Relative Timing of Activity

Direct contrasts of tasks are typically motivated by cognitive theories that suggest a key process distinction; however, these theories also sometimes suggest different temporal profiles for different processes. For example, retrieval mode has often been defined as a tonic state or mental set, and as such can be expected to have an extended temporal response (Lepage et al., 2000; Rugg & Wilding, 2000). Although PET studies are severely limited with respect to disambiguating the temporal profiles of different cognitive operations, fMRI is somewhat more capable while still enabling precise spatial localization. Consistent with the assertions that retrieval mode constitutes an extended neurocognitive set or state, ERP studies of recognition have suggested that a relatively tonic neural response underlies the establishment of retrieval mode. For example, using ERP techniques, Duzel et al. (1999)

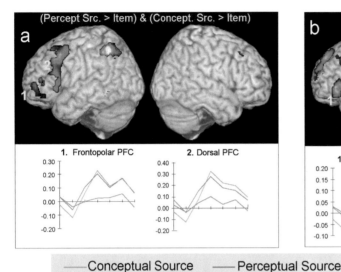

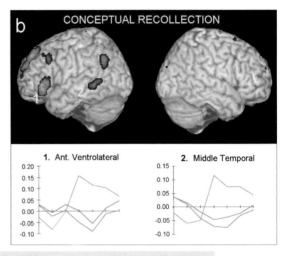

Conceptual Source ———— Perceptual Source ———— Novelty Detection

Figure 8.9
Activation data of Dobbins and Wagner (2005). (*a*) Regions demonstrating greater activation for source recollection in comparison to novelty detection, regardless of target domain (conceptual or perceptual). SPM is overlaid on a canonical brain using MRIcro and depicts the overlap between regions demonstrating a greater response during perceptual source versus novelty detection and a greater response during conceptual source versus novelty detection (joint probability .001). Regions demonstrating any appreciable difference between the two source conditions are excluded from the map (exclusive masking .1). Hemodynamic response functions are depicted for representative regions of interest (ROIs), with the ordinate representing percent signal change and tick marks on abscissa representing 2-sec time increments following stimulus onset. (*b*) Regions showing a greater response to the pleasant/unpleasant rating task than the living/nonliving rating task at encoding, and a greater response during conceptual than perceptual source retrieval (joint probability .001). This pattern is consistent with a role in the conceptual elaboration of probes. (*c*) Regions showing a greater response during perceptual compared with conceptual source retrieval (.001), consistent with a role in the perceptual elaboration of probes. See plate 16 for color version.

demonstrated a sustained DC shift that accrued over 10 sec retrieval lists during episodic but not semantic retrieval. This shift was most prominent over frontal electrode sites, and a parallel PET investigation further implicated frontopolar regions. (figure 8.10).

In response to event-related fMRI data suggesting that frontopolar responses may be atypical in their temporal delay or dispersion (Schacter et al., 1997), several research groups have modified fMRI modeling techniques in order to disentangle trial-specific versus statelike BOLD responses. These new techniques mix the modeling of blocks versus trial events, allowing one to potentially isolate regions responsive to changes in individual task elements (e.g., old versus new items) versus those more related to global differences across periods (e.g., easy versus difficult blocks).

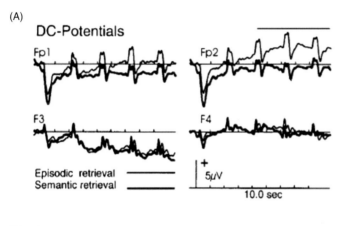

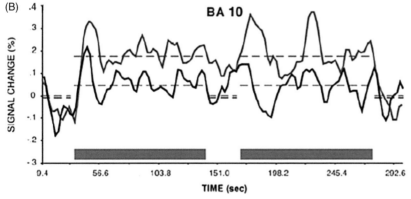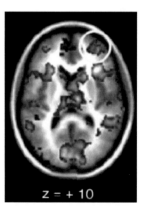

Figure 8.10
(*a*) ERP results from Duzel et al. (1999) indicating a DC shift in frontopolar activity during the course of 10-sec retrieval epochs. (*b*) fMRI data demonstrating tonic block differences between more and less demanding retrieval in Velanova et al. (2003).

(A)

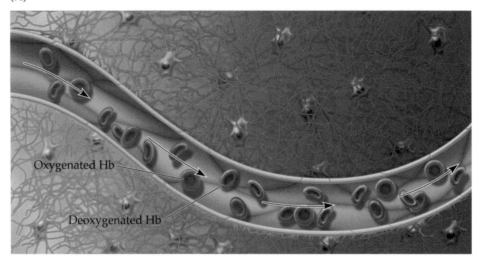

Oxygenated Hb

Deoxygenated Hb

(B)

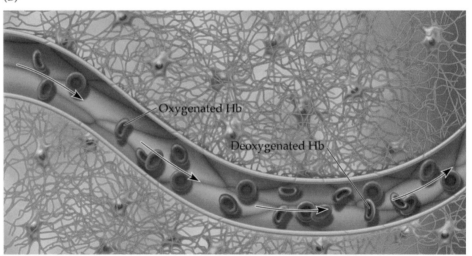

Oxygenated Hb

Deoxygenated Hb

Plate 1 Summary of BOLD signal generation. Under normal conditions, oxygenated hemoglobin is converted to deoxygenated hemoglobin at a constant rate within the capillary bed (*A*). However, when neurons become active, there is an increase in the supply of oxygenated hemoglobin above that needed by the neurons. This results in a relative decrease in the amount of deoxygenated hemoglobin (*B*) and a corresponding decrease in the signal loss due to T2* effects. The fMRI signal thus increases in areas of neuronal activity. See chapter 2.

tions, as we have hypothesized, the similarity space (and thus the adaptation effects) should reflect this shift.

Connecting the Dots

In the opening pages of his book on networks, Albert-László Barabási considers the effect of reductionism on scientific progress: "The assumption is that once we understand the parts, it will be easy to grasp the whole. Divide and conquer; the devil is in the details. Therefore for decades we have been forced to see the world through its constituents.... Now we are close to knowing just about everything there is to know about the pieces. But we are as far as we have ever been from understanding nature as a whole" (Barabási, 2002, 6).

For much of this chapter, we have been taking apart semantic memory. Although we are not quite in the position to say we know "just about everything there is to know" about the pieces that make up our semantic memory networks, the contributions of neuroimaging to that enterprise are on the rise. The next step—or a parallel venture—will be to study the network properties of semantic memory, including how it develops and how it degrades. We have already seen the influence of "network thinking" on cognitive models of semantic memory; one such example is the work of McClelland and Rogers described earlier (McClelland & Rogers, 2003), and there are many others. However, most neuroimaging studies of semantic memory are still largely reductionist, even if the results describe "networks of activation." This will change.

Emerging neuroimaging methods are making it easier to describe the structural networks that provide the scaffolding for semantic memory and the correlated patterns that emerge: Studies that invasively trace anatomical projections in monkeys (Petrides & Pandya, 2002) can now be approximated in humans using diffusion tensor imaging (DTI) and functional connectivity analyses. For example, DTI-derived estimates of white matter density can be used to predict the magnitude of the fMRI response in adjacent gray matter during working memory tasks (Olesen et al., 2003). Patterns of task-dependent correlated activity between anterior and posterior cortical regions have been used to describe functions of PFC (Bokde et al., 2001). These methods are beginning to be used to describe networks that could give rise to the sorts of computational principles proposed by cognitive theorists (McClelland & Rogers, 2003). Perhaps these inquiries will lead to the discovery that semantic networks—like networks that describe the Internet, the economy, and the cell—have the same "hublike" properties that govern many evolving networks and that give those networks both resilience and vulnerability in predictable ways (Barabási, 2002). Networks are everywhere, and we will be hearing more about them in the functional neuroimaging of semantic memory.

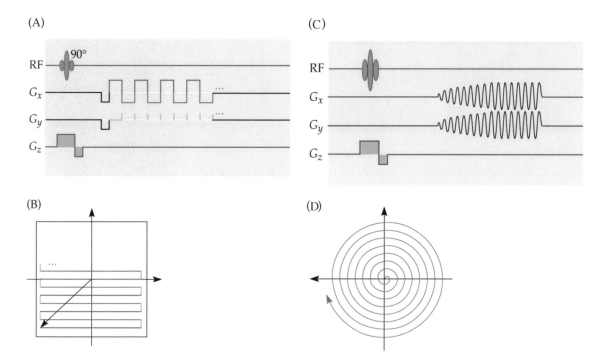

(A)

RF — 90°

G_x

G_y

G_z

(C)

RF

G_x

G_y

G_z

(B)

(D)

Plate 2 (A, B) Pulse sequences used in fMRI. Most common for fMRI are pulse sequences using echo-planar imaging (EPI). In an EPI pulse sequence (A), the spatial gradients are rapidly cycled on and off in a stair-step pattern following the initial excitation pulse. This results in a back-and-forth trajectory through k-space (B). Pulse sequences used in fMRI. Recently developed spiral imaging sequences use sinusoidally changing gradients (C) to generate a curving path through k-space (B). See chapter 2.

Plate 3 (opposite, top) Experiment illustrating the contamination of data by the movement of mass within the magnetic field. A spherical phantom remained completely stationary during a series of T2*-weighted scans. Four 1-kg bags of saline solution were mounted on a wooden pole to approximate the mass of a human arm. Every 30 sec, the mass moved between the left and right side of the phantom and then remained stationary for the remainder of the interval. (A) A comparison between the signal when the mass was to the right versus the left of the phantom illustrates widespread false "activation." (B) The time course within a region denoted by the black box in the third slice of (A) is shown by the black line. Note the changes in overall signal level and the brief spikes whenever the external mass changed position. The reference time course used to generate the map in (A) is indicated by the blue line. (C) A statistical map showing regions where spiking occurred at the time of movement. (D) The time course within the region indicated by the black box in the third slice of (C) is shown by the black line. The reference time course used to generate the map in (C) is indicated by the blue line. (E) The comparison between the signal with the mass at each position is shown after motion correction was applied. There is no reduction of false activation. (F) Output of a motion detection and correction algorithm (in Brain Voyager, with similar results from Statistical Parametric Mapping software). The resulting three translation parameters are shown by blue lines, and the three rotation parameters are shown by red lines. Note that although there was no movement whatsoever in the phantom, the algorithm detected and falsely attempted to correct for spurious motion created by the moving external mass. See chapter 3.

Plate 4 (opposite, bottom) Cue-related activity. Group-averaged data for brain regions significantly activated to attention-directing cues, overlaid onto a brain rendered in 3D. Areas activated in response to location cues are shown in blue, to color cues are shown in red, and areas activated by both cues are shown in green. Maps are displayed using a height threshold of $p < 0.005$ (uncorrected) and an extent threshold of 10 contiguous voxels. See chapter 4.

A. Pre-corrected Statistical Map 1:

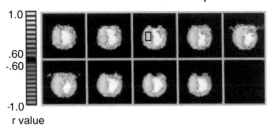

1.0
.60
-.60
-1.0
r value

B. Time Course 1:

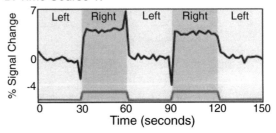

C. Pre-corrected Statistical Map 2:

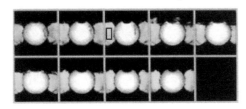

D. Time Course 2:

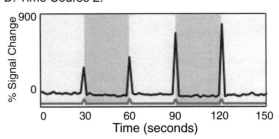

E. Post-corrected Statistical Map 1:

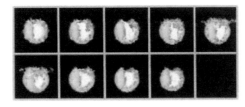

F. Motion Correction Parameters

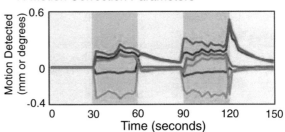

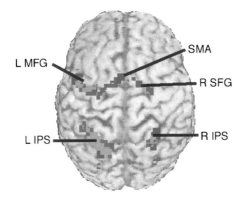

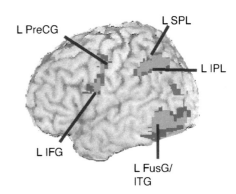

● Location Cues
● Color Cues
● Both Cues

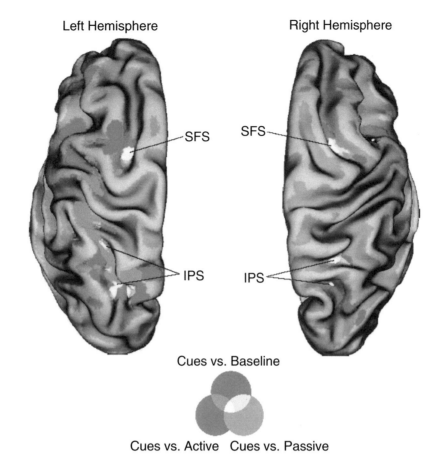

Plate 5 Anatomical overlap between the three categories of contrasts. Each focus was categorized into the Cue vs. Baseline (red), Cue vs. Passive (green), or Cue vs. Active (blue) group; projected onto the inflated brain; smoothed (8 mm); and painted onto the surface. White represents the intersection of all three categories. (Reprinted from *Neurobiology of Attention*, L. Itti, G. Rees, & J. Tsotsos (Eds). "Identifying the neural systems of top-down attentional control: A meta-analytic approach," pp. 63–68, Copyright 2005, with permission from Elsevier.) See chapter 4.

Plate 6 Group-average data for brain regions more active to location cues than color cues overlaid onto key slices of a single subject's anatomical image cutting through superior cortex (z = 45, 50, and 55 mm). See chapter 4.

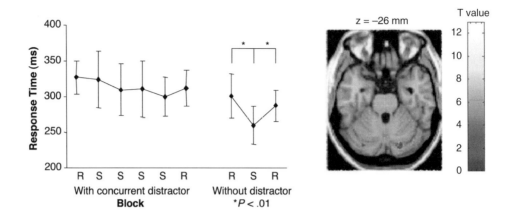

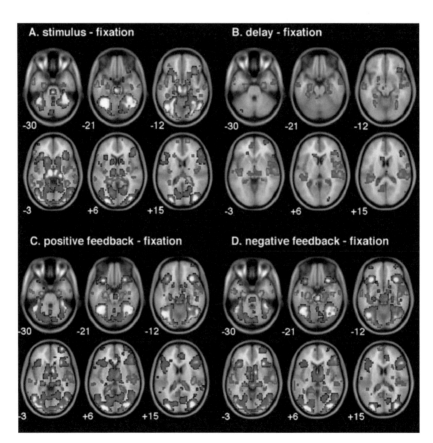

Plate 7 Behavioral and neuroimaging results adapted from from Seidler et al. (2002). Behavioral results (left) show that during training with a concurrent distractor task, subjects show no evidence of sequence learning. However, once the secondary task is removed, they show robust sequence knowledge. Cerebellar activity was associated only with the expression of learning at transfer (right), but not with learning. See chapter 5.

Plate 8 Results from Aron et al. (2004), depicting activation during each trial component of a probabilistic classification task. See chapter 5.

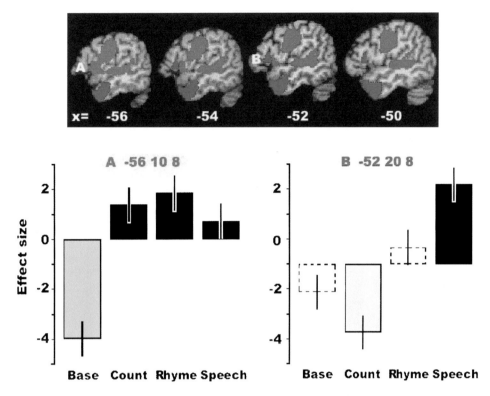

Plate 9 Results from a PET study of speech production on 12 subjects (Blank et al., 2002; 2003). Two contrasts are displayed: in red, the contrast of all speech conditions—propositional speech, the recitation of overlearned nursery rhymes, and counting—with a baseline condition of low-level auditory attention; and in blue, the contrast of propositional speech with counting. The results are displayed on sagittal single-subject MR slices. The peak in pars opercularis (A) for the first contrast (–56 10 8) lies only 12 mm away from the peak in pars triangularis (B) in the second contrast (–52 20 8). See chapter 7.

Plate 10 *(opposite, top)* This PET study (Mummery et al., 1999) investigated the brain responses to listening to increasing rates of single, unrelated, bisyllabic nouns (range 1–75 words/min) and signal-correlated noise (SCN) at the same rates (SCN comprises the time-amplitude envelopes of the words with all spectrotemporal detail removed by filling the envelopes with white noise). Voxels in which there was a linear increase in activity to both SCN and words were identified separately from voxels where the response was to words and not to SCN. These were coregistered, in yellow and red, respectively, onto an averaged T1-weighted MRI template. The slices are 4 mm apart, displayed posterior-anterior for the coronal slices and dorsal-ventral for the axial slices. The "speech-specific" (at least specific relative to SCN) extended forward along both left and right superior temporal gyri. Two plots of activity (arbitrary units centered around zero) for SCN and words at the different rates of presentation are shown, one taken from a voxel in the left anterior superior temporal gyrus (stereotactic coordinates –54 4 –8) and the other from the left planum temporale (–50 –36 12). In the latter region, the responses to SCN and words were indistinguishable. See chapter 7.

Plate 11 *(opposite, bottom)* This result is taken from the PET study of Scott and colleagues (2000). The subjects "passively" heard normal speech (Sp), degraded but intelligible speech (VCSp), spectrally rotated normal speech (RotSp; unintelligible, but closely matched the acoustic complexity of normal speech) and spectrally rotated degraded speech (RotVCSp). The response (displayed on successive posterior-anterior coronal and dorsal-ventral axial MR templates, spaced 4 mm apart) in the left anterior superior temporal sulcus (–54 6 –16, in red) corresponded to the intelligibility of the stimulus, whereas the signal in the right superior temporal gyrus (66 –12 0, in yellow) corresponded to acoustic complexity. See chapter 7.

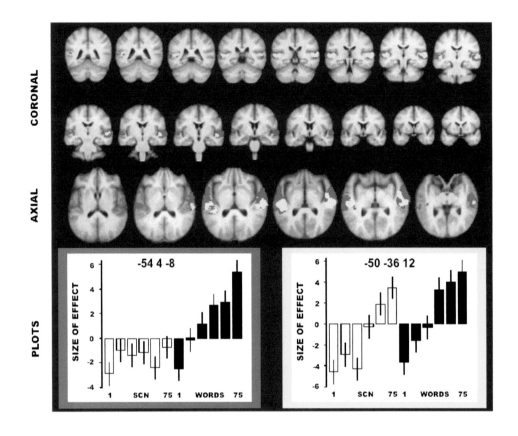

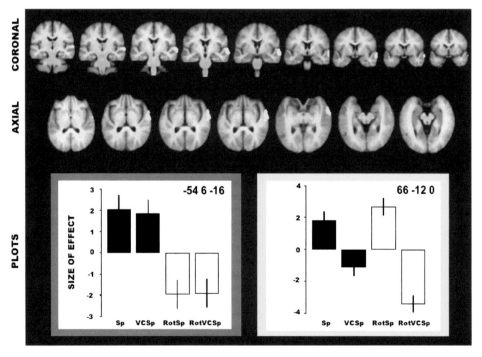

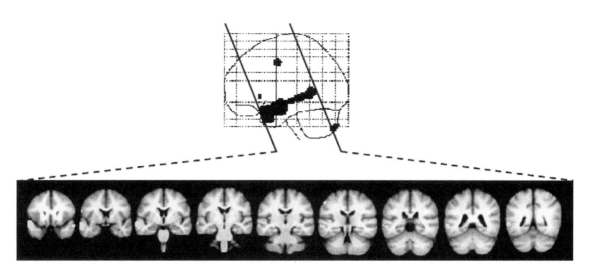

Plate 12 This result from an unpublished PET study included reading narratives contrasted with reading illegible textlike arrays of pseudo script. The contrast showed activity along the length of the left superior temporal sulcus. Activity displayed on the sagittal statistical parametric map has also been displayed on coronal MR slices, in the same manner as in plates 10 and 11. See chapter 7.

Plate 13 *(opposite, top)* (*A*) Results of Wagner et al. (1998) showing greater activation in the anterior lateral inferior prefrontal cortex (LIPC) and left parahippocampal gyrus during encoding for items that are later recognized with high confidence compared to those later forgotten. Percent signal change is shown in line graphs, and locations from which time course data are drawn are highlighted on coronal and horizontal brain sections. (*B*) Results from Brewer et al. (1998). Displayed are three graphs depicting the MR signal intensity change over time during encoding for trials later given a "remember" response (in red), a "familiar" response (in green) and those later forgotten (in blue). Right frontal and bilateral parahippocampal regions show encoding activation that is greatest for items later "remembered," intermediate for items later "familiar," and least active for items later forgotten. See chapter 8.

Plate 14 *(opposite, bottom)* (*A*) Results from Davachi et al. (2003) showing encoding activation during scene imagery correlated with later source recollection in the hippocampus and later item recognition in the perirhinal cortex. (*B*) Results from Ranganath et al. (2004) showing increased encoding activation during size and animacy judgments in rhinal cortex correlated with later recognition confidence. Activation in hippocampus and posterior parahippocampal gyrus correlated with later source recollection (color in which word was presented). (*C*) Results from Kirwan and Stark (2004) demonstrating encoding-related activation during face-name associative encoding dependent on later associative recognition. They found that activation in both hippocampus and parahippocampal gyrus correlated with later associative recognition. Regions of interest are displayed on sagittal section as well as on coronal sections. See chapter 8.

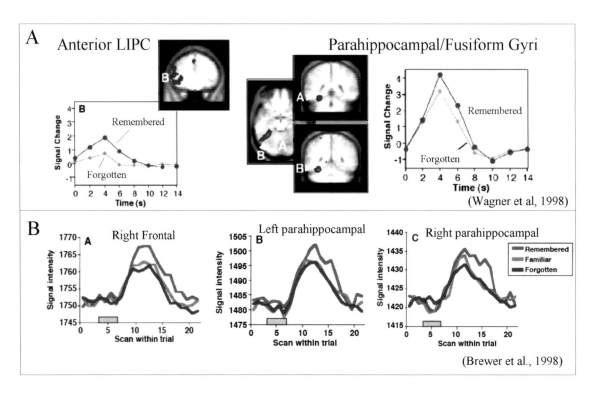

(Wagner et al, 1998)

(Brewer et al., 1998)

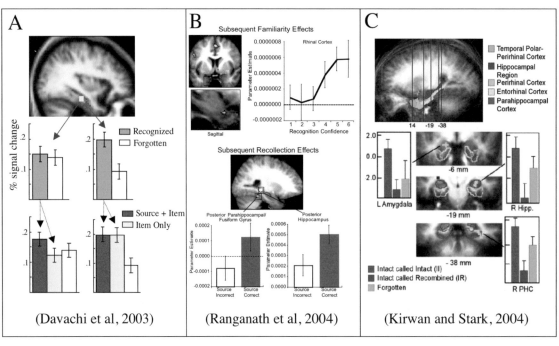

(Davachi et al, 2003)

(Ranganath et al, 2004)

(Kirwan and Stark, 2004)

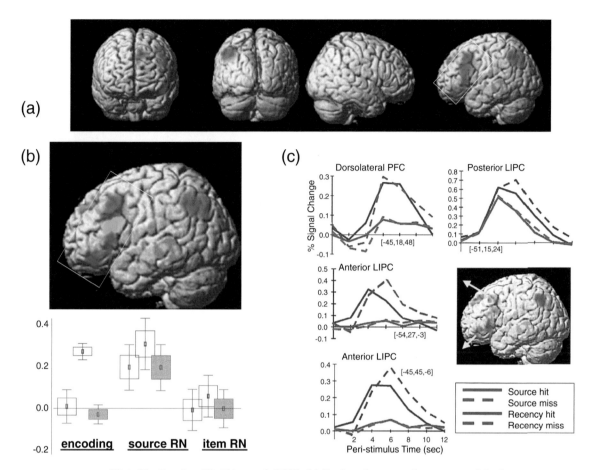

Plate 15 Results of Dobbins et al. (2002). (*a*) Regions demonstrating greater activity for source versus item memory on matched retrieval probes. (*b*) Regions implicated in source memory displayed different functional characteristics. Whereas dorsal and frontopolar regions (red) were selectively active during source memory, anterior ventrolateral PFC (blue) was active during both source memory and semantic processing (but not item memory). (*c*) Regions implicated in source memory were insensitive to the outcome of the source memory trial, and in fact displayed slightly higher signal during failed source retrieval attempts. See chapter 8.

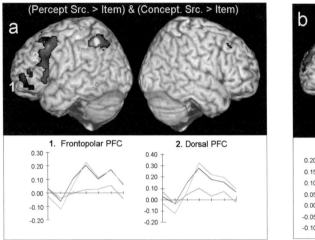

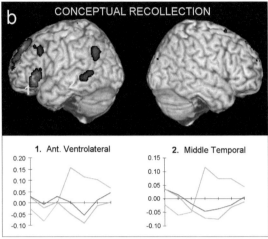

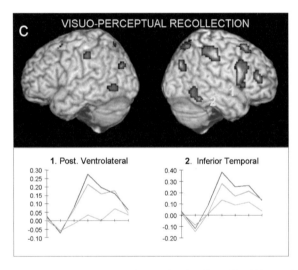

Plate 16 Activation data of Dobbins and Wagner (2005). (*a*) Regions demonstrating greater activation for source recollection in comparison to novelty detection, regardless of target domain (conceptual or perceptual). SPM is overlaid on a canonical brain using MRIcro and depicts the overlap between regions demonstrating a greater response during perceptual source versus novelty detection and a greater response during conceptual source versus novelty detection (joint probability .001). Regions demonstrating any appreciable difference between the two source conditions are excluded from the map (exclusive masking .1). Hemodynamic response functions are depicted for representative regions of interest (ROIs), with the ordinate representing percent signal change and tick marks on abscissa representing 2-sec time increments following stimulus onset. (*b*) Regions showing a greater response to the pleasant/unpleasant rating task than the living/nonliving rating task at encoding, and a greater response during conceptual than perceptual source retrieval (joint probability .001). This pattern is consistent with a role in the conceptual elaboration of probes. (*c*) Regions showing a greater response during perceptual compared with conceptual source retrieval (.001), consistent with a role in the perceptual elaboration of probes. See chapter 8.

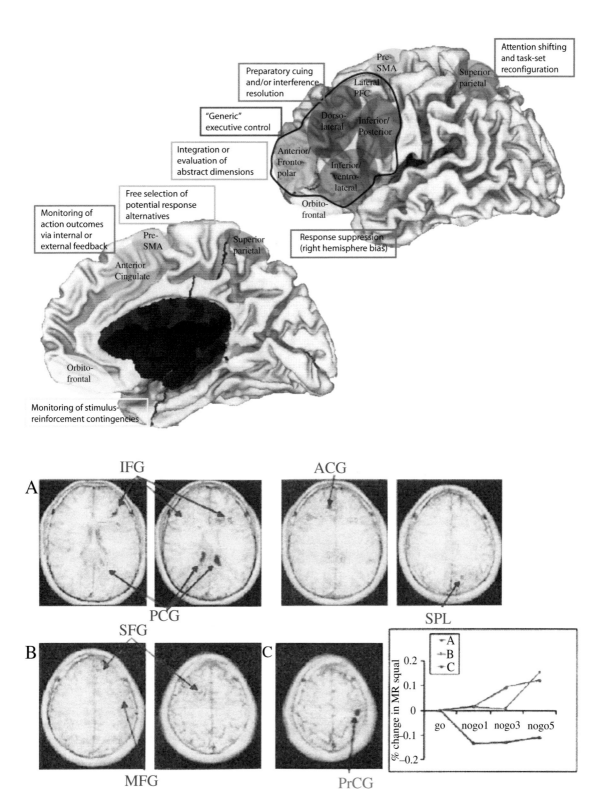

Plate 17 *(opposite, top)* Anatomical designations of brain areas that are part of the network for executive control and the task conditions or factors that reliably activate them. Shown are lateral (upper) and medial (lower) brain surfaces. Color codes represent different brain regions discussed in the review and the corresponding task conditions or factors that appear to activate them. Lateral PFC region (outlined in black) is subdivided into inferior/posterior, inferior/ventrolateral, dorsolateral, and anterior/frontopolar regions. See chapter 10.

Plate 18 *(opposite, bottom)* Differential patterns of activation in a parametric manipulation of the number of go trials preceding nogo trials. (*A*) Brain regions showing the context effect. (*B*) Brain regions showing an increase in activation only to nogo trials following five go trials. (*C*) Brain regions showing a response to the go trials. (*D*) Three patterns observed for the comparison of go trials with nogo trials after one, three, or five preceding go trials. (Adapted with permission from Durston, Thomas et al., 2002.) See chapter 11.

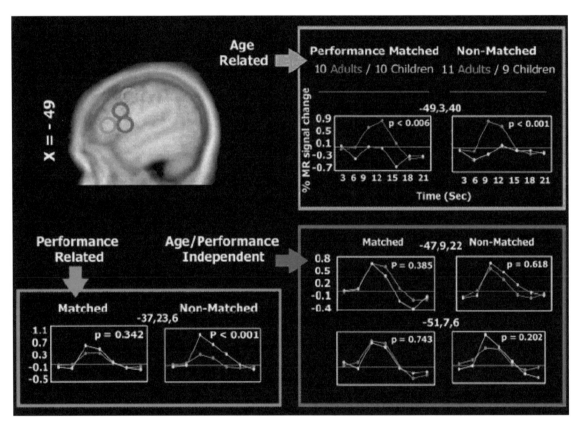

Plate 19 One of the alternatives available to developmental cognitive neuroscientists to distinguish activation differences that are performance-, as opposed to age-related, involves separating groups of adults and children in terms of their performance on a task. Schlaggar et al. employed this approach in a simple word-reading task. "Matched" groups of adults and children produced equivalent behavioral performances, in contrast to "nonmatched" groups. Frontal and extrastriate foci displayed activity that was either (1) performance- and age-independent, with adults and children producing similar activation in both the matched and the nonmatched group; (2) performance-dependent, with adults and children producing similar activation in the matched but not the nonmatched group; and (3) age-dependent, with dissimilar activity in adults and children for both the matched and the nonmatched group. (Adapted with permission from Schlaggar et al., 2002.) See chapter 11.

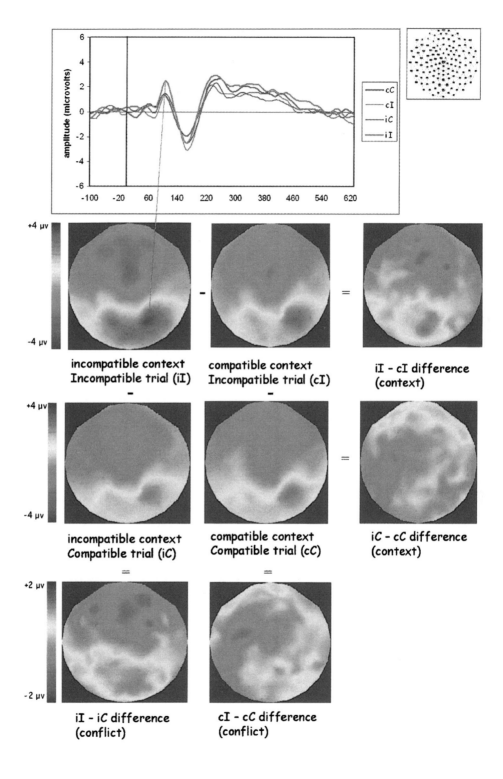

Plate 20 *(opposite)* Event-related potentials are locked to stimulus presentation in an adaptation of the flanker task (Eriksen and Eriksen, 1974) designed to investigate effects of previous response context (compatible or incompatible flanker arrays) on early stimulus processing of compatible and incompatible flanker arrays. Averaged waveforms across a number of posterior channels and scalp topographies across conditions at 112 msec post stimulus onset indicate an interaction between previous context and current stimulus array on very early stimulus processing, as indexed by a positive deflection in the visual P1 for incompatible flanker arrays preceded by incompatible flanker arrays only. (Reprinted with permission.) cI, incompatible trial preceded by compatible context; iI, incompatible trial preceded by incompatible context; iC, compatible trial preceded by incompatible context; cC, compatible trial preceded by compatible context. (Adapted from Scerif et al., in press.) See chapter 11.

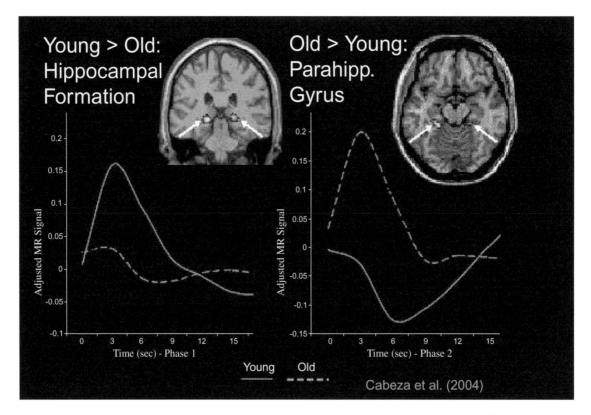

Plate 21 Dissociation between two medial temporal lobe regions. The hippocampal formation, bilaterally, was more activated in YAs than in OAs during all tasks (task-independent age effect), whereas the parahippocampal gyrus, bilaterally, was more activated in OAs than in YAs during the ER task (task-specific age effect). The age-related increase in parahippocampal gyrus was positively correlated with the number of Know responses, consistent with the idea that OAs rely more on familiarity during recognition (Cabeza et al., 2004). See chapter 12.

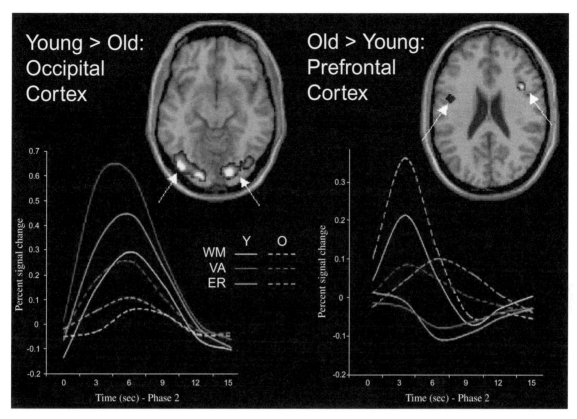

Plate 22 Task-independent age effects. Compared with YAs, OAs showed weaker activity in occipital cortex but greater activity in frontal regions (Cabeza et al., 2004). See chapter 12.

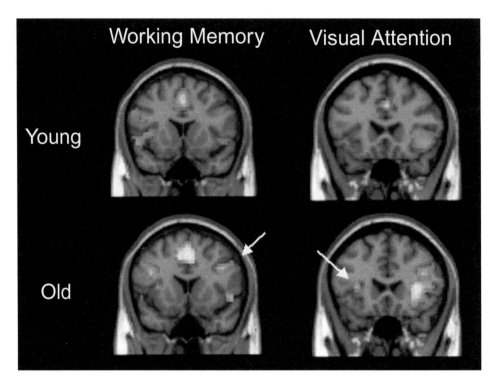

Plate 23 OAs showed contralateral recruitment in right PFC during WM and in left PFC during VA. As a result of these changes, activity in certain PFC regions was more bilateral in OAs than in YAs (Hemispheric Asymmetry Reduction in Older Adults, or HAROLD) (Cabeza et al., 2004). See chapter 12.

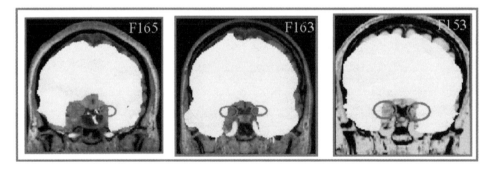

Plate 24 Signal voids in the vicinity of the amygdala due to magnetic susceptibility artifacts. Images depict thresholded signal-to-noise maps overlaid onto each subject's structural scan in a coronal section through the amygdala (outlined in red). For all three subjects, the medial aspect of the left and right amygdalae are located outside the sensitivity map, indicating insufficient signal-to-noise for a *t*-test comparison based on an expected 1% peak signal change. None of these participants showed significant amygdala activation during the encoding of emotionally aversive complex scenes. Data were acquired from a 1.5 T Siemens Vision scanner using conventional whole-brain gradient-echo echoplanar imaging. (Adapted from LaBar et al., 2001.) See chapter 13.

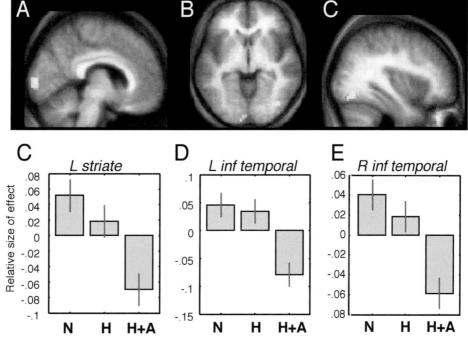

Plate 25 Statistical parametric maps of emotion x group interaction (*A–C*) across the whole brain showing the main effect for fearful vs. neutral faces differed between patient groups in the left striate cortex (*A*), left and right inferior temporal lobe (*B*), and right inferior temporal lobe (*C*). Parameter estimates for the relative size of effect in this ANOVA (arbitrary units, mean centered) for peaks in left striate cortex, left inferior temporal lobe, and right inferior temporal lobe show increased activation to fearful faces in both normal controls (N) and patients with damage confined to the hippocampus (H), but not patients with both hippocampal and amygdala damage (A + H). (Adapted from Vuilleumier et al., 2004.) See chapter 13.

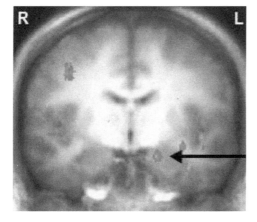

Plate 26 A statistical map presented in the coronal plane showing significant signal increases in the left amygdala (arrow) for the contrast of negative vs. positively cues surprise faces. (Adapted from Kim et al., 2004.) See chapter 13.

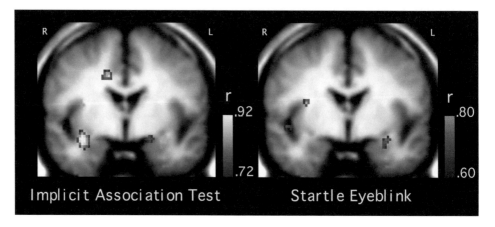

Plate 27 Correlation maps indicating brain regions where the relative differential BOLD response to black vs. white unfamiliar faces is significantly correlated with implicit measures of race bias for white American subjects. The implicit measures are (*left*) the Implicit Association Test (IAT), a reaction time measurement designed to measure conflict in evaluative judgments (Greenwald et al., 1998) and startle eyeblink (*right*) a physiological measure that assesses the strength of the startle reflex as it is modulated by emotional valence (Grillon et al., 1991). For both implicit measures of race bias, negative bias toward black is correlated with differential BOLD responses in the right amygdala. (Adapted from Phelps et al., 2000.) See chapter 13.

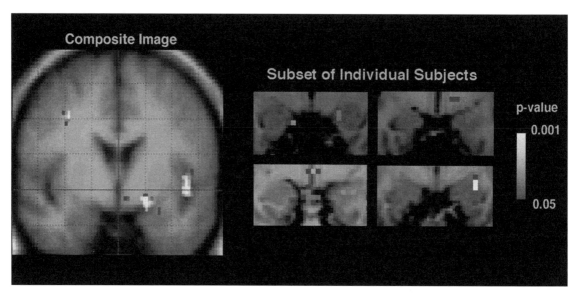

Plate 28 Group composite (*left*) and selected individual (*right*) statistical maps showing left amygdala activation to a colored square verbally linked to the possibility of a mild shock ("threat") versus another colored square not linked to shock ("safe"), demonstrating left amygdala involvement in instructed fear. (Adapted from Phelps et al., 2001.) See chapter 13.

Using these techniques, Velanova et al. (2003) demonstrated an apparently sustained, tonic increase in the response of right frontopolar PFC during demanding retrieval blocks (compared with less demanding blocks), and suggested that this tonic response is critically tied to establishing a retrieval set or mode (see also McDermott et al., 1999). (figure 8.10).

Instead of characterizing activity as item- or state-related, an alternative way of characterizing activity during retrieval is with respect to whether it appears reliably linked to the retrieval question (cue) or the retrieval probes. Several long-standing cognitive models suggest that a critical element in retrieval, particularly contextual retrieval, is planning or describing what one wants to retrieve (CD. A. Norman & Bobrow, 1979; Raaijmakers & Shiffrin, 1981; Schacter et al., 1998). More specifically, these models suggest that efficient search of episodic memory depends on the construction and maintenance of a coarse description of the kind or amount of desired memory content that will suffice as an answer. These contextual descriptions are often referred to as retrieval plans, and their construction or maintenance may be compromised in the elderly (e.g. Johnson et al., 2004).

Comparisons of source versus item memory have suggested that left dorsal and frontopolar PFC are generally engaged in the former, and thus these regions are potential candidates for the instantiation of retrieval planning. Interestingly, however, right frontopolar responses are often not evident in comparisons of source and item recognition despite the central role afforded this region with respect to retrieval mode. One possibility is that both source and item recognition tasks are riding upon a tonic increase in the right frontopolar region, and therefore direct comparisons do not isolate this region (i.e., they equally rely upon retrieval mode). An alternative possibility is suggested by the ERP research of Herron & Wilding (2004). As noted earlier, these researchers observed similar elevated responses to different types of source recognition questions over right frontopolar electrode sites. Critically, this response was time-locked to the appearance of the retrieval question (source recognition > semantic process), which appeared 2300 msecs prior to the onset of the actual retrieval probe. Given the millisecond response accuracy of ERPs, this strongly suggests that right frontopolar activity may actually precede contextual memory retrieval attempts. Thus mixed fMRI designs such as that of Velanova et al. (2003) may be capturing anticipatory or preparatory responses that precede item presentation, and that are more heavily represented during demanding retrieval blocks.

Nascent fMRI studies attempting to isolate cue from probe activity provide some initial evidence for this hypothesis. One method of isolating cue from probe activity, used by Simons and colleagues, is to present null trials following some source recognition cues (J. S. Simons et al., 2005). Using this technique, retrieval task cues were presented 1 sec in advance of the probes. On most trials, cues were followed by previously studied probe items, requiring a memory search and judgment. However, on null trials, a response indicator simply appeared, instructing the subjects which button to press. Hence, on these trials, no active retrieval could occur because probes were never presented. Simons et al. (in press) found that a left frontopolar region (BA 10) was more active during recovery of previous semantic operations versus recovery of list/recency information during standard trials (see also Dobbins et al., 2003). Furthermore, this retrieval orientation effect was present even when probes did not follow the retrieval cues (as indicated by a conjunction analysis). Thus, preparatory responses in the left but not the right frontopolar region anteceded active retrieval operations.

Dobbins and Han (in prep.) took an alternative approach to disentangling cue and probe activity. Using a design similar to that employed in visual attention research (e.g., Hopfinger et al., 2000), Dobbins and Han disentangled cue from probe activity by temporally jittering the relative onset of retrieval cues (both source and item) from their matched retrieval probes (6, 8, or 10 sec delay). These delayed retrieval conditions were interspersed with standard trials in which the cue and probes appeared simultaneously. Consistent with prior research, the contrast of source and item recognition during simultaneous presentation revealed the expected left-lateralized and midline PFC regions (figure 8.11). However, when the analysis was restricted to the retrieval cue activity during the delayed cuing condition, several PFC regions displayed increased activity in response to source questions compared with item questions that anteceded the appearance of retrieval probes. These regions included left dorsal and posterior ventrolateral PFC, anterior cingulate/SMA, and right frontopolar PFC.

Thus these regions demonstrated a preparatory response that was largely exclusive to upcoming active source retrieval operations (figure 8.11). Importantly, although a right frontopolar response isolating subsequent source from item trials was evident for the cues, source and item responses did not differ in response to the later probes in isolation, or when cues and probes were presented simultaneously. These data suggest that right frontopolar cortex may play a critical role preceding active retrieval attempts that is disrupted when probe processing is initiated.

Verdicality of Memory Report
We have been largely silent regarding differences in accuracy across the various tasks we have discussed. Somewhat surprisingly, this is because there is sparse evidence that PFC responses during contextual retrieval tasks directly reflect the outcome of retrieval. In the case of right frontopolar PFC, this is perhaps not surprising, given its apparent anticipatory or statelike tonic responses. However, direct comparisons of correct and incorrect source memory trials have failed to demonstrate retrieval outcome differences in left PFC regions that clearly differentiate

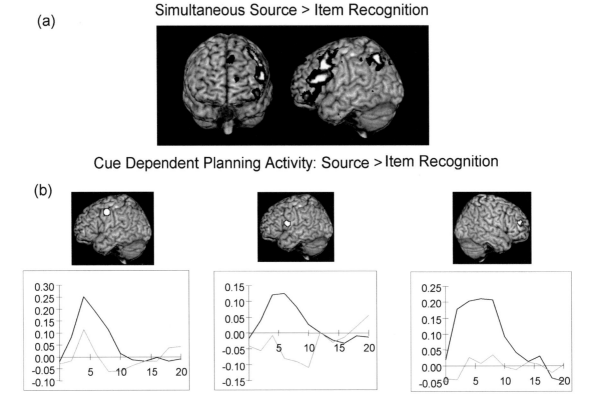

Figure 8.11
Data from Dobbins and Han (in prep). (*a*) During simultaneous presentation of cues and probes, a familiar left-lateralized network is observed demonstrating greater activity during source versus item recognition. (*b*) Using a manipulation that delayed probe onset relative to the retrieval cues, demonstrated differential source versus item activation during the anteceding cue phase of retrieval trials, suggesting that source memory entails planning or anticipatory responses.

source and item recognition trials. For example, although Dobbins et al. (2003) found that the left MTL demonstrated greater activity for correct versus incorrect source attributions, the numerous PFC regions that were reliably linked to source memory instead failed to display similar success effects; in fact, activity was numerically greater during failed retrieval attempts (see figure 8.3c). This makes sense from the standpoint of elaborative or monitoring operations, since these would be required even if the attempt was unsuccessful. Likewise, in a highly similar network of PFC regions, Kahn et al. (2004) also failed to find differences in prefrontal responses as a function of source retrieval outcome, although these regions were generally more active during trials of old items than trials of new items.

Although these null success effects in PFC make sense in light of proposed controlled retrieval operations thought to support source memory, they potentially conflict with previous characterizations of basic recognition imaging data. More specifically, a contrast frequently employed in event-related fMRI studies of item recognition is the comparison of correct responses to old items (hits) and correct responses to new items (correct rejections) (figure 8.1). When compared, left PFC regions very similar to those seen during comparisons of source and item recognition are implicated, demonstrating greater activity for old items (e.g., D. I. Donaldson et al., 2001; Henson et al., 1999; Konishi et al., 2000; McDermott et al., 2000). This comparison is often termed a "retrieval success" contrast, given that the level of memory evidence should clearly differ for correctly identified old and new items. Recently however, finer-grained manipulations raise doubts about this interpretation. For example, Wheeler and Buckner (2003) found that highly rehearsed items which were easily identified as old (figure 8.12, 20x) yielded activations in left posterior and mid-ventrolateral regions (BA 44, BA 45/47) virtually identical to those observed for new items and generated less, not more, activity than items that were rehearsed only once (1x). This is exactly the opposite pattern that would be expected if activity in these regions signified the recovery, or operations dependent on the recovery, of episodic information.

Overall, this led Wheeler and Buckner (2003) to suggest a positive relationship between left ventrolateral activity and the need for controlled processing during demanding retrieval. From this perspective, the recruitment of left PFC regions during contrasts of source versus item recognition, and during contrasts of old versus

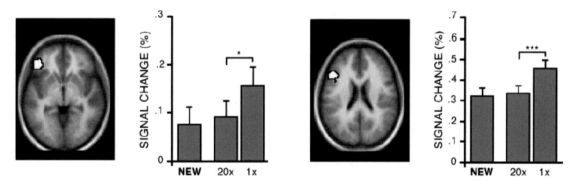

Figure 8.12
Data from Wheeler and Buckner (2003) suggesting that left PFC activity during recognition reflects controlled retrieval processes and not retrieval success effects. Items viewed 20 times prior to testing demonstrated the same low level of activity as entirely new items that were correctly rejected. Furthermore, items that were less well encoded (seen once), demonstrated increased activity in left PFC regions also implicated in source memory.

new items within item recognition, likely identifies a network enabling controlled search or monitoring processes. In the case of old/new recognition, poorly encoded items may engender a moderate, and hence ambiguous, sense of familiarity that results in the subject continuing the search in an attempt to confirm the item's status. For example, in figure 8.1, items in the vicinity of where the old and new item distributions overlap yield highly ambiguous memory evidence. Given this, subjects may continue to monitor for more conclusive episodic content before assigning a response to the item. In contrast, items yielding high evidence signals (20x) and low evidence signals (new) can often be quickly and confidently classified. Similarly, Kahn et al. (2004) suggested that in tests of source memory which include new items, subjects may engage in familiarity-gated recollection attempts, such that the attempt to recover source information, and hence activity in left PFC involved in controlled elaboration or monitoring, is contingent upon the item's familiarity. Items that are perceived as unfamiliar or novel are rejected outright, whereas those engendering a sense of familiarity potentially consistent with prior study are subjected to a more thorough evaluation in the attempt to recover source information (see also Atkinson & Juola, 1974; Kahn et al., 2004).

Although there is little evidence suggesting the presence of retrieval success effects in PFC, there are reports demonstrating success or success-related effects in posterior perceptual association areas and the MTL. With respect to the former, it has been hypothesized that remembering an event results in some degree of recapitulation of the sensory and perceptual experiences of the original. Evidence for this recapitulation hypothesis has come from event-related studies in which subjects attempt to recover the perceptual characteristics of prior encounters with probe items. For example, Wheeler et al. (2000) paired verbal descriptors with either sounds or pictures during an extensive two-day study period. Following this, subjects were tested during retrieval requiring a source attribution for the presented verbal descriptors; that is, they were required to decide if the descriptor (e.g., "dog") was previously paired with a sound or a picture of a dog. Consistent with the recapitulation hypothesis, activity levels in left fusiform and superior temporal gyrus differed as a function of an item's previous perceptual association.

Following the work of Wheeler et al. (2000) other studies have also reported sensory-specific activations related to the qualities of prior experiences (e.g. Gottfried et al., 2004; Kahn et al., 2004). Although these studies fit nicely with the idea that episodic memory involves some form of recovery of the constituents of the original experiences, some caution is warranted with respect to whether recapitulation effects are the cause or the consequence of remembering. More specifically, as pointed out by Kahn et al. (2004), activity in sensory-specific areas may arise following recovery of symbolic information specifying contextual elements, in which case subjects may then selectively attend to certain representational domains or may engage in imagery that elicits activity in sensory-specific regions. Under such a model, the recollection of context and the imagining of its properties would be separable processes.

Although recent evidence implicates recapitulation during episodic remembering, it appears that sometimes cortical activation differences between targets and lures can occur below the limen of consciousness, particularly when using paradigms, such as the Roediger/McDermott/Deese false memory paradigm, that are constructed to yield high rates of false alarms to lures. During the Roediger/McDermott/Deese false memory paradigm, subjects are shown a series of words (e.g., pillow, nighttime, blanket) that converge on a critical lure not presented during study (e.g., sleep) (Roediger & McDermott, 1995). Although the critical lures are not presented at study, subjects often falsely and confidently claim to remember having seen them. Cabeza et al. (2001) ported the false memory paradigm to the fMRI environment and found an interesting dissociation in the left MTL region. Anterior left MTL demonstrated a similar and elevated BOLD activity to both studied targets (hits) and incorrectly endorsed critical lures (false alarms) in comparison to correctly rejected lures unrelated to study list items (correct rejections). In contrast, left posterior MTL demonstrated an elevated response that was selective to studied targets; critical lures and lures unrelated to previously studied items demonstrated similar diminished responses (Cabeza et al., 2001). This led Cabeza et al. to conclude that the anterior-posterior MTL differences reflected different efferent connections to the MTL regions from semantic and sensory cortices, respectively.

From this perspective, posterior MTL regions distinguished the related critical lures from the targets because the semantically related lures were accompanied by recovery of less perceptual content than the previously viewed targets. This is consistent with cognitive studies demonstrating that although subjects often incorrectly endorse critical lures, they tend to report recovery of less perceptual content when doing so (e.g., K. A. Norman & Schacter, 1997). If correct, this suggests that cortical responses which directly or indirectly reflect recovery of encoded sensory-specific content do not necessarily contribute to the overt endorsement of items (see also Slotnick & Schacter 2004).

Given the focus of this section on the veridicality of report, it is perhaps surprising that a greater emphasis has not been placed upon activations occurring in the hippocampus and surrounding regions known to be essential for episodic memory. Although differential MTL responses are now common for comparisons of correct versus incorrect memory responses across various retrieval paradigms, there remains considerable variability in the location of these activations from study to study. For reviews with a heavy or exclusive emphasis on hippocampal and surrounding MTL responses during episodic retrieval, we point the reader toward Schacter & Wagner (1999) and Henson (2005).

Qualia Versus Continua in Memory Evidence

The consistency of paradigms contrasting source and item recognition suggests that when subjects try to recover the qualitative characteristics of prior experiences, there is consistent recruitment of left PFC and parietal and midline regions. From within the source monitoring framework, some of this activity is presumed to reflect monitoring for systematic or deliberative aspects of one's prior cognitive processes, whereas assessing the novelty of an item is presumed to rely upon a more heuristic monitoring process. Similarly, a dual-process characterization of these findings suggests that the attempt to recollect specific characteristics of a prior event will heavily engage left PFC regions, perhaps for some of the same reasons that left PFC regions are recruited during other conceptual classification or working memory tasks. However, one can assess the past in a fashion that seems less categorical and more continuous in nature. Similar distinctions are routinely made in research on perception and imagery. For example, Kosslyn and colleagues (1989) distinguish between categorical and coordinate representations of spatial relations, and have conducted research linking these with the left and right cerebral hemispheres, respectively. Likewise, one might suspect that memory engrams can be assessed for both categorical (i.e., recollection) and continuous (i.e., familiarity/fluency) properties.

Evidence supporting this or a similar distinction during episodic retrieval is relatively sparse. However, there appear to be certain types of memory judgments that, unlike source memory judgments, preferentially recruit right PFC regions, particularly dorsal PFC. For example, in an early PET study by Cabeza et al. (1997), subjects were scanned during two different, two-alternative forced-choice (2AFC) memory judgments for verbal stimuli. During simple recognition, subjects were presented with one old item and one new item, and simply selected the previously seen item. In contrast, during relative recency judgments, the two words in a pair differed in terms of their recency of prior exposure (i.e., study list position), and the subject's task was to select the most recently viewed item. A direct contrast of recency versus recognition judgments revealed increases in PFC regions that were considerably more prominent in right dorsal PFC areas (see also Cabeza et al., 2000; Cabeza et al., 1997). A more recent fMRI-based study also found differential recruitment of right dorsal and frontopolar PFC during recency judgments when compared directly with a source discrimination task (Dobbins et al., 2003), and this pattern of laterality appears to generalize to recency and source attributions conducted in the context of a working memory (WM) paradigm (Mitchell et al., 2004).

Importantly, the recruitment of right PFC regions does not appear solely confined to judgments of temporal recency. Dobbins et al. (2004) examined judgments of prior exposure frequency (JOF) under the hypothesis that these judgments similarly rely upon assessments of item familiarity, as opposed to prior qualitative processing differences, across targets and lures. During the paradigm, subjects had to decide whether previously viewed pictures had been seen 6 or 2 times (JOF) or whether the current test picture was identical to that studied or a different exemplar (e.g., a different type of telephone). This latter same/different judgment was included as a reference task. Restricting analyses to those items which remained the same between study and test, there was a prominent asymmetry during retrieval, with both right dorsal and frontopolar regions activated during the JOF but showing minimal response during the same/different judgment (figure 8.13).

Finally, research employing the Remember/Know report technique also potentially supports the notion that right PFC is involved in the monitoring or evaluation of heuristic or familiarity-based item information. For example, in the Remember/Know studies of Henson et al. (1999) and Eldridge et al. (2000), greater activity was observed in right dorsal middle frontal regions during "know" responses versus "remember" responses. Under a dual-process interpretation, this would suggest that memory attributions based solely upon item familiarity rely predominantly upon right PFC. Alternatively, Henson et al. (1999) suggested that the right PFC responses were a function of postretrieval monitoring based on the idea that items which evoke "know" responses incur repeated evaluation or monitoring operations, given their close proximity to the old/new decision criterion (see also Henson et al., 2000).

Overall, retrieval paradigms based on judgments of recency and frequency, and those employing the Remember/Know procedure, suggest that recruitment of right dorsal, and perhaps frontopolar, regions is most prominent when the tasks either target quantitative characteristics of prior experiences (e.g., how recent? how frequent?) or when recollection fails and the response is based primarily upon item familiarity ("know" responses). However, more research directly contrasting different types of retrieval tasks is clearly warranted before firm conclusions can be drawn, particularly since performance during recency, frequency, and "knowing" judgments is often quite low.

Issues

Relative to its cognitive counterpart, the functional imaging of episodic encoding and retrieval is still in its infancy. Despite this, even a partial review such as the one conducted here suggests room for considerable optimism. Although cognitive research has firmly established certain task dissociations, such as that between semantic and nonsemantic processing and source and item memory, the nature and extent of those dissociations has often been difficult to delineate further, owing to the limitations of accuracy and reaction time measures. For example, do source and

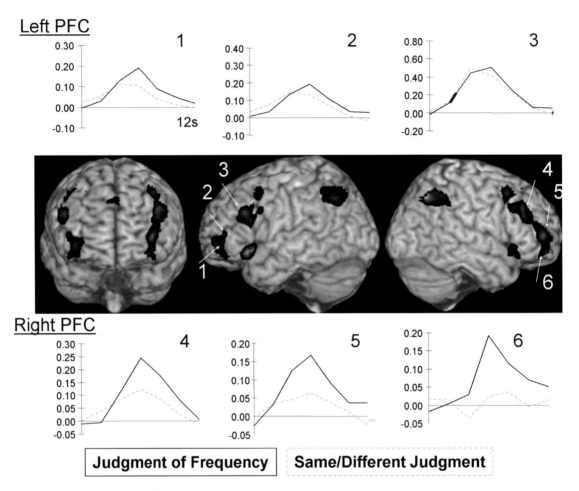

Figure 8.13

Hemispheric differences in response to judgments of frequency (JOF). Although comparisons of source and item memory often implicate left PFC, Dobbins et al. (2004) demonstrated increased recruitment of right PFC regions when subjects were required to estimate the frequency of prior exposures to items versus when they were to judge whether the item was a same or different exemplar than previously viewed (activity shown for items that remained the same from study to test).

item tasks rely upon different evidence, decision systems, or some combination of both? It is just these types of questions that functional imaging will help to resolve. For example, fMRI comparisons of source and item retrieval have already clearly implicated a network of left-lateralized PFC, posterior parietal, and midline responses that are heavily recruited during source but not item recognition. Furthermore, with respect to PFC, these responses appear insensitive to source retrieval outcome, and the differentiation of source and item memory activity may temporally precede the processing of the retrieval probes in several key regions, suggesting a key role in planning retrieval intentions. In contrast to these patterns in PFC, MTL regions often display differential activation for correct and incorrect source attributions, so presumably their role in retrieval is less strategic and perhaps more evidence-based and involuntary (Moscovitch, 1992). Furthermore, the distinctions that are being drawn now between contributions of distinct MTL regions to episodic encoding were not possible without functional imaging technology.

Regardless of these and similar functional imaging advances, defining the precise functional contribution of different areas, or their interactions, to episodic encoding and retrieval still remains a daunting task, although steps are now being taken to provide such initial component process models of episodic retrieval (Burgess et al., 2005; Moscovitch & Winocur, 2002; J. S. Simons & Spiers, 2003). Hopefully, these initial advances will culminate in the ability to specify regression-like multiregional models that maximize the prediction of memory behavior across individuals or conditions, and that are capable of numerically elucidating the different relative contributions of different cortical regions to the prediction of bias, accuracy, confidence, reaction time, and other key behavioral indices of different types of memory experiences.

References

Alexander, M. P., Stuss, D. T., & Fansabedian, N. (2003). California Verbal Learning Test: Performance by patients with focal frontal and non-frontal lesions. *Brain* 126, 1493–1503.

Atkinson, R. C., & Juola, J. G. (1974). Search and decision processes in recongnition memory. In R. C. Atkinson, R. D. Luce, D. H. Krantz, & P. Suppes (Eds.), *Contemporary Developments in Mathematical Psychology*, vol. 1, *Learning, Memory, and Thinking*, 243–293. San Francisco: Freeman.

Awh, E., Jonides, J., Smith, E. E., Schumacher, E. H., Koeppe, R. A., & Katz, S. (1996). Dissociation of storage and rehearsal in verbal working memory: Evidence from positron emission tomography. *Psychological Science* 7, 25–31.

Bauer, P. J. (2004). Getting explicit memory off the ground: Steps toward construction of a neuro-developmental account of changes in the first two years of life. *Developmental Review* 24, 347–373.

Brewer, J. B., Zhao, Z., Desmond, J. E., Glover, G. H., & Gabrieli, J. D. E. (1998). Making memories: Brain activity that predicts how well visual experience will be remembered. *Science* 281, 1185–1187.

Brown, M. W., & Aggleton, J. P. (2001). Recognition memory: What are the roles of the perirhinal cortex and hippocampus? *Nature Reviews Neuroscience* 2, 51–61.

Buckner, R. L. (1996). Beyond HERA: Contributions of specific prefrontal brain areas to long-term memory retrieval. *Psychonomic Bulletin and Review* 3, 149–158.

Buckner, R. L. & Logan, J. M. (2001). Functional neuroimaging methods: PET and fMRI. In R. Cabeza & A. Kingstone (Eds.), *Handbook of Functional Neuroimaging of Cognition*, 27–48. Cambridge, MA: MIT Press.

Burgess, P. W., Simons, J. S., Dumontheil, I., & Gilbert, S. J. (2005). The gateway hypothesis of rostral prefrontal cortex (area 10) function. In J. Duncan, L. Phillips, & P. Mc Leod (Eds.), *Speed, Control and Age: In Honour of Patrick Rabbitt*. Oxford: Oxford University Press.

Cabeza, R., Anderson, N. D., Houle, S., Mangels, J. A., & Nyberg, L. (2000). Age-related differences in neural activity during item and temporal-order memory retrieval: A positron emission tomography study. *Journal of Cognitive Neuroscience* 12, 197–206.

Cabeza, R., Mangels, J., Nyberg, L., Habib, R., Houle, S., McIntosh, A. R., & Tulving, E. (1997). Brain regions differentially involved in remembering what and when: A PET study. *Neuron* 19, 863–870.

Cabeza, R., & Nyberg, L. (1997). Imaging cognition: An empirical review of PET studies with normal subjects. *Journal of Cognitive Neuroscience* 9, 1–26.

Cabeza, R., Rao, S. M., Wagner, A. D., Mayer, A. R., & Schacter, D. L. (2001). Can medial temporal lobe regions distinguish true from false? An event-related functional MRI study of veridical and illusory recognition memory. *Proceedings of the National Academy of Sciences USA* 98, 4805–4810.

Cansino, S., Maquet, P., Dolan, R. J., & Rugg, M. D. (2002). Brain activity underlying encoding and retrieval of source memory. *Cerebral Cortex* 12, 1048–1056.

Chein, J. M., & Fiez, J. A. (2001). Dissociation of verbal working memory system components using a delayed serial recall task. *Cerebral Cortex* 11, 1003–1014.

Cohen, N. J., Eichenbaum, H., Deacedo, B. S., & Corkin, S. (1985). Different memory systems underlying acquisition of procedural and declarative knowledge. *Annals of the New York Academy of Sciences* 444, 54–71.

Craik, F. I. M., & Lockhart, R. S. (1972). Levels of processing: A framework for memory research. *Journal of Verbal Learning and Verbal Behavior* 11, 671–684.

Davachi, L., Maril, A., & Wagner, A. D. (2001). When keeping in mind supports later bringing to mind: Neural markers of phonological rehearsal predict subsequent remembering. *Journal of Cognitive Neuroscience* 13, 1059–1070.

Davachi, L., Mitchell, J. P., & Wagner, A. D. (2003). Multiple routes to memory: Distinct medial temporal lobe processes build item and source memories. *Proceedings of the National Academy of Sciences USA* 100, 2157–2162.

Davachi, L., & Wagner, A. D. (2002). Hippocampal contributions to episodic encoding: Insights from relational and item-based learning. *Journal of Neurophysiology* 88, 982–990.

Dobbins, I. G., Foley, H., Schacter, D., & Wagner, A. (2002). Executive control during retrieval: Multiple prefrontal processes subserve source memory. *Neuron* 35, 989–996.

Dobbins, I. G., & Han, S. (in prep). Cue- versus probe-dependent prefrontal cortex activity during contextual remembering.

Dobbins, I. G., Kroll, N. E., & Yonelinas, A. (2004). Dissociating familiarity from recollection using rote rehearsal. *Memory & Cognition* 32, 932–944.

Dobbins, I. G., Rice, H. J., Wagner, A. D., & Schacter, D. L. (2003). Memory orientation and success: Separable neurocognitive components underlying episodic recognition. *Neuropsychologia* 41, 318–333.

Dobbins, I. G., Schnyer, D. M., Verfaellie, M., & Schacter, D. L. (2004). Cortical activity reductions during repetition priming can result from rapid response learning. *Nature* 428, 316–319.

Dobbins I., G., & Wagner, A. D. (2005). Domain-general and domian-sensitive prefrontal mechanisms for recollecting events and detecting novelty. *Cerebral Cortex* 23 [Epub ahead of print].

Dolan, R. J., & Fletcher, P. C. (1997). Dissociating prefrontal and hippocampal function in episodic memory encoding. *Nature* 388, 582–585.

Donaldson, D. I., Petersen, S. E., Ollinger, J. M., & Buckner, R. L. (2001). Dissociating state and item components of recognition memory using fMRI. *NeuroImage* 13, 129–142.

Donaldson, W. (1996). The role of decision processes in remembering and knowing. *Memory & Cognition* 24, 523–533.

Duzel, E., Cabeza, R., Picton, T. W., Yonelinas, A. P., Scheich, H., Heinze, H. J., & Tulving, E. (1999). Task-related and item-related brain processes of memory retrieval. *Proceedings of the National Academy of Sciences USA* 96, 1794–1799.

Eldridge, L. L., Knowlton, B. J., Furmanski, C. S., Bookheimer, S. Y., & Engel, S. A. (2000). Remembering episodes: A selective role for the hippocampus during retrieval. *Nature Neuroscience* 3, 1149–1152.

Fiez, J. A. (1997). Phonology, semantics, and the role of the left inferior prefrontal cortex. *Human Brain Mapping* 5, 79–83.

Fletcher, P. C., & Henson, R. N. (2001). Frontal lobes and human memory: Insights from functional neuroimaging. *Brain* 124 (Pt 5), 849–881.

Fletcher, P. C., Shallice, T., & Dolan, R. J. (1998). The functional roles of prefrontal cortex in episodic memory. I. Encoding. *Brain* 121, 1239–1248.

Foster, J. K., & Jelicic, M. (Eds.), (1999). *Memory: Systems, Process, or Function?* New York: Oxford University Press.

Gabrieli, J. D. E., Brewer, J. B., Desmond, J. E., & Glover, G. H. (1997). Separate neural bases of two fundamental memory processes in the human medial temporal lobe. *Science* 276, 264–266.

Gardiner, J. M., & Java, R. I. (1993a). Recognising and remembering. In A. F. Collins, S. E. Gathercole, and et al. (Eds.), *Theories of Memory*, 143–188. Hillsdale, NJ: Erlbaum.

Gardiner, J. M., & Java, R. I. (1993b). Recognition memory and awareness: An experiential approach. *European Journal of Cognitive Psychology* 5, 337–346.

Gold, B. T., & Buckner, R. L. (2002). Common prefrontal regions coactivate with dissociable posterior regions during controlled semantic and phonological tasks. *Neuron* 35, 803–812.

Gottfried, J. A., Smith, A. P., Rugg, M. D., & Dolan, R. J. (2004). Remembrance of odors past: Human olfactory cortex in cross-modal recognition memory. *Neuron* 42, 687–695.

Hamann, S. B., & Squire, L. R. (1997). Intact perceptual memory in the absence of conscious memory. *Behavioral Neuroscience* 111, 850–854.

Henson, R. (2005). A mini-review of fMRI studies of human medial temporal lobe activity associated with recognition memory. *Quarterly Journal of Experimental Psychology* 58B, 340–360.

Henson, R. N., Rugg, M. D., Shallice, T., & Dolan, R. J. (2000). Confidence in recognition memory for words: Dissociating right prefrontal roles in episodic retrieval. *Journal of Cognitive Neuroscience* 12, 913–923.

Henson, R. N. A., Rugg, M. D., Shallice, T., Josephs, O., & Dolan, R. J. (1999). Recollection and familiarity in recognition memory: An event-related functional magnetic resonance imaging study. *Journal of Neuroscience* 19, 3962–3972.

Herron, J. E., & Wilding, E. L. (2004). An electrophysiological dissociation of retrieval mode and retrieval orientation. *NeuroImage* 22, 1554–1562.

Hopfinger, J. B., Buonocore, M. H., & Mangun, G. R. (2000). The neural mechanisms of top-down attentional control. *Nature Neuroscience* 3, 284–291.

Jackson, O. III, & Schacter, D. L. (2004). Encoding activity in anterior medial temporal lobe supports subsequent associative recognition. *NeuroImage* 21, 456–462.

Johnson, M. K., Hashtroudi, S., & Lindsay, D. S. (1993). Source monitoring. *Psychological Bulletin* 114, 3–28.

Johnson, M. K., Mitchell, K. J., Raye, C. L., & Greene, E. J. (2004). An age-related deficit in prefrontal cortical function associated with refreshing information. *Psychological Science* 15, 127–132.

Jonides, J., Schumacher, E. H., Smith, E. E., Koeppe, R. A., Awh, E., Reuter-Lorenz, P. A., Marshuetz, C., & Willis, C. R. (1998). The role of parietal cortex in verbal working memory. *Journal of Neuroscience* 18, 5026–5034.

Kahn, I., Davachi, L., & Wagner, A. (2004). Functional-neuroanatomic correlates of recollection: Implications for models of recognition memory. *Journal of Neuroscience* 24, 4172–4180.

Kelley, W. M., Miezin, F. M., McDermott, K. B., Buckner, R. L., Raichle, M. E., Cohen, N. J., Ollinger, J. O., Akbudak, E., Conturo, T. E., Snyder, A. Z., & Petersen, S. E., (1998). Hemispheric specialization in human dorsal frontal cortex and medial temporal lobe for verbal and nonverbal memory encoding. *Neuron* 20, 927–936.

Kensinger, E. A., Clarke, R. J., & Corkin, S. (2003). What neural correlates underlie successful encoding and retrieval? A functional magnetic resonance imaging study using a divided attention paradigm. *Journal of Neuroscience* 23, 2407–2415.

Kirchhoff, B. A., Wagner, A. D., Maril, A., & Stern, C. E. (2000). Prefrontal-temporal circuitry for episodic encoding and subsequent memory. *Journal of Neuroscience* 20, 6173–6180.

Kirwan, C. B., & Stark, C. E. (2004). Medial temporal lobe activation during encoding and retrieval of novel face-name pairs. *Hippocampus* 14, 919–930.

Klein, D., Olivier, A., Milner, B., Zatorre, R. J., Johnsrude, I., Meyer, E., & Evans, A. C. (1997). Obligatory role of the LIFG in synonym generation: Evidence from PET and cortical stimulation. *NeuroReport* 8, 3275–3279.

Konishi, S., Wheeler, M. E., Donaldson, D. I., & Buckner, R. L. (2000). Neural correlates of episodic retrieval success. *NeuroImage* 12, 276–286.

Kosslyn, S. M., Koenig, O., Barrett, A., Cave, C. B., Tang, J., & Gabrieli, J. D. (1989). Evidence for two types of spatial representations: Hemispheric specialization for categorical and coordinate relations. *Journal of Experimental Psychology: Human Perception and Performance* 15, 723–735.

Lepage, M., Ghaffar, O., Nyberg, L., & Tulving, E. (2000). Prefrontal cortex and episodic memory retrieval mode. *Proceedings of the National Academy of Sciences USA* 97, 506–511.

Lepage, M., Habib, R., & Tulving, E. (1998). Hippocampal PET activations of memory encoding and retrieval: The HIPER model. *Hippocampus* 8, 313–322.

Levin, D. T., Simons, D. J., Angelone, B. L., & Chabris, C. F. (2002). Memory for centrally attended changing objects in an incidental real-world change detection paradigm. *British Journal of Psychology* 93, 289–302.

Macmillan, N. A., & Creelman, C. D. (1991). *Detection Theory: A User's Guide.* New York: Cambridge University Press.

Marr, D. (1971). Simple memory: A theory for archicortex. *Philosophical Transactions of the Royal Society of London* B262, 23–81.

Mayes, A. R., & Downes, J. J., (Eds.). (1997). *Theories of Organic Amnesia.* Hove, UK: Psychology Press.

Mayes, A. R., Holdstock, J. S., Isaac, C. L., Montaldi, D., Grigor, J., Gummer, A., Cariga, P., Downes, J. J., Tsivilis, D., Gaffan, D., et al. (2004). Associative recognition in a patient with selective hippocampal lesions and relatively normal item recognition. *Hippocampus* 14, 763–784.

McClelland, J. L., McNaughton, B. L., & O'Reilly, R. C. (1995). Why there are complementary learning systems in the hippocampus and neocortex: Insights from the successes and failures of connectionist models of learning and memory. *Psychological Review* 102, 419–437.

McDermott, K. B., Buckner, R. L., Petersen, S. E., Kelley, W. M., & Sanders, A. L. (1999). Set-specific and code-specific activation in frontal cortex: An fMRI study of encoding and retrieval of faces and words. *Journal of Cognitive Neuroscience* 11, 631–640.

McDermott, K. B., Jones, T. C., Petersen, S. E., Lageman, S. K., & Roediger, H. L. III. (2000). Retrieval success is accompanied by enhanced activation in anterior prefrontal cortex during recognition memory: An event-related fMRI study. *Journal of Cognitive Neuroscience* 12, 965–976.

Meunier, M., Bachevalier, J., Mishkin, M., & Murray, E. A. (1993). Effects on visual recognition of combined and separate ablations of the entorhinal and perirhinal cortex in rhesus monkeys. *Journal of Neuroscience* 13, 5418–5432.

Mitchell, K. J., Johnson, M. K., Raye, C. L., & Greene, E. J. (2004). Prefrontal cortex activity associated with source monitoring in a working memory task. *Journal of Cognitive Neuroscience* 16, 921–934.

Montaldi, D., Mayes, A. R., Barnes, A., Pirie, H., Hadley, D. M., Patterson, J., & Wyper, D. J. (1998). Associative encoding of pictures activates the medial temporal lobes. *Human Brain Mapping* 6, 85–104.

Morcom, A. M., & Rugg, M. D. (2002). Getting ready to remember: The neural correlates of task set during recognition memory. *NeuroReport* 13, 149–152.

Morris, D. C., Bransford, J. D., & Franks, J. J. (1977). Levels of processing versus transfer appropriate processing. *Journal of Verbal Learning and Verbal Behavior* 16, 519–533.

Moscovitch, M. (1992). Memory and working-with-memory: A component process model based on modules and central systems. *Journal of Cognitive Neuroscience* 4, 257–267.

Moscovitch, M., Goshen Gottstein, Y., & Vriezen, E. (1994). Memory without conscious recollection: A tutorial review from a neuropsychological perspective. In Carlo Umiltà & Morris Moscovitch (Eds.), *Attention and Performance XV: Conscious and Nonconscious Information Processing*, 619–660. Cambridge, MA: MIT Press.

Moscovitch, M., & Winocur, G. (2002). The frontal cortex and working with memory. In Donald T. Stuss & Robert T. Knight (Eds.), *Principles of Frontal Lobe Function*, 188–209. New York: Oxford University Press.

Nolde, S. F., Johnson, M. K., & D'Esposito, M. (1998). Left prefrontal activation during episodic remembering: An event-related fMRI study. *NeuroReport* 9, 3509–3514.

Norman, D. A., & Bobrow, D. G. (1979). Descriptions: An intermediate stage in memory retrieval. *Cognitive Psychology* 11, 107–123.

Norman, K. A., & O'Reilly, R. C. (2003). Modeling hippocampal and neocortical contributions to recognition memory: A complementary-learning-systems approach. *Psychological Review* 110, 611–646.

Norman, K. A., & Schacter, D. L. (1997). False recognition in younger and older adults: Exploring the characteristics of illusory memories. *Memory & Cognition* 25, 838–848.

Nyberg, L., Cabeza, R., & Tulving, E. (1996). PET studies of encoding and retrieval: The HERA model. *Psychonomic Bulletin & Review* 3, 135–148.

O'Reilly, R. C., & Rudy, J. W. (2000). Computational principles of learning in the neocortex and hippocampus. *Hippocampus* 10, 389–397.

Otten, L. J., Henson, R. N., & Rugg, M. D. (2001). Depth of processing effects on neural correlates of memory encoding: Relationship between findings from across- and within-task comparisons. *Brain* 124, 399–412.

Otten, L. J., & Rugg, M. D. (2001). Task-dependency of the neural correlates of episodic encoding as measured by fMRI. *Cerebral Cortex* 11, 1150–1160.

Owen, A. M. (2003). HERA today, gone tomorrow? *Trends in Cognitive Sciences* 7, 383–384.

Paller, K. A., Kutas, M., & Mayes, A. R. (1987). Neural correlates of encoding in an incidental learning paradigm. *Electroencephalography and Clinical Neurophysiology* 67, 360–371.

Parkinson, J. K., Murray, E. A., & Mishkin, M. (1988). A selective mnemonic role for the hippocampus in monkeys: Memory for the location of objects. *Journal of Neuroscience* 8, 4159–4167.

Paulesu, E., Frith, C. D., & Frackowiak, R. S. J. (1993). The neural correlates of the verbal component of working memory. *Nature* 362, 342–345.

Petersen, S. E., van Mier, H., Fiez, J. A., & Raichle, M. E. (1998). The effects of practice on the functional anatomy of task performance. *Proceedings of the National Academy of Sciences USA* 95, 853–860.

Poldrack, R. A., Wagner, A. D., Prull, M. W., Desmond, J. E., Glover, G. H., & Gabrieli, J. D. E. (1999). Functional specialization for semantic and phonological processing in the left inferior prefrontal cortex. *NeuroImage* 10, 15–35.

Prince, S. E., Daselaar, S. M., & Cabeza, R. (2005). Neural correlates of relational memory: Successful encoding and retrieval of semantic and perceptual associations. *Journal of Neuroscience* 25, 1203–1210.

Raaijmakers, J. G., & Shiffrin, R. M. (1981). Search of associative memory. *Psychological Review* 88, 93–134.

Ranganath, C., Johnson, M. K., & D'Esposito, M. (2000). Left anterior prefrontal activation increases with demands to recall specific perceptual information. *Journal of Neuroscience* 20, RC108.

Ranganath, C., Yonelinas, A. P., Cohen, M. X., Dy, C. J., Tom, S. M., & D'Esposito, M. (2004). Dissociable correlates of recollection and familiarity within the medial temporal lobes. *Neuropsychologia* 42, 2–13.

Raye, C. L., Johnson, M. K., Mitchell, K. J., Nolde, S. F., et al. (2000). fMRI investigations of left and right PFC contributions to episodic remembering. *Psychobiology* 28, 197–206.

Roediger, H. L. (1990). Implicit memory: Retention without remembering. *American Psychologist* 45, 1043–1056.

Roediger, H. L. III. (2000). Why retrieval is the key process in understanding human memory. In *E. Tulving (Ed.), Memory, Consciousness, and the Brain: The Tallinn Conference*, 52–75. Philadelphia: Psychology Press.

Roediger, H. L., & McDermott, K. B. (1995). Creating false memories: Remembering words not presented in lists. *Journal of Experimental Psychology: Learning, Memory, and Cognition* 21, 803–814.

Rombouts, S. A., Machielsen, W. C., Witter, M. P., Barkhof, F., Lindeboom, J., & Scheltens, P. (1997). Visual association encoding activates the medial temporal lobe: A functional magnetic resonance imaging study. *Hippocampus* 7, 594–601.

Rugg, M. D. (1995). Event-related potential studies of human memory. In M. S. Gazzaniga (Ed.), *The Cognitive Neurosciences*, 789–801. (Cambridge, MA: MIT Press).

Rugg, M. D., Allan, K., & Birch, C. S. (2000). Electrophysiological evidence for the modulation of retrieval orientation by depth of study processing. *Journal of Cognitive Neuroscience* 12, 664–678.

Rugg, M. D., Otten, L. J., & Henson, R. N. (2002). The neural basis of episodic memory: Evidence from functional neuroimaging. *Philosophical Transactions of the Royal Society of London* B357, 1097–1110.

Rugg, M. D., & Wilding, E. L. (2000). Retrieval processing and episodic memory. *Trends in Cognitive Sciences* 4, 108–115.

Sanquist, T. F., Rohrbaugh, J. W., Syndulko, K., & Lindsley, D. B. (1980). Electrocortical signs of levels of processing: Perceptual analysis and recognition memory. *Psychophysiology* 17, 568–576.

Schacter, D. L., Buckner, R. L., Koutstaal, W., Dale, A. M., & Rosen, B. R. (1997). Late onset of anterior prefrontal activity during true and false recognition: An event-related fMRI study. *NeuroImage* 6, 259–269.

Schacter, D. L., Curran, T., Galluccio, L., Milberg, W. P., & Bates, J. F. (1996). False recognition and the right frontal lobe: A case study. *Neuropsychologia* 34, 793–808.

Schacter, D. L., & Graf, P. (1986). Preserved learning in amnesic patients: Perspectives from research on direct priming. *Journal of Clinical & Experimental Neuropsychology* 8, 727–743.

Schacter, D. L., Norman, K. A., & Koutstaal, W. (1998). The cognitive neuroscience of constructive memory. *Annual Review of Psychology* 49, 289–318.

Schacter, D. L., & Tulving, E. (1994). What are the memory systems of 1994? In D. L. Schacter & E. Tulving (Eds.), *Memory Systems 1994*, 1–38. Cambridge, MA: MIT Press.

Schacter, D. L., & Wagner, A. D. (1999). Medial temporal lobe activations in fMRI and PET studies of episodic encoding and retrieval. *Hippocampus* 9, 7–24.

Scoville, W. B., & Milner, B. (1957). Loss of recent memory after bilateral hippocampal lesions. *Journal of Neurology, Neurosurgery, and Psychiatry* 20, 11–21.

Shallice, T., Fletcher, P., Frith, C. D., Grasby, P., Frackowiak, R. S., & Dolan, R. J. (1994). Brain regions associated with acquisition and retrieval of verbal episodic memory. *Nature* 368, 633–635.

Simons, D. J., & Rensink, R. A. (2005). Change blindness: Past, present, and future. *Trends in Cognitive Sciences* 9, 16–20.

Simons, J. S., Gilbert, S. J., Owen, A. M., Fletcher, P. C., & Burgess, P. W. (2005). Distinct roles for lateral and medial anterior prefrontal cortex in the control of contextual recollection. *Journal of Neurophysiology* 94(1), 813–820.

Simons, J. S., & Spiers, H. J. (2003). Prefrontal and medial temporal lobe interactions in long-term memory. *Nature Reviews Neuroscience* 4, 637–648.

Slotnick, S. D., & Schacter, D. L. (2004) A sensory signature that distinguishes true from false memories. Nature Neuroscience 7(6), 664–672. Epub 2004 May 23.

Small, S. A., Nava, A. S., Perera, G. M., De La Paz, R., Mayeux, R., & Stern, Y. (2001). Circuit mechanisms underlying memory encoding and retrieval in the long axis of the hippocampal formation. *Nature Neuroscience* 4, 442–449.

Sperling, R., Chua, E., Cocchiarella, A., Rand-Giovannetti, E., Poldrack, R., Schacter, D. L., & Albert, M. (2003). Putting names to faces: Successful encoding of associative memories activates the anterior hippocampal formation. *NeuroImage* 20, 1400–1410.

Sperling, R. A., Bates, J. F., Cocchiarella, A. J., Schacter, D. L., Rosen, B. R., & Albert, M. S. (2001). Encoding novel face-name associations: A functional MRI study. *Human Brain Mapping* 14, 129–139.

Squire, L. R. (1992a). Declarative and nondeclarative memory: Multiple brain systems supporting learning and memory. *Journal of Cognitive Neuroscience* 4, 232–243.

Squire, L. R. (1992b). Memory and the hippocampus: A synthesis from findings with rats, monkeys, and humans. *Psychological Review* 99, 195–231.

Squire, L. R., & Butters, N. (Eds.). (1992). *Neuropsychology of Memory*, 2nd ed. New York: Guilford Press.

Squire, L. R., Stark, C. E., & Clark, R. E. (2004). The medial temporal lobe. *Annual Review of Neuroscience* 27, 279–306.

Stark, C. E., & Squire, L. R. (2001). Simple and associative recognition memory in the hippocampal region. *Learning and Memory* 8, 190–197.

Stark, C. E., & Squire, L. R. (2003). Hippocampal damage equally impairs memory for single items and memory for conjunctions. *Hippocampus* 13, 281–292.

Stern, C. E., Corkin, S., Gonzalez, R. G., Guimaraes, A. R., Baker, J. R., Jennings, P. J., Carr, C. A., Sugiura, R. M., Vedantham, V., & Rosen, B. R. (1996). The hippocampal formation participates in novel picture encoding: Evidence from functional magnetic resonance imaging. *Proceedings of the National Academy of Sciences USA* 93, 8660–8665.

Strange, B. A., Fletcher, P. C., Henson, R. N., Friston, K. J., & Dolan, R. J. (1999). Segregating the functions of human hippocampus. *Proceedings of the National Academy of Sciences USA* 96, 4034–4039.

Strange, B. A., Otten, L. J., Josephs, O., Rugg, M. D., & Dolan, R. J. (2002). Dissociable human perirhinal, hippocampal, and parahippocampal roles during verbal encoding. *Journal of Neuroscience* 22, 523–528.

Swick, D., & Knight, R. T. (1999). Contributions of prefrontal cortex to recognition memory: Electrophysiological and behavioral evidence. *Neuropsychology* 13, 155–170.

Teng, E., & Squire, L. R. (1999). Memory for places learned long ago is intact after hippocampal damage. *Nature* 400, 675–677.

Thompson-Schill, S. L., D'Esposito, M., Aguirre, G. K., & Farah, M. J. (1997). Role of left inferior prefrontal cortex in retrieval of semantic knowledge: A reevaluation. *Proceedings of the National Academy of Sciences USA* 94, 14792–14797.

Tulving, E. (1983). *Elements of Episodic Memory.* New York: Oxford University Press.

Tulving, E. (1985). Memory and consciousness. *Canadian Psychology* 26(1), 1–12.

Tulving, E., Kapur, S., Craik, F. I. M., Moscovitch, M., & Houle, S. (1994). Hemispheric encoding/retrieval asymmetry in episodic memory: Positron emission tomography findings. *Proceedings of the National Academy of Sciences USA* 91, 2016–2020.

Tulving, E., Markowitsch, H. J., Kapur, S., Habib, R., & Houle, S. (1994). Novelty encoding networks in the human brain: Positron emission tomography data. *NeuroReport* 5, 2525–2528.

Tulving, E., Schacter, D. L., McLachlan, D. R., & Moscovitch, M. (1988). Priming of semantic autobiographical knowledge: A case study of retrograde amnesia. *Brain & Cognition* 8, 3–20.

Tulving, E., Schacter, D. L., & Stark, H. A. (1982). Priming effects in word-fragment completion are independent of recognition memory. *Journal of Experimental Psychology: Learning, Memory, and Cognition* 8, 336–342.

Velanova, K., Jacoby, L. L., Wheeler, M. E., McAvoy, M. P., Petersen, S. E., & Buckner, R. L. (2003). Functional-anatomic correlates of sustained and transient processing components engaged during controlled retrieval. *Journal of Neuroscience* 23, 8460–8470.

Wagner, A. D., Koutstaal, W., & Schacter, D. L. (1999). When encoding yields remembering: Insights from event-related neuroimaging. Philosophical Transactions of the Royal Society of London B354, 1307–1324.

Wagner, A. D., Pare-Blagoev, E. J., Clark, J., & Poldrack, R. A. (2001). Recovering meaning: Left prefrontal cortex guides controlled semantic retrieval. *Neuron* 31, 329–338.

Wagner, A. D., Poldrack, R. A., Eldridge, L. E., Desmond, J. E., Glover, G. H., & Gabrieli, J. D. E. (1998). Material-specific lateralization of prefrontal activation during episodic encoding and retrieval. *NeuroReport* 9, 3711–3717.

Wagner, A. D., Schacter, D. L., Rotte, M., Koutstaal, W., Maril, A., Dale, A. M., Rosen, B. R., & Buckner, R. L. (1998). Building memories: Remembering and forgetting of verbal experiences as predicted by brain activity. *Science* 281, 1188–1191.

Warrington, E. K., & Weiskrantz, L. (1974). The effect of prior learning on subsequent retention in amnestic patients. *Neuropsychologia* 12, 419–428.

Wheeler, M. E., & Buckner, R. L. (2003). Functional dissociation among components of remembering: Control, perceived oldness, and content. *J Neuroscience* 23(9), 3869–3880.

Wheeler, M. E., Petersen, S. E., & Buckner, R. L. (2000). Memory's echo: Vivid remembering reactivates sensory-specific cortex. *Proceedings of the National Academy of Sciences USA* 97(20), 11125–11129.

Wilding, E. L. (1999). Separating retrieval strategies from retrieval success: An event-related potential study of source memory. *Neuropsychologia* 37, 441–454.

Wixted, J. T., & Stretch, V. (2004). In defense of the signal detection interpretation of remember/know judgments. *Psychonomic Bulletin and Review* 11, 616–641.

Yonelinas, A. P. (2002). The nature of recollection and familiarity: A review of 30 years of research. *Journal of Memory and Language* 46, 441–517.

Yonelinas, A. P., Hopfinger, J. B., Buonocore, M. H., Kroll, N. E. A., & Baynes, K. (2001). Hippocampal, parahippocampal and occipital-temporal contributions to associative and item recognition memory: An fMRI study. *NeuroReport* 12, 359–363.

Zola-Morgan, S., & Squire, L. R. (1986). Memory impairment in monkeys following lesions limited to the hippocampus. *Behavioral Neuroscience* 100, 155–160.

Zola-Morgan, S., & Squire, L. R. (1992). The components of the medial temporal lobe memory system. In L. R. Squire & N. Butters (Eds.), *Neuropsychology of Memory*, 2nd ed., 325–335. New York: Guilford Press.

9 Functional Neuroimaging of Working Memory

Clayton E. Curtis and Mark D'Esposito

Working memory is an evolving concept that refers to the short-term storage of information that is not accessible in the environment and to the set of processes that keep this information active for later use. From a psychological perspective, working memory has been conceptualized as comprising multiple components, such as executive control and active maintenance processes. This chapter will review functional neuroimaging studies (PET and fMRI) which have provided evidence that prefrontal cortex is a critical node in the functional neural network supporting working memory. Also, recent data will be reviewed regarding the functional organization of prefrontal cortex.

Introduction

Working memory refers to the temporary representation of information that was just experienced or just retrieved from long-term memory but no longer exists in the external environment. These internal representations are short-lived, but can be maintained for longer periods of time through active rehearsal strategies, and can be subjected to operations that manipulate the information in such a way that it becomes useful for goal-directed behavior. Working memory is a system that is critically important in cognition and seems necessary in the course of performing many other cognitive functions, such as reasoning, language comprehension, planning, and spatial processing. Although working memory is an evolving construct, most often its definitions include both storage and (executive) control components (Miyake & Shah, 1999). Cognitive neuroscientists are searching for ways to dissociate the separable components of working memory in such a way that these separate functions can be localized within separate brain regions (i.e., *brain mapping*). Equally important is the goal of engineering models of the mechanisms by which the brain supports high-level cognitive processes such as working memory.

The prefrontal cortex (PFC) appears to be the most important brain region necessary for working memory (figure 9.1). Two consistent findings from studies of
monkeys performing delayed response tasks suggest a critical role for the PFC in
working memory. First, experimental lesions of the principal sulcus in the dorsolateral prefrontal cortex (DLPFC) impair performance on working memory tasks
(Jacobsen, 1936; Fuster, 1997; Curtis & D'Esposito, 2004) and exacerbate with
increasing memory retention intervals (Miller & Orbach, 1972; Bauer & Fuster,
1976; Funahashi et al., 1993). That is, forgetting increases not only when a delay is
imposed but also increases with the length of the delay. Second, electophysiological
single-unit recordings from the DLPFC often show persistent, sustained levels of
neuronal firing during the retention interval of delayed-response tasks (Fuster &
Alexander, 1971; Kubota & Niki, 1971; Funahashi et al., 1989). This sustained activity
is thought to provide a bridge between the stimulus cue—for instance, the location
of a flash of light—and its contingent response—for instance—a saccade to the
remembered location. Persistent activity during blank memory intervals is a very
powerful observation and has established a strong link implicating the DLPFC as
a critical node supporting working memory.

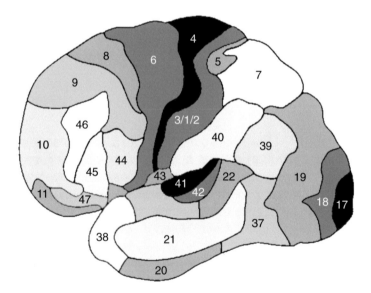

Figure 9.1
Schematic parcellation of the human brain based on cytoarchitecture divisions of Brodmann (1909). In
the frontal cortex, premotor areas (6 and 44) include the frontal eye fields bilaterally and Broca's area
in the left hemisphere. Multimodal association frontal cortex includes dorsolateral prefrontal cortex
(DLPFC), which refers to areas 46 and 9, ventrolateral prefrontal cortex (VLPFC), which refers to areas
45 and 47 and frontopolar or anterior PFC, which refers to area 10.

Subcomponents of Working Memory

A solid understanding of how working memory processes are implemented in the brain may hinge on our ability to resolve the nature of stored representations in addition to the types of operations performed on such representations that are necessary for guiding behavior (Curtis & D'Esposito, 2003a; Wood & Grafman, 2003). This is essentially restating, in traditional cognitive science terminology, that we must be able to dissociate storage functions (representations) and executive control functions (operations). *Representations* are symbolic codes for information stored either transiently or permanently in neuronal networks. Maintenance and storage are not synonymous. Storage, in the context of working memory, is the representation of memoranda through neuronal activity, that is, an activity-based definition (Miller & Cohen, 2001). The term "maintenance" is used more broadly to describe both the active representation and any processes that influence which items survive passive decay and distraction. *Operations* are processes or computations performed on representations. Examples of control processes or operations include the modification, transformation, integration, and manipulation of the originally encoded item.

Besides the representation-operation distinction, another key way to fractionate working memory into subcomponents is by considering the type of information that is being represented. This separation is essentially a further fractionation of the representation or storage subcomponent. In this regard, separate working memory subsystems selectively process and store different domains of information (e.g., space, object, verbal, visual, auditory, etc.). The most important distinction that has been made is between spatial and nonspatial visual information, given the extensive literature showing segregated processing streams of visual information. A ventral "what" pathway primarily performs analyses of visual features, eventually leading to object recognition as information from V1 travels through the occipital lobe to the inferior temporal lobe (Ungerleider & Mishkin, 1982). A dorsal "where" pathway primarily processes signals relating to motion and space, often in service of visually guided actions, as information travels from V1 through MT and the posterior parietal cortex, finally reaching M1 and the dorsal premotor cortex (Milner & Goodale, 1995).

Models of working memory (Baddeley, 1986; Miyake & Shah, 1999) and models of PFC function (Goldman-Rakic, 1987; Passingham, 1993; D'Esposito, Postle et al., 2000; E. K. Miller, 2000; Petrides, 2000a; Fuster, 2001; E. K. Miller & Cohen, 2001) vary substantially in the relative importance given to representations and operations (Curtis & D'Esposito, 2003a; Wood & Grafman, 2003). For example, Baddeley's model (Baddeley, 1986) of working memory proposes that information is represented in various storage buffers, depending on the form of the information (e.g., verbal or visuospatial). A central executive, similar to Norman and Shallice's supervisory attentional scheduler (Shallice & Burgess, 1996), is proposed to coordinate operations performed on the contents of information represented in memory. Some models attribute storage functions or representations to posterior cortical areas (e.g., premotor, parietal, and temporal cortex) and reserve the collection of "executive" operations for the PFC (Smith & Jonides, 1999; D'Esposito, Postle et al., 2000; Petrides, 2000a).

Models of Dorsolateral Prefrontal Cortical Function

Founded on experimental lesion and unit recording data in awake-behaving monkeys, Goldman-Rakic (1987) formalized her highly influential theory of PFC function. In this model, lesions of Brodmann's area 46 in the DLPFC impair the ability to maintain online sensory representations that are no longer present in the environment but are necessary for adaptive performance. Damage to the DLPFC results in the *forgetting* of relevant information. Persistent delay-period activity reflects the temporary storage of some stimulus feature such as its position or shape (Funahashi et al., 1993; Chafee & Goldman-Rakic, 1998; Constantinidis et al., 2001). Although local operations permit the feeding of sensory representations to neurons that control effectors, for example, the primary function of the DLPFC is proposed to be creation and maintenance of internal representations of relevant sensory information. E. K. Miller and Cohen (2001) extend this idea by suggesting that in addition to recent sensory information, integrated representations of task contingencies and even abstract rules (e.g., if this object, then this later response) are also maintained in the prefrontal cortex. This notion is similar to what Fuster (1997) has emphasized: that the PFC is critically responsible for temporal integration, the mediation of events separated in time but contingent on one another. Sustained delay-period activity may reflect the maintenance of several goal-directed representations, including past sensory events (i.e., a retrospective code), but also representations of anticipated action and preparatory set (i.e., prospective codes) (Quintana & Fuster, 1999; D'Esposito, Ballard et al., 2000). All of these models emphasize that the DLPFC plays a prominent storage role in the temporary maintenance of relevant information through persistent neural activity.

However, other models place less emphasis on a storage role for the DLPFC and instead (or additionally) emphasize its role in providing top-down control over more posterior regions where information is actually stored (Smith & Jonides, 1999; D'Esposito, Postle et al., 2000; Petrides, 2000b; Miller & Cohen, 2001). Thus, the sustained activity in the DLPFC does not reflect the storage of representations *per se*; it reflects some maintenance operation or top-down process that influences which aspects of our external or internal milieu are actively maintained in other posterior areas. Studies showing the enhancement of task performance and changes in the properties of extrastriate cortex attributable to the focusing of visual attention have been influential in developing this viewpoint (Desimone & Duncan, 1995; Kastner & Ungerleider, 2001).

Although clearly we are able to perform a variety of high-level tasks that require "executive" control processes, this does not imply that a homunculus-like entity exists in the brain. In fact, among researchers a strong sentiment against the notion that an "executive control" module exists in the brain is best summarized by Goldman-Rakic: "Based on anatomical, physiological, and lesion evidence in both monkeys and humans, 'a central-executive' in the form of an all-purpose polymodal processor may not exist, and to the contrary, a strong case can be made for the view that the substrates of cognition reside in the parallelism of the brain's modularized information processing systems" (Goldman-Rakic, 1996a, 13473; but also see 1996b). Therefore, we must not confuse postulating that the PFC plays an important role in "executive control" processes and postulating that the PFC is the site of the central executive.

In summary, working memory is not a unitary system, and can be viewed as a set of properties that characterize how this cognitive system makes use of temporarily activated representations to guide behavior. These properties may be behaviorally and neurally dissociable. Many methods exist to examine the neural basis of working memory in humans. The lesion method, for example, has been helpful in establishing the necessity of PFC in working memory function (for a review, see D'Esposito & Postle, 1999). However, since injury to PFC in humans is rarely restricted in its location, testing ideas about the necessity of a specific region of PFC for specific components of working memory by using lesion studies in humans is difficult. Functional neuroimaging, such as positron emission tomography (PET) or functional MRI (fMRI), provides another means of testing such ideas and in fact is currently the best method we have for investigating the physiology of the human brain (reviewed in the next section). It is important to realize, however, that unlike lesion studies, imaging studies support inferences about the *engagement* of a particular brain system by a cognitive process, but not about its *necessity* to these processes (Sarter et al., 1996). That is, neuroimaging studies cannot, alone, tell us whether the function of a neural system represents a neural substrate of that function or a nonessential process associated with that function. Moreover, this observation applies equally to all methods of physiological measurement, such as single- and multiunit electrophysiology, EEG, and MEG. Thus, data derived from neuroimaging studies provide one piece of converging evidence that is being accumulated to determine the neural basis of working memory.

Functional Neuroimaging Studies of Working Memory

Maintenance Processes

There is now a critical mass of studies (more than 100) that have used functional neuroimaging in humans to investigate brain regions engaged during working memory tasks (for a review, see Curtis & D'Esposito, 2003a; D'Esposito, Ballards et al., 1998). Review of the details of each of these studies is beyond the scope of this chapter, but those studies which highlight the critical advancements to our understanding of the neural basis of working memory will be considered. For example, Jonides and colleagues (1993) performed the first imaging study, using PET, which showed that PFC was activated during performance of a spatial working memory task that was analogous to the one used in the monkey studies. In this study, subjects were presented with two types of trials. In the memory condition, subjects were required to maintain the spatial location of three dots appearing on a visual display across a 3 sec delay. After this delay, a probe for location memory consisted of a single outline circle that either encircled the location of one of the previous dots or did not. In the perception condition, the three dots were again presented on a visual display, but immediately following their presentation, a probe circle appeared simultaneously with the dots, and the subject made a perceptual judgment as to whether or not the probe encircled a dot.

The rationale of this study was that "subtraction" of images obtained during the perceptual condition from images obtained from the memory condition would reveal brain regions that require the storage of spatial information during the retention interval, and not sensorimotor components of the task. Comparison of the block of trials with a delay period and a block of trials without a delay period produced activation within PFC as well as occipital, parietal, and premotor cortices. The location of the PFC activation in this study was within right Brodmann's area 47 (inferior frontal gyrus), which is inferior to the proposed homologous region in the principal sulcus (area 46), the site of spatial working memory in monkeys (Funahashi et al., 1989; Funahashi et al., 1993). Nevertheless, this study was an important demonstration that human PFC, like monkey PFC, may be critical for maintaining internal representations across time.

Subsequently, numerous other imaging studies have utilized delayed-response tasks with requirements for storage of spatial (Jonides et al., 1993; McCarthy et al., 1994; Goldberg et al., 1996; McCarthy et al., 1996; Smith et al., 1996; Sweeney et al., 1996; Belger et al., 1998; Courtney et al., 1998; Petit et al., 1998; Awh et al., 1999; Postle & D'Esposito, 1999; Nystrom et al., 2000; Postle, Berger et al., 2000; Rowe et al., 2000; Zarahn et al., 2000; Pochon et al., 2001; Rowe & Passingham, 2001; Corbetta et al., 2002; Glahn et al., 2002; Leung et al., 2002; Sakai et al., 2002; Simon et al., 2002; Zald et al., 2002; Postle & D'Esposito, 2003; Brown et al., 2004; Curtis et al., 2004; Postle et al., 2004) as well as nonspatial (i.e., letters, words, faces, objects) information (Paulesu et al., 1993; Petrides et al., 1993; Awh et al., 1996; Fiez et al., 1996; Schumacher et al., 1996; Smith et al., 1996; Braver et al., 1997; Desmond et al., 1997; Jonides et al., 1997; Jonides et al., 1998; Rypma et al., 1999; Nystrom et al., 2000; Chein & Fiez, 2001; Davachi et al., 2001; Barde & Thompson-Schill, 2002; Chein et al., 2002; Gruber & von Cramon, 2003; Walter et al., 2003; Crottaz-Herbette et al., 2004). Also, many other studies have been performed using more complex types of working memory tasks, such as n-back tasks (e.g., Petrides et al., 1993; Cohen et al., 1994; McCarthy et al., 1994; Owen et al., 1996; Salmon et al., 1996; Smith et al., 1996). Consistent across these studies is the demonstration of lateral PFC activation in a comparison between blocks of trials designed to have greater memory requirements than a matched control task.

A potential problem in interpretation of an imaging study such as that of Jonides, or the many others that were subsequently reported, is that they rely on the assumptions of the method of cognitive subtraction. Cognitive subtraction attempts to correlate brain activity with specific processes by pairing two tasks that are assumed to be matched perfectly for every sensory, motor, and cognitive process except the process of interest (Posner et al., 1988). For example, in the Jonides study it was assumed that the only difference between the two experimental conditions was the delay period (and therefore the process of memory storage). Although the application of cognitive subtraction to imaging was a major innovation when originally introduced (Petersen et al., 1988), it has become clear that it is a potentially flawed methodology that may lead to erroneous interpretation of imaging data.

The assumptions that must be relied upon for cognitive subtraction methodology can be faulty for at least two reasons. First, it involves the assumption of *additivity* (or *pure insertion*), the idea that a cognitive process can be added to a preexisting set of cognitive processes without affecting them (Sternberg, 1969). For example, the delayed-response paradigm typically used to study working memory is composed of a memory delay period between a "perceptual" process (the perception of the item[s] to be stored) and a "choice" process (a required decision based upon the item that was stored). The neural substrates of the memory process are proposed to be revealed by a subtraction of the integrated (i.e., averaged, summed, or totaled) functional hemodynamic signal during a no-delay condition (i.e., a block of trials without a delay period) from that during a delay condition (i.e., a block of trials with a delay period). In this example, failure to meet the assumptions of cognitive subtraction will occur if the insertion of a delay period between the "perceptual" and "choice" processes interacts with these other behavioral processes in the task. The nonmemory processes may be different in delay trials compared with no-delay trials; for example, more activation may be expected during the perceptual encoding epoch when the subjects are aware that they are going to have to remember the spatial locations over a delay period.

A second reason that cognitive subtraction methodology can be faulty is that in neuroimaging, an additional requirement must be met in order for cognitive subtractive methodology to yield nonartifactual results: the transform between the neural signal and the neuroimaging signal must be linear. In two studies thus far using functional MRI (fMRI), some nonlinearities have been observed in this system (Boynton et al., 1996; Vazquez & Noll, 1998). In our example of a delayed-response paradigm, failure will occur if the sum of the transform of neural activity to hemodynamic signal for the "perceptual" and "choice" processes differs when a delay is inserted as compared with when it is not present. In this example, artifacts of cognitive subtraction might lead to the inference that a region displayed delay-correlated increases in neural activity when in actuality it did not.

To overcome these potential problems, "event-related" fMRI designs were developed that do not rely on cognitive subtraction (for review, see D'Esposito, Aguirre, Zarahn, Ballard et al., 1998; Rosen et al., 1998). These designs allow one to detect changes in fMRI signal evoked by neural events associated with single behavioral trials as opposed to blocks of such trials or, as we will see, even specific events within a trial. Event-related fMRI designs are somewhat analogous to designs employed in event-related potential (ERP) studies, in that the functional responses occurring during different temporal portions within a trial can be analyzed.

As mentioned, spatial delayed-response tasks typically have a stimulus presentation period, an ensuing delay (of a few seconds), and a choice period. Changes in single-unit neural activity have been observed during each of these task components in electrophysiological studies of nonhuman primates. For example, Fuster and colleagues (1982), using a visual delayed-response task, observed that responses of single PFC neurons to the initial stimulus presentation ended within a few hundred milliseconds of stimulus offset. They also observed changes in firing rate in single neurons in lateral PFC during the delay period that were sustained for several seconds. If these results also characterize human PFC function, it should be possible with an event-related fMRI design to temporally resolve functional changes correlated with the delay period from those correlated with the stimulus presentation/ early delay period.

The logic of one implementation of an event-related fMRI design is as follows (Zarahn et al., 1997; Postle, Zarahn, et al., 2000) and is illustrated in figure 9.2. A single behavioral trial may be hypothesized to be associated with one brief neural event, or several brief neural events that are subcomponent processes which are engaged within a trial (i.e., encoding or retrieval in a delayed-response task). A neural event will cause a brief fMRI signal change, which is called the hemodynamic response. If we wish to detect and differentiate the fMRI signal evoked by a series

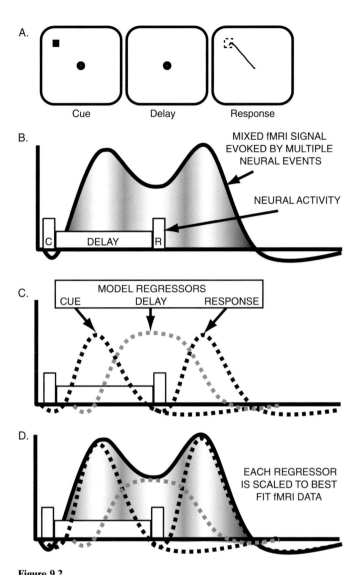

Figure 9.2

Delayed-response task and modeling within trial components of event-related fMRI data. (*A*) A proto-typic oculomotor delayed-response task, like all delayed-response tasks, has three main epochs: a sample cue period where stimuli to be remembered are presented, an unfilled delay period where stimuli are retained in memory, and finally a response period where a memory-guided response (i.e., saccade) is required. Event-related designs for fMRI have the ability to statistically disambiguate the hemodynamic signals specifically related to encoding the cue stimuli and generating memory-guided responses from the maintenance-related activity present in the retention interval. (*B*) When multiple sequential neural events occur within a trial, the resulting fMRI response is a mixture of signals emanating from more than one time and more than one trial component. The gradient under the curve schematically represents the mixing or temporal overlap of the various signal components. For example, the white region at the peak of the first hump is almost exclusively evoked from neural processing during the cue phase of the task. However, just a few seconds later, in the darker portion just to the right, the signal is a mixture of processing at the cue phase and the beginning of the delay period. (*C*) In order to resolve the individual components of the mixed fMRI signal, separate regressors can be used to independently model the cue, delay, and response phases of the trial. (*D*) The magnitudes of the regressors scale with the degree to which they account for variance in the observed time series data. The magnitude of the delay regressor can be used as an index for maintenance-related activity.

of sequential neural events (such as the presentation of the stimulus and, seconds later, the execution of the response), one method would be to statistically model the evoked fMRI signal using a pair of hemodynamic responses as covariates, each shifted to the appropriate time period in which the event of interest is thought to occur. Importantly, covariates shaped like hemodynamic response functions could theoretically be used to model any neural event, even if the event is sustained, such as delay period activity.

Analyzing in the manner described above, we observed during the performance of a spatial delayed-response task that several brain regions, including PFC, consistently displayed activity that correlated with the delay period across subjects (Zarahn et al., 1996, 1999). This finding suggests that these regions may be involved in temporary maintenance of spatial representations in humans. With this event-related fMRI design, we could be confident that activity observed was not due to differences in other components of the task (i.e., presentation of the cue or motor response) during the behavioral trials. Most important, these results do not rely on the assumptions of cognitive subtraction. An example of the time series of the fMRI signal averaged across trials for a PFC region displaying delay-correlated activity is shown in figure 9.3a.

In this same study, we also found direct evidence for the failure of cognitive subtraction (see figure 9.3b). We found a region in PFC that did not display sustained activity during the delay (in an event-related analysis), yet showed greater activity

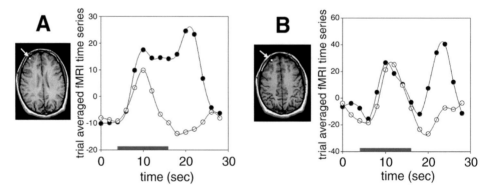

Figure 9.3
(*A*) An example of the time series of the fMRI signal averaged across trials for a PFC region that displayed delay-correlated activity is shown. Filled black circles represent activity for delay trials and open circles are trials without a delay. (*B*) An example of a time series where the integrated activity for the presentation of the cue and response during the delay trials (filled black circles) is greater than that observed during the combined presentation of the cue and response in the no-delay trials (open circles). This reflects a violation of the assumptions of cognitive subtraction that are made by most block design experiments. The solid gray bar represents the duration of the delay period of the behavioral task.

in the delay trials compared with the trials without a delay. In any blocked neuro-imaging study, such as those reviewed above, that compare delay versus no-delay trials with subtraction, such a region would be detected and likely assumed to be a "memory" region. Thus, this result provides empirical grounds for adopting a healthy doubt regarding the inferences drawn from imaging studies that have relied on cognitive subtraction.

Other studies using event-related designs have also investigated the temporal dynamics of neural activity, but during working memory tasks using nonspatial information. For example, Courtney and colleagues (1997) utilized a delayed-response task that required the maintenance of faces. Ventral occipitotemporal regions exhibited predominantly transient responses to the stimuli, consistent with a role in perceptual processing, whereas PFC demonstrated sustained activity over the memory delay, consistent with a role in active maintenance of face information. We now briefly summarize major findings from imaging studies of working memory categorized by the type of information that is being maintained (i.e., verbal, spatial, object). We focus on studies that used event-related designs which allowed the investigators to separate maintenance activity during delay periods from the encoding and response periods of delayed-response type tasks.

Spatial Working Memory Maintenance

Past human neuroimaging studies have generally implicated widespread and distributed frontal-parietal networks during the performance of spatial working memory tasks (Jonides et al., 1993; McCarthy et al., 1994; Goldberg et al., 1996; McCarthy et al., 1996; Smith et al., 1996; Sweeney et al., 1996; Belger et al., 1998; Courtney et al., 1998; Petit et al., 1998; Awh et al., 1999; Postle & D'Esposito, 1999; Nystrom et al., 2000; Postle, Berger et al., 2000; Rowe et al., 2000; Zarahn et al., 2000; Pochon et al., 2001; Rowe and Passingham, 2001; Corbetta et al., 2002; Glahn et al., 2002; Leung et al., 2002; Sakai et al., 2002; Simon et al., 2002; Zald et al., 2002; Postle & D'Esposito, 2003; Brown et al., 2004; Curtis et al., 2004; Postle et al., 2004). Event-related fMRI studies that have isolated delay-period activity have provided consistent evidence that signals in the frontal eye fields (FEF), nearby posterior portions of superior frontal sulcus (area 8), and the intraparietal sulcus (IPS) persist throughout the entire delay period (Courtney et al., 1998; Zarahn et al., 1999; Postle, Berger et al., 2000; Rowe et al., 2000; Zarahn et al., 2000; Leung et al., 2002; Sakai et al., 2002; Brown et al., 2004; Curtis et al., 2004). For example, Curtis et al. (2004) scanned subjects while they performed oculomotor delayed-response tasks that required maintenance of the spatial position of a single dot of light over a delay period after which a memory-guided saccade was generated. Both the FEF and IPS time courses showed activity that spanned the entire delay period (figure 9.4). Importantly, we

a.

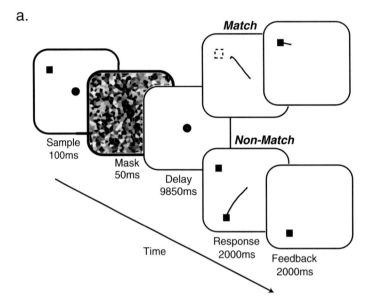

b.

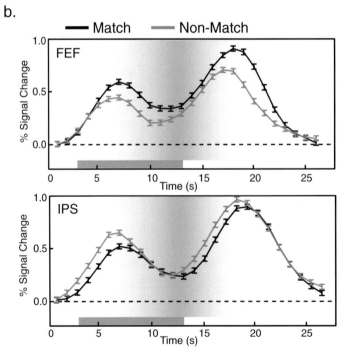

Figure 9.4 a, b

C.

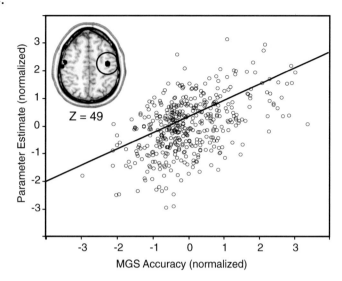

Figure 9.4

Event-related study of spatial working memory by Curtis et al. (2004). (*a*) Schematic depiction of the oculomotor delayed-response tasks where subjects used the cue's location to make a memory-guided saccade. Both the matching-to-sample (top) and non-matching-to-sample (bottom) tasks began with the brief presentation of a small square target. During matching trials, the subject made a memory-guided saccade (depicted by the thin black line) after the disappearance of the fixation cue marking the end of the delay. Feedback was provided by the re-presentation of the cue. At this point, the subject corrected any errors by shifting gaze to the cue. The difference between the end point fixation after the memory-guided saccade and the fixation to acquire the feedback cue was used as an index of memory accuracy. During non-matching trials, the subject made a saccade to the square that did not match the location of the sample cue. (*b*) Average (±S.E. bars) BOLD time series data for matching- (black) and non-matching-to-sample (gray) oculomotor delayed-response tasks. The solid gray bar represents the delay interval. The gray gradient in the background depicts the probability that the BOLD signal is emanating from the delay period, where darker gray indicates that it is more probable. The frontal eye fields (FEF) show greater delay period activity during the matching task where an oculomotor strategy is efficient. The right intraparietal sulcus (IPS) shows greater delay period activity during the non-matching task when subjects are biased from using such a strategy. (*c*) Scatter plot showing the correlation between memory-guided saccade (MGS) accuracy and the magnitude of the delay period parameter estimates in the right FEF. More accurate MGS was associated with greater delay-period activity.

were also able to demonstrate that the magnitude of FEF and IPS delay-period activity predicted the accuracy of the memory-guided saccade generated after the delay. This relationship suggests that the fidelity of the stored location is reflected in the delay-period activity. Therefore, both the FEF and the IPS may be involved in the storage of spatial information.

Findings from monkey (Bruce & Goldberg, 1985; Schlag & Schlag-Rey, 1987; Schall & Thompson, 1999; Andersen & Buneo, 2002) and human (Sweeney et al., 1996; Luna et al., 1998; Grosbras et al., 2001; Connolly et al., 2002; Cornelissen et al., 2002; Curtis & D'Esposito, 2003b; DeSouza et al., 2003) studies suggest that the FEF contains representations of saccadic intentions. The FEF contains an organized map of visual space defined in oculomotor coordinates (Bruce & Goldberg, 1985). Therefore, the activity in the FEF during spatial working memory tasks could reflect the activity of neurons that are responsible for moving the eyes to the remembered location, referred to as a *prospective motor code*. This type of coding of space could be used in memory tasks even when no eye movement is made because the saccade can be suppressed. Curtis et al. (2004) provide evidence for this type of motor coding of space by comparing two conditions in which subjects were biased toward or against the use of a prospective motor code. In one condition (match), subjects can plan a saccade to acquire the target as soon as it appears and can delay the initiation of the saccade until after the delay. Delay-period activity should reflect this strategy, the maintenance of a prospective motor code or motor intention. In a comparison condition, a saccade was made after the retention interval to an unpredictable location that did not match the location of the sample (nonmatch-to-sample). The subjects still had to remember the location of the sample so that they could discern between the matching and nonmatching targets. But because a saccade was never made to the sample location and the nonmatching location was unpredictable, we reasoned that this manipulation biased the subject away from maintaining a motor code during the delay. Instead, it encouraged the maintenance of a retrospective sensory code, or sustained spatial attention.

Delay-period activity was greater for the match compared with nonmatch conditions in the FEF, suggesting a plausible mechanism by which the FEF contributes to spatial working memory. The sustained activity in the FEF likely reflects the representation of the saccade vector to acquire the target location of the sample. Support for this interpretation comes from monkey (Bruce & Goldberg, 1985; Schlag and Schlag-Rey, 1987; Schall & Thompson, 1999; Andersen & Buneo, 2002) and human (Sweeney et al., 1996; Luna et al., 1998; Grosbras et al., 2001; Connolly et al., 2002; Cornelissen et al., 2002; Curtis & D'Esposito, 2003b; DeSouza et al., 2003; Brown et al., 2004) studies which suggest that the FEF contains representations of saccade intentions. Indeed, FEF contains an organized map of visual space defined in oculomotor coordinates (Bruce & Goldberg, 1985). Delay-period activity was greater for the nonmatch compared with match trials in the IPS, suggesting that when a motor intention cannot be maintained, another mechanism is enacted, such as maintenance of spatially directed covert attention. Activity in posterior parietal cortex has consistently been linked to the representation of space in electrophysiological studies of monkeys (Gnadt & Andersen, 1988; Constantinidis & Steinmetz, 1996; Gottlieb & Goldberg, 1999; Goldberg et al., 2002) and imaging studies of humans (Heide et al., 2001; Sereno et al., 2001; Merriam et al., 2003; Brown et al., 2004).

Again, activity in the FEF was greater during the delay period on trials when subjects knew the direction of the memory-guided saccade (match) compared with trials when subjects did not know the direction of the memory-guided saccade (nonmatch; see figure 9.4). Therefore, a plausible mechanism for spatial maintenance is the sustained activation of oculomotor neurons whose response field matches the location of the memory cue. Another possibility exists that must also be considered. The activation of the FEF neurons could be a form of spatial rehearsal, similar to the way that Broca's area is thought to support verbal rehearsal with subvocal motor articulations that refresh phonological representations stored in posterior parietal cortex. The FEF could refresh the spatial representations stored in posterior parietal cortex via subthreshold activation of FEF neurons coding for tagged portions of space. Importantly, humans with lesions in the FEF have impaired visually guided (Rivaud et al., 1994) and memory-guided saccades (Pierrot-Deseilligny et al., 1991).

Verbal Working Memory Maintenance

In no other area of working memory research has Baddeley's model (1986) been more influential than with the study of verbal working memory. This stems from the fact that the most formalized aspect of their model is the *phonological loop*, a subsystem of working memory that is proposed to maintain verbal information. The phonological loop is thought to operate via two mechanisms. First, a *phonological store* is thought to contain representations of speech sounds (phonemes) whose activations decay passively and rapidly over time. Second, an *articulatory rehearsal process* is thought to actively refresh the phonological representations that need to be maintained and is primarily a subvocal process that can be observed though introspection. Data from both PET and fMRI studies suggest that separate frontal and parietal regions may support these separate storage and rehearsal processes. Inferior posterior parietal cortex (areas 39 and 40) is thought to be the most important substrate for phonological storage of verbal information, while cortical areas that support the motor aspects of speech production (Broca's area 44, SMA, and cerebellum) are thought to be critical for articulatory rehearsal (Paulesu et al., 1993;

Petrides et al., 1993; Awh et al., 1996; Fiez et al., 1996; Schumacher et al., 1996; Smith et al., 1996; Braver et al., 1997; Desmond et al., 1997; Jonides et al., 1997; Jonides et al., 1998; Rypma et al., 1999; Nystrom et al., 2000; Chein & Fiez, 2001; Davachi et al., 2001; Barde & Thompson-Schill, 2002; Chein et al., 2002; Gruber & von Cramon, 2003; Walter et al., 2003; Crottaz-Herbette et al., 2004). Although the evidence linking the frontal premotor areas with articulatory rehearsal processes is particularly consistent, establishing that the inferior parietal cortex does indeed serve as a phonological storage area, consistent with Baddeley's model, continues to be debatable. Several studies have failed to find predicted activation in the left inferior posterior parietal cortex (Jonides et al., 1998; Becker et al., 1999; Chein & Fiez, 2001). Nonetheless, much of the data support such a relationship. Using an event-related design, Chein and Fiez (2001) reported that Broca's area and area 40 of the inferior parietal cortex showed a pattern of sustained activity during the delay period of a verbal working memory task (figure 9.5). This was a critical demonstration that was required if these regions are indeed involved in verbal storage during the memory delay.

The investigators also tested two other important predictions that are made by Baddeley's model, that states that the phonological loop is actually composed of distinct storage and rehearsal mechanisms. Performance on tests of verbal working memory is better for phonologically distinct words compared with performance when the words are phonologically similar (e.g., toy, boy, joy). The *word-similarity effect* is thought to stem from confusions in the storage of overlapping representations and is predicted to tax the phonological storage system. Performance on verbal working memory tasks is also worse when words that are longer, or have more syllables, are used. The *word-length effect* is thought to stem from the increased time it takes to subvocalize the words, allowing more time for passive decay of the stored representations. Thus, the word-length effect is predicted to tax articulatory rehearsal processes.

Chein and Fiez (2001) showed that the signal in Broca's area was greater during the delay period on trials in which subjects were maintaining 3-syllable words compared with 1-syllable words. The sustained activity in Broca's area was consistent with articulatory rehearsal because it showed a word-length effect. The left inferior parietal cortex (area 40) showed a word-similarity effect—activity was greater on trials when the words were phonologically related compared with when they were distinct. The increased signal for pseudo words (e.g., blick, rame, scote) is also consistent with a phonological storage role because increased demands are placed on phonological storage when semantic representations are absent (Jonides et al., 1998). Therefore, frontal premotor regions, especially Broca's area, and the inferior parietal cortex are the key substrates implicated in processes necessary for the maintenance of verbal material.

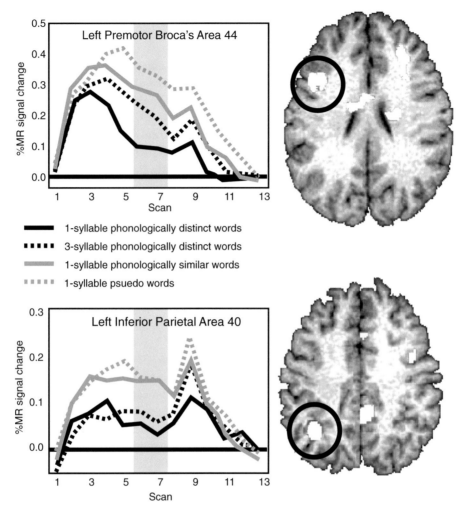

Figure 9.5
Main results from Chein and Fiez (2001) study of verbal working memory. The circled regions on the right depict Broca's and inferior parietal cortex. On the left are time series data from these regions. Both Broca's area and inferior parietal cortex show sustained activity during the maintenance of verbal material. Consistent with an important role in articulatory rehearsal processes, Broca's area showed a word-length effect—activity was greater during the delay period on trials in which subjects were maintaining three-syllable words compared with one-syllable words. The left inferior parietal cortex (area 40) showed a word-similarity effect—activity was greater on trials when the words were phonologically related compared with when they were distinct.

Object Working Memory Maintenance

A number of studies have accumulated that investigated the maintenance of objects, mostly visually presented faces, houses, and line drawings that are not easily verbalizable (Courtney et al., 1994; Haxby et al., 1994; Smith et al., 1995; Courtney et al., 1996; McCarthy et al., 1996; Courtney et al., 1997; Belger et al., 1998; Cullen et al., 1998; Postle & D'Esposito, 1999; Curtis, Zald, lee et al., 2000; Curtis, Zald et al., 2000; Haxby et al., 2000; Jha & McCarthy, 2000; Jiang et al., 2000; Mecklinger et al., 2000; Pollmann & von Cramon, 2000; Postle, Stern et al., 2000; Druzgal & D'Esposito, 2001; Rama et al., 2001; Mecklinger et al., 2002; Druzgal & D'Esposito, 2003; Linden et al., 2003; Postle et al., 2003; Sala et al., 2003). Consistently, posterior cortical areas along the inferior temporal lobe that normally respond to the visual presentation of select objects also tend to activate during object working memory tasks. Therefore, the temporal lobe appears to play an important role in short-term storage of object features. For example, the fusiform gyrus, the ventral convexity surface of the temporal lobe, activates to a greater extent when a subject is shown pictures of faces compared with other types of complex visual stimuli, such as pictures of houses or scenes or household objects (Kanwisher et al., 1997), and, given its somewhat selective response properties, has been termed the "fusiform face area" (FFA).

There are four important findings which indicate that posterior extrastriate cortical regions such as the FFA play an important role in the mnemonic storage of object features. First, the FFA shows persistent delay-period activity (Druzgal & D'Esposito, 2001; Rama et al., 2001; Druzgal & D'Esposito, 2003; Postle et al., 2003) during working memory tasks. Second, the activity in the FFA is somewhat selective for faces; it is greater during delays in which subjects are maintaining faces compared with other objects (Sala et al., 2003). Third, as the number of faces that are being maintained increases, the magnitude of the delay period activity increases in the FFA (Jha & McCarthy, 2000; Druzgal & D'Esposito, 2001, 2003). Such *load effects* strongly suggest a role in short-term storage because as the number of items that must be represented increases, so should the storage demands and the measured fMRI signals. Fourth, using a delayed paired associates task, Ranganath et al. (2004) has shown that the FFA responds during an unfilled delay interval following the presentation of a house that the subject has learned is associated with a certain face. Therefore, the delay period for FFA activity likely reflects the reactivated image of the associated face that was retrieved from long-term memory (figure 9.6) even though no face was actually presented before the delay. Together, these studies suggest that posterior regions of visual association cortex, such as the FFA, participate in the internal storage of specific classes of visual object features. Most likely, the mechanisms used to create internal representations of objects that are no longer

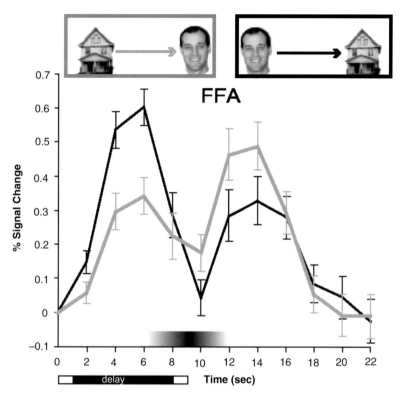

Figure 9.6
Human inferior temporal activity during visual associative memory retrieval and maintenance from Ranganath et al. (2004). In this event-related fMRI study, subjects were scanned while they were shown a face or a house that was previously learned in a face-house pair, and were asked to recall and maintain its associate across a delay period. Activity during the initial cue phase in the fusiform face area (FFA) was greater when the cue was a face compared with when it was a house. However, during the delay period, activity reflected the type of information that was active in memory, rather than the previously presented cue stimulus—that is, delay activity in the FFA was greater when a face was recalled in response to a house cue. Gray lines represent time series from FFA when a house was presented at cue and its face pair was tested at the probe phase. Black lines represent the face-house pairing order.

in the environment are similar to the mechanisms used to represent objects that exist in the external environment.

There have been several reports of delay period specific activations in the PFC during object working memory tasks as well (Smith et al., 1995; Courtney et al., 1996; McCarthy et al., 1996; Smith et al., 1996; Courtney et al., 1997; Manoach et al., 1997; Belger et al., 1998; Cohen et al., 1998; Courtney et al., 1998; Postle & D'Esposito, 1999; Jha & McCarthy, 2000; Nystrom et al., 2000; Postle, Stern et al., 2000; Stern et al., 2000; Rama et al., 2001; Munk et al., 2002; Pessoa et al., 2002; Druzgal & D'Esposito, 2003; Ranganath et al., 2003; Sala et al., 2003). However, the localization of the delay-period activity appears varied across the dorsal, ventral, and medial portions of the PFC. The most consistent finding in that regard may be a greater bias toward right hemisphere activation for object working memory compared with verbal working memory.

Issues

What Is the Meaning of Persistent Activity During Working Memory Delays?

Working memory allows animals to use information that is not currently present in the environment but is vital to adaptive behavior. Internal representations must be formed and sustained such that the cross-temporal contingencies can be established. Sustained neural activity during the delay period between a sensory cue, such as the position of a briefly flashed spot of light, and a later motor response, such as a shift of gaze to the remembered location, is compelling evidence that this activity is a memory representation (Fuster & Alexander, 1971; Kubota & Niki, 1971; Gnadt & Andersen, 1988; Funahashi et al., 1989). Over 30 years has elapsed since these initial observations, but the nature of these signals remains elusive. What is actually being represented in various brain regions during working memory delays? For example, during a memory delay, one may need to look back to a past perceptual event in order to maintain a *retrospective* sensory code, or may need to look forward to a future action to maintiain a *prospective* motor code, in order to link events that are separated in time but are contingent upon one another (Boussaoud & Wise, 1993; Funahashi et al., 1993; Quintana & Fuster, 1999; Rainer et al., 1999; D'Esposito, Balland et al., 2000; Curtis et al., 2004). It is likely that different brain regions represent different types of memory codes. As Fuster has written, ongoing behavior can be thought of as a stage of a chained perception-action cycle, and the brain represents information at many different levels. There are several different strategies that functional neuroimaging studies can use to attempt determine the code represented in different brain regions.

A good example of one strategy has already been discussed. The Curtis et al. study (2004) (see figure 9.4) experimentally manipulated factors that biased subjects toward or against the use of a prospective motor code. The nature of the persistent signals could be inferred from brain areas that were sensitive to this manipulation. That example demonstrates how one might begin to test hypotheses about the mechanisms that give rise to delay-period activity. Another method is to systematically manipulate factors that affect storage and evaluate whether or not delay activity is similarly affected. This idea has been explored through increasing the memory load by increasing the number of items to represent in memory, which should tax storage mechanisms. Several studies have manipulated load to test whether the persistent activity in the dorsolateral PFC that has been repeatedly noted reflects the storage of visually presented material. Three event-related fMRI studies that manipulated memory load have failed to find that the delay-period activity was affected by load (Rypma & D'Esposito, 1999; Jha & McCarthy, 2000; Postle, Berger et al., 2000).

For example, Jha and McCarthy (2000) reported that remembering 3 faces did not evoke greater delay-period activity in the DLPFC than remembering 1 face at any point during 15 or 24 sec memory delays. These findings, thus, are contrary to the view that the DLPFC simply maintains task-relevant representations. However, Leung, Gore, and Goldman-Rakic (Leung et al., 2002) demonstrated that the DLPFC does not sustain a significant level of activity throughout an 18 sec delay when maintaining 3 faces in memory, but does so if 5 faces are required to be remembered. Two recent studies from our laboratory have also detected significant effects of memory load on delay-period DLPFC activity during face (Druzgal & D'Esposito, 2003) and letter (Rypma et al., 2002) working memory tasks.

Although results are mixed, some studies find that DLPFC activity increases when the number of items to be maintained increases. This seems to support the conclusion that the DLPFC plays an important role in memory storage—since increasing the demands of storage should be expected to increase BOLD signal in a region where representations are being actively stored—but there are equally plausible explanations that need to be investigated. First, the DLPFC activity may reflect top-down biasing signals to more posterior regions where the representations are actually stored (E. K. Miller & Cohen, 2001; Curtis & D'Esposito, 2003a). Second, the large memory loads could be beyond the capacity of working memory and might invoke strategic changes in the way information is represented (Cowan, 2001). Rypma et al. (Rypma & D'Esposito, 1999; Rypma et al., 2002) have argued that the increased signal changes with increased load in the DLPFC are the consequence of the strategic process of data compression (e.g., chunking) because these effects are most prominent during the cue period when encoding takes place. Strategic organization of memoranda is a control process that is distinct from raw storage of representations.

Another method for determining the nature of the representations in different brain regions is to disrupt maintenance and look for dissociations of brain activity. For example, the level of activity in area 46 correlates with how resistant the memory representation is to performance degradation caused by distraction (Sakai et al., 2002). Subjects first encoded the order and spatial position of 5 cues, then before memory was tested, they performed a secondary spatial distraction task. In area 46, but not premotor area 6/8 or IPS, the level of persistent activity prior to the distraction correlated with memory performance after the distraction (figure 9.7). The increased level of activity may have reflected the amount of rehearsal or

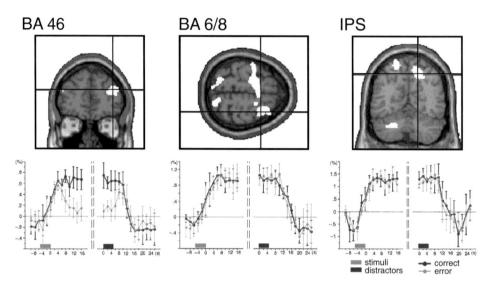

Figure 9.7
An event-related study by Sakai et al. (2002) had subjects first encode the order and spatial positions of five cues (gray bar). Subjects had to maintain this information for several seconds and then encountered a secondary spatial distraction task (black bar). Then memory performance was tested. On correct trials, when the subjects successfully maintained the stimuli, the activity in area 46 was greater, as can be seen by the average (±S.E. bars) BOLD time series data. In area 46, but not premotor area 6/8 or IPS, the level of persistent activity prior to the distraction correlated with memory performance after the distraction.

some other process that transformed the representations into a form that was less susceptible to distraction. Overall, the goal of future research in this area should focus on the meaning of persistent signals in the PFC, since these signals are key to understanding the implementation of working memory in the brain.

What Is the Functional Organization of the Lateral PFC?

While there is strong support for the view that lateral PFC is critical for working memory maintenance processes, it is unclear whether functional subdivisions within PFC exist. Goldman-Rakic and colleagues first put forth a proposal that different PFC regions are critical for active maintenance of different types of information. Based on monkey electrophysiological and lesion studies (Funahashi et al., 1989; Wilson et al., 1993), it was proposed that persistent activity within ventrolateral PFC reflects the temporary maintenance of nonspatial codes (such as an object's color and shape), whereas dorsolateral PFC activity reflects maintenance of spatial codes (such as the location of an object in space). This hypothesis had the appeal of parsimony, because a similar organization exists in the visual system, which is segregrated into "what" and "where" pathways (Ungerleider & Haxby, 1994). Also, anatomical studies in monkeys have demonstrated that parietal cortex (i.e., spatial vision regions) predominantly projects to a dorsal region of lateral PFC (Petrides & Pandya, 1984; Cavada & Goldman-Rakic, 1989), whereas temporal cortex (i.e., object vision regions) projects more ventrally within lateral PFC (Barbas, 1988).

Numerous functional neuroimaging studies of humans have attempted to test this hypothesis regarding PFC organization (for a review, see D'Esposito, Aguirre, Zarahn et al., 1998). For example, in a blocked design PET study of delayed-response tasks using faces and locations of faces as stimuli (Courtney et al., 1996), it was found that a direct comparison of the two memory conditions revealed that the spatial working memory task resulted in greater activation within left superior frontal sulcus (Brodmann's areas 8, 6) and the face working memory task resulted in greater activation in a more ventral right PFC region (areas 9, 45, 46). In a follow-up study using an event-related fMRI design (Courtney et al., 1998), a double dissociation was found between face and spatial working memory. It was observed that within the superior frontal sulcus in both hemispheres, there was significantly more sustained activity during spatial than during face working memory delay periods. By contrast, left inferior frontal gyrus showed significantly more sustained activity during face than during spatial working memory delay periods.

Another possible axis along which human lateral PFC may be organized is according to the type of operations performed upon information being actively maintained, rather than the type of information being maintained. For example, Petrides proposed that there are two processing systems, one dorsal and the other ventral, within lateral PFC (Petrides & Pandya, 1994). It was proposed that ventral PFC (Brodmann's areas 45, 47) is the site where information is initially received from posterior association areas and where active comparisons of maintained information are made. In contrast, dorsal PFC (areas 9, 46, 9/46) is recruited only when "monitoring" and "manipulation" of this information is required.

This model received initial support from an empirical PET study performed by Owen and colleagues (1996) in which dorsal PFC activation was found during three spatial working memory tasks thought to require greater monitoring of remembered information than two other memory tasks, which activated only ventral PFC. We also tested this model of process-specific PFC organization using event-related fMRI (D'Esposito et al., 1999). In our study, subjects were presented two types of trials in random order in which they were required either to (1) *maintain* a sequence of letters across a delay period or (2) *manipulate* (alphabetize) this sequence during the delay in order to respond correctly to a probe. In every subject, delay-period activity was found in both dorsal and ventral PFC in both types of trials. However, dorsal PFC activity was greater in trials during which actively maintained information was manipulated. These findings suggest that dorsal PFC may exhibit greater recruitment during conditions where additional processing of actively maintained information is required supporting a process-specific PFC organization.

On the surface, these two models of PFC organization seem incompatible, and to this day papers continue to be published pitting one against the other. However, a closer look at the empirical data from human functional imaging and monkey physiology studies since the mid-1990s leads to the conclusion that both models accurately describe PFC organization. Part of the reason for the persistence of the notion that these models are orthogonal to one another resulted from a lack in preciseness of the anatomical definitions of dorsal and ventral PFC that were being used. For example, as reviewed above, the principal evidence cited to support the "domain-specific" PFC organization (Goldman-Rakic & Leung, 2002) derives from studies by Courtney and colleagues, who found that the superior frontal sulcus (area 6/8) appears to be specific to spatial working memory, whereas regions within inferior frontal gyrus (areas 45, 47) appear to be specific to nonspatial information (e.g., faces). Unquestionably, the superior frontal sulcus is anatomically "dorsal" to the inferior frontal gyrus, Thus, on the surface these data provide strong support for a dorsal-what vs. ventral-where, domain-specific PFC organization.

However, other evidence from monkey physiological and human functional imaging studies seems inconsistent with the domain-specific hypothesis because it provides evidence that certain dorsal and ventral PFC regions do not appear specific to one domain of information. For example, several single-unit recording studies during delayed-response tasks have found a mixed population of neurons throughout dorsal and ventral regions of lateral PFC that are not clearly segregated by the type of information (i.e., spatial versus nonspatial) that is being stored (Rosenkilde et al., 1981; Fuster et al., 1982; Quintana et al., 1988; Rao et al., 1997). Also, cooling of PFC (Fuster & Bauer, 1974; Bauer & Fuster, 1976; Quintana & Fuster, 1993) and dorsal PFC lesions cause impairments on nonspatial working memory tasks (Mishkin et al., 1969; Petrides, 1995), and ventral PFC lesions cause spatial impairments (Mishkin et al., 1969; Iversen & Mishkin, 1970; Butters et al., 1973). Finally, another study found that ventral PFC lesions in monkeys did not cause delay-dependent defects on a visual pattern association task and a color matching task (Rushworth et al., 1997). Also, there are numerous human functional imaging studies that have failed to find different patterns of PFC activation during spatial vs. nonspatial working memory tasks (e.g., Owen et al., 1998; Postle et al., 1999; Nystrom et al., 2000).

How can we reconcile all of these findings? The answer emerges from a close examination of the particular PFC regions that do, or do not, exhibit persistent activity that is specific to a particular type of information. Thus, domain specificity may exist within the superior frontal sulcus (area 6/8) and portions of the inferior frontal gyrus (areas 44, 45, 47), but other lateral PFC regions, such as middle frontal gyrus (areas 9, 46, 9/46) may not show domain specificity. Thus, a coarse subdivision of PFC into dorsal and ventral regions fails to account for the possibility that both domain-specific and process-specific organization may exist. Thus, a hybrid model of PFC organization could accommodate the empirical findings (Postle & D'Esposito, 2000).

A problem with a hybrid model is that it is extremely difficult to capture, in cognitive or neural terms, the specific type of processes that are being attributed to the middle frontal gyrus (areas 9, 46, 9/46). Are the processes attributed to this region, such as "monitoring" and "manipulation," distinct from active maintenance processes? For example, one possibility is that "monitoring" and "manipulation" tasks recruit middle frontal gyrus because they require active maintenance of more abstract relations (e.g., semantic, temporal, etc.) between items (Wendelken, 2001). In this view, the PFC is not organized by different types of processing modules, but by the abstractness of the representations being actively maintained. This organization could be hierarchic, ranging from features of an object (e.g., red), to more abstract dimensions (e.g., color), to superordinate representations such as goals or task context (e.g., color-naming task). Recent evidence from functional neuroimaging studies has begun to provide support for this idea.

Considerable evidence exists that premotor cortex (BA 6) is involved in the selection of responses when guided by simple stimulus features (Schumacher & D'Esposito, 2002; Jiang & Kanwisher, 2003a, 2003b; Schumacher et al., 2003). For example, Schumacher and D'Esposito (2002) manipulated the difficulty of response selection based on two factors: the compatibility of a spatial location with a manual response and the ease with which a cue stimulus could be perceptually discriminated from surrounding distractor stimuli. In contrast to ventral PFC regions, which showed little sensitivity to either manipulation, and to the dorsal PFC, which was exclusively sensitive to compatibility, premotor cortex was additively sensitive to both spatial and visual manipulations of the cue features. Similarly, evidence from single-unit recordings of monkeys suggests that premotor cortex, and not dorsal PFC, encodes simple stimulus-response mappings (Weinrich et al., 1984; Wallis & Miller, 2003). In contrast to premotor cortex, several studies have shown that dorsal PFC encodes the abstract relationship between a stimulus and a response based on a contextual cue (Bunge et al., 2003; Wallis & Miller, 2003; Boettiger & D'Esposito, 2005).

And finally, frontopolar cortex (BA 10; FPC) has been implicated in relying on a high-level goal or task context in order to interpret a cue during selection of an action. Such processing is critical to the extent that a cue does not map directly to a response, but requires the subject to reflect on additional, remembered contextual information or goals to interpret the cue (Koechlin et al., 1999; Koechlin et al., 2003;

Sakai & Passingham, 2003). For example, Badre and Wagner (2004) observed greater FPC activation when a cue for the response was symbolic and arbitrary, in contrast to directly naming the response, and thus had to be verified with respect to the remembered trial context (in this case the serial order in which the appropriate response had been presented). Furthermore, this activation in FPC was evident even when simpler order-response selection demands were minimal, because the appropriate response had been prepared in advance.

A recent neuroimaging study has tested this model of hierarchical PFC organization within one set of experiments (Koechlin et al., 2003). In this fMRI study, the frequency of to-be-selected representations was manipulated in an effort to impact levels of PFC processing. Manipulation of the number of responses within a block primarily affected premotor cortex. Manipulation of the number of relevant stimulus dimensions within a block impacted dorsolateral PFC. Finally, manipulation of the across-block frequency of cue-to-response or cue-to-dimension mappings impacted FPC responses. Interestingly, structural equation modeling of the fMRI data revealed path coefficients from FPC to dorsal PFC to premotor cortex (but not in the opposite direction), broadly consistent with a hierarchic organization. An important contribution from this study is that it considers the entire frontal cortex, from premotor regions to the most anterior portion of prefrontal cortex (area 10), an area that has been relatively ignored in working memory research. This type of PFC organization is also consistent with data derived from a connectionist model that possessed both a concrete feature level and an abstract dimension level in its "PFC" and could produce the double dissociations reported in the monkey data (O'Reilly et al., 2002).

E. K. Miller and Cohen (2001) have presented a synthesis of empirical findings with a theoretical model regarding how basic maintenance processes subserved by the PFC can exert cognitive control. They propose that PFC delay activity is specific to those representations which are behaviorally relevant, enabling an animal or human to prospectively integrate across time when selecting an action. Automatic behaviors can be mediated by computations in posterior neocortices with little influence from internal goals maintained by the PFC. When "bottom-up" processes are insufficient for or in conflict with current goals, available cues may be insufficient to uniquely specify a response. Under such circumstances, the active maintenance of relevant behavioral representations permits the appropriate selection for action.

The PFC has extensive reciprocal connections with most of the brain and is situated at the apex of mnemonic, affective, perceptual, and motor pathways arising from posterior and subcortical processors. Thus, it is in a privileged position to store behaviorally relevant representations and exert cognitive control. Frontal cortex appears to be hierarchically organized, not simply in a dorsal/ventral fashion but in a posterior/anterior direction from premotor regions to frontopolar cortex (figure 9.8). Future research must continue to determine the regional distinctions that define functional topography of frontal cortex and the principles by which these regions interact to produce controlled behavior. A critical mass of human functional imaging studies, combined with monkey lesion and physiological studies of monkeys, have begun to call into question traditional distinctions in PFC organization. A newer framework suggests there is flexibility in functional boundaries and that function versus content theoretical accounts may fail to be mutually exclusive where boundaries exist (Badre & Wagner, 2004).

In summary, goal-directed behavior, which is both intentional and flexible, requires the active maintenance of a broad range of perceptual, mnemonic, and motor representations. For example, imagine hitting a golf ball. If your ball is in the woods, you may need to maintain the location of the flag in the distance as you keep your eye on the ball. As you prepare to hit your ball, you also have to maintain the rules of the game, since any movement of the ball as you address it may result in a penalty stroke. And finally, if you are playing poorly, it is important to maintain the original goal for taking up the game—to exercise and enjoy yourself.

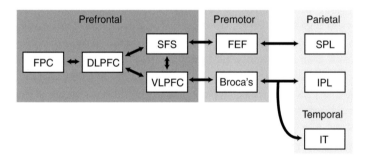

Figure 9.8
Simplified schematic depicting the hierarchical organization of key areas critical for working memory. The frontal cortex appears hierarchically organized, not simply in a dorsal/ventral fashion but in a posterior/anterior direction from premotor regions to anterior frontopolar cortex. Nonspatial, especially verbal, working memory depends on a network of ventral cortical regions including the ventrolateral PFC (VLPFC, areas 45 and 47), Broca's area (area 44), and posterior parietal and temporal cortex. This network maintains information by the activation of stored semantic representations and subvocal articulatory rehearsal processes. Similarly, spatial working memory depends on a network of dorsal cortical regions including the superior frontal sulcus (SFS, area 8), FEF (area 6), and the superior portions of parietal cortex (SPL, area 7). This network maintains positional information through the shifting and maintenance of spatial attention and motor intention. Anterior PFC regions such as the dorsolateral PFC (DLPFC, area 46) and frontopolar cortex (FPC, area 10) interact with both of these networks and appear to maintain more abstract representations, such as task goals and behaviorally relevant contexts.

How Does the PFC Interact with Other Brain Regions to Support Working Memory?

The first step in neuroimaging is necessarily one of localization of function, in which we often attempt to ascribe a particular cognitive function, such as a component of working memory, to a brain region. Nonetheless, neuroimaging scientists are at the same time well aware that the implementations of discrete cognitive functions are almost surely distributed across many nodes in a network. One of the next steps in a functional neuroimaging is likely to be attempts to characterize networks of cortical activity associated with cognition. Importantly, fMRI has the unique ability to simultaneously image multiple regions of the brain. Thus, it has the often-touted potential, just being realized, (McIntosh, 2000; Friston, 2002; Sun et al., 2004) to characterize interactions between the nodes in neural networks, such as the network that supports working memory.

For example, we described above how different cortical areas might maintain relatively different codes across a memory delay in an oculomotor spatial delayed-response task (Curtis et al., 2004). Recall that the frontal eye fields (FEF), for example, were more active during the delay when the direction of the memory-guided saccade was known compared with when it was not known throughout the delay. Other areas showed the opposite pattern. Despite these task-dependent differences in regional activity, we could assume, but not address, the functional interactions between the identified nodes of the putative network. Standard univariate analysis of fMRI data, in which each brain voxel is analyzed independently of all others, reveals no more than independent activity within these regions. In a follow-up study, we used a multivariate technique, coherence, to formally characterize functional interactions between the FEF and other brain areas (Curtis et al., 2005). Coherence is a statistic that is analogous to correlation, but is performed on the time-series data once it has been fast-Fourier-transformed into frequency space (Sun et al., 2004). Using coherence, we found that the type of representational codes being maintained in working memory biases frontal-parietal interactions and therefore influences network dynamics. For example, coherence between FEF and other oculomotor areas was greater when a motor representation was an efficient strategy to bridge the delay period. However, coherence between the FEF and higher-order multimodal areas (e.g., dorsolateral prefrontal cortex) was greater when a sensory representation must be maintained in working memory.

With similar goals, Gazzaley, Rissman, and D'Esposito (Gazzaley et al., 2004) utilized another type of multivariate analysis that allowed them to explore functional connectivity between brain regions during the distinct stages of a delayed face recognition task. They modeled the individual trial components of the task for every trial separately, not averaged across the whole trial as is usually done. In order to assess network interactions, they correlated the parameter estimates for every trial derived from the FFA with all other brain voxels. High correlations indicate that the trial-to-trial variability in the magnitude of the parameter estimates between two regions was high, suggesting functional connectivity. This analysis revealed a network of brain regions with significant correlations with the FFA during the retention interval. This maintenance network included the dorsolateral and ventrolateral PFC, premotor cortex, intraparietal sulcus, caudate nucleus, thalamus, hippocampus, and occipitotemporal regions.

Functional MRI is uniquely suited to measure network dynamics because it simultaneously records correlates of neural activity throughout the functioning brain with high spatial resolution. Together, the findings from these initial studies (Gazzaley et al., 2004; Curtis et al., 2005) support the notion that the coordinated functional interaction between nodes of a widely distributed network underlies the active maintenance of internal representations. Moreover, they may signal the beginning of a new generation of multivariate studies that use fMRI to characterize network dynamics.

Summary and Conclusions

Elucidation of the cognitive and neural architectures underlying human working memory has been an important focus of cognitive neuroscience for much of the period since the mid-1990s. One conclusion that arises from this research is that working memory, a faculty that enables temporary storage and manipulation of information in the service of behavioral goals, can be viewed as neither a unitary nor a dedicated system. Data from numerous imaging studies has been reviewed and has demonstrated that a network of brain regions, including the PFC, is critical for the active maintenance of internal representations. Moreover, it appears that the PFC has functional subdivisions that are organized by the abstractness of these representations (e.g., features, rules, goals). Finally, working memory function is not localized to a single brain region but likely is an emergent property of the functional interactions between the PFC and other posterior regions. Numerous questions remain regarding the neural basis of this complex cognitive system, but imaging studies such as those reviewed in this chapter should continue to provide converging evidence for such questions.

References

Andersen, R. A., & Buneo, C. A. (2002). Intentional maps in posterior parietal cortex. *Annual Review of Neuroscience* 25, 189–220.

Awh, E., Jonides, J., Smith, E. E., Buxton, R. B., Frank, L. R., Love, T., Wong, E. C., & Gmeindl, L. (1999). Rehearsal in spatial working memory: Evidence from neuroimaging. *Psychological Science* 10, 433–437.

Awh, E., Jonides, J., Smith, E. E., Schumacher, E. H., Koeppe, R. A., & Katz, S. (1996). Dissociation of storage and rehearsal in verbal working memory: Evidence from PET. *Psychological Science* 7, 25–31.

Baddeley, A. (1986). *Working Memory*. New York: Oxford University Press.

Badre, D., & Wagner, A. D. (2004). Selection, integration, and conflict monitoring: Assessing the nature and generality of prefrontal cognitive control mechanisms. *Neuron* 41, 473–487.

Barbas, H. (1988). Anatomic organization of basoventral and mediodorsal visual recipient prefrontal regions in the rhesus monkey. *Journal of Comparative Neurology* 276, 313–342.

Barde, L. H., & Thompson-Schill, S. L. (2002). Models of functional organization of the lateral prefrontal cortex in verbal working memory: Evidence in favor of the process model. *Journal of Cognitive Neuroscience* 14, 1054–1063.

Bauer, R. H., & Fuster, J. M. (1976). Delayed-matching and delayed-response deficit from cooling dorsolateral prefrontal cortex in monkeys. *Journal of Comparative and Physiological Psychology* 90, 293–302.

Becker, J. T., MacAndrew, D. K., & Fiez, J. A. (1999). A comment on the functional localization of the phonological storage subsystem of working memory. *Brain and Cognition* 41, 27–38.

Belger, A., Puce, A., Krystal, J. H., Gore, J. C., Goldman-Rakic, P., & McCarthy, G. (1998). Dissociation of mnemonic and perceptual processes during spatial and nonspatial working memory using fMRI. *Human Brain Mapping* 6, 14–32.

Boettiger, C. A., & D'Esposito, M. (2005). Frontal networks for learning and executing arbitrary stimulus-response associations. *Journal of Neuroscience* 25, 2723–2732.

Boussaoud, D., & Wise, S. P. (1993). Primate frontal cortex: Neuronal activity following attentional versus intentional cues. *Experimental Brain Research* 95, 15–27.

Boynton, G. M., Engel, S. A., Glover, G. H., & Heeger, D. J. (1996). Linear systems analysis of functional magnetic resonance imaging in human V1. *Journal of Neuroscience* 16, 4207–4221.

Braver, T. S., Cohen, J. D., Nystrom, L. E., Jonides, J., Smith, E. E., & Noll, D. C. (1997). A parametric study of prefrontal cortex involvement in human working memory. *NeuroImage* 5, 49–62.

Brodmann, K. (1909). *Vergleichende Lokalisationslehre der Grosshirnrinde.* Leipzig: Barth.

Brown, M. R., DeSouza, J. F., Goltz, H. C., Ford, K., Menon, R. S., Goodale, M. A., & Everling, S. (2004). Comparison of memory- and visually guided saccades using event-related fMRI. *Journal of Neurophysiology* 91, 873–889.

Bruce, C. J., & Goldberg, M. E. (1985). Primate frontal eye fields. I. Single neurons discharging before saccades. *Journal of Neurophysiology* 53, 603–635.

Bunge, S. A., Kahn, I., Wallis, J. D., Miller, E. K., & Wagner, A. D. (2003). Neural circuits subserving the retrieval and maintenance of abstract rules. *Journal of Neurophysiology* 90, 3419–3428.

Butters, N., Butter, C., Rosen, J., & Stein, D. (1973). Behavioral effects of sequential and one-stage ablations of orbital prefrontal cortex in monkey. *Experimental Neurology* 39, 204–214.

Cavada, C., & Goldman-Rakic, P. S. (1989). Posterior parietal cortex in rhesus monkey: II. Evidence for segregated corticocortical networks linking sensory and limbic areas with frontal lobe. *Journal of Comparative Neurology* 287, 422–445.

Chafee, M. V., & Goldman-Rakic, P. S. (1998). Matching patterns of activity in primate prefrontal area 8a and parietal area 7ip neurons during a spatial working memory task. *Journal of Neurophysiology* 79, 2919–2940.

Chein, J. M., & Fiez, J. A. (2001). Dissociation of verbal working memory system components using a delayed serial recall task. *Cerebral Cortex* 11, 1003–1014.

Chein, J. M., Fissell, K., Jacobs, S., & Fiez, J. A. (2002). Functional heterogeneity within Broca's area during verbal working memory. *Physiology & Behavior* 77, 635–639.

Cohen, J. D., Forman, S. D., Braver, T. S., Casey, B. J., Servan-Schreiber, D., & Noll, D. C. (1994). Activation of prefrontal cortex in a nonspatial working memory task with functional MRI. *Human Brain Mapping* 1, 293–304.

Cohen, J. D., Nystrom, L. E., Braver, T. S., Sabb, F. W., Delgado, M. R., & Noll, D. C. (1998). fMRI studies of the topographic organization of working memory representations in prefrontal cortex. *Cognitive Neuroscience Society Abstracts* 5, 87.

Connolly, J. D., Goodale, M. A., Menon, R. S., & Munoz, D. P. (2002). Human fMRI evidence for the neural correlates of preparatory set. *Nature Neuroscience* 5, 1345–1352.

Constantinidis, C., Franowicz, M. N., & Goldman-Rakic, P. S. (2001). The sensory nature of mnemonic representation in the primate prefrontal cortex. *Nature Neuroscience* 4, 311–316.

Constantinidis, C., & Steinmetz, M. A. (1996). Neuronal activity in posterior parietal area 7a during the delay periods of a spatial memory task. *Journal of Neurophysiology* 76, 1352.

Corbetta, M., Kincade, J. M., & Shulman, G. L. (2002). Neural systems for visual orienting and their relationships to spatial working memory. *Journal of Cognitive Neuroscience* 14, 508–523.

Cornelissen, F. W., Kimmig, H., Schira, M., Rutschmann, R. M., Maguire, R. P., Broerse, A., Den Boer, J. A., & Greenlee, M. W. (2002). Event-related fMRI responses in the human frontal eye fields in a randomized pro- and antisaccade task. *Experimental Brain Research* 145, 270–274.

Courtney, S. M., Petit, L., Maisog, J. M., Ungerleider, L. G., & Haxby, J. V. (1998). An area specialized for spatial working memory in human frontal cortex. *Science* 279, 1347–1351.

Courtney, S. M., Ungerleider, L. G., Keil, K., & Haxby, J. V. (1994). Dissociation and interaction of human neural systems for object and spatial working memory: A PET rCBF study. *Society for Neuroscience Abstracts* 20, 6.

Courtney, S. M., Ungerleider, L. G., Keil, K., & Haxby, J. V. (1996). Object and spatial visual working memory activate separate neural systems in human cortex. *Cerebral Cortex* 6, 39–49.

Courtney, S. M., Ungerleider, L. G., Keil, K., & Haxby, J. V. (1997). Transient and sustained activity in a distributed neural system for human working memory. *Nature* 386, 608–611.

Cowan, N. (2001). The magical number 4 in short-term memory: A reconsideration of mental storage capacity. *Behavioral and Brain Sciences* 24, 87–114.

Crottaz-Herbette, S., Anagnoson, R. T., & Menon, V. (2004). Modality effects in verbal working memory: Differential prefrontal and parietal responses to auditory and visual stimuli. *NeuroImage* 21, 340–351.

Cullen, C. M., Oster, M. N., Bucci, J., Snow, M., Miller, E. K., & Corkin, S. (1998). fMRI activation during performance of object and spatial components of a working memory task. *NeuroImage* 7, S876.

Curtis, C. E., & D'Esposito, M. (2003a). Persistent activity in the prefrontal cortex during working memory. *Trends in Cognitive Sciences* 7, 415–423.

Curtis, C. E., & D'Esposito, M. (2003b). Success and failure suppressing reflexive behavior. *Journal of Cognitive Neuroscience* 15, 409–418.

Curtis, C. E., & D'Esposito, M. (2004). The effects of prefrontal lesions on working memory performance and theory. *Cognitive, Affective, and Behavioral Neuroscience* 4, 528–539.

Curtis, C. E., Rao, V. Y., & D'Esposito, M. (2004). Maintenance of spatial and motor codes during oculomotor delayed response tasks. *Journal of Neuroscience* 24, 3944–3952.

Curtis, C. E., Sun, F. T., Miller, L. M., & D'Esposito, M. (2005). Coherence between fMRI time-series distinguishes two spatial working memory networks. *NeuroImage* 26, 177–183.

Curtis, C. E., Zald, D. H., Lee, J. T., & Pardo, J. V. (2000). Object and spatial alternation tasks with minimal delays activate the right anterior hippocampus proper in humans. *NeuroReport* 11, 2203–2207.

Curtis, C. E., Zald, D. H., & Pardo, J. V. (2000). Organization of working memory within the human prefrontal cortex: A PET study of self-ordered object working memory. *Neuropsychologia* 38, 1503–1510.

Davachi, L., Maril, A., & Wagner, A. D. (2001). When keeping in mind supports later bringing to mind: Neural markers of phonological rehearsal predict subsequent remembering. *Journal of Cognitive Neuroscience* 13, 1059–1070.

D'Esposito, M., Aguirre, G. K., Zarahn, E., Ballard, D., et al. (1998). Functional MRI studies of spatial and nonspatial working memory. *Cognitive Brain Research* 7, 1–13.

D'Esposito, M., Aguirre, G. K., Zarahn, E., Ballard, D., Shin, R. K., & Lease, J. (1998). Functional MRI studies of spatial and nonspatial working memory. *Cognitive Brain Research* 7, 1–13.

D'Esposito, M., Ballard, D., Zarahn, E., & Aguirre, G. K. (2000). The role of prefrontal cortex in sensory memory and motor preparation: An event-related fMRI study. *NeuroImage* 11, 400–408.

D'Esposito, M., & Postle, B. R. (1999). The dependence of span and delayed-response performance on prefrontal cortex. *Neuropsychologia* 37, 1303–1315.

D'Esposito, M., Postle, B. R., Ballard, D., & Lease, J. (1999). Maintenance and manipulation of information held in working memory: An event-related fMRI study. *Brain and Cognition* 41, 66–86.

D'Esposito, M., Postle, B. R., & Rypma, B. (2000). Prefrontal cortical contributions to working memory: Evidence from event-related fMRI studies. *Experimental Brain Research* 133, 3–11.

Desimone, R., & Duncan, J. (1995). Neural mechanisms of selective visual attention. *Annual Review of Neuroscience* 18, 193–222.

Desmond, J. E., Gabrieli, J. D., Wagner, A. D., Ginier, B. L., & Glover, G. H. (1997). Lobular patterns of cerebellar activation in verbal working-memory and finger-tapping tasks as revealed by functional MRI. *Journal of Neuroscience* 17, 9675–9685.

DeSouza, J. F., Menon, R. S., & Everling, S. (2003). Preparatory set associated with pro-saccades and anti-saccades in humans investigated with event-related fMRI. *Journal of Neurophysiology* 89, 1016–1023.

Druzgal, T. J., & D'Esposito, M. (2001). Activity in fusiform face area modulated as a function of working memory load. *Cognitive Brain Research* 10, 355–364.

Druzgal, T. J., & D'Esposito, M. (2003). Dissecting contributions of prefrontal cortex and fusiform face area to face working memory. *Journal of Cognitive Neuroscience* 15, 771–784.

Fiez, J. A., Raife, E. A., Balota, D. A., Schwarz, J. P., Raichle, M. E., & Petersen, S. E. (1996). A positron emission tomography study of the short-term maintenance of verbal information. *Journal of Neuroscience* 16, 808–822.

Friston, K. (2002). Beyond phrenology: What can neuroimaging tell us about distributed circuitry? *Annual Review of Neuroscience* 25, 221–250.

Funahashi, S., Bruce, C. J., & Goldman-Rakic, P. S. (1989). Mnemonic coding of visual space in the monkey's dorsolateral prefrontal cortex. *Journal of Neurophysiology* 61, 331–349.

Funahashi, S., Bruce, C. J., & Goldman-Rakic, P. S. (1993). Dorsolateral prefrontal lesions and oculomotor delayed-response performance: Evidence for mnemonic "scotomas." *Journal of Neuroscience* 13, 1479–1497.

Fuster, J. (1997). *The Prefrontal Cortex: Anatomy, Physiology, and Neuropsychology of the Frontal Lobes*, 3rd ed. New York: Raven Press.

Fuster, J. M. (2001). The prefrontal cortex—an update: Time is of the essence. *Neuron* 30, 319–333.

Fuster, J. M., & Alexander, G. E. (1971). Neuron activity related to short-term memory. *Science* 173, 652–654.

Fuster, J. M., & Bauer, R. H. (1974). Visual short-term memory deficit from hypothermia of frontal cortex. *Brain Research* 81, 393–400.

Fuster, J. M., Bauer, R. H., & Jervey, J. P. (1982). Cellular discharge in the dorsolateral prefrontal cortex of the monkey in cognitive tasks. *Experimental Neurology* 77, 679–694.

Gazzaley, A., Rissman, J., & D'Esposito, M. (2004). Functional connectivity during working memory maintenance. *Cognitive, Affective, and Behavioral Neuroscience* 4, 580–599.

Glahn, D. C., Kim, J., Cohen, M. S., Poutanen, V. P., Therman, S., Bava, S., Van Erp, T. G., Manninen, M., Huttunen, M., Lonnqvist, J., Standertskjold-Nordenstam, C. G., & Cannon, T. D. (2002). Maintenance and manipulation in spatial working memory: Dissociations in the prefrontal cortex. *NeuroImage* 17, 201–213.

Gnadt, J. W., & Andersen, R. A. (1988). Memory related motor planning activity in posterior parietal cortex of macaque. *Experimental Brain Research* 70, 216–220.

Goldberg, M. E., Bisley, J., Powell, K. D., Gottlieb, J., & Kusunoki, M. (2002). The role of the lateral intraparietal area of the monkey in the generation of saccades and visuospatial attention. *Annals of the New York Academy of Sciences* 956, 205–215.

Goldberg, T. E., Berman, K. F., Randolph, C., Gold, J. M., & Weinberger, D. R. (1996). Isolating the mnemonic component in spatial delayed response: A controlled PET ^{15}O-labeled water regional cerebral blood flow study in normal humans. *NeuroImage* 3, 69–78.

Goldman-Rakic, P. S. (1987). Circuitry of the prefrontal cortex and the regulation of behavior by representational memory. In: F. Plum & V. Mountcastle (Eds.), *Handbook of Physiology, sec. 1, The Nervous System, vol. 5, Higher Functions of the Brain*, 373–417. Bethesda, MD: American Physiological Society.

Goldman-Rakic, P. S. (1996a). Regional and cellular fractionation of working memory. *Proceedings of the National Academy of Sciences USA* 93, 13473–13480.

Goldman-Rakic, P. S. (1996b). The prefrontal landscape: Implications of functional architecture for understanding human mentation and the central executive. *Philosophical Transactions of the Royal Society of London* B351, 1445–1453.

Goldman-Rakic, P. S., & Leung, H.-C. (2002). Functional architecture of the dorsolateral prefrontal cortex in monkeys and humans. In R. T. Knight (Ed.), *Principles of Frontal Lobe Function* New York: Oxford University Press.

Gottlieb, J., & Goldberg, M. E. (1999). Activity of neurons in the lateral intraparietal area of the monkey during an antisaccade task. *Nature Neuroscience* 2, 906–912.

Grosbras, M. H., Leonards, U., Lobel, E., Poline, J. B., LeBihan, D., & Berthoz, A. (2001). Human cortical networks for new and familiar sequences of saccades. *Cerebral Cortex* 11, 936–945.

Gruber, O., & von Cramon, D. Y. (2003). The functional neuroanatomy of human working memory revisited: Evidence from 3-T fMRI studies using classical domain-specific interference tasks. *NeuroImage* 19, 797–809.

Haxby, J. V., Horwitz, B., Ungerleider, L. G., Maisog, J. M., et al. (1994). The functional organization of human extrastriate cortex: A PET-rCBF study. *Journal of Neuroscience* 14, 6336–6353.

Haxby, J. V., Petit, L., Ungerleider, L. G., & Courtney, S. M. (2000). Distinguishing the functional roles of multiple regions in distributed neural systems for visual working memory. *NeuroImage* 11, 145–156.

Heide, W., Binkofski, F., Seitz, R. J., Posse, S., Nitschke, M. F., Freund, H. J., & Kompf, D. (2001). Activation of frontoparietal cortices during memorized triple-step sequences of saccadic eye movements: An fMRI study. *European Journal of Neuroscience* 13, 1177–1189.

Iversen, S. D., & Mishkin, M. (1970). Perseverative interference in monkeys following selective lesions of the inferior prefrontal convexity. *Experimental Brain Research* 11, 376–386.

Jacobsen, C. F. (1936). The functions of the frontal association areas in monkeys. *Comparative Psychology Monographs* 13, 1–60.

Jha, A. P., & McCarthy, G. (2000). The influence of memory load upon delay-interval activity in a working-memory task: An event-related functional MRI study. *Journal of Cognitive Neuroscience* 12(Supp. 2), 90–105.

Jiang, Y., Haxby, J. V., Martin, A., Ungerleider, L. G., & Parasuraman, R. (2000). Complementary neural mechanisms for tracking items in human working memory. *Science* 287, 643–646.

Jiang, Y., & Kanwisher, N. (2003a). Common neural mechanisms for response selection and perceptual processing. *Journal of Cognitive Neuroscience* 15, 1095–1110.

Jiang, Y., & Kanwisher, N. (2003b). Common neural substrates for response selection across modalities and mapping paradigms. *Journal of Cognitive Neuroscience* 15, 1080–1094.

Jonides, J., Schumacher, E. H., Smith, E. E., Koeppe, R. A., Awh, E., Reuter-Lorenz, P. A., Marshuetz, C., & Willis, C. R. (1998). The role of parietal cortex in verbal working memory. *Journal of Neuroscience* 18, 5026–5034.

Jonides, J., Schumacher, E. H., Smith, E. E., Lauber, E., Awh, E., Minoshima, S., & Koeppe, R. A. (1997). Verbal working memory load affects regional brain activation as measured by PET. *Journal of Cognitive Neuroscience* 9, 462–475.

Jonides, J., Smith, E. E., Koeppe, R. A., Awh, E., Minoshima, S., & Mintun, M. A. (1993). Spatial working memory in humans as revealed by PET. *Nature* 363, 623–625.

Kanwisher, N., McDermott, J., & Chun, M. M. (1997). The fusiform face area: A module in huma extrastriate cortex specialized for face perception. *Journal of Neuroscience* 17, 4302–4311.

Kastner, S., & Ungerleider, L. G. (2001). The neural basis of biased competition in human visual cortex. *Neuropsychologia* 39, 1263–1276.

Koechlin, E., Basso, G., Pietrini, P., Panzer, S., & Grafman, J. (1999). The role of the anterior prefrontal cortex in human cognition. *Nature* 399, 148–151.

Koechlin, E., Ody, C., & Kouneiher, F. (2003). The architecture of cognitive control in the human prefrontal cortex. *Science* 302, 1181–1185.

Kubota, K., & Niki, H. (1971). Prefrontal cortical unit activity and delayed alternation performance in monkeys. *Journal of Neurophysiology* 34, 337–347.

Leung, H. C., Gore, J. C., & Goldman-Rakic, P. S. (2002). Sustained mnemonic response in the human middle frontal gyrus during on-line storage of spatial memoranda. *Journal of Cognitive Neuroscience* 14, 659–671.

Linden, D. E., Bittner, R. A., Muckli, L., Waltz, J. A., Kriegeskorte, N., Goebel, R., Singer, W., & Munk, M. H. (2003). Cortical capacity constraints for visual working memory: Dissociation of fMRI load effects in a fronto-parietal network. *NeuroImage* 20, 1518–1530.

Luna, B., Thulborn, K. R., Strojwas, M. H., McCurtain, B. J., Berman, R. A., Genovese, C. R., & Sweeney, J. A. (1998). Dorsal cortical regions subserving visually guided saccades in humans: An fMRI study. *Cerebral Cortex* 8, 40–47.

Manoach, D. S., Schlaug, G., Siewert, B., Darby, D. G., Bly, B. M., Benfield, A., Edelman, R. R., & Warach, S. (1997). Prefrontal cortex fMRI signal changes are correlated with working memory load. *NeuroReport* 8, 545–549.

McCarthy, G., Blamire, A. M., Puce, A., Nobre, A. C., Bloch, G., Hyder, F., Goldman-Rakic, P., & Shulman, R. G. (1994). Functional magnetic resonance imaging of human prefrontal cortex activation during a spatial working memory task. *Proceedings of the National Academy of Sciences USA* 91, 8690–8694.

McCarthy, G., Puce, A., Constable, R. T., Krystal, J. H., Gore, J. C., & Goldman-Rakic, P. (1996). Activation of human prefrontal cortex during spatial and nonspatial working memory tasks measured by functional MRI. *Cerebral Cortex* 6, 600–611.

McIntosh, A. R. (2000). Towards a network theory of cognition. *Neural Networks* 13, 861–870.

Mecklinger, A., Bosch, V., Gruenewald, C., Bentin, S., & von Cramon, D. Y. (2000). What have Klingon letters and faces in common? An fMRI study on content-specific working memory systems. *Human Brain Mapping* 11, 146–161.

Mecklinger, A., Gruenewald, C., Besson, M., Magnie, M. N., & von Cramon, D. Y. (2002). Separable neuronal circuitries for manipulable and non-manipulable objects in working memory. *Cerebral Cortex* 12, 1115–1123.

Merriam, E. P., Genovese, C. R., & Colby, C. L. (2003). Spatial updating in human parietal cortex. *Neuron* 39, 361–373.

Miller, E. K. (2000). The prefrontal cortex and cognitive control. *Nature Reviews Neuroscience* 1, 59–65.

Miller, E. K., & Cohen, J. D. (2001). An integrative theory of prefrontal cortex function. *Annual Review of Neuroscience* 24, 167–202.

Miller, M. H., & Orbach, J. (1972). Retention of spatial alternation following frontal lobe resections in stump-tailed macaques. *Neuropsychologia* 10, 291–298.

Milner, A. D., & Goodale, M. A. (1995). *The Visual Brain in Action.* New York: Oxford University Press.

Mishkin, M., Vest, B., Waxler, M., & Rosvold, H. E. (1969). A re-examination of the effects of frontal lesions on object alternation. *Neuropsychologia* 7, 357–363.

Miyake, A., & Shah, P. (Eds.) (1999). *Models of Working Memory.* New York: Cambridge University Press.

Munk, M. H., Linden, D. E., Muckli, L., Lanfermann, H., Zanella, F. E., Singer, W., & Goebel, R. (2002). Distributed cortical systems in visual short-term memory revealed by event-related functional magnetic resonance imaging. *Cerebral Cortex* 12, 866–876.

Nystrom, L. E., Braver, T. S., Sabb, F. W., Delgado, M. R., Noll, D. C., & Cohen, J. D. (2000). Working memory for letters, shapes, and locations: fMRI evidence against stimulus-based regional organization in human prefrontal cortex. *NeuroImage* 11, 424–446.

O'Reilly, R. C., Noelle, D. C., Braver, T. S., & Cohen, J. D. (2002). Prefrontal cortex and dynamic categorization tasks: Representational organization and neuromodulatory control. *Cerebral Cortex* 12, 246–257.

Owen, A. M., Evans, A. C., & Petrides, M. (1996). Evidence for a two-stage model of spatial working memory processing within the lateral frontal cortex: A positron emission tomography study. *Cerebral Cortex* 6, 31–38.

Owen, A. M., Stern, C. E., Look, R. B., Tracey, I., Rosen, B. R., & Petrides, M. (1998). Functional organization of spatial and nonspatial working memory processing within the human lateral frontal cortex. *Proceedings of the National Academy of Sciences USA* 95, 7721–7726.

Passingham, R. (1993). *The Frontal Lobes and Voluntary Action.* New York: Oxford University Press.

Paulesu, E., Frith, C. D., & Frackowiak, R. S. J. (1993). The neural correlates of the verbal component of working memory. *Nature* 362, 342–345.

Pessoa, L., Gutierrez, E., Bandettini, P., & Ungerleider, L. (2002). Neural correlates of visual working memory: fMRI amplitude predicts task performance. *Neuron* 35, 975–987.

Petersen, S. E., Fox, P. T., Posner, M. I., Mintun, M. I., & Raichle, M. E. (1988). Positron emission tomographic studies of the cortical anatomy of single-word processing. *Nature* 331, 585–589.

Petit, L., Courtney, S. M., Ungerleider, L. G., & Haxby, J. V. (1998). Sustained activity in the medial wall during working memory delays. *Journal of Neuroscience* 18, 9429–9437.

Petrides, M. (1995). Impairments on nonspatial self-ordered and externally ordered working memory tasks after lesions of the mid-dorsal lateral part of the lateral frontal cortex of monkey. *Journal of Neuroscience* 15, 359–375.

Petrides, M. (2000a). Dissociable roles of mid-dorsolateral prefrontal and anterior inferotemporal cortex in visual working memory. *Journal of Neuroscience* 20, 7496–7503.

Petrides, M. (2000b). The role of the mid-dorsolateral prefrontal cortex in working memory. *Experimental Brain Research* 133, 44–54.

Petrides, M., Alivisatos, B., Meyer, E., & Evans, A. C. (1993). Functional activation of the human frontal cortex during the performance of verbal working memory tasks. *Proceedings of the National Academy of Sciences USA* 90, 878–882.

Petrides, M., & Pandya, D. N. (1984). Projections to the frontal cortex from the posterior parietal region in the rhesus monkey. *Journal of Comparative Neurology* 228, 105–116.

Petrides, M., & Pandya, D. N. (1994). Comparative architectonic analysis of the human and macaque frontal cortex. In J. Grafman (Ed.), *Handbook of Neuropsychology*, 17–58. Amsterdam: Elsevier.

Pierrot-Deseilligny, C., Rivaud, S., Gaymard, B., & Agid, Y. (1991). Cortical control of memory-guided saccades in man. *Experimental Brain Research* 83, 607–617.

Pochon, J. B., Levy, R., Poline, J. B., Crozier, S., Lehericy, S., Pillon, B., Deweer, B., Le Bihan, D., & Dubois, B. (2001). The role of dorsolateral prefrontal cortex in the preparation of forthcoming actions: An fMRI study. *Cerebral Cortex* 11, 260–266.

Pollmann, S., & von Cramon, D. Y. (2000). Object working memory and visuospatial processing: Functional neuroanatomy analyzed by event-related fMRI. *Experimental Brain Research* 133, 12–22.

Posner, M. I., Petersen, S. E., Fox, P. T., & Raichle, M. E. (1988). Localization of cognitive operations in the human brain. *Science* 240, 1627–1631.

Postle, B. R., Awh, E., Jonides, J., Smith, E. E., & D'Esposito, M. (2004). The where and how of attention-based rehearsal in spatial working memory. *Cognitive Brain Research* 20, 194–205.

Postle, B. R., Berger, J. S., & D'Esposito, M. (1999). Functional neuroanatomical double dissociation of mnemonic and executive control processes contributing to working memory performance. *Proceedings of the National Academy of Sciences USA* 96, 12959–12964.

Postle, B. R., Berger, J. S., Taich, A. M., & D'Esposito, M. (2000). Activity in human frontal cortex associated with spatial working memory and saccadic behavior. *Journal of Cognitive Neuroscience* 12(supp. 2), 2–14.

Postle, B. R., & D'Esposito, M. (1999). "What"-Then-"Where" in visual working memory: An event-related fMRI study. *Journal of Cognitive Neuroscience* 11, 585–597.

Postle, B. R., & D'Esposito, M. (2000). Evaluating models of the topographical organization of working memory function in frontal cortex with event-related fMRI. *Psychobiology* 28, 132–145.

Postle, B. R., & D'Esposito, M. (2003). Spatial working memory activity of the caudate nucleus is sensitive to frame of reference. *Cognitive, Affective, and Behavioral Neuroscience* 3, 133–144.

Postle, B. R., Druzgal, T. J., & D'Esposito, M. (2003). Seeking the neural substrates of visual working memory storage. *Cortex* 39, 927–946.

Postle, B. R., Stern, C. E., Rosen, B. R., & Corkin, S. (2000). An fMRI investigation of cortical contributions to spatial and nonspatial visual working memory. *NeuroImage* 11, 409–423.

Postle, B. R., Zarahn, E., & D'Esposito, M. (2000). Using event-related fMRI to assess delay-period activity during performance of spatial and nonspatial working memory tasks. *Brain Research Brain Research Protocol* 5, 57–66.

Quintana, J., & Fuster, J. M. (1993). Spatial and temporal factors in the role of prefrontal and parietal cortex in visuomotor integration. *Cerebral Cortex* 3, 122–132.

Quintana, J., & Fuster, J. M. (1999). From perception to action: Temporal integrative functions of prefrontal and parietal neurons. *Cerebral Cortex* 9, 213–221.

Quintana, J., Yajeya, J., & Fuster, J. (1988). Prefrontal representation of stimulus attributes during delay tasks. I. Unit activity in cross-temporal integration of motor and sensory-motor information. *Brain Research* 474, 211–221.

Rainer, G., Rao, S. C., & Miller, E. K. (1999). Prospective coding for objects in the primate prefrontal cortex. *Journal of Neuroscience* 19, 5493–5505.

Rama, P., Sala, J. B., Gillen, J. S., Pekar, J. J., & Courtney, S. M. (2001). Dissociation of the neural systems for working memory maintenance of verbal and nonspatial visual information. *Cognitive, Affective, and Behavioral Neuroscience* 1, 161–171.

Ranganath, C., Cohen, M. X., Dam, C., & D'Esposito, M. (2004). Inferior temporal, prefrontal, and hippocampal contributions to visual working memory maintenance and associative memory retrieval. *Journal of Neuroscience* 24, 3917–3925.

Ranganath, C., Johnson, M. K., & D'Esposito, M. (2003). Prefrontal activity associated with working memory and episodic long-term memory. *Neuropsychologia* 41, 378–389.

Rao, S. C., Rainer, G., & Miller, E. K. (1997). Integration of what and where in the primate prefrontal cortex. *Science* 276, 821–824.

Rivaud, S., Muri, R. M., Gaymard, B., Vermersch, A. I., & Pierrot-Deseilligny, C. (1994). Eye movement disorders after frontal eye field lesions in humans. *Experimental Brain Research* 102, 110–120.

Rosen, B. R., Buckner, R. L., & Dale, A. M. (1998). Event-related functional MRI: Past, present, and future. *Proceedings of the National Academy of Sciences USA* 95, 773–780.

Rosenkilde, C. E., Bauer, R. H., & Fuster, J. M. (1981). Single cell activity in ventral prefrontal cortex of behaving monkeys. *Brain Research* 209, 375–394.

Rowe, J. B., & Passingham, R. E. (2001). Working memory for location and time: Activity in prefrontal area 46 relates to selection rather than maintenance in memory. *NeuroImage* 14, 77–86.

Rowe, J. B., Toni, I., Josephs, O., Frackowiak, R. S., & Passingham, R. E. (2000). The prefrontal cortex: Response selection or maintenance within working memory? *Science* 288, 1656–1660.

Rushworth, M. F. S., Nixon, P. D., Eacott, M. J., & Passingham, R. E. (1997). Ventral prefrontal cortex is not essential for working memory. *Journal of Neuroscience* 17, 4829–4838.

Rypma, B., Berger, J. S., & D'Esposito, M. (2002). The influence of working-memory demand and subject performance on prefrontal cortical activity. *Journal of Cognitive Neuroscience* 14, 721–731.

Rypma, B., & D'Esposito, M. (1999). The roles of prefrontal brain regions in components of working memory: Effects of memory load and individual differences. *Proceedings of the National Academy of Sciences USA* 96, 6558–6563.

Rypma, B., Prabhakaran, V., Desmond, J. E., Glover, G. H., & Gabrieli, J. D. E. (1999). Load-dependent roles of frontal brain regions in the maintenance of working memory. *NeuroImage* 9, 216–226.

Sakai, K., & Passingham, R. E. (2003). Prefrontal interactions reflect future task operations. *Nature Neuroscience* 6, 75–81.

Sakai, K., Rowe, J. B., & Passingham, R. E. (2002). Active maintenance in prefrontal area 46 creates distractor-resistant memory. *Nature Neuroscience* 5, 479–484.

Sala, J. B., Rama, P., & Courtney, S. M. (2003). Functional topography of a distributed neural system for spatial and nonspatial information maintenance in working memory. *Neuropsychologia* 41, 341–356.

Salmon, E., Van der Linden, M., Collette, F., Delfiore, G., Maquet, P., Degueldre, C., Luxen, A., & Franck, G. (1996). Regional brain activity during working memory tasks. *Brain* 119, 1617–1625.

Sarter, M., Bernston, G., & Cacioppo, J. (1996). Brain imaging and cognitive neuroscience: Toward strong inference in attributing function to structure. *American Psychologist* 51, 13–21.

Schall, J. D., & Thompson, K. G. (1999). Neural selection and control of visually guided eye movements. *Annual Review of Neuroscience* 22, 241–259.

Schlag, J., & Schlag-Rey, M. (1987). Evidence for a supplementary eye field. *Journal of Neurophysiology* 57, 179–200.

Schumacher, E. H., & D'Esposito, M. (2002). Neural implementation of response selection in humans as revealed by localized effects of stimulus-response compatibility on brain activation. *Human Brain Mapping* 17, 193–201.

Schumacher, E. H., Elston, P. A., & D'Esposito, M. (2003). Neural evidence for representation-specific response selection. *Journal of Cognitive Neuroscience* 15, 1111–1121.

Schumacher, E. H., Lauber, E., Awh, E., Jonides, J., Smith, E. E., & Koeppe, R. A. (1996). PET evidence for an amodal verbal working memory system. *NeuroImage* 3, 79–88.

Sereno, M. I., Pitzalis, S., & Martinez, A. (2001). Mapping of contralateral space in retinotopic coordinates by a parietal cortical area in humans. *Science* 294, 1350–1354.

Shallice, T., & Burgess, P. (1996). The domain of supervisory processes and temporal organization of behaviour. *Philosophical Transactions of the Royal Society of London* B351, 1405–1411 (discussion 1411–1412).

Simon, S. R., Meunier, M., Piettre, L., Berardi, A. M., Segebarth, C. M., & Boussaoud, D. (2002). Spatial attention and memory versus motor preparation: Premotor cortex involvement as revealed by fMRI. *Journal of Neurophysiology* 88, 2047–2057.

Smith, E. E., & Jonides, J. (1999). Storage and executive processes in the frontal lobes. *Science* 283, 1657–1661.

Smith, E. E., Jonides, J., & Koeppe, R. A. (1996). Dissociating verbal and spatial working memory using PET. *Cerebral Cortex* 6, 11–20.

Smith, E. E., Jonides, J., Koeppe, R. A., Awh, E., Schumacher, E. H., & Minoshima, S. (1995). Spatial versus object working memory: PET investigations. *Journal of Cognitive Neuroscience* 7, 337–356.

Stern, C. E., Owen, A. M., Tracey, I., Look, R. B., Rosen, B. R., & Petrides, M. (2000). Activity in ventro-lateral and mid-dorsolateral prefrontal cortex during nonspatial visual working memory processing: Evidence from functional magnetic resonance imaging. *NeuroImage* 11, 392–399.

Sternberg, S. (1969). The discovery of processing stages: Extensions of Donders' method. *Acta Psychologica* 30, 276–315.

Sun, F. T., Miller, L. M., & D'Esposito, M. (2004). Measuring interregional functional connectivity using coherence and partial coherence analyses of fMRI data. *NeuroImage* 21, 647–658.

Sweeney, J. A., Mintun, M. A., Kwee, S., Wiseman, M. B., Brown, D. L., Rosenberg, D. R., & Carl, J. R. (1996). Positron emission tomography study of voluntary saccadic eye movements and spatial working memory. *Journal of Neurophysiology* 75, 454–468.

Ungerleider, L. G., & Haxby, J. V. (1994). "What" and "where" in the human brain. *Current Opinion in Neurobiology* 4, 157–165.

Ungerleider, L. G., & Mishkin, M. (1982). Two cortical visual systems. In D. J. Ingle, M. A. Goodale, & R. J. W. Mansfield (Eds.), *Analysis of Visual Behavior*, 549–586. Cambridge, MA: MIT Press.

Vazquez, A. L., & Noll, D. C. (1998). Nonlinear aspects of the BOLD response in functional MRI. *NeuroImage* 7, 108–118.

Wallis, J. D., & Miller, E. K. (2003). From rule to response: Neuronal processes in the premotor and prefrontal cortex. *Journal of Neurophysiology* 90, 1790–1806.

Walter, H., Bretschneider, V., Gron, G., Zurowski, B., Wunderlich, A. P., Tomczak, R., & Spitzer, M. (2003). Evidence for quantitative domain dominance for verbal and spatial working memory in frontal and parietal cortex. *Cortex* 39, 897–911.

Weinrich, M., Wise, S. P., & Mauritz, K. H. (1984). A neurophysiological study of the premotor cortex in the rhesus monkey. *Brain* 107(2), 385–414.

Wendelken, C. (2001). The role of mid-dorsolateral prefrontal cortex in working memory: A connectionist model. *Neurocomputing* 44–46, 1009–1016.

Wilson, F. A. W., O'Scalaidhe, S. P., & Goldman-Rakic, P. S. (1993). Dissociation of object and spatial processing domains in primate prefrontal cortex. *Science* 260, 1955–1958.

Wood, J. N., & Grafman, J. (2003). Human prefrontal cortex: Processing and representational perspectives. *Nature Reviews Neuroscience* 4, 139–147.

Zald, D. H., Curtis, C. E., Folley, B. S., & Pardo, J. V. (2002). Prefrontal contributions to delayed spatial and object alternation: A positron emission tomography study. *Neuropsychology* 16, 182–189.

Zarahn, E., Aguirre, G. K., & D'Esposito, M. (1996). Delay-specific activity within prefrontal cortex demonstrated during a working memory task: A functional MRI study. *Society Neuroscience Abstracts* 22, 968.

Zarahn, E., Aguirre, G. K., & D'Esposito, M. (1997). A trial-based experimental design for functional MRI. *NeuroImage* 6, 122–138.

Zarahn, E., Aguirre, G. K., & D'Esposito, M. (1999). Temporal isolation of the neural correlates of spatial mnemonic processing with functional MRI. *Cognitive Brain Research* 7, 255–268.

Zarahn, E., Aguirre, G., & D'Esposito, M. (2000). Replication and further studies of neural mechanisms of spatial mnemonic processing in humans. *Cognitive Brain Research* 9, 1–17.

10

Functional Neuroimaging of Executive Functions

Todd S. Braver and Hannes Ruge

Introduction

For humans, the most prized of all our mental faculties is likely our capability for directing our thoughts and actions in accordance with internal goals, and for flexibly readjusting these goals when necessary. The term "executive function" is typically used to describe these regulatory and goal-directed components of cognition. However, the term itself, with its implicit reference to a hidden homunculus, indicates the difficulty of understanding how such executive functions might arise in the brain. Thus, a fundamental challenge for cognitive neuroscience is to determine the underlying representations, computations, and neural specializations that enable cognition and action to appear coordinated, purposeful, and self-regulatory. Cognitive neuroscience investigations of executive functions have accelerated in an amazingly rapid fashion within the last decade, due in large part to the development of sophisticated neuroimaging methods for noninvasively monitoring human brain activity. Indeed, a striking example of this accelerating growth is the observation that studies of executive processes are currently one of the largest components of the cognitive neuroimaging literature, yet in the previous edition of this book (published in 2001) there was no chapter devoted to executive function as a distinct area.

Although neuroimaging contributions to executive control research have only been very recent, there has been a long tradition of study in this area within neuropsychology, behavioral neuroscience, and cognitive science. Neuropsychological research has focused attention on the critical role of the frontal lobes in self-regulatory behavior, starting from the earliest case studies of individuals such as Phineas Gage (e.g., Harlow, 1848; Macmillan, 2000), to the more focused and systematic reports of Luria (1966). Starting with the seminal work of Milner (1963), experimental neuropsychology investigations have been instrumental in developing task paradigms that provide sensitive and objective probes for assessing executive function and its relationship to underlying brain areas. For example, studies with the Wisconsin Card Sort Task (WCST) indicated that frontal patients were more likely than other brain-damaged groups to show "perseverative" type behavior, staying with an old card-sorting rule even after repeated feedback that the rule was no longer correct. In addition, the experimental neuropsychology literature has contributed a number of other tasks for studying executive functions developed in the context of work with brain-damaged populations. These include tests of verbal fluency, planning (the Tower of London), attention switching (Trail Making), inhibition (go-no go), and sustained/selective attention (continuous performance test).

In parallel with the human neuropsychological research, behavioral neuroscience studies have provided strong confirmation and elaboration of the importance of the prefrontal cortex (PFC) in executive control. Early studies demonstrated fairly convincingly that frontal lesions markedly increased distractability in delayed-response tasks (which require holding a reward-eliciting behavior in check for a short period of time following presentation of an environmental cue) by impairing the ability to maintain goal-relevant information or context in mind even when such information is no longer perceptually available (e.g., Jacobsen, 1935). Later electro-physiological studies in awake behaving monkeys showed that during such delayed-response tasks, prefrontal neurons showed stimulus-specific increases in activity that were sustained throughout the delay interval and correlated with correct performance (Fuster, 1989; Goldman-Rakic, 1987). These studies have been of critical importance for establishing the role of PFC in active maintenance functions, and in specifying the representational and dynamic properties of this brain region. More recent work has emphasized how these properties of PFC might subserve cognitive control functions by representing rule-like information, enabling the learning of temporal associations between stimuli and response, filtering perceptual information in accordance with task goals, and exerting a top-down bias on action and perceptual systems (E. K. Miller & Cohen, 2001).

These types of neuropsychological and neurophysiological findings influenced the development of general theoretical models of cognition, starting with early work on planning (G. A. Miller et al., 1960) and progressing to more recent computational cognitive architectures (Anderson, 1983; Meyer & Kieras, 1997; Newell, 1990). In these models, a central role was given to a working memory structure where goal-related representations could be temporarily activated to bias sequences of thought and action. Ideas regarding the top-down biasing effects of goal information on action selection were more firmly crystallized in the supervisory attentional system (SAS) theory of Norman and Shallice (1986), which specified a control mechanism selectively invoked when automatic stimulus-response sequences are inappropriate or inadequate for completing actions in a goal-compatible fashion.

The SAS theory explicitly suggested that this control structure was located in the frontal lobes, and further specified the types of tasks situations most dependent upon frontal integrity: (a) when the task requires that a habitual response be suppressed; (b) when the task is novel and unpracticed; (c) when the task is dangerous or technically difficult; (d) when planning is required; and (e) when errors need to be monitored or corrected. Consequently, the SAS model has been very influential in guiding modern cognitive neuroscience investigations regarding the decomposition of different executive functions, as described below. Similarly, the SAS account has influenced more neuroscience-based theoretical models of control. For example, the models of Cohen and colleagues show how active maintenance of goal-like representations can occur in PFC via local recurrent connectivity, and how simple feedback connections allow these PFC representations to serve as a top-down bias on local competitive interactions within direct task pathways, thus achieving a simple form of control in cognitive tasks such as the Stroop (Cohen et al., 1996; Cohen et al., 1990).

Notions of executive function have also strongly influenced more domain-specific cognitive theories, in particular theories of memory. The classic information-processing theory of Atkinson and Shiffrin (1971) suggested that control processes play a significant role in how information gets into and out of the short-term and long-term stores, via modulation of encoding, rehearsal, decision, and retrieval strategies. This basic idea has been elaborated in more recent theories postulating that PFC may serve as this control interface, "working with memory" by strategically filtering retrieved content (Moscovitch, 1992; Shimamura, 1995, 2000).

Baddeley, in his influential model of working memory (WM), reinterpreted the Atkinson and Shiffrin view of short-term memory by suggesting that (a) short-term storage occurs in qualitatively distinct buffers for verbal (the phonological loop) and visuospatial (the visuospatial scratch pad) information, and (b) that these buffers serve as a "mental blackboard" for complex cognition (Baddeley, 1986). Critically, the Baddeley model cast a specific role for a "central executive" that appropriately utilized the stored information in the service of task-related processing. Baddeley's structurally based account provided a strong impetus for cognitive neuroscience-based research programs aimed at dissociating storage and control functions within WM in terms of their underlying neural substrates (D'Esposito et al., 1998; Smith & Jonides, 1999).

Nevertheless, a limitation of the Baddeley model, repeatedly acknowledged by Baddeley himself, is that the theory did not clearly specify what constituted an executive function within WM. Thus, it has not been clear whether the central executive referred to a single, monolithic mechanism or to a collection of distinct subprocesses subserved by multiple separate mechanisms. This major gap in theorizing regarding executive control has begun to be remedied (Baddeley, 1996). However, there is still no consensus as to exactly what are the functions that should be termed "executive," and how many distinct functions there are (Miyake et al., 2000).

The lack of conceptual clarity regarding the components of executive control is especially noticeable when surveying the large and ever-growing neuroimaging literature in this domain. Thus, there is some ambiguity as to how to structure a review of the literature in a chapter such as this one. In the following section, we have decided to organize the literature into categories according to what seem to be natural groupings of studies and tasks, rather than arguing for strict conceptual divisions.

Functional Neuroimaging Studies of Executive Functions

Given the vastness of the literature, it is beyond the scope of this chapter to provide an exhaustive review of all neuroimaging studies of executive function. Rather, in this section we hope to provide a road map or overview of the existing literature, pointing out the emerging trends and themes in different subareas, and thus provide a starting point for further study. Likewise, because of the very nature of executive functions, neuroimaging studies in this domain have a strong overlap with many others, especially WM, episodic memory, attention, and emotion. Since these other domains are the focus of different chapters, we will restrict our coverage to studies that are explicitly targeted toward examining the interaction of executive control with domain-specific processes. Finally, given the focus in the literature on the frontal lobes as the critical neural substrate of executive control, we will pay special attention to PFC-relevant findings. However, it should go without saying that a full understanding of executive function will likely involve a network of multiple interacting brain systems, of which the PFC is just one component.

Below, we review seven distinct categories of executive function that have been examined in the neuroimaging literature. These categories are summarized in table 10.1, which provides an organizing structure regarding the nomenclature we have adopted for each category and the associated task paradigms discussed.

Strategic Control of Memory

As mentioned above, much of the attention given to executive functions in cognitive psychology and neuroscience has emerged from the memory literature. Thus, many of the earliest neuroimaging studies focusing on executive control functions and PFC occurred in the context of examining WM and episodic memory tasks. Moreover,

Table 10.1
Executive functions and associated tasks

Category	Tasks Reviewed
Strategic control of memory	source memory, prospective memory, recency memory, tip-of-the-tongue (TOT), divided-attention encoding, manipulation and updating in WM, "recent negative" Sternberg, n-back (+lures)
Stimulus-response interference	Stroop, Eriksen, Simon
Response inhibition	go nogo, stop signal, antisaccade
Underdetermined responding	verb generation, random number generation, manual "free selection" tasks
Performance monitoring	WCST, error-processing tasks, reward/penalty feedback tasks
Task management	task switching, dual-task coordination, psychological refractory period (PRP)
Higher cognition	Tower of London (ToL), Raven's Progressive Matrices (RPM), logical reasoning tasks, integration tasks

in recent years there has been a growing appreciation of the notion that many putative WM or episodic memory tasks actually more strongly tap into executive processes (for review, see Fletcher & Henson, 2001). Thus, in the n-back, a now standard WM task in the neuroimaging literature, the activation of lateral PFC regions is thought by many investigators to reflect executive operations on stored information rather than active maintenance processes per se (Smith & Jonides, 1999; Veltman et al., 2003). Likewise, the activation of anterior PFC regions (BA 10) that is so commonly observed in episodic retrieval tasks, is now thought to reflect control operations acting to structure how retrieval occurs, via engagement of a sustained retrieval mode (Duzel et al., 2001; Lepage et al., 2000; Velanova et al., 2003) or through transient activation of postretrieval monitoring and decision processes (Ranganath et al., 2000).

Neuroimaging studies of memory have also broadened considerably, and now a significant subset of these studies are explicitly focused on elucidating the role of control processes within different memory domains. In particular, there are now neuroimaging studies focused on memory tasks that are thought to predominantly tap into the strategic control of mnemonic processes, such as recency memory (determining which of two items was more recently encountered), source memory (determining the specific context, such as where or when an item was encountered), and prospective memory (retrieving previously encoded action goals at a specific time or when a specific event occurs).

These studies have confirmed the basic assumption that PFC is engaged to subserve such strategic processes, but have also provided more detailed information. For example, source memory tasks appear to engage anterior PFC regions, suggesting a specific role for a retrieval mode or postretrieval processes establishing recollection (e.g., Dobbins et al., 2003). Similar observations have been made regarding prospective memory (Burgess et al., 2003). In contrast, recency memory may involve only dorsolateral PFC regions, particularly within the right hemisphere (Dobbins et al., 2003; Konishi et al., 2002). Another interesting study examined executive control in semantic memory, focusing on the so-called tip-of-the-tongue (TOT) phenomenon, when facts that are familiar and known cannot be appropriately retrieved. In this study (Maril et al., 2001), TOT events were associated with a distinct pattern of brain activity, involving activation within dorsolateral PFC and anterior cingulate cortex (ACC), that was interpreted as a sign of the cognitive conflict elicited in such situations, and the need to resolve it (see "Stimulus-Response Interference" and "Performance Monitoring," below).

Other memory studies have focused on how changes in the encoding context influence the demands on control processes. For example, dividing attention during intentional encoding (typically by adding a secondary task requirement) reduces the activity within lateral PFC regions, and also impairs memory performance (Iidaka et al., 2000; Kensinger et al., 2003). This suggests that PFC control processes are an important component of how encoding occurs. For verbal stimuli, PFC-mediated control may be especially critical for enabling elaborative phonological and semantic processing, which have a strong impact on encoding and later memory. This idea has been suggested by findings in which item-level activity in lateral PFC (particularly in the left hemisphere) during encoding tasks involving elaborative phonological or semantic processing is correlated with later memory performance (Wagner et al., 1998). Interestingly, these left frontal regions may be involved not only in controlling how each item is encoded but also in instantiating and updating the relevant task or instructional context when needed (see "Task Management," below).

In a study by Reynolds et al. (2004) testing this hypothesis, trial-by-trial switching of encoding contexts (i.e., two different semantic classification tasks) led to increased activity in left lateral PFC, but this activity appeared to reduce the activation available to support elaborative item-level processes that are associated with successful encoding. Thus, a consensus appears to be emerging that left lateral PFC, particularly in inferior regions, is critical for enabling controlled access to task-relevant phonological and semantic representations of verbal stimuli, especially in situations where such task-relevant representations are not automatically evoked by the stimulus (Fletcher et al., 2000; Thompson-Schill et al., 1997; Wagner et al., 2001). Moreover, there has been quite a bit of research consistent with the idea that left inferior PFC is subdivided into posterior and anterior portions that are selectively involved in controlling access to phonological and semantic representations, respectively (e.g., Poldrack et al., 1999).

Within the domain of WM, much attention has been directed toward the role of executive processes in "manipulating" actively maintained information in accordance with task demands. Thus, in studies conducted by D'Esposito and colleagues, verbal WM conditions involving manipulation (e.g., alphabetic reordering of verbal materials) appear to engage dorsolateral PFC regions more than tasks involving simple maintenance (e.g., Postle et al., 1999). Similar results have been observed in studies examining manipulation in spatial WM (e.g., vertical flipping of stored spatial locations; Glahn et al., 2002). However, it has been notoriously difficult to demonstrate this dissociation in an unambiguous fashion, especially when considering confounds such as task difficulty (e.g., Veltman et al., 2003). This may be partly due to the problems of defining exactly what constitutes manipulation, in mechanistic terms, and of determining whether generic manipulation processes exist (rather than having special-purpose mechanisms devoted to different types of manipulation).

A similar issue examined in the literature is whether WM updating—deactivating previously stored information to enable new information to gain access to storage—represents a unique executive process specialized brain region (Collette & Van der Linden, 2002). One way this issue has been investigated is through a focus on the dynamics of brain activity, since active maintenance processes are likely to be sustained throughout the storage interval, while updating processes should be engaged only transiently. A study of the n-back task supported this dissociation, with dorsolateral PFC regions showing sustained activity and WM load-sensitive activity, while inferior PFC regions showed transient activity (Cohen et al., 1997). Similarly, a study comparing the n-back task and the WCST task found that these same inferior PFC regions were also transiently engaged in the WCST when the card-sorting rule had to be updated (Konishi et al., 1999).

Other work has suggested that the inferior PFC activity may not reflect updating per se, but a more generic inhibitory process operating on WM contents. A task paradigm that has been gaining rapid popularity for investigating this issue is the "recent negative" variant of the Sternberg item recognition task (e.g., Jonides et al., 1998). In this task, recognition probes on some trials are "recent negatives," which indicate an item that was not part of the memory set maintained in WM for the current trial, but was part of the memory set from the previous trial. On "recent negative" trials, successful responding requires both a strong WM trace of the current trial memory set and inhibition of the misleading familiarity cues evoked by the probe. In a series of neuroimaging studies of with the "recent negative" Sternberg task, Jonides and colleagues observed that "recent negative" trials were selectively associated with activation in the left inferior PFC region associated with updating in the n-back task (Brodmann's area 45), with activation occurring following probe onset (Jonides et al., 2002). This result seems to suggest that "recent negative" probes elicit transient inhibitory (or interference resolution; see

"Stimulus-Response Interference," below) processes to allow WM content to compete more effectively with probe-evoked (but misleading) familiarity traces. However, a study by Bunge et al. (2001) found that "recent negative" effects were associated with increased activity in the same (wider set of) brain regions showing sensitivity to WM load. This finding suggests a more complex interpretation of the relationship between WM maintenance and probe-related interference.

More recent studies of the n-back task may also support the notion that interference resolution is an important component of task performance. In a study by Gray et al. (2003), analyses focused on "lure" trials, in which the item was a nontarget because it was not an n-back repeat, but was a repetition of a recently presented item (e.g., a 2-back repeat in a 3-back task). These items were assumed to require the same types of inhibitory or interference resolution processes as "recent negative" trials in the Sternberg task. It was found that transient activation on lure trials in the same lateral inferior PFC regions (among others) was selectively associated with performance on these trials—and, moreover, with individual differences in fluid intelligence. Thus, high-ability individuals may be more likely to be able to resolve lure-trial interference by transiently engaging specific PFC mechanisms that combat this interference.

Stimulus-Response Interference

A second category of neuroimaging studies on executive functions derives from the cognitive literature on attention control. In particular, a major focus of this literature is on the mechanisms of selective attention: keeping attention focused on task-relevant stimulus-and-response information in the face of irrelevant and distracting stimulus-and-response features. Neuroimaging methods provide a means of determining what neural mechanisms are critical for selective attention control, and in particular how instances of stimulus-response interference can be resolved when encountered. The paradigmatic example of stimulus-response interference in a selective attention task is the Stroop task, probably the most familiar and well-used task in all of experimental psychology. Thus it is not surprising that since the mid-1990s, the Stroop task has also become one of the most frequently studied neuroimaging tasks, with over 100 papers published at the time of writing this chapter. Many of these studies have used the Stroop task to probe brain function changes in different populations (e.g., schizophrenics; Carter et al., 1997).

However, the critical issue regarding the Stroop task that captures the interest of cognitive neuroscientists studying executive function is what neural control processes become engaged to suppress interference arising from incongruent word-name information. This question has been examined in numerous ways, across various neuroimaging studies, by (1) comparing incongruent trials or task blocks against *neutral* trial or block controls (e.g., Banich et al., 2000); (2) comparing incongruent trials or blocks against congruent trial or block controls (e.g., Carter et al., 2000); (3) manipulating the frequency of different trial types (e.g., congruent vs. incongruent; Leung et al., 2000); (4) comparing different forms of incongruent stimuli (e.g., those which directly conflict with the response vs. those which conflict only at a semantic level; Milham et al., 2003); (5) comparing different types of relevant and irrelevant stimulus dimensions (e.g., COLOR-word, PICTURE-word; Milham et al., 2001) or response modalities (e.g., verbal vs. manual; Barch et al., 2001); and (6) by comparing the effects of practice (e.g., Bush et al., 1998).

In general, across all of these studies a few common themes have emerged. First, the lateral PFC and anterior cingulate cortex are reliably more active under conditions involving high interference relative than conditions involving low interference. Further, the activity level in lateral PFC has been found to be positively associated with successful performance (e.g., MacDonald et al., 2000). However, many other brain regions have also been implicated, such as the posterior parietal cortex and extrastriate cortex (Carter et al., 1995; Pardo et al., 1990). These types of findings have led to the development of further questions, regarding the various subprocesses associated with interference suppression. For example, an important issue in the attention literature revolves around the distinction between the source of attention control and the site at which attention control modulates ongoing processing. It has been postulated by some authors that the lateral PFC serves as the source of Stroop attentional control, whereas extrastriate cortical regions serve as the site of attentional modulation (Carter et al., 1995). Yet a further question remains as to whether the processes occurring at the site of attentional modulation reflect attention-based enhancement of the task-relevant dimension or attention-based suppression of the irrelevant dimension.

A study by Banich et al. (2000) investigated this issue by altering, in various conditions, either the information contained in the task-relevant dimension (color, location) or the information contained in the irrelevant dimension (word, picture). They observed that holding the relevant dimension constant while manipulating the irrelevant dimension led to modulations of activity within parietal and extrastriate cortex. Conversely, manipulating the relevant dimension while holding the irrelevant one constant modulated activity within the lateral PFC and precuneus. This result seems to suggests that the PFC and precuneus form a network involved in attention-based enhancement, whereas the parietal and extrastriate cortex may form a network for attention-based inhibition. Further studies will be needed to determine more conclusively whether these regions form functionally connected networks, with one serving as the source and the other the site of attentional modulation (e.g., by focusing on the temporal dynamics of activity, as in Corbetta et al., 2000).

The Stroop task is not the only paradigm used to examine stimulus-response interference. In fact, many task situations have "Strooplike" characteristics arising from a form of stimulus-response interference. Relevant examples include the Eriksen flanker and Simon tasks. Moreover, theoretical analyses have suggested that these tasks and others can be taxonomized according to how such interference arises (Kornblum et al., 1990). In the Simon paradigm, interference arises when the irrelevant spatial location of an object conflicts with the response required for the object, if the response also has a spatial component to it (e.g., making a left-hand response to the shape of an object located in the right side of a display). In the Eriksen task, interference arises when irrelevant flanking stimuli conflict on some dimension with the features of a task-relevant central stimulus. The similarities and differences among these paradigms have captured the interest of neuroimaging researchers studying attention control. Thus, a number of imaging studies have begun to focus on other Strooplike tasks, such as the Eriksen and Simon tasks—and, moreover, have begun to compare brain activation patterns across tasks, to better understand their underlying commonalities and differences (e.g., Peterson et al., 2002). In terms of commonalities across tasks, a generally reliable finding in this literature is that interference conditions are associated with increases in lateral PFC activity, along with other related brain areas such as the ACC.

One interesting examination of cross-task differences has been in examining different types of interference present within the Flanker task. In particular, in this task, interference between flanking stimuli and the response (stimulus-response or S-R interference) can be dissociated from interference between the central and flanking stimuli (stimulus-stimulus, or S-S interference, which occurs when the two stimuli differ but are both associated with the same response). A study by Van Veen et al. (2001) directly examined brain activity across these two types of interference, and found that only S-R interference was associated with ACC activity, even though both types affected behavioral performance. In contrast, left inferior PFC showed increased activity to both types of interference (though activity was greater for S-R). No region showed selective activation to S-S interference. Other studies have confirmed the selective engagement of ACC in S-R interference in both the Stroop (e.g., Milham et al., 2001) and "recent negative" Sternberg tasks (Nelson et al., 2003). Such results are consistent with a general action-monitoring function ascribed to the ACC in various theories (Ridderinkhof et al., 2004). (See "Performance Monitoring," below).

Response Inhibition

A third category of executive function examined in neuroimaging studies is that of response inhibition. A common observation in the clinical and neuropsychological literatures is that many types of disorders appear to involve impairments in the ability to withhold strong response tendencies that are contextually or socially inappropriate. Thus, individuals exhibiting a "disinhibition" syndrome (frequently due to traumatic brain injury) often cannot stop themselves from making inappropriate social actions (e.g., making offensive comments in conversation). Likewise, disorders such as ADHD seem to be associated with a strong tendency to act impulsively or without normal restraints on behavior. Classically, neuropsychologists have studied failures of inhibition via well-known tasks such as Luria's tapping task or the go-no go paradigm. These and other tasks from the experimental literature have also been examined in neuroimaging studies. In these studies, the central question of interest is, What neural processes become engaged when inappropriate actions must be suppressed, and how are these inhibitory processes affected by various task factors?

The go-nogo has become a favorite tool for investigating these questions in neuroimaging studies, because the stimuli and responses can be very simple and frequently repeated. The basic paradigm involves a class of stimuli to which the participant is to respond as quickly as possible (go), and another class that, when presented, requires a withholding of the response (nogo). With the advent of event-related imaging techniques it is very simple to analyze brain activation on go and nogo trials separately, and to examine activation differences between successful and unsuccessful inhibition. Across a number of studies the most common theme reported is that the pattern of brain activity associated with inhibition (e.g., nogo > go trials) is right-hemisphere-dominant with distinct foci within prefrontal and parietal cortex, along with additional reliable activity in the ACC (e.g., Garavan et al., 1999; Konishi, Nakajima, Uchida, Sekihara et al., 1998). However, this typical pattern does not seem to be absolute; many studies have observed a bilateral pattern of activity, at least in dorsolateral and inferior PFC regions (e.g., Durston et al., 2002; Menon et al., 2001).

A secondary issue that has been frequently examined is how activity in these regions is affected by manipulations of the relative frequency of go vs. nogo trials. Interestingly, activation in nogo-sensitive PFC and ACC regions was greatest under conditions when nogo frequency was the lowest (Braver et al., 2001), or following a sequence of go trials (e.g., Durston et al., 2003). Under these conditions, inhibitory processes might be thought to be the most challenged, since inhibitory events are rare, and thus potentially surprising. Some investigators have argued from these results that response frequency is the primary factor driving nogo activity rather than inhibition per se, whereas others have shown that even when frequency is controlled, the same brain regions are active. For example, Braver et al. (2001) found that the ACC, right dorsolateral PFC, and right inferior PFC were equally active for both low-frequency nogo trials and low-frequency go trials. Yet Liddle et al. (2001) kept go and nogo trials at equal frequency but found these same regions were more strongly activated on nogo trials. A potential resolution of the issue may involve whether and how participants prioritize go and nogo responses (i.e., which category is more salient or more strongly in the focus of attention). Future studies will need to investigate this question more directly.

A related paradigm for studying response inhibition is the stop-signal task (Logan, 1994). An attractive feature of this task is that it provides a method for estimating the time required to stop a response, as well as a means of manipulating the tendency for inhibitory failure, through the timing of when the stop signal occurs. Thus, under these conditions it has been examined whether activity in any brain region adequately predicts inhibitory success or failure (Garavan et al., 2002; Rubia et al., 2003). Rubia et al. found that right inferior PFC was significantly more active on successful stop-signal trials, further suggesting that this region plays a central role in the inhibition process. A similar result was observed in a study by Hester et al. (2004) in a go/nogo task which also showed that lateral PFC regions increased activity when a preceding cue predicted future inhibitory demands. Finally, a focused neuropsychological investigation found that right inferior PFC damage was selectively associated with inhibitory deficits in the stop-signal task, with the extent of tissue damage correlated with the magnitude of inhibitory deficit (Aron et al., 2003).

A final class of inhibitory task that has been widely used is the anti-saccade (Guitton et al., 1985). This task differs from the other two in that it typically involves a distinct response modality (eye movements instead of hand movements). The key requirement of the task is that following the onset of a briefly presented peripheral cue, the subject must make a saccade to a location 180 degrees opposite from the cue. Such a saccade strongly conflicts with the innate and prepotent tendency to move the eyes directly to the location of the cue (known as a pro-saccade). Thus, inhibitory processes are thought to be engaged to override the automatic response tendency, such that oculomotor control systems can be utilized in a voluntary and task-driven manner. Although similar to the other inhibitory paradigms, the anti-saccade offers the opportunity to study inhibitory processes within the context of a motor system whose neuroanatomy and neurophysiology have been extensively examined and characterized in primates. For example, it is well understood that the frontal and supplementary eye fields (FEF and SEF) play key roles in voluntary saccade generation, through interactions with posterior parietal (LIP) and subcortical systems such as the superior colliculus (Dorris et al., 1997).

Human neuroimaging studies of the anti-saccade task have thus standardly focused attention on the role of the FEF and SEF in suppressing reflexive eye movement (e.g., Sweeney et al., 1996). Event-related fMRI studies have offered the opportunity to examine and dissociate preparatory activity during anti-saccade trials from response-related activity (Curtis & D'Esposito, 2003; DeSouza et al., 2003). For example, a study by Curtis and D'Esposito (2003) provided more specific evidence that increased activity in the FEF and SEF is critical for appropriate oculomotor preparation, by demonstrating that activity levels in these areas are related to anti-saccade success. Interestingly, however, these results actually suggest that the FEF and SEF regions involved in anti-saccade responses appear to be the same ones that subserve normal memory-guided saccades in the absence of inhibition. Thus, appropriate anti-saccade behavior appears to be due to the preparatory engagement of systems required for the facilitation of saccades in a planned direction rather than the engagement of specific regions needed to inhibit incorrect response tendencies. Indeed, this may be a general principle of cognitive control, in which top-down frontal signals enhance activation in task-relevant perceptual and motor pathways rather than directly suppressing irrelevant information (e.g., Desimone & Duncan, 1995).

Underdetermined Responding

A hallmark of executive control is the ability to respond freely on the basis of an endogenously generated decision, goal, or intention. This captures the sense that much of our behavior is truly voluntary or willed. This characteristic of executive control is best seen in situations where responses to be generated are only weakly determined by the current environment and context. Such underdetermined response situations contrast with others in which the available responses are strongly constrained by the properties of the eliciting stimulus (i.e., its "affordance")—which we typically refer to as stimulus-response associations—or by the specific task to be performed (i.e., given the task context, there is only one correct response). Thus, to examine underdetermined responding, it is necessary to devise conditions in which multiple actions may be equally appropriate to a given stimulus or at a given moment in time. The assumption then is that under these conditions, an endogenous control mechanism is engaged to select a specific response on the basis of some internal criteria, even if those criteria reflect the (abstract) goal of randomness.

A large number of neuroimaging studies have attempted to examine the neural mechanisms underlying underdetermined responding (or "willed action" or "free selection"). These studies have been examined in both manual responding and language production. Studies of language production have a long history, beginning with the first verb generation tasks studied by Petersen and colleagues (1989). In the verb generation paradigm, participants are required to verbally generate an appropriate action to a visually presented noun (e.g., say "BAKE" if the word "CAKE" is presented). Similar paradigms involve fluency tasks, such as thinking of words beginning with a particular letter or in a particular semantic category (e.g.,

Frith et al., 1991) and stem completion tasks (Buckner et al., 1995). A common finding across all of these tasks is activation in medial frontal regions such as the anterior cingulate and pre-SMA, and in left lateral PFC.

Other studies have directly examined the effect of selection in these tasks by examining differences in brain activation related to changes in generative constraints, such as the number of response options possible on a given trial (Barch et al., 2000; Desmond et al., 1998; Thompson-Schill et al., 1997). For example, in an event-related fMRI study of the verb generation task, Barch et al. (2000) examined activation on trials where the noun was associated with many possible verbs in comparison with trials in which there were few possible associates. Activity in left inferior frontal cortex (BA 44) and ACC was greater when there were many possible associates (low-constraint nouns), and thus a higher demand on selection. Additionally, the ACC also showed greater activity on trials in which the participant produced a verb that was only weakly associated with the noun, and this effect was enhanced for nouns for which there was a strongly associated verb (that was not selected). Interestingly, the left inferior frontal cortex was not sensitive to these latter effects. This finding and others (e.g., Wagner et al., 2001), suggest that the left inferior frontal cortex may be engaged primarily to provide goal-based facilitation of semantic or lexical retrieval when stimulus cues are insufficient by themselves (as discussed in "Strategic Control of Memory," above). Conversely, the ACC may have served to detect the high degree of response conflict or stimulus-response interference evoked by the target noun (see "Stimulus-Response Interference," above, and "Performance Monitoring," below).

Probably the most extreme form of verbal underdetermined response task is the random-number generation paradigm (Baddeley et al., 1998). There have been many variants of this task studied over the years (Jahanshahi & Dirnberger, 1999; Petrides et al., 1993), but all require participants to verbally generate, at a relatively quick rate, a nonrepetitive, nonstereotyped sequence of digits. These studies have all tended to observe the same pattern of dorsolateral PFC activity associated with generation, as well as that activity patterns show sensitivity to counting rate (Daniels et al., 2003). The pattern of results suggests that dorsolateral PFC may serve as a response controller, monitoring for and suppressing tendencies to respond according to habitual patterns. Support for this hypothesis has come from studies using transcranial magnetic stimulation (TMS) techniques to temporarily deactivate the PFC (Jahanshahi & Dirnberger, 1999; Jahanshahi et al., 1998). During TMS stimulation occurring over the dorsolateral PFC, the tendency for participants to generate stereotyped sequences increased. Interestingly, the pattern has been observed only during left hemisphere stimulation, with right hemisphere stimulation producing no behavioral changes.

The initiation, selection, and generation of "willed actions" has been studied with tasks requiring manual responses. Most of these tasks require participants to move a joystick in one of multiple directions or to press one of multiple responses, according to a pattern of their own choosing (e.g., Frith et al., 1991). The pattern of results appears to be similar to that observed in verbal generation tasks, with both dorsolateral PFC, and medial frontal cortex, including the ACC and SMA, being reliably engaged. However, in this domain, more recent work has enabled further functional dissociation of these two regions. For example, in a study conducted by Lau et al. (2004), dorsolateral PFC activity was found to be equivalent in a random selection task and in cued-selection task with a high number of potential targets. In contrast, a region of pre-SMA was found to be engaged only by random selection, and activation in the region was significantly correlated with reaction time latency. Lau et al. suggested that pre-SMA might be specifically involved in the endogenous generation of potential response options, while the dorsolateral PFC might be involved in selecting one of these options for execution.

Performance Monitoring

An important feature of many task situations is the need to dynamically monitor and adjust one's own behavior in order to optimally achieve task goals. Performance monitoring and adjustment seem to rely upon a number of component executive processes: (a) sensitivity to either environmental or internal cues that indicate performance success or failure; (b) maintenance and integration of such cues over time, to assess and confirm subtle trends; and (c) translation of performance information into an adaptive adjustment of cognitive or response strategy. Since the mid-1990s there has been a rapidly accelerating pace of neuroimaging research geared toward understanding the neural mechanisms underlying performance monitoring.

The relationship of performance monitoring to executive control has been classically studied within the neuropsychological literature through examination of the Wisconsin Card Sort Task (WCST). Although this task is multicomponent in nature, the greatest demands on executive function may center around the requirement to adjust an internal task set or decision rule, based upon somewhat ambiguous feedback information. The perseverative errors reliably observed by patients with PFC damage and other patient groups with executive control impairments appear to involve a failure to appropriately process or utilize such feedback signals to adjust cognitive strategy. Neuroimaging studies of the WCST have long confirmed the role of PFC in global performance (e.g., Berman et al., 1995), but more recently have also focused attention on the feedback processing components of the task itself. For example, Konishi and colleagues (Konishi, Nakajima, Uchida, Kameyama, et al.,

1998) used event-related fMRI to isolate activation on trials with negative feedback. This analysis revealed selective activation in bilateral regions of inferior PFC (BA 45).

A similar study by Monchi et al. (2001) also observed feedback-related activation in lateral PFC that included both inferior and dorsolateral regions, along with activation in the ACC. Another study by Konishi and colleagues (2003) attempted to dissociate the affective component of negative feedback (i.e., signaling an inappropriate response) from the informational content (i.e., signaling the need to adjust the task set). They found that the medial frontal lobe was associated primarily with the affective component of feedback, whereas right-lateralized inferior (BA 47) and dorsolateral PFC regions (BA 9/45/46) were associated with the informational component.

A somewhat different theme in the investigation of performance monitoring processes emerged in the early 1990s from studies in the ERP literature. In particular, this research identified a specific ERP (event-related potential) component, known as the ERN (error-related negativity), that was elicited following commission of an error in simple cognitive tasks. The ERN was first observed in tasks where no explicit feedback was provided to participants, but the task was simple enough (and speeded, to produce a high error rate) that errors were likely detected internally with high reliability (Falkenstein et al., 1990; Gehring et al., 1993). Later studies also detected the presence of an ERN-like component linked to explicit (i.e., external) error feedback, under conditions where internal error detection was much more difficult (Miltner et al., 1997). These studies suggested that the source of the ERN was in the medial frontal cortex, around the location of the ACC (Dehaene et al., 1994). Thus, an interpretation of the results was that the ACC served as a neural system invoked to detect and respond to error-related information through corrections in behavior, such as slowing of responses (a performance pattern frequently observed following errors; e.g., Laming, 1979).

The error-related research on the ERN has been subsequently confirmed with fMRI, with event-related imaging studies clearly indicating increased ACC activity during error commission (e.g., Kiehl et al., 2000). Interestingly, at the same time these neuroimaging findings were coming out, a somewhat different theory was emerging which suggested that the ACC played a more general performance-monitoring function that involved the detection of conflict during the course of response generation, even under conditions where the eventual response was correct (Botvinick et al., 1999; Carter et al., 1998). The conflict-monitoring theory suggested that error detection was a special case of conflict, and provided a computational account that appeared to integrate many disparate results (such as explaining why the same pattern of ACC activity is commonly observed across response inhibition, stimulus-response interference, and underdetermined response tasks). Importantly, a component of this theory specifies the relationship between conflict detection and subsequent performance adjustment by postulating that ACC activity feeds into control mechanisms, such as those in lateral PFC, that implement a change in task goals, response speed, or attentional bias (Botvinick et al., 2001).

The conflict-monitoring and error detection hypotheses of ACC function have together spawned a large and growing literature not only from ERP and fMRI methods, but also involving ACC or frontal lesion patients (e.g. Gehring & Knight, 2000; Swick & Turken, 2002). A number of studies have sought to test whether error-related signals in ACC might be anatomically distinct from those associated with conflict (e.g., Garavan et al., 2003; Ullsperger & von Cramon, 2001). Other studies have focused on whether explicit error feedback also produces activity within the same ACC regions (e.g., Holroyd et al., 2004). Still other studies have focused on the relationship between errors and subsequent changes in cognitive control or behavioral performance (Garavan et al., 2002). The literature is rapidly evolving, and a growing theme is that the ACC and related medial frontal areas may play a generalized performance-monitoring function, of integrating both internal and external cues regarding performance, that could be used to adjust response selection strategies (Ridderinkhof et al., 2004).

A final theme in the neuroimaging literature on performance monitoring has been to focus on feedback-related brain activity within the context of gambling or decision-making tasks involving monetary rewards and penalties (e.g., Elliott et al, 2000). One prominent finding in this literature is the involvement of the orbitofrontal cortex (OFC) under conditions involving trial-by-trial monetary feedback information. This has led to a general idea that the OFC may be important for keeping track of the valence of such feedback (Krawczyk, 2002; Rolls, 2000).

A study by O'Doherty and colleagues (2001) examined this hypothesis, using event-related fMRI to compare the neural response on reward vs. penalty feedback trials. Distinct OFC regions were engaged by positive and negative monetary feedback, with medial regions showing more responsivity to rewards and lateral regions showing greater sensitivity to punishments. Moreover, the magnitude of activity in each of these regions was correlated with the magnitude of reward and penalty. A follow-up study by O'Doherty, Dayan, et al. (2003) provided evidence that activity in these regions does not merely track reinforcement values over time, but may also signal whether such information will be used to bias changes in behavioral choices. Thus, activity levels in the medial and lateral OFC was greater for trials in which reward or punishment did not lead to a change in behavior, relative to trials in which a behavioral switch occurred. The dorsal ACC (a similar region to that activated in conflict and error studies) was found to be selectively active under conditions in which penalties were associated with a subsequent shift in behavioral choice.

Other studies employing similar task designs have suggested that a region at the intersection of the anterior insula and caudolateral OFC might be involved in linking penalties or reduction in reward with a switch in behavioral choice (e.g., Cools et al., 2002). Interestingly, a recent study has suggested that activity in dorsal ACC and in lateral OFC could be doubly dissociated on the basis of whether feedback information was given after a response that was freely selected or made according to an externally specified instruction (Walton et al., 2004). The task was a response-switching paradigm in which one of three stimulus-response mapping rules was in place at any time. Participants were intermittently given a cue to switch response rules, but were not told which rule was now appropriate, and had to determine this through feedback information. In one condition, following a switch cue, participants had to freely select the next response and evaluate the subsequent feedback, while in another condition participants had to make a prespecified (by the experimenter) response before evaluating the feedback. ACC activity was selectively associated with feedback monitoring under free-choice conditions, whereas OFC activity was linked to feedback-monitoring when the response was prespecified. This result was interpreted as suggesting that ACC monitors the feedback relationship between freely generated actions and their associated outcomes, whereas OFC tracks the outcome of externally guided actions in order to adjust internal representations of stimulus-reward associations.

Task Management

A central notion of many theories of executive control is that individuals are able to internally represent "task sets" or "task rules" (a set of goals and constraints for behavior within a task context) that collectively provide a regulating force on information processing and action selection (Bunge, 2004). These task-set representations (and the processes that act on them) are postulated to be distinct from the task-specific representations and processes themselves, and thus serve a managerial function in coordinating task flow. Theorists have suggested that the best approach for tapping into these task management processes is by studying performance in multitask environments (Monsell & Driver, 2000). Under these conditions, cross-task interference is thought to be a central limiting factor in performance, and thus control processes may be invoked to minimize or resolve this interference. Two types of experimental paradigms have emerged in the behavioral literature for studying these processes: task-switching and dual-task coordination. Neuroimaging researchers have adapted both of these paradigms to understand the neural mechanisms underlying task management.

Task-switching paradigms require rapid switching among two (or sometimes more) tasks, in either a predictable but uncued, or random and cued, sequence. The central finding is that performance suffers on trials where the task switches relative to when it repeats (e.g., Allport et al., 1994; Meiran, 1996). This finding has been classically interpreted as suggesting that a distinct process is required to accomplish the "switch" or reconfiguration of internal task representations. Although this original interpretation has become much more complex, it has served as the theoretical basis for a quickly growing neuroimaging literature. Thus, a number of studies have compared activity in task-switch trials relative to task-repeat trials, using event-related fMRI (e.g., Dove et al., 2000; Sohn et al., 2000). Although, as is typical in the executive control literature, many of these studies were focused on the role of lateral PFC, the results have been somewhat ambiguous.

Studies using less sensitive blocked designs have suggested PFC activity is increased during task-switching blocks (e.g., Dreher et al., 2002). However, event-related fMRI studies do not typically find switch-selective activity in lateral PFC—that is, the same regions are also activated on task-repeat trials (e.g., Kimberg et al., 2000). Moreover, the studies that have reported switch-related lateral PFC increases observe this pattern only under specific (and potentially contradictory) conditions, such as when advance preparatory cues are provided (e.g., Sohn et al., 2000) or when insufficient preparatory time is given (e.g., Ruge et al., 2005). Instead, the most reliable region for observing switch-related activity seems to be the superior parietal cortex (for review, see Wager et al., 2004).

Lateral PFC, particularly posterior PFC regions (e.g., the inferior frontal junction, BA 44/6), does seem to play an important role in task-switching environments, but the activity appears to index more general processes associated with cued task preparation or interference resolution that may not be specific to task switches (Brass & von Cramon, 2002; Derrfuss et al., 2004). For example, PFC activity is greater (a) when task sequences are random rather than predictable (Dreher et al., 2002); (b) following an explicit preparatory cue (Braver et al., 2003); (c) when a previously suppressed task set has to be activated again (Dreher & Berman, 2002); and (d) when the task-set representation increases in complexity, i.e., task rules are more complicated (Bunge et al., 2003). Interestingly, anterior (BA 10) rather than dorsolateral regions of PFC were found to show sustained activation during task-switch blocks relative to single-task blocks, and this activity was associated with the "mixing cost" (the performance effect due specifically to performing in multitask relative to single-task environments) (Braver et al., 2003). The activity in this region was interpreted as potentially reflecting a high-order subgoal monitoring or preparatory attentional process that detects cues indicating a switch in task.

An interesting issue that has not been fully explored in this literature is the exact distinction between task switching and other forms of attention switching, such as switching between: response mappings (e.g., Dove et al., 2000), different perceptual features (e.g., Rushworth et al., 2002), different perceptual dimensions (e.g., Pollman,

2001), or the focus of attention within working memory (e.g., Garavan et al., 2000). Do these other situations activate the same brain areas as task-switching studies? One meta-analysis (Wager et al., 2004) suggests that the commonalities across different types of switching tasks are greater than the differences, with the parietal cortex showing the most reliable effects of all switching conditions.

Studies involving dual-task paradigms differ from those involving task-switching in that multiple tasks are presented, and have to be performed, within an overlapping time interval. Thus, dual-task performance requires the coordination, scheduling, and segregation of task representations rather than simply rapid updating (Baddeley, 1996). Neuroimaging researchers have sought to determine the brain regions selectively engaged under dual-task conditions, under the assumption that such regions might serve as the central "task coordinator" that enables successful performance. In the first study to make this claim, D'Esposito suggested that dorsolateral PFC was selectively activated by requirements to perform a spatial and a semantic task concurrently, and that the activation could not be purely due to the increase in task difficulty itself (D'Esposito et al., 1995). However, later studies provided more equivocal results, with PFC and other regions showing increased dual-task activity but in the same location as regions activated during single-task conditions (e.g., Bunge et al., 2000). Thus, these studies argued against the presence of "dual-task-specific" brain areas. Yet other dual-task studies have drawn conclusions more similar to the early D'Esposito work (e.g., Szameitat et al., 2002). Still, no definitive demonstration of selective dual-task-related activity has been presented at this time.

A different set of questions has been addressed by other researchers in this domain: How, why, and under what conditions do two tasks interfere with one another when performed simultaneously? One idea, investigated by Klingberg and colleagues, is that two tasks will interfere with one another if they both engage the same region of cortex (Klingberg & Roland, 1997). Thus, under dual-task conditions, the activation level in certain task-related brain regions has been found to be less than the sum of activity occurring in each of the single-task conditions (i.e., a subadditive interaction; see "Interactive Effects" under "Issues," below; Just et al., 2001). Such findings suggest some kind of constraint on task-related activation, due to inhibitory processes or limited processing capacity, or a combination of the two.

Other studies have focused on finding out the processing stage at which interference occurs. These studies have examined the temporal characteristics of task overlap, relying on a phenomenon known as the psychological refractory period (PRP) effect (Pashler, 1994; Welford, 1952). The PRP effect is a slowing of reaction time when a second task is presented while the first task is still in a particular stage of completion, but not if it has already passed that stage. Thus, PRP tasks standardly manipulate temporal overlap between the two tasks by varying the SOA (stimulus onset asynchrony) for the second task relative to the first. Neuroimaging studies examining the PRP effect have suggested that inferior PFC, typically right-lateralized, shows increased activity during short SOAs (when temporal overlap between the tasks is high), but not during long SOAs (when task overlap is low; e.g., Herath et al., 2001). This activity has been interpreted as reflecting the presence of cross-task interference (and the need to resolve it) either at the response selection stage (Herath et al., 2001) or during perceptual attention (Jiang & Kanwisher, 2003). It will be important for future studies to investigate the relationship between these forms of cross-task interference resolution process, and the simpler forms of stimulus-response interference resolution processes discussed above (under "Stimulus-Response Interference").

Higher Cognition

There are certain mental processes that seem to represent the pinnacle of human cognitive skills and achievement, and that most strongly set our species apart from others. These mental processes, which include planning, novel problem-solving, and abstract reasoning, have long been the subject of intense research interest because they are typically thought to reflect the essence of intelligence and higher cognition. Likewise, these higher cognitive skills may be the ones that most strongly require the engagement of executive processes, to ensure that complex chains of thought can be appropriately directed toward highly abstract behavioral goals. Within the neuroimaging literature growing attention has been given to the underlying cognitive and neural processes associated with the higher cognitive domains of planning, problem solving, and reasoning. Two research strategies have emerged for investigations within this domain. One approach has been to directly utilize or adapt classic experimental tasks drawn from the neuropsychological or intelligence testing literature, such as Raven's Progressive Matrices, the Tower of Hanoi/London, analogy problems, and logical reasoning tasks (e.g., syllogisms). A second approach has been to develop new experimental paradigms (or novel variants of existing tasks) that attempt to get at the essential cognitive elements of the standard tasks within a more simplified framework, such that critical task factors can be isolated and manipulated more selectively .

The most popular of the classic experimental tasks studied in higher-cognitive neuroimaging studies is the Tower of London (ToL) planning task, adapted from the well-known Tower of Hanoi problem in cognitive psychology. An attractive feature of the ToL is that it enables the presentation of multiple planning problems that can be incrementally graded in complexity and difficulty. A number of studies have directly examined the effect of difficulty manipulations on brain activity (e.g., Baker et al., 1996; Fincham et al., 2002). These studies have tended to find that increased planning complexity is associated with corresponding increases in a widespread network including parietal, prefrontal, and medial frontal regions. This network is highly overlapping with that observed in a range of visuospatial WM tasks. However, Baker et al. (1996) established that in a direct comparison of the two types of tasks (ToL vs. visual WM), the ToL was associated with selectively increased activity in anterior PFC regions (BA 10). Other studies have tended to confirm this pattern (e.g., van den Heuvel et al., 2003). Conversely, a study by Beauchamp found that increased practice with ToL problems led to automatization in task performance that was associated with decreased activity in dorsolateral and anterior PFC but an increase in activity within basal ganglia regions (Beauchamp et al., 2003).

A similar pattern of findings has been observed in studies with a different problem-solving task—Raven's Progressive Matrices—that has been employed experimentally as a probe of general fluid (i.e., knowledge-independent) intelligence. As with the ToL, neuroimaging studies with Raven's task have varied problem complexity to examine the effect of this manipulation on brain activity (e.g., Prabhakaran et al., 1997). This work has suggested that the most difficult Raven's problems, which demand integrating relationships among various stimulus dimensions (e.g., shape, texture, etc.), selectively engage anterior PFC regions. The pattern has been found to remain selective even when controlling for effects due to task difficulty (Kroger et al., 2002) or changes in performance (i.e., slower response latencies; Christoff et al., 2001).

A third type of higher-cognitive task studied in the neuroimaging literature is logical reasoning. Many of these types of studies have been carried out by Goel and colleagues (Goel, in press). A number of different types of logic problems have been examined, including inductive vs. deductive and transitive inference. As might be expected, a wide variety of logic problems all commonly activate lateral PFC regions (e.g., Knauff et al., 2003). Some studies have attempted to specifically dissociate the executive mechanisms that support different reasoning processes. For example, a common distinction in the reasoning literature is between judging logical validity and judging plausibility. Deductive arguments attempt to demonstrate logical validity or necessity, while inductive arguments attempt only to demonstrate plausibility. In two imaging studies directly comparing matched inductive and deductive reasoning tasks (Goel & Dolan, 2004; Goel et al., 1997), left inferior PFC (BA 44) was more strongly activated in the deductive condition, whereas left dorsolateral PFC (BA 9) was more strongly engaged by induction. The results were interpreted as suggesting that deductive reasoning makes strong demands on verbal working memory and the phonological loop, whereas inductive reasoning requires the evaluation of propositions against background knowledge, and thus may engage specific executive monitoring processes.

A review of the neuroimaging literature on higher cognitive tasks conducted by Christoff & Gabrieli (2000) argued that many of these tasks tend to activate anterior or polar regions of PFC (BA 10). Likewise, these authors have suggested that a common cognitive component of these types of tasks is that they require internally generated (i.e., abstract) monitoring or evaluation representations (Christoff et al., 2003). For example, in the Tower of London task, one has to internally generate several possible moves and then evaluate which of these is most promising in terms of progress toward a goal. Thus, Christoff and Gabrieli postulated that frontopolar PFC might be selectively engaged to carry out these monitoring or evaluation functions in a wide variety of cognitive task contexts, including episodic retrieval (see "Strategic Control of Memory," above). The ideas proposed by Christoff and Gabrieli were very similar to an account put forward by Koechlin et al. (1999) in a study reported at around the same time. Koechlin et al. provided results that demonstrated the selective activation of frontopolar cortex (lateral BA 10) under conditions requiring cognitive "branching." This term was invoked to describe the process of maintaining information in working memory while performing a second task, such that the two sources of information can be evaluated or integrated. Koechlin et al., like Christoff and Gabrieli, claimed that branching operations form a core component of many higher cognitive tasks.

The development of specific functional hypotheses regarding the role of anterior PFC in higher cognition has led to an increased and more focused interest in both "branching" or integration-type computations and how they engage anterior PFC (Ramnani & Owen, 2004). A number of studies have now investigated integration effects within working memory, demonstrating that such requirements also tend to engage anterior PFC regions (e.g., Badre & Wagner, 2004; Braver & Bongiolatti, 2002; Prabhakaran et al., 2000). For example, in Prabhakaran et al. (2000), anterior PFC was selectively engaged by conditions requiring participants to integrate the location and identity of spatially arranged letters in working memory, in comparison with conditions requiring the same numbers of letters and locations to be maintained (but letters and locations were segregated). Similarly, Braver & Bongiolatti demonstrated that right frontopolar cortex was engaged by the requirement to integrate the contents of working memory with the results of a subgoal task (semantic classification), but not by a matched working memory or semantic classification task performed in isolation (Braver & Bongiolatti, 2002). Finally, related work has also shown that anterior PFC regions are also engaged by integration effects within analogical reasoning (Bunge et al., 2004). In this study, judging whether two word pairs were related along the same semantic dimension (i.e., analogous) engaged left anterior PFC, whereas just judging semantic relatedness of a single word pair did not lead to increased activation. Taken together, these findings suggest that anterior PFC involvement might be a critical feature of many higher cognitive tasks, since such tasks often require the integration of abstract sources of information within working memory.

Issues

As the above review indicates, the neuroimaging literature on executive function is vibrant, vital, and rapidly expanding. Indeed, it is fair to say that we may look back at the first decade of the twenty-first century as a "golden age" in executive function research. However, the rapidity with which new studies have emerged over the last few years makes it very difficult to keep pace with, and adequately summarize, the progress of the field. Nevertheless, it is clear that a few themes and trends have emerged in the last few years regarding the neural basis of specific control functions (see figure 10.1, plate 17):

• Task conditions involving the preparatory cuing of attention or the use of attentional control to resolve interference tend to activate posterior and inferior regions of lateral PFC.

• Task conditions requiring the temporary suppression of ongoing responses tend to activate right inferior PFC regions.

• Task conditions requiring rapid shifting of attention to different dimensions or reconfiguration of task sets reliably engage the superior parietal cortex.

• Task conditions involving the free selection of potential response alternatives engage superior medial frontal areas near the SMA.

• Task conditions involving the processing of internal or external feedback related to the outcome of generated actions reliably engage the ACC and nearby medial frontal areas

• Task conditions that require the tracking of changing stimulus-reinforcement contingencies elicit activation in the OFC.

• Complex cognitive activities (such as planning, analogy verification, and controlled episodic retrieval) that involve the evaluation or integration of abstract dimensions maintained in working memory tend to engage the anteriormost regions of PFC (BA 10).

Despite the excitement stemming from these new discoveries regarding the neural substrates of executive control, a reader of this review might find it difficult to not be discouraged by the diverse set of tasks and studies that appear to engage a common set of brain regions, such as the lateral PFC and ACC. Indeed, a fair

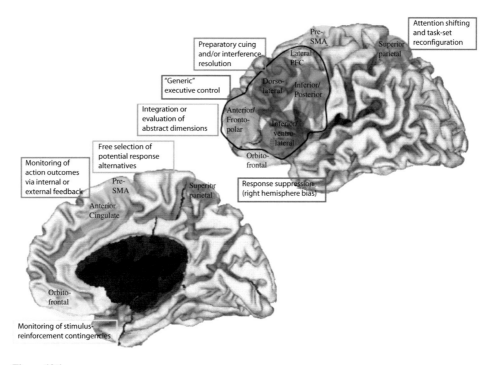

Figure 10.1
Anatomical designations of brain areas that are part of the network for executive control and the task conditions or factors that reliably acti1vate them. Shown are lateral (upper) and medial (lower) brain surfaces. Color codes represent different brain regions discussed in the review and the corresponding task conditions or factors that appear to activate them. Lateral PFC region (outlined in black) is subdivided into inferior/posterior, inferior/ventrolateral, dorsolateral, and anterior/frontopolar regions. See plate 17 for color version.

summary of the neuroimaging literature is that lateral PFC, and dorsolateral regions in particular, will be engaged during the performance of any task that requires the invocation of executive control. Thus, on the basis of such a literature survey one might reasonably conclude that the lateral PFC and similar regions, such as the ACC, serve as neural substrates of a monolithic and mysterious "central executive" that is ubiquitously engaged whenever a task requires the invocation of executive control. In fact, similar conclusions have been drawn by a number of investigators (Dehaene et al., 1998; Duncan & Owen, 2000). While such interpretations do seem reasonable, given the bulk of the literature, they nevertheless feel somewhat unsatisfying to the cognitive neuroscientist seeking to decompose executive functions into their most basic elements and fundamental components.

What, exactly, is the lateral PFC doing that gives it such importance in executive control? In particular, a fundamental challenge for the field seems to be to determine the particular processing mechanisms, representational specializations, and organizing properties of this brain area that give rise to its involvement in such a wide range of control processes and tasks. Likewise, even if certain specific regions within and outside of lateral PFC are coming into greater focus in terms of their particular roles in executive control, a better understanding needs to emerge regarding the "division of labor" among distinct control process, and how such processes interact to produce coordinated behavior in complex cognitive tasks. In the text that follows, we provide our own opinions, recommendations, and illustrative examples about how best to make further progress in this domain.

Processes vs. Tasks

A common approach utilized in neuroimaging studies of executive control is to directly import tasks developed in the neuropsychological or cognitive literature to examine particular executive processes (e.g., Stroop and interference, go-no go and inhibition, Tower of London and planning). In this approach, patterns of brain activity evoked during task performance (relative to a control condition) serve as a window into the neural systems subserving such processes. However, a truism from cognitive psychology is that no task is "process pure," which indicates that classical subtractive design approaches (e.g., Posner et al., 1988) will be insufficiently selective for isolating control processes of interest in executive function research.

Within cognitive psychology, a standard research strategy is to develop an underlying process model, based upon detailed task analysis, that specifies how the process of interest will be engaged in various tasks and be affected by various task variables. This translates into an experimental approach in which complex, multifactor, or parametric designs are utilized to provide a range of control conditions. Likewise, multiple, convergent experiments are conducted to confirm predictions regarding a complete pattern of behavior. Thus, we would argue that a similar approach is the one most likely to be successful in neuroimaging studies attempting to isolate and identify neural substrates of specific executive processes. Indeed, it is heartening to see that such approaches are starting to be the norm rather than the exception within the literature. For example, Banich and colleagues have provided an extended neuroimaging analysis of the Stroop task across multiple studies that has revealed how various task factors influence interference detection and resolution processes within lateral PFC, ACC, and interacting posterior brain regions (Banich et al., 2001).

A similar type of process-oriented research strategy might be to understand the commonalities and differences in neural activity across superficially distinct tasks that may nevertheless all engage the same underlying control functions, albeit in potentially different ways. For example, Braver et al. (2001) demonstrated that a common network of brain regions, including the ACC, were equivalently activated by low-frequency events across three different tasks—oddball, go/nogo, and two-alternative forced choice—suggesting that low-frequency responding may involve specific control functions regardless of task context.

In addition, such approaches might reveal hidden factors that are linked to the activation of control-associated brain regions across tasks but tend to be overlooked by researchers. Thus, in the Braver et al. study, there was a suggestive hint that the right-lateralized PFC activity typically associated with response inhibition (as in the go/nogo), might be more strongly linked to the frequency of inhibitory events rather than to the demands on inhibition per se. Thus, response frequency (or a related construct, such as the violation of a local sequential pattern; e.g., Huettel et al., 2002) might be an important factor influencing right lateral PFC that could be more thoroughly explored across a wider range of task contexts. It is likely that there are other types of similar critical, but "undiscovered," task variables which may modulate control processes in multiple task contexts.

Double Dissociations

Currently, the strongest evidence within neuroimaging for establishing the presence of regional brain specialization in cognitive function is the double dissociation (Smith et al., 1995). Importantly, firm conclusions regarding the presence of a double dissociation can be drawn only when it is successfully demonstrated that the dissociation pattern is statistically reliable. The most rigorous statistical criterion is the presence of a full region x condition crossover interaction (or more complex variants), whereby condition A is significantly greater than condition B in Region 1, while in Region 2 condition B is significantly greater than condition A. Thus, although it is seemingly obvious, we would recommend that more effort be extended toward the establishment of double dissociation among control-related brain regions before drawing inferences regarding functional specialization. Moreover, we would suggest that further emphasis be given to pairs of regions for which double dissociations have already been established as a focus of further systematic research efforts. Thankfully, there have been a number of such dissociations demonstrated in the literature (many of which we have discussed above), and these have led to important advances in our conceptual understanding of the neural organization of executive control. For example, in MacDonald et al. (2000) a double dissociation between lateral PFC and ACC was clearly demonstrated in a task-switching variant of the Stroop. In this study ACC was found to be selectively engaged by the detection of response conflict (i.e., the presentation of an incongruent trial), whereas the lateral PFC was selectively engaged by the demand for preparatory attentional control (i.e., the presentation of a task cue specifying an upcoming color-naming trial).

Interactive Effects of Task Factors

A definitional characteristic of executive processes is that they are not an embedded component of task-specific processing networks, but serve to modulate the flow of processing within such networks, in accordance with behavioral goals. Consequently, it is likely that the presence of specific executive processes will be best revealed not through direct manipulation of experimental factors affecting task-specific processes, but instead by determining how such factors interact with other factors that influence the demand on such control processes. In other words, it is likely that executive control processes are going to be most sensitive to the interaction of two or more task factors rather than to single factors. This may be especially true when considering processes that are involved in integrating diverse sets of information. For example, Ramnani & Owen (2004) argued that anterior PFC regions will be engaged only by the coordination of multiple subtasks, and thus should be revealed in terms of a superadditive interaction of factors affecting the difficulty of completing each task. Likewise, Gray et al. (2002) postulated that if lateral PFC was selectively involved in the integration of affective states and cognitive task goals, then this brain region should show a mood state x cognitive task interaction, but no main effect of either mood or task itself (i.e., a full crossover or subadditive interaction). Such a pattern was observed in bilateral anterior PFC (BA 46/10). These results suggest that studies of executive control should utilize factorial designs wherever possible, and in particular in experimental contexts where theoretical significance can be attributed to the interaction effect in terms of its relevance for executive control.

Brain-Behavior Relationships

Although it is seemingly obvious, inferences regarding the control functions thought to be subserved by specific brain regions can be most strongly tested by linking activity in these regions to behavior. In particular, one would ideally observe a selective relationship between the activity level in the putative neural control region and performance in task components thought to be most dependent on the specific control function subserved by the region. Of course in standard neuroimaging studies the kinds of relationships that can be established are purely correlational rather than causal. Nevertheless, even correlational relationships, if specific enough, can greatly strengthen inferences regarding causality. Thus, as is occurring with greater frequency in the literature, testing for activity-performance correlations in putative neural control regions should form an essential part of the neuroimaging analysis procedure.

The types of correlations that can be examined might be both between individuals and within individuals. For example, MacDonald et al. (2000) found a negative between-subject correlation between cue-related preparatory activity in lateral PFC and the size of the Stroop interference effect. This suggested that individuals who more strongly activated PFC prior to a Stroop stimulus showed a greater ability to combat the interfering effects of stimulus incongruence. In contrast, Braver et al. (2003) found a within-subject negative correlation between cue-related lateral PFC activity and the magnitude of task-switching reaction time costs. This indicated that trials with small switch costs were associated with greater preparatory PFC activity. Thus, both trial-related and subject-related variability in task performance appear to be linked to corresponding variations in lateral PFC activity following the presentation of preparatory attention cues.

Individual Differences

An issue closely linked to the one just discussed is that executive control processes may be highly variable across individuals. In particular, there may be many different routes or strategies available for achieving executive control during cognitive task performance. Such control-related variability may be an intrinsic or stable characteristic of individuals, and linked to constructs such as domain-specific cognitive skills, domain-general cognitive capabilities, or dispositional traits Thus, it may become increasingly important to consider these sources of individual difference when interpreting the results of neuroimaging studies. As an example, Gray and colleagues observed that activation of lateral PFC and ACC during performance of the n-back WM task was negatively correlated with trait levels of dispositional extraversion (Gray & Braver, 2002; Gray et al., 2005). This finding was interpreted as suggesting that extraverted individuals exhibited greater neural efficiency (mediated by personality-linked changes in dopamine function) that enabled successful performance even with reduced control-related brain activity (Braver et al., in press). The important take-home point is that without measuring and controlling for such sources of individual variation, misleading interpretations of neuroimaging data may occur.

Consideration of Affective-Motivational Variables

Related to the previous point, it is worth pointing out the emerging relationship between imaging studies of emotion and those of executive control. There have now been imaging studies of working memory that have examined the role not only of personality and emotion on working memory, as discussed above (Gray & Braver,

2002; Gray et al., 2002), but also of the impact of reward and motivational manipulations on brain activity (Pochon et al., 2002; Taylor et al., 2004). All of these studies have shown that critical neural systems of executive control (e.g., lateral PFC and ACC) are also influenced by affective-motivational variables. Indeed, it is rapidly becoming appreciated that there may be a tight relationship between the neural systems involved in executive control and those involved in emotion processing and regulation. This view has been strengthened by studies in the emotion literature which have demonstrated that exerting self-control over emotional reactions to events or reward feedback recruits lateral PFC and ACC, along with more "traditional" emotion-related brain systems such as the striatum, orbitofrontal cortex, and amygdala (e.g., Beauregard et al., 2001; Ochsner et al., 2002). Although studies of this type are in their infancy, the second decade of the twenty-first century will likely see an accelerating pace of research examining the intersection of emotion and cognition. For example, imaging studies are beginning to compare the relationship between emotional conflict or interference and the more traditional stimulus-response interference examined in Strooplike tasks (Compton et al., 2003). Additional systematic investigations of this type are needed. More generally, we encourage investigators conducting neuroimaging studies of executive control to more closely consider affective-motivational processes when interpreting the results of their studies. In particular, we suspect that successful theories of the neural mechanisms of executive control will provide an account in which the specialized contributions of specific brain systems are described in terms of integrated cognitive and affective components.

Temporal Dynamics of Neural Activity

The primate neurophysiology literature has strongly suggested that a critical characteristic of PFC neurons is their ability to sustain changes in activity levels over extended temporal intervals and distractor stimuli (Miller et al., 1996). This finding serves as the core evidence regarding the involvement of PFC in the active maintenance functions of WM. Nevertheless, in human neuroimaging studies, it is controversial whether PFC activity truly represents active maintenance processes, and under what conditions such processes occur (e.g., Postle et al., 1999; Sakai et al., 2002). Thus, in some WM studies, PFC activity is transient rather than sustained, and occurs at the time of response selection rather than active maintenance (Rowe et al., 2000). Indeed, for some theorists, the role of PFC in executive functions rather than WM per se is defined by the transient engagement of this region when control demands temporarily increase (Smith & Jonides, 1999).

In our own work, we have been developing a theoretical framework which suggests that the temporal dynamics and types of control functions subserved by PFC regions might be highly variable (Braver et al., in press). In particular, we have suggested the dual mechanisms of control (DMC) account, whereby control processes can be either proactive (i.e., anticipatory and sustained) or reactive (i.e., demand-driven and transient), depending on both situational and individual factors. As an example, we have observed that in the Stroop task, when the expectancy for Stroop interference is low (mostly congruent trials), activity in lateral PFC and ACC transiently increases during performance of interference trials (Braver & Hoyer, 2003). Conversely, when interference expectancy is high (mostly incongruent trials), lateral PFC activity is observed that is sustained across trials (i.e., present during intertrial intervals) and not modulated by the presence of interference. We interpreted this result as suggesting that interference expectancy can modulate the temporal dynamics of PFC activity and, moreover, that the type of executive control is implemented during task performance. Based on this framework, we suggest that executive control studies should focus on the temporal dynamics of activity within critical brain areas such as the PFC and, in particular, examine both transient and sustained types of effects. Moreover, careful attention needs to be paid to the potentially subtle task factors (and individual difference characteristics of the studied sample) that might influence whether executive control is occurring in a reactive or proactive manner.

Connectivity Approaches

Executive control almost certainly involves the widespread interaction and coordination of processing from multiple neural systems. Moreover, it is likely that critical mechanisms of control will be revealed not only through changes in activation of individual brain regions but also in how one brain region influences the activation of another. Analyses of cross-regional interactions in brain activation, typically referred to as "functional and effective connectivity," can be studied through a number of different approaches, from simple correlation to more complex and specialized techniques, such as structural equation modeling, partial least squares, dynamic causal modeling, and independent components analysis (Nyberg & McIntosh, 2001; Penny et al., 2004).

   Although the application of such techniques is still not widespread within neuroimaging studies of executive control, it is growing, and will likely have a strong influence on the future direction of the field. Connectivity approaches are likely to be most critical in understanding how changes in executive control function, both across individuals (e.g., group or individual difference effects) and across time within individuals (e.g., strategy or learning effects), are reflected in changed information flow through critical nodes of the brain control network. Indeed, the utilization of functional connectivity analyses has already provided intriguing findings related to these questions in related areas, such as the relationship between PFC and posterior and subcortical brain regions in working memory (Glabus et al., 2003), episodic memory (Grady et al., 2003), and attention tasks (Rowe et al., 2002). We hope that investigators will incorporate such connectivity approaches more regularly into studies of executive function.

Model-Based Neuroimaging

A final suggestion we would like to make is that neuroimaging studies of executive control are likely to be most informative when designed with explicit reference to an existing theoretical or computational model. Models provide a basis from which to make strong predictions and inferences regarding the nature of specific control mechanisms. In particular, models can specify the conditions under which specific control processes might be engaged, how these will interact with other processes, and, most important, how they should influence behavior. There are now a number of examples in which different types of formal or computational models have been used to design and interpret neuroimaging studies of executive control. Some of the models are based on high-level symbolic or production system frameworks (Anderson et al., 2003; Newman et al., 2003), others on neural network architectures (Botvinick et al., 2001; Holroyd & Coles, 2002), and still others on mathematical formalisms (O'Doherty et al., 2003).

An important component of such work is that it drives a tighter integration between the accumulation of neuroimaging results and the development and refinements of specific executive control theories. For example, in Jones et al (2002), simulations with a computational model of the ACC conflict monitoring theory led to predictions regarding trial-by-trial fluctuations in ACC activity that were tested (and confirmed) in a reanalysis of previously published neuroimaging data. Likewise, Brown and Braver (2005) recently developed a novel computational model of ACC function in which ACC serves as a prediction-learning system regarding the likelihood of error commission in specific contexts. This model was used to derive counterintuitive predictions regarding ACC activity that were tested and confirmed in a subsequent imaging study.

Models can also be used to test predictions regarding how different neural mechanisms of executive control interact to influence behavior during cognitive task performance. Thus, Kerns et al. (2004) conducted an fMRI study of the Stroop to test a prediction of the conflict-monitoring theory regarding how fluctuations in ACC activity produce subsequent shifts in lateral PFC activity, and also corresponding changes in behavioral performance. Similarly, computational models can provide a formal mathematical basis from which to understand how large-scale activity might propagate in a distributed neural control network (Deco et al., 2004; Horwitz et al.,

2000). In short, it is our firm belief that formal theoretical models will be essential for making substantial progress in understanding how large-scale interactions in a distributed network of specialized neural mechanisms can give rise to the emergent phenomena of executive control. Thus, we hope that the synergistic linkage of modeling and imaging will enable the next decade to become a true "golden age" in the cognitive neuroscience of executive control.

References

Allport, D. A., Styles, E. A., & Hsieh, S. (1994). Shifting intentional set: Exploring the dynamic control of tasks. In C. Umiltà & M. Moscovitch (Eds.), *Conscious and Nonconscious Information Processing: Attention and Performance*, vol. 15, 421–452. New York: Oxford University Press.

Anderson, J. R. (1983). *The Architecture of Cognition.* Cambridge, MA: Harvard University Press.

Anderson, J. R., Qin, Y., Sohn, M. H., Stenger, V. A., & Carter, C. S. (2003). An information-processing model of the BOLD response in symbol manipulation tasks. *Psychonomic Bulletin & Review* 10(2), 241–261.

Aron, A. R., Fletcher, P. C., Bullmore, E. T., Sahakian, B. J., & Robbins, T. W. (2003). Stop-signal inhibition disrupted by damage to right inferior frontal gyrus in humans. *Nature Neuroscience* 6(2), 115–116.

Atkinson, R. C., & Shiffrin, R. M. (1971). The control of short-term memory. *Scientific American* 225, 82–90.

Baddeley, A. (1986). *Working Memory.* New York: Oxford University Press.

Baddeley, A. (1996). Exploring the central executive. *Quarterly Journal of Experimental Psychology* 49(1), 5–28.

Baddeley, A., Emslie, H., Kolodny, J., & Duncan, J. (1998). Random generation and the executive control of working memory. *Quarterly Journal of Experimental Psychology* A51(4), 819–852.

Badre, D., & Wagner, A. D. (2004). Selection, integration, and conflict monitoring: Assessing the nature and generality of prefrontal cognitive control mechanisms. *Neuron* 41(3), 473–487.

Baker, S. C., Rogers, R. D., Owen, A. M., Frith, C. D., Dolan, R. J., Frackowiak, R. S., et al. (1996). Neural systems engaged by planning: A PET study of the Tower of London task. *Neuropsychologia* 34(6), 515–526.

Banich, M. T., Milham, M. P., Atchley, R., Cohen, N. J., Webb, A., Wszalek, T., et al. (2000a). fMRI studies of Stroop tasks reveal unique roles of anterior and posterior brain systems in attentional selection. *Journal of Cognitive Neuroscience* 12(6), 988–1000.

Banich, M. T., Milham, M. P., Atchley, R. A., Cohen, N. J., Webb, A., Wszalek, T., et al. (2000b). Prefrontal regions play a predominant role in imposing an attentional "set": Evidence from fMRI. *Cognitive Brain Research* 10(1–2), 1–9.

Banich, M. T., Milham, M. P., Jacobson, B. L., Webb, A., Wszalek, T., Cohen, N. J., et al. (2001). Attentional selection and the processing of task-irrelevant information: Insights from fMRI examinations of the Stroop task. *Progress in Brain Research* 134, 459–470.

Barch, D. M., Braver, T. S., Akbudak, E., Conturo, T., Ollinger, J., & Snyder, A. (2001). Anterior cingulate cortex and response conflict: Effects of response modality and processing domain. *Cerebral Cortex* 11(9), 837–848.

Barch, D. M., Braver, T. S., Sabb, F. W., & Noll, D. C. (2000). Anterior cingulate and the monitoring of response conflict: Evidence from an fMRI study of overt verb generation. *Journal of Cognitive Neuroscience* 12(2), 298–309.

Beauchamp, M. H., Dagher, A., Aston, J. A., & Doyon, J. (2003). Dynamic functional changes associated with cognitive skill learning of an adapted version of the Tower of London task. *NeuroImage* 20(3), 1649–1660.

Beauregard, M., Levesque, J., & Bourgouin, P. (2001). Neural correlates of conscious self-regulation of emotion. *Journal of Neuroscience* 21(18), RC165.

Berman, K. F., Ostrem, J. L., Randolph, C., Gold, J., Goldberg, T. E., Coppola, R., et al. (1995). Physiological activation of a cortical network during performance of the Wisconsin Card Sorting Test: A positron emission tomography study. *Neuropsychologia* 33(8), 1027–1046.

Botvinick, M., Nystrom, L. E., Fissell, K., Carter, C. S., & Cohen, J. D. (1999). Conflict monitoring versus selection-for-action in anterior cingulate cortex. *Nature* 402(6758), 179–181.

Botvinick, M. M., Braver, T. S., Barch, D. M., Carter, C. S., & Cohen, J. D. (2001). Conflict monitoring and cognitive control. *Psychological Review* 108(3), 624–652.

Brass, M., & von Cramon, D. Y. (2002). The role of the frontal cortex in task preparation. *Cerebral Cortex* 12(9), 908–914.

Braver, T. S., Barch, D. M., Gray, J. R., Molfese, D. L., & Snyder, A. (2001). Anterior cingulate cortex and response conflict: Effects of frequency, inhibition and errors. *Cerebral Cortex* 11(9), 825–836.

Braver, T. S., & Bongiolatti, S. R. (2002). The role of frontopolar cortex in subgoal processing during working memory. *NeuroImage* 15(3), 523–536.

Braver, T. S., Gray, J. R., & Burgess, G. C. (in press). Explaining the many varieties of working memory variation: Dual mechanisms of cognitive control. In A. Conway, C. Jarrold, M. Xaue, A. Miyake, & J. Towse (Eds.), *Variation in Working Memory*. New York: Oxford University Press.

Braver, T. S., & Hoyer, C. M. (2003). *Transient vs. sustained cognitive control during Stroop performance.* Paper presented at the Forty-second Annual Meeting of the Psychonomics Society, Vancouver, B.C.

Braver, T. S., Reynolds, J. R., & Donaldson, D. I. (2003). Neural mechanisms of transient and sustained cognitive control during task switching. *Neuron* 39(4), 713–726.

Brown, J. W., & Braver, T. S. (2005). Learned predictions of error likelihood in the anterior cingulate cortex. *Science* 307(5712), 1118–1121.

Buckner, R. L., Raichle, M. E., & Petersen, S. E. (1995). Dissociation of human prefrontal cortical areas across different speech production tasks and gender groups. *Journal of Neurophysiology* 74(5), 2163–2173.

Bunge, S. A. (2004). How we use rules to select actions: A review of evidence from cognitive neuroscience. *Cognitive, Affective, and Behavioral Neuroscience* 4(4), 564–579.

Bunge, S. A., Kahn, I., Wallis, J. D., Miller, E. K., & Wagner, A. D. (2003). Neural circuits subserving the retrieval and maintenance of abstract rules. *Journal of Neurophysiology* 90(5), 3419–3428.

Bunge, S. A., Klingberg, T., Jacobsen, R. B., & Gabrieli, J. D. (2000). A resource model of the neural basis of executive working memory. *Proceedings of the National Academy of Sciences USA* 97(7), 3573–3578.

Bunge, S. A., Ochsner, K. N., Desmond, J. E., Glover, G. H., & Gabrieli, J. D. (2001). Prefrontal regions involved in keeping information in and out of mind. *Brain* 124(10), 2074–2086.

Bunge, S. A., Wendelken, C., Badre, D., & Wagner, A. D. (2005). Analogical reasoning and prefrontal cortex: Evidence for separable retrieval and integration mechanisms. *Cerebral Cortex.* 15(3), 239–249.

Burgess, P. W., Scott, S. K., & Frith, C. D. (2003). The role of the rostral frontal cortex (area 10) in prospective memory: A lateral versus medial dissociation. *Neuropsychologia* 41(8), 906–918.

Bush, G., Whalen, P. J., Rosen, B. R., Jenike, M. A., McInerney, S. C., & Rauch, S. L. (1998). The counting Stroop: An interference task specialized for functional neuroimaging—validation study with functional MRI. *Human Brain Mapping* 6(4), 270–282.

Carter, C. S., Braver, T. S., Barch, D. M., Botvinick, M. M., Noll, D., & Cohen, J. D. (1998). Anterior cingulate cortex, error detection, and the online monitoring of performance. *Science* 280(5364), 747–749.

Carter, C. S., Macdonald, A. M., Botvinick, M., Ross, L. L., Stenger, V. A., Noll, D., et al. (2000). Parsing executive processes: Strategic vs. evaluative functions of the anterior cingulate cortex. *Proceedings of the National Academy of Sciences USA* 97(4), 1944–1948.

Carter, C. S., Mintun, M., & Cohen, J. D. (1995). Interference and facilitation effects during selective attention: An $H_2^{15}O$ PET study of Stroop task performance. *NeuroImage* 2(4), 264–272.

Carter, C. S., Mintun, M., Nichols, T., & Cohen, J. D. (1997). Anterior cingulate gyrus dysfunction and selective attention deficits in schizophrenia: [^{15}O]H$_2$O PET study during single-trial Stroop task performance. *American Journal of Psychiatry* 154(12), 1670–1675.

Christoff, K., & Gabrieli, J. D. (2000). The frontopolar cortex and human cognition: Evidence for a rostrocaudal hierarchical organization within the human prefrontal cortex. *Psychobiology* 28, 168–186.

Christoff, K., Prabhakaran, V., Dorfman, J., Zhao, Z., Kroger, J. K., Holyoak, K. J., et al. (2001). Rostrolateral prefrontal cortex involvement in relational integration during reasoning. *NeuroImage* 14(5), 1136–1149.

Christoff, K., Ream, J. M., Geddes, L. P., & Gabrieli, J. D. (2003). Evaluating self-generated information: Anterior prefrontal contributions to human cognition. *Behavioral Neuroscience* 117(6), 1161–1168.

Cohen, J. D., Braver, T. S., & O'Reilly, R. C. (1996). A computational approach to prefrontal cortex, cognitive control and schizophrenia: Recent developments and current challenges. *Philosophical Transactions of the Royal Society of London* B351(1346), 1515–1527.

Cohen, J. D., Dunbar, K., & McClelland, J. L. (1990). On the control of automatic processes: A parallel distributed processing account of the Stroop effect. *Psychological Review* 97(3), 332–361.

Cohen, J. D., Perlstein, W. M., Braver, T. S., Nystrom, L. E., Noll, D. C., Jonides, J., et al. (1997). Temporal dynamics of brain activation during a working memory task. *Nature* 386(6625), 604–608.

Collette, F., & Van der Linden, M. (2002). Brain imaging of the central executive component of working memory. *Neuroscience and Biobehavioral Reviews* 26(2), 105–125.

Compton, R. J., Banich, M. T., Mohanty, A., Milham, M. P., Herrington, J., Miller, G. A., et al. (2003). Paying attention to emotion: An fMRI investigation of cognitive and emotional Stroop tasks. *Cognitive, Affective, and Behavioral Neuroscience* 3(2), 81–96.

Cools, R., Clark, L., Owen, A. M., & Robbins, T. W. (2002). Defining the neural mechanisms of probabilistic reversal learning using event-related functional magnetic resonance imaging. *Journal of Neuroscience* 22(11), 4563–4567.

Corbetta, M., Kincade, J. M., Ollinger, J. M., McAvoy, M. P., & Shulman, G. L. (2000). Voluntary orienting is dissociated from target detection in human posterior parietal cortex. *Nature Neuroscience* 3, 292–297.

Curtis, C. E., & D'Esposito, M. (2003). Success and failure suppressing reflexive behavior. *Journal of Cognitive Neuroscience* 15(3), 409–418.

Daniels, C., Witt, K., Wolff, S., Jansen, O., & Deuschl, G. (2003). Rate dependency of the human cortical network subserving executive functions during generation of random number series—a functional magnetic resonance imaging study. *Neuroscience Letters* 345(1), 25–28.

D'Esposito, M., Aguirre, G. K., Zarahn, E., Ballard, D., Shin, R. K., & Lease, J. (1998). Functional MRI studies of spatial and nonspatial working memory. *Cognitive Brain Research* 7(1), 1–13.

D'Esposito, M., Detre, J. A., Alsop, D. C., Shin, R. K., Atlas, S., & Grossman, M. (1995). The neural basis of the central executive system of working memory. *Nature* 378(6554), 279–281.

Deco, G., Rolls, E. T., & Horwitz, B. (2004). "What" and "where" in visual working memory: A computational neurodynamical perspective for integrating fMRI and single-neuron data. *Journal of Cognitive Neuroscience* 16(4), 683–701.

Dehaene, S., Kerszberg, M., & Changeux, J. P. (1998). A neuronal model of a global workspace in effortful cognitive tasks. *Proceedings of the National Academy of Sciences USA* 95(24), 14529–14534.

Dehaene, S., Posner, M. I., & Tucker, D. M. (1994). Localization of a neural system for error detection and compensation. *Psychological Science* 5(5), 303–306.

Derrfuss, J., Brass, M., & von Cramon, D. Y. (2004). Cognitive control in the posterior frontolateral cortex: Evidence from common activations in task coordination, interference control, and working memory. *NeuroImage* 23(2), 604–612.

Desimone, R., & Duncan, J. (1995). Neural mechanisms of selective visual attention. *Annual Review of Neuroscience* 18, 193–222.

Desmond, J. E., Gabrieli, J. D., & Glover, G. H. (1998). Dissociation of frontal and cerebellar activity in a cognitive task: Evidence for a distinction between selection and search. *NeuroImage* 7(4, pt. 1), 368–376.

DeSouza, J. F., Menon, R. S., & Everling, S. (2003). Preparatory set associated with pro-saccades and anti-saccades in humans investigated with event-related fMRI. *Journal of Neurophysiology* 89(2), 1016–1023.

Dobbins, I. G., Rice, H. J., Wagner, A. D., & Schacter, D. L. (2003). Memory orientation and success: Separable neurocognitive components underlying episodic recognition. *Neuropsychologia* 41(3), 318–333.

Dorris, M. C., Pare, M., & Munoz, D. P. (1997). Neuronal activity in monkey superior colliculus related to the initiation of saccadic eye movements. *Journal of Neuroscience* 17(21), 8566–8579.

Dove, A., Pollmann, S., Schubert, T., Wiggins, C. J., & von Cramon, D. Y. (2000). Prefrontal cortex activation in task switching: An event-related fMRI study. *Cognitive Brain Research* 9(1), 103–109.

Dreher, J. C., & Berman, K. F. (2002). Fractionating the neural substrate of cognitive control processes. *Proceedings of the National Academy of Sciences USA* 99(22), 14595–14600.

Dreher, J. C., Koechlin, E., Ali, S. O., & Grafman, J. (2002). The roles of timing and task order during task switching. *NeuroImage* 17(1), 95–109.

Duncan, J., & Owen, A. M. (2000). Common regions of the human frontal lobe recruited by diverse cognitive demands. *Trends in Neurosciences* 23(10), 475–483.

Durston, S., Davidson, M. C., Thomas, K. M., Worden, M. S., Tottenham, N., Martinez, A., et al. (2003). Parametric manipulation of conflict and response competition using rapid mixed-trial event-related fMRI. *NeuroImage* 20(4), 2135–2141.

Durston, S., Thomas, K. M., Worden, M. S., Yang, Y., & Casey, B. J. (2002). The effect of preceding context on inhibition: An event-related fMRI study. *NeuroImage* 16(2), 449–453.

Duzel, E., Picton, T. W., Cabeza, R., Yonelinas, A. P., Scheich, H., Heinze, H. J., et al. (2001). Comparative electrophysiological and hemodynamic measures of neural activation during memory-retrieval. *Human Brain Mapping* 13(2), 104–123.

Elliott, R., Friston, K. J., & Dolan, R. J. (2000). Dissociable neural responses in human reward systems. *Journal of Neuroscience* 20(16), 6159–6165.

Falkenstein, M., Hohnsbein, J., Hoormann, J., & Blanke, L. (1990). Effects of errors in choice reaction tasks on the ERP under focused and divided attention. In C. H. M. Brunia, A. W. K. Gaillard, & A. Kok (Eds.), *Psychophysiological Brain Research* 192–195. Tilburg, The Netherlands: Tilburg University Press.

Fincham, J. M., Carter, C. S., van Veen, V., Stenger, V. A., & Anderson, J. R. (2002). Neural mechanisms of planning: A computational analysis using event-related fMRI. *Proceedings of the National Academy of Sciences USA* 99(5), 3346–3351.

Fletcher, P. C., & Henson, R. N. (2001). Frontal lobes and human memory: Insights from functional neuroimaging. *Brain* 124(5), 849–881.

Fletcher, P. C., Shallice, T., & Dolan, R. J. (2000). "Sculpting the response space"—an account of left prefrontal activation at encoding. *NeuroImage* 12(4), 404–417.

Frith, C. D., Friston, K., Liddle, P. F., & Frackowiak, R. S. (1991). Willed action and the prefrontal cortex in man: A study with PET. *Proceedings of the Royal Society of London* B244(1311), 241–246.

Fuster, J. M. (1989). *The Prefrontal Cortex*, 2nd ed. New York: Raven Press.

Garavan, H., Ross, T. J., Kaufman, J., & Stein, E. A. (2003). A midline dissociation between error-processing and response-conflict monitoring. *NeuroImage* 20(2), 1132–1139.

Garavan, H., Ross, T. J., Li, S. J., & Stein, E. A. (2000). A parametric manipulation of central executive functioning. *Cerebral Cortex* 10(6), 585–592.

Garavan, H., Ross, T. J., Murphy, K., Roche, R. A., & Stein, E. A. (2002). Dissociable executive functions in the dynamic control of behavior: Inhibition, error detection, and correction. *NeuroImage* 17(4), 1820–1829.

Garavan, H., Ross, T. J., & Stein, E. A. (1999). Right hemispheric dominance of inhibitory control: An event-related functional MRI study. *Proceedings of the National Academy of Sciences USA* 96(14), 8301–8306.

Gehring, W. J., Goss, B., Coles, M. G. H., Meyer, D. E., & Donchin, E. (1993). A neural system for error detection and compensation. *Psychological Science* 4, 385–390.

Gehring, W. J., & Knight, R. T. (2000). Prefrontal-cingulate interactions in action monitoring. *Nature Neuroscience* 3, 516–520.

Glabus, M. F., Horwitz, B., Holt, J. L., Kohn, P. D., Gerton, B. K., Callicott, J. H., et al. (2003). Interindividual differences in functional interactions among prefrontal, parietal and parahippocampal regions during working memory. *Cerebral Cortex* 13(12), 1352–1361.

Glahn, D. C., Kim, J., Cohen, M. S., Poutanen, V. P., Therman, S., Bava, S., et al. (2002). Maintenance and manipulation in spatial working memory: Dissociations in the prefrontal cortex. *NeuroImage* 17(1), 201–213.

Goel, V. (in press). Cognitive neuroscience of deductive reasoning. In K. Holyoak & R. Morrison (Eds.), *Cambridge Handbook of Thinking & Reasoning.* New York: Cambridge University Press.

Goel, V., & Dolan, R. J. (2004). Differential involvement of left prefrontal cortex in inductive and deductive reasoning. *Cognition* 93(3), B109–121.

Goel, V., Gold, B., Kapur, S., & Houle, S. (1997). The seats of reason? An imaging study of deductive and inductive reasoning. *NeuroReport* 8(5), 1305–1310.

Goldman-Rakic, P. S. (1987). Circuitry of the prefrontal cortex and the regulation of behavior by representational memory. In F. Plum & V. Mountcastle (Eds.), *Handbook of Physiology, sec. 1, The Nervous System,* vol. 5, *Higher Functions of the Brain,* 373–417. Bethesda, MD: American Physiological Society.

Grady, C. L., McIntosh, A. R., & Craik, F. I. (2003). Age-related differences in the functional connectivity of the hippocampus during memory encoding. *Hippocampus* 13(5), 572–586.

Gray, J. R., & Braver, T. S. (2002). Personality predicts working-memory-related activation in the caudal anterior cingulate cortex. *Cognitive, Affective, and Behavioral Neuroscience* 2(1), 64–75.

Gray, J. R., Braver, T. S., & Raichle, M. E. (2002). Integration of emotion and cognition in the lateral prefrontal cortex. *Proceedings of the National Academy of Sciences USA* 99(6), 4115–4120.

Gray, J. R., Burgess, G. C., Schaefer, A., Yarkoni, T., Larsen, R. L., & Braver, T. S. (2005). Personality differences in neural processing efficiency revealed using fMRI. *Cognitive, Affective, and Behavioral Neuroscience,* 5, 182–190.

Gray, J. R., Chabris, C. F., & Braver, T. S. (2003). Neural mechanisms of general fluid intelligence. *Nature Neuroscience* 6(3), 316–322.

Guitton, D., Buchtel, H. A., & Douglas, R. M. (1985). Frontal lobe lesions in man cause difficulties in suppressing reflexive glances and in generating goal-directed saccades. *Experimental Brain Research* 58, 455–472.

Harlow, J. M. (1848). Passage of an iron bar through the head. *Boston Medical and Surgical Journal* 39, 389–393.

Herath, P., Klingberg, T., Young, J., Amunts, K., & Roland, P. (2001). Neural correlates of dual task interference can be dissociated from those of divided attention: An fMRI study. *Cerebral Cortex* 11(9), 796–805.

Hester, R. L., Murphy, K., Foxe, J. J., Foxe, D. M., Javitt, D. C., & Garavan, H. (2004). Predicting success: Patterns of cortical activation and deactivation prior to response inhibition. *Journal of Cognitive Neuroscience* 16(5), 776–785.

Holroyd, C. B., & Coles, M. G. (2002). The neural basis of human error processing: Reinforcement learning, dopamine, and the error-related negativity. *Psychological Review* 109(4), 679–709.

Holroyd, C. B., Nieuwenhuis, S., Yeung, N., Nystrom, L., Mars, R. B., Coles, M. G., et al. (2004). Dorsal anterior cingulate cortex shows fMRI response to internal and external error signals. *Nature Neuroscience* 7(5), 497–498.

Horwitz, B., Friston, K. J., & Taylor, J. G. (2000). Neural modeling and functional brain imaging: An overview. *Neural Networks* 13(8–9), 829–846.

Huettel, S. A., Mack, P. B., & McCarthy, G. (2002). Perceiving patterns in random series: Dynamic processing of sequence in prefrontal cortex. *Nature Neuroscience* 5(5), 485–490.

Iidaka, T., Anderson, N. D., Kapur, S., Cabeza, R., & Craik, F. I. (2000). The effect of divided attention on encoding and retrieval in episodic memory revealed by positron emission tomography. *Journal of Cognitive Neuroscience* 12(2), 267–280.

Jacobsen, C. E. (1935). Functions of the frontal association area in primates. *Archives of Neurological Psychiatry* 33, 558–569.

Jahanshahi, M., & Dirnberger, G. (1999). The left dorsolateral prefrontal cortex and random generation of responses: Studies with transcranial magnetic stimulation. *Neuropsychologia* 37(2), 181–190.

Jahanshahi, M., Profice, P., Brown, R. G., Ridding, M. C., Dirnberger, G., & Rothwell, J. C. (1998). The effects of transcranial magnetic stimulation over the dorsolateral prefrontal cortex on suppression of habitual counting during random number generation. *Brain* 121(8), 1533–1544.

Jiang, Y., & Kanwisher, N. (2003). Common neural mechanisms for response selection and perceptual processing. *Journal of Cognitive Neuroscience* 15(8), 1095–1110.

Jones, A. D., Cho, R. Y., Nystrom, L. E., Cohen, J. D., & Braver, T. S. (2002). A computational model of anterior cingulate function in speeded response tasks: Effects of frequency, sequence, and conflict. *Cognitive, Affective, and Behavioral Neuroscience* 2(4), 300–317.

Jonides, J., Badre, D., Curtis, C., Thompson-Schill, S. L., & Smith, E. E. (2002). Mechanisms of conflict resolution in prefrontal cortex. In D. T. Stuss & R. T. Knight (Eds.), *Principles of Frontal Lobe Function*, 233–245. New York: Oxford University Press.

Jonides, J., Smith, E. E., Marshuetz, C., Koeppe, R. A., & Reuter-Lorenz, P. A. (1998). Inhibition in verbal working memory revealed by brain activation. *Proceedings of the National Academy of Sciences USA* 95(14), 8410–8413.

Just, M. A., Carpenter, P. A., Keller, T. A., Emery, L., Zajac, H., & Thulborn, K. R. (2001). Interdependence of nonoverlapping cortical systems in dual cognitive tasks. *NeuroImage* 14(2), 417–426.

Kensinger, E. A., Clarke, R. J., & Corkin, S. (2003). What neural correlates underlie successful encoding and retrieval? A functional magnetic resonance imaging study using a divided attention paradigm. *Journal of Neuroscience* 23(6), 2407–2415.

Kerns, J. G., Cohen, J. D., MacDonald, A. W. III, Cho, R. Y., Stenger, V. A., & Carter, C. S. (2004). Anterior cingulate conflict monitoring and adjustments in control. *Science* 303(5660), 1023–1026.

Kiehl, K. A., Liddle, P. F., & Hopfinger, J. B. (2000). Error processing and the rostral anterior cingulate: An event-related fMRI study. *Psychophysiology* 37(2), 216–223.

Kimberg, D. Y., Aguirre, G. K., & D'Esposito, M. (2000). Modulation of task-related neural activity in task-switching: An fMRI study. *Cognitive Brain Research* 10(1–2), 189–196.

Klingberg, T., & Roland, P. E. (1997). Interference between two concurrent tasks is associated with activation of overlapping fields in the cortex. *Cognitive Brain Research* 6(1), 1–8.

Knauff, M., Fangmeier, T., Ruff, C. C., & Johnson-Laird, P. N. (2003). Reasoning, models, and images: Behavioral measures and cortical activity. *Journal of Cognitive Neuroscience* 15(4), 559–573.

Koechlin, E., Basso, G., Pietrini, P., Panzer, S., & Grafman, J. (1999). The role of the anterior prefrontal cortex in human cognition. *Nature* 399(6732), 148–151.

Konishi, S., Jimura, K., Asari, T., & Miyashita, Y. (2003). Transient activation of superior prefrontal cortex during inhibition of cognitive set. *Journal of Neuroscience* 23(21), 7776–7782.

Konishi, S., Kawazu, M., Uchida, I., Kikyo, H., Asakura, I., & Miyashita, Y. (1999). Contribution of working memory to transient activation in human inferior prefrontal cortex during performance of the Wisconsin Card Sorting Test. *Cerebral Cortex* 9(7), 745–753.

Konishi, S., Nakajima, K., Uchida, I., Kameyama, M., Nakahara, K., Sekihara, K., et al. (1998). Transient activation of inferior prefrontal cortex during cognitive set shifting. *Nature Neuroscience* 1(1), 80–84.

Konishi, S., Nakajima, K., Uchida, I., Sekihara, K., & Miyashita, Y. (1998). No-go dominant brain activity in human inferior prefrontal cortex revealed by functional magnetic resonance imaging. *European Journal of Neuroscience* 10(3), 1209–1213.

Konishi, S., Uchida, I., Okuaki, T., Machida, T., Shirouzu, I., & Miyashita, Y. (2002). Neural correlates of recency judgment. *Journal of Neuroscience* 22(21), 9549–9555.

Kornblum, S., Hasbroucq, T., & Osman, A. (1990). Dimensional overlap: Cognitive basis for stimulus-response compatibility—a model and taxonomy. *Psychological Review* 97(2), 253–270.

Krawczyk, D. C. (2002). Contributions of the prefrontal cortex to the neural basis of human decision making. *Neuroscience and Biobehavioral Reviews* 26(6), 631–664.

Kroger, J. K., Sabb, F. W., Fales, C. L., Bookheimer, S. Y., Cohen, M. S., & Holyoak, K. J. (2002). Recruitment of anterior dorsolateral prefrontal cortex in human reasoning: A parametric study of relational complexity. *Cerebral Cortex* 12(5), 477–485.

Laming, D. (1979). Choice reaction performance following an error. *Acta Psychologica* 43, 199–224.

Lau, H. C., Rogers, R. D., Ramnani, N., & Passingham, R. E. (2004). Willed action and attention to the selection of action. *NeuroImage* 21(4), 1407–1415.

Lepage, M., Ghaffar, O., Nyberg, L., & Tulving, E. (2000). Prefrontal cortex and episodic memory retrieval mode. *Proceedings of the National Academy of Sciences USA* 97(1), 506–511.

Leung, H. C., Skudlarski, P., Gatenby, J. C., Peterson, B. S., & Gore, J. C. (2000). An event-related functional MRI study of the Stroop color-word interference task. *Cerebral Cortex* 10(6), 552–560.

Liddle, P. F., Kiehl, K. A., & Smith, A. M. (2001). Event-related fMRI study of response inhibition. *Human Brain Mapping* 12(2), 100–109.

Logan, G. D. (1994). On the ability to inhibit thought and action: A user's guide to the stop signal paradigm. In D. Dagebach & T. H. Carr (Eds.), *Inhibitory Processes in Attention, Memory, and Language*, 189–239. San Diego: Academic Press.

Luria, A. R. (1966). *Higher Cortical Functions in Man.* London: Tavistock.

MacDonald, A. W. III, Cohen, J. D., Stenger, V. A., & Carter, C. S. (2000). Dissociating the role of the dorsolateral prefrontal and anterior cingulate cortex in cognitive control. *Science* 288(5472), 1835–1838.

Macmillan, M. (2000). Restoring Phineas Gage: A 150th retrospective. *Journal of the History of the Neurosciences* 9(1), 46–66.

Maril, A., Wagner, A. D., & Schacter, D. L. (2001). On the tip of the tongue: An event-related fMRI study of semantic retrieval failure and cognitive conflict. *Neuron* 31(4), 653–660.

Meiran, N. (1996). Reconfiguration of processing mode prior to task performance. *Journal of Experimental Psychology: Leraning, Memory, and Cognition* 22, 1423–1442.

Menon, V., Adleman, N. E., White, C. D., Glover, G. H., & Reiss, A. L. (2001). Error-related brain activation during a Go/NoGo response inhibition task. *Human Brain Mapping* 12(3), 131–143.

Meyer, D. E., & Kieras, D. E. (1997). A Computational Theory of Executive Cognitive Processes and Multiple-Task Performance, Part I Basic Mechanisms. *Psychological Review* 104(1), 3–65.

Milham, M. P., Banich, M. T., & Barad, V. (2003). Competition for priority in processing increases prefrontal cortex's involvement in top-down control: An event-related fMRI study of the Stroop task. *Cognitive Brain Research* 17(2), 212–222.

Milham, M. P., Banich, M. T., Webb, A., Barad, V., Cohen, N. J., Wszalek, T., et al. (2001). The relative involvement of anterior cingulate and prefrontal cortex in attentional control depends on nature of conflict. *Cognitive Brain Research* 12(3), 467–473.

Miller, E. K., & Cohen, J. D. (2001). An integrative theory of prefrontal cortex function. *Annual Review of Neuroscience* 24, 167–202.

Miller, E. K., Erickson, C. A., & Desimone, R. (1996). Neural mechanisms of visual working memory in prefrontal cortex of the macaque. *Journal of Neuroscience* 16, 5154–5167.

Miller, G. A., Galanter, E., & Pribram, K. H. (1960). *Plans and the Structure of Behavior.* New York: Holt, Rinehart and Winston.

Milner, B. (1963). Effects of different brain lesions on card sorting. *Archives of Neurology* 9, 90–100.

Miltner, W. H. R., Braun, C. H., & Coles, M. G. H. (1997). Event-related brain potentials following incorrect feedback in a time-estimation task: Evidence for a "generic" neural system for error-detection. *Journal of Cognitive Neuroscience* 9, 788–798.

Miyake, A., Friedman, N. P., Emerson, M. J., Witzki, A. H., Howerter, A., & Wager, T. D. (2000). The unity and diversity of executive functions and their contributions to complex "frontal lobe" tasks: A latent variable analysis. *Cognitive Psychology* 41, 49–100.

Monchi, O., Petrides, M., Petre, V., Worsley, K., & Dagher, A. (2001). Wisconsin Card Sorting revisited: Distinct neural circuits participating in different stages of the task identified by event-related functional magnetic resonance imaging. *Journal of Neuroscience* 21(19), 7733–7741.

Monsell, S., & Driver, J., eds. (2000). *Control of Cognitive Processes*, vol. 18. Cambridge, MA: MIT Press.

Moscovitch, M. (1992). Memory and working-with-memory: A component process model based on modules and central systems. *Journal of Cognitive Neuroscience* 4, 257–267.

Nelson, J. K., Reuter-Lorenz, P. A., Sylvester, C. Y., Jonides, J., & Smith, E. E. (2003). Dissociable neural mechanisms underlying response-based and familiarity-based conflict in working memory. *Proceedings of the National Academy of Sciences USA* 100(19), 11171–11175.

Newell, A. (1990). *Unified Theories of Cognition* New York: Cambridge University Press.

Newman, S. D., Carpenter, P. A., Varma, S., & Just, M. A. (2003). Frontal and parietal participation in problem solving in the Tower of London: fMRI and computational modeling of planning and high-level perception. *Neuropsychologia* 41(12), 1668–1682.

Norman, D. A., & Shallice, T. (1986). Attention to action: Willed and automatic control of behavior. In R. J. Davidson, G. E. Schwartz, & D. Shapiro (Eds.), *Consciousness and Self-regulation*, vol. 4, 1–18. New York: Plenum Press.

Nyberg, L., & McIntosh, A. R. (2001). Functional neuroimaging: Network analyses. In R. Cabeza & A. Kingstone (Eds.), *Handbook of Functional Neuroimaging of Cognition*, 49–72. Cambridge, MA: MIT Press.

O'Doherty, J., Critchley, H., Deichmann, R., & Dolan, R. J. (2003). Dissociating valence of outcome from behavioral control in human orbital and ventral prefrontal cortices. *Journal of Neuroscience* 23(21), 7931–7939.

O'Doherty, J., Kringelbach, M. L., Rolls, E. T., Hornak, J., & Andrews, C. (2001). Abstract reward and punishment representations in the human orbitofrontal cortex. *Nature Neuroscience* 4(1), 95–102.

O'Doherty, J. P., Dayan, P., Friston, K., Critchley, H., & Dolan, R. J. (2003). Temporal difference models and reward-related learning in the human brain. *Neuron* 38(2), 329–337.

Ochsner, K. N., Bunge, S. A., Gross, J. J., & Gabrieli, J. D. E. (2002). Rethinking feelings: An fMRI study of the cognitive regulation of emotion. *Journal of Cognitive Neuroscience* 14(8), 1215–1229.

Pardo, J. V., Pardo, P. J., Janer, K. W., & Raichle, M. E. (1990). The anterior cingulate cortex mediates processing selection in the Stroop attentional conflict paradigm. *Proceedings of the National Academy of Sciences USA* 87(1), 256–259.

Pashler, H. (1994). Dual-Task Interference in Simple Tasks: Data and Theory. *Psychological Bulletin* 116(2), 220–244.

Penny, W. D., Stephan, K. E., Mechelli, A., & Friston, K. J. (2004). Modelling functional integration: A comparison of structural equation and dynamic causal models. *NeuroImage* 23(supp. 1), S264–S274.

Petersen, S. E., Fox, P. T., Posner, M. I., Mintun, M., & Raichle, M. E. (1989). Positron emission tomographic studies of the processing of single words. *Journal of Cognitive Neuroscience* 1(2), 153–170.

Peterson, B. S., Kane, M. J., Alexander, G. M., Lacadie, C., Skudlarski, P., Leung, H. C., et al. (2002). An event-related functional MRI study comparing interference effects in the Simon and Stroop tasks. *Cognitive Brain Research* 13(3), 427–440.

Petrides, M., Alivisatos, B., Meyer, E., & Evans, A. C. (1993). Functional activation of the human frontal cortex during the performance of verbal working memory tasks. *Proceedings of the National Academy of Sciences USA* 90(3), 878–882.

Pochon, J. B., Levy, R., Fossati, P., Lehericy, S., Poline, J. B., Pillon, B., et al. (2002). The neural system that bridges reward and cognition in humans: An fMRI study. *Proceedings of the National Academy of Sciences USA* 99(8), 5669–5674.

Poldrack, R. A., Wagner, A. D., Prull, M. W., Desmond, J. E., Glover, G. H., & Gabrieli, J. D. E. (1999). Functional specialization for semantic and phonological processing in the left inferior prefrontal cortex. *NeuroImage* 10(1), 15–35.

Pollman, S. (2001). Switching between dimensions, locations, and responses: The role of the left fronto-polar cortex. *Journal of Cognitive Neuroscience* 14, S118-S124.

Posner, M. I., Petersen, S. E., Fox, P. T., & Raichle, M. E. (1988). Localization of cognitive operations in the human brain. *Science* 240, 1627–1631.

Postle, B. R., Berger, J. S., & D'Esposito, M. (1999). Functional neuroanatomical double dissociation of mnemonic and executive control processes contributing to working memory performance. *Proceedings of the National Academy of Sciences USA* 96(22), 12959–12964.

Prabhakaran, V., Narayanan, K., Zhao, Z., & Gabrieli, J. D. (2000). Integration of diverse information in working memory within the frontal lobe. *Nature Neuroscience* 3(1), 85–90.

Prabhakaran, V., Smith, J. A., Desmond, J. E., Glover, G. H., & Gabrieli, J. D. (1997). Neural substrates of fluid reasoning: An fMRI study of neocortical activation during performance of the Raven's Progressive Matrices Test. *Cognitive Psychology* 33(1), 43–63.

Ramnani, N., & Owen, A. M. (2004). Anterior prefrontal cortex: Insights into function from anatomy and neuroimaging. *Nature Reviews Neuroscience* 5(3), 184–194.

Ranganath, C., Johnson, M. K., & D'Esposito, M. (2000). Left anterior prefrontal activation increases with demands to recall specific perceptual information. *Journal of Neuroscience* 20(22), RC108.

Reynolds, J. R., Donaldson, D. I., Wagner, A. D., & Braver, T. S. (2004). Item- and task-level processes in the left inferior prefrontal cortex: Positive and negative correlates of encoding. *NeuroImage* 21(4), 1472–1483.

Ridderinkhof, K. R., Ullsperger, M., Crone, E. A., & Nieuwenhuis, S. (2004). The role of the medial frontal cortex in cognitive control. *Science* 306(5695), 443–447.

Rolls, E. T. (2000). The orbitofrontal cortex and reward. *Cerebral Cortex* 10(3), 284–294.

Rowe, J., Friston, K., Frackowiak, R., & Passingham, R. (2002). Attention to action: Specific modulation of corticocortical interactions in humans. *NeuroImage* 17(2), 988–998.

Rowe, J. B., Toni, I., Josephs, O., Frackowiak, R. S., & Passingham, R. E. (2000). The prefrontal cortex: Response selection or maintenance within working memory? *Science* 288(5471), 1656–1660.

Rubia, K., Smith, A. B., Brammer, M. J., & Taylor, E. (2003). Right inferior prefrontal cortex mediates response inhibition while mesial prefrontal cortex is responsible for error detection. *NeuroImage* 20(1), 351–358.

Ruge, H., Brass, M., Koch, I., Rubin, O., Meiran, N., & von Cramon, D. Y. (2005). Advance preparation and stimulus-induced interference in cued task switching: Further insights from BOLD fMRI. *Neuropsychologia* 43(3), 340–355.

Rushworth, M. F., Hadland, K. A., Paus, T., & Sipila, P. K. (2002). Role of the human medial frontal cortex in task switching: A combined fMRI and TMS study. *Journal of Neurophysiology* 87(5), 2577–2592.

Sakai, K., Rowe, J. B., & Passingham, R. E. (2002). Active maintenance in prefrontal area 46 creates distractor-resistant memory. *Nature Neuroscience* 5(5), 479–484.

Shimamura, A. P. (1995). Memory and frontal lobe function. In M. S. Gazzaniga (Ed.), *The Cognitive Neurosciences*, 803–813. Cambridge, MA: MIT Press.

Shimamura, A. P. (2000). Toward a cognitive neuroscience of metacognition. *Consciousness and Cognition* 9(2, pt. 1), 313–323; discussion 324–326.

Smith, E. E., & Jonides, J. (1999). Storage and executive processes in the frontal lobes. *Science* 283(5408), 1657–1661.

Smith, E. E., Jonides, J., Koeppe, R. A., Awh, E., Schumacher, E. H., & Minoshima, S. (1995). Spatial versus object working memory: PET investigations. *Journal of Cognitive Neuroscience* 7(3), 337–356.

Sohn, M. H., Ursu, S., Anderson, J. R., Stenger, V. A., & Carter, C. S. (2000). Inaugural article: The role of prefrontal cortex and posterior parietal cortex in task switching. *Proceedings of the National Academy of Sciences USA* 97(24), 13448–13453.

Sweeney, J. A., Mintun, M. A., Kwee, S., Wiseman, M. B., Brown, D. L., Rosenberg, D. R., et al. (1996). Positron emission tomography study of voluntary saccadic eye movements and spatial working memory. *Journal of Neurophysiology* 75(1), 454–468.

Swick, D., & Turken, A. U. (2002). Dissociation between conflict detection and error monitoring in the human anterior cingulate cortex. *Proceedings of the National Academy of Sciences USA* 99(25), 16354–16359.

Szameitat, A. J., Schubert, T., Muller, K., & von Cramon, D. Y. (2002). Localization of executive functions in dual-task performance with fMRI. *Journal of Cognitive Neuroscience* 14(8), 1184–1199.

Taylor, S. F., Welsh, R. C., Wager, T. D., Phan, K. L., Fitzgerald, K. D., & Gehring, W. J. (2004). A functional neuroimaging study of motivation and executive function. *NeuroImage* 21(3), 1045–1054.

Thompson-Schill, S. L., D'Esposito, M., Aguirre, G. K., & Farah, M. J. (1997). Role of left inferior prefrontal cortex in retrieval of semantic knowledge: A reevaluation. *Proceedings of the National Academy of Sciences USA* 94(26), 14792–14797.

Ullsperger, M., & von Cramon, D. Y. (2001). Subprocesses of performance monitoring: A dissociation of error processing and response competition revealed by event-related fMRI and ERPs. *NeuroImage* 14(6), 1387–1401.

van den Heuvel, O. A., Groenewegen, H. J., Barkhof, F., Lazeron, R. H., van Dyck, R., & Veltman, D. J. (2003). Frontostriatal system in planning complexity: A parametric functional magnetic resonance version of Tower of London task. *NeuroImage* 18(2), 367–374.

van Veen, V., Cohen, J. D., Botvinick, M. M., Stenger, V. A., & Carter, C. S. (2001). Anterior cingulate cortex, conflict monitoring, and levels of processing. *NeuroImage* 14(6), 1302–1308.

Velanova, K., Jacoby, L. L., Wheeler, M. E., McAvoy, M. P., Petersen, S. E., & Buckner, R. L. (2003). Functional-anatomic correlates of sustained and transient processing components engaged during controlled retrieval. *Journal of Neuroscience* 23(24), 8460–8470.

Veltman, D. J., Rombouts, S. A., & Dolan, R. J. (2003). Maintenance versus manipulation in verbal working memory revisited: An fMRI study. *NeuroImage* 18(2), 247–256.

Wager, T. D., Jonides, J., & Reading, S. (2004). Neuroimaging studies of shifting attention: A meta-analysis. *NeuroImage* 22(4), 1679–1693.

Wagner, A. D., Pare-Blagoev, E. J., Clark, J., & Poldrack, R. A. (2001). Recovering meaning: Left prefrontal cortex guides controlled semantic retrieval. *Neuron* 31(2), 329–338.

Wagner, A. D., Schacter, D. L., Rotte, M., Koutstaal, W., Maril, A., Dale, A. M., et al. (1998). Building memories: Remembering and forgetting of verbal experiences as predicted by brain activity. *Science* 281(5380), 1188–1191.

Walton, M. E., Devlin, J. T., & Rushworth, M. F. (2004). Interactions between decision making and performance monitoring within prefrontal cortex. *Nature Neuroscience* 7, 1259–1265.

Welford, A. T. (1952). The "Psychological Refractory Period" and the Timing of High-Speed Performance—a Review and a Theory. *British Journal of Psychology* 43, 2–19.

III DEVELOPMENTAL, SOCIAL, AND CLINICAL APPLICATIONS

11

Functional Neuroimaging of Early Cognitive Development

Gaia Scerif, Eleni Kotsoni, and B. J. Casey

Introduction

Integrating our knowledge of the normal functional anatomy in the adult with that of the developing brain is a basic objective of developmental neuroscience because it enables a mechanistic understanding of how functional circuits become established over time. It also provides a framework in which neurodevelopmental disorders can be studied in terms of the atypical developmental trajectories that they impose on brain development. Imaging techniques discussed in the current volume provide converging sources of information on the neural correlates of *adult* cognitive processes. However, progress in these technologies has offered tools to study changes in functional brain specialization during early development. The various imaging techniques differ in terms of relative spatial and temporal resolution, depth of recording, relative invasiveness, expense, and ease of use with developmental populations. Thus, only a small number of them are currently being used to investigate the neural bases of development across cognitive domains, from acoustic and phonemic processing, to the processing of faces, to the development of literacy and numeracy, to improvements in attentional and inhibitory control. We refer the reader to Casey and de Haan (2002) and Casey and Munakata (2002) for recent articles reviewing these findings in detail for specific cognitive domains.

This chapter focuses on two techniques (functional magnetic resonance imaging and event-related potentials) that have been most commonly used to study processes of neurocognitive development across the life span. An overview of these techniques and their methodological challenges is presented, together with currently available solutions. Second, we discuss how the combination of the two methods may provide unique information on developmental changes in brain function, pointing out some of the difficulties facing their full integration. Future directions including the combination of these techniques and others will complement our current understanding of the development of distributed neural networks involved in cognitive processes.

Functional Neuroimaging of Early Cognitive Development

Both event-related brain potentials (ERPs) and functional magnetic resonance imaging (fMRI) have been applied to neurodevelopmental questions. Although both techniques measure functional brain activation, they are not identical because each reflects different aspects of neuronal function at a physiological level: ERPs provide a remote measurement of the electric potential generated by neuronal activity, and fMRI measures slower changes in blood oxygenation secondary to neuronal activity. They also ask distinct but complementary questions of brain functional specialization in the adult: fMRI focuses on localization, and ERP on fast temporal processing. Within a developmental context, the former is more appropriate in identifying structures or circuits involved in cognition through development, while the latter is very powerful in outlining the temporal sequence of processes implementing cognitive functions across age groups. We provide a brief description of each method and illustrate the challenges facing their application to the study of development.

Functional Magnetic Resonance Imaging

fMRI is based on the assumption that regional changes in neural activity are associated with magnetic differences between oxygenated and deoxygenated blood (Ogawa et al., 1992; Kwong et al., 1992). In short, fMRI measures a blood-oxygenation-level-dependent (BOLD) response, which reflect, among other things, the concentration of deoxygenated hemoglobin, blood flow, and blood volume. More specifically, this technique relies on the observation that hemoglobin becomes strongly paramagnetic in its deoxygenated state and therefore can be used as a naturally occurring contrast agent; highly oxygenated brain regions produce a larger magnetic resonance (MR) signal than less oxygenated areas. It is assumed that maps of the MR signal intensity reflect changes in neuronal activity during the activated state. However, this hemodynamic change is not instantaneous; rather, it is temporally delayed by approximately 6 sec following the activation or presentation of the stimulus. With the development of new experimental designs such as event-related or selective trial averaging, it has been possible to measure activation over events just 2 sec apart (Rosen et al., 1998). This has increased the versatility of the technique and expanded the possibilities for experimental applications, but the temporal resolution of fMRI remains considerably inferior to the millisecond accuracy of ERPs. fMRI, however, has better spatial resolution than ERP, typically on the order of

2–4 mm in plane. It is therefore advantageous when assessing developmental changes in the functioning of small or deep subcortical structures such as the amygdala and the basal ganglia.

With its lack of need for ionizing radiation or exogenous contrast agents, functional magnetic resonance imaging provides an excellent tool for testing how cognitive and neural processes develop. However, due to both the technical difficulties reviewed below and its relatively greater perceived invasiveness (e.g., elevated noise levels, reliance on an enclosed testing environment), magnetic resonance imaging has been used less for research in infants and very young children than ERPs, especially without clear clinical concerns motivating the need to scan individual children. This concern is pervasive in developmental studies, despite the fact that safety requirements (e.g., care in not introducing metallic items in the scanner room, etc.) do not change across age groups. Therefore the majority of published studies focus either on investigating typical brain development in older children (6–7 years or older) or on pediatric populations (e.g., preterm infants; Peterson, 2003). For patient groups, many imaging studies focus predominantly on the neurocognitive outcomes of early insults, but only much later in childhood rather than during infancy (e.g., children affected by early-onset lesions, Liegeois et al., 2004; outcome at eight years of age for children born preterm, Peterson, 2003).

Nevertheless, exciting recent studies have successfully investigated functional activation very early in life, in infants and even in neonates. For example, Dehaene-Lambertz et al. (2002) scanned healthy 2- to 3-month-olds while they listened to either forward or backward speech or silence. Speech activated a large section of the right temporal lobe, and activation was significantly greater at the level of the right compared with the left planum temporale, a finding that mirrors the left-hemispheric dominance found in adults. However, the comparison between forward and backward speech highlighted higher activation for the former in the left angular gyrus and precuneus, and not the temporal lobe, as is characteristic of adults performing the same task. Furthermore, when the infants who were awake during the session were compared with those who were deeply asleep, dorsolateral prefrontal cortex showed greater activation for forward compared with backward speech for awake infants, but not in sleeping ones.

The findings suggest that while areas devoted to speech processing in adults are already engaged by speech in infancy, these patterns of activation are less specific in infancy than they are in later life. Processing also involves cortical areas that are not normally recruited by adults during similar tasks, but are involved when retrieving information from verbal working memory, suggesting intriguing developmental similarities and differences in the processing of simple speech. These findings have been interpreted as supporting a view of language acquisition as progressive specialization of a left-hemisphere network of areas under the influence of attentional biases (Dehaene-Lambertz et al., 2002), illustrating how functional imaging can inform theories of neurocognitive development. With regard to functional imaging through later development, a number of studies have shown both stable and changing patterns of functional activity in older children compared with adults within the context of working memory (e.g., Casey et al., 1995; Thomas et al., 1999; Nelson et al., 2000; Klingberg et al., 2002), inhibitory control (e.g., Casey et al., 1997; Luna et al., 2001; Bunge et al., 2002; Durston et al., 2002), and reading (e.g., Schlaggar et al., 2002).

Meaningful quantitative comparisons of areas of functional activation, from infancy into adulthood, are complicated by differences in data acquisition and experimental design, as well as difficulties with data analysis. We review these challenges in turn. These issues are not simply trivial methodological difficulties related to measuring developmental changes in brain activity, but truly constrain the inferences that can be made about the neural bases of cognitive development. One cannot conclude that similarities or differences in activity are attributable to precise patterns of cognitive processing across age groups unless other potential confounding factors are well understood and controlled for.

Applying fMRI to any population different from normal adult subjects introduces a number of problems that need to be addressed, from data acquisition to analysis and interpretation. Beginning with image acquisition, motion represents a particular challenge for direct comparisons across groups, because the number of activated voxels is expected to be strongly influenced by motion artifacts (Hajnal et al., 1994). This is particularly a problem at high field strengths, because higher field strengths amplify the MR signal (e.g., it measures only 1% to 2% change in a 1.5 Tesla ambient field) and ultimately contrast-to-noise, but they also amplify the signal artifacts such as those due to motion or magnetic susceptibility. This issue is a concern for pediatric studies, where children under 8 years and those presenting certain pediatric disorders (e.g., children with ADHD) have difficulty staying still during a scan. Gradually, researchers have developed child-friendly head restraint techniques (e.g., painted masks, foam padding) that limit motion.

Another challenge for image acquisition with developing populations of all age groups is the elevated noise in the scanning environment, which is louder at higher field strengths. Sound attenuation by shielding the magnet tunnel with foam, placing a noise protection helmet on the ears, and then covering the helmet with a foam mold has been used with participants as young as infants (Dehaene-Lambertz et al., 2002) and is partially successful in eliminating sounds of up to 100 dB. Some researchers have resorted to scanning infants while they are asleep, or sedating the infants, but this limits the kinds of processes or responses that can be meaningfully tested, and may actually obscure intriguing effects that are found only in awake infants. Greater need for sound attenuation measures in children may also interfere with assessing fine auditory processing because auditory stimuli may have to be delivered suboptimally through loudspeakers inserted in the noise protection earphones.

An important adaptation to developmental imaging studies has been the use of simulators, which reproduce the look, feel, and noise levels of the scanner and can significantly reduce anxiety during scanning. The simulator session also allows the child the opportunity to practice head and body control that are so important to reduce motion during the testing session. Prescan visits during which the child enters the actual scanner environment prior to the day of the scan serve a similar purpose.

Beyond potential difficulties with data acquisition, comparisons between child and adult data are complicated by a number of factors related to analytic assumptions. Given their smaller capillaries, faster heart rate and respiration, greater synaptic density, and immature myelination, one may well expect differences in the BOLD response in infants and children compared with adults. However, the characteristics of the BOLD response in children and adolescents appear to be similar to those in adults, in terms of both the time course and peak amplitude, as a number of recent studies have tested directly (e.g., Schlaggar et al., 2002; Kang et al., 2003; Burgund et al., 2002). Findings with infants are contradictory, with some studies showing a time course compatible with the adult response (e.g., Dehaene-Lambertz et al., 2002) and others showing a reversal at variable ages, depending on regions of interest (e.g., Seghier et al., 2004). These differences are problematic, because the available analytic tools employ the shape of the adult hemodynamic response to model random and experimental effects.

There are a number of further considerations that may significantly affect the ability to interpret patterns of brain activity between developing populations, from spatial normalization to the potential effects of age-related structural differences on the locations of functional foci. Spatial normalization to a common template may affect age groups' data differently and potentially introduce spurious functional differences. These differences could account for some of the reported findings across ages, because age-dependent differences in proportional brain region sizes may result in distortions when transforming children's brain images into adult standard atlases, and thus influence comparisons across ages (Gaillard et al., 2001). This represents a potentially serious difficulty in interpreting similarities and differences in functional activation, as well as direct voxelwise comparisons across age groups.

Burgund et al. (2002) systematically investigated the effects of transforming structural images of 7- and 8-year-old children and adult brains to Talairach space (Tailarach & Tournoux, 1988). After image normalization, 10 consistently identifiable sulci were chosen for comparison across child and adult brains. In terms of location differences, three of these sulci revealed significant differences (superior temporal, parieto-occipital and olfactory sulcus), and variability was greater in children than adults for the central sulcus but none of the others differed. The differences observed between child and adult brains were small, albeit systematic. Importantly, when Burgund et al. (2002) modeled the extent to which these differences may affect functional data, they found a critical threshold for misregistration, given 5 mm fMRI image resolution, beyond which spurious functional effects may be seen. This should therefore be taken into consideration when investigating developmental differences in particularly small regions. More recently, Kang et al. (2003) found that in the majority of functional foci, time courses and peak amplitude of the BOLD response were similar in 7- and 8-year-olds compared with adults. Differences in the location of the foci were negligible, supporting the validity of direct statistical comparisons in a common stereotactic space for children as young as 7 to adulthood.

Beside spatial normalization and its potential effects on the location of activation foci, experimental design also presents challenges for developmental neuroscientists. A crucial factor is related to performance differences across age groups. Observed differences in brain activity between adults, children, and infants (and therefore the conclusions that can be drawn about neural recruitment for various cognitive functions) may be confounded by differences in task performance between groups. Some of the first imaging studies illustrate this challenge clearly. Casey et al. (1995) scanned children between the ages of 9 and 11 while they performed a working memory task that had been validated previously with adults (Cohen et al., 1994). The task required children to observe sequentially presented letters and respond when the current letter matched the letter occurring two trials back (2-back memory task), overcoming the interference of the intervening letter. In a comparison condition children monitored the stream of letters for the occurrence of a predetermined letter, to control for the stimulus processing and response requirements of the task.

Results showed reliably higher activity in dorsolateral prefrontal cortex (inferior frontal gyrus and middle frontal gyrus) and anterior cingulate cortex in children for the working memory condition. The distribution of activity across frontal gyri for children and adults was strikingly similar. However, the percent change in signal observed for children was on average two or three times higher than that observed in adults. Could this be an indication of developmental changes in prefrontal activity recruited by similar working memory demands? Critical considerations caution against drawing such an inference prematurely. Children's accuracy on the task was lower (70–75%) than for adults (at or above 90%), suggesting that children found the task more demanding. Thus, differences in activation could be maturational, strategic, or both.

A number of approaches have been utilized to address the problem of performance differences. First, it is possible to independently examine brain regions that correlate with behavioral performance versus those which correlate with age. In a typical fMRI experiment, participants are asked to perform behavioral tasks that differ along some construct of interest. In general, a subtraction is then performed, comparing task conditions that isolate the construct of interest and presumably the neural substrate. In this first approach, correlational analyses are performed to examine how the magnitude or degree of activation during performance of the task relates to behavioral performance (mean reaction times or accuracy). This allows one to consider performance and age-related differences independently, to help distinguish between developmental and individual differences.

For example, Casey et al. (1997) examined the relation between changes in the BOLD signal and individual differences in performance on a go/nogo task versus changes associated with age. This study highlighted correlations between activity in ventral prefrontal cortex and successful inhibition of go responses that were independent of age. Additionally and critically, children activated dorsolateral prefrontal cortex more than adults when performing this task, and this difference could not be accounted for simply by variability in performance because children who performed best on the task (at the level of adults in the number of errors committed) activated this area more than the other children. Klingberg et al. (2002) used a similar strategy in a working memory task: older children showed greater activation of the superior frontal and parietal cortices than younger children. Furthermore, individual working memory capacity correlated with activity in these regions (left superior frontal sulcus and left intraparietal sulcus), suggesting that the amplitude of the BOLD signal was enhanced as a function of age and that this change may reflect enhanced memory capacity and efficiency through adolescence. Thus this approach helps to disentangle developmental and individual differences in cognitive functioning and their neural bases.

A second approach to tease apart performance and age-related influences on brain activity involves carefully equating performance between children and adults by titrating task difficulty. This approach has been used with a number of tasks including a n-back task (Thomas et al., 1999), a flanker task (Durston, Tottenham, et al., 2003) and go/nogo task (Durston, Thomas, Worden, et al., 2002). For example, Thomas et al. (1999) investigated the patterns of cortical activity during a spatial working memory task similar to that of Casey et al. (1995) and validated with adults across multiple testing sites (Braver et al., 1997; Casey et al., 1998). Subjects monitored a linear array of four boxes for the location of a dot that appeared every 2 sec for 500 msec. In memory blocks (compared with control visual inspection and motor response blocks). Participants were required to indicate the location at which the dot had appeared a given number of trials previously (from 1 trial back or 2 back) and were tested before scanning to assess which memory load would be necessary to obtain accuracy between 75 and 95%, in order to equate performance across age groups. This resulted in some participants being scanned while performing a 2-back load and others with the 1-back load. Results were fairly consistent with those obtained by Casey and colleagues (1995), supporting the suggestion that, regardless of task difficulty, children rely on prefrontal recruitment more than adults when engaging working memory. Similarly, in a go/nogo task, the number of go responses preceding a nogo response were parametrically manipulated to increase the degree of interference between the two response choices (go or nogo). Children and adults made more errors as a function of the number of go trials preceding a nogo trial, but the children had difficulty even when only a single go trial preceded a nogo trial (Durston, Thomas, Yang, et al., 2002). They also maximally activated prefrontal and parietal regions that adults recruited monotonically as a function of the number of preceding go trials. Figure 11.1 (see plate 18) illustrates and summarizes the findings. The parametric manipulation allowed equating performance across groups by examining different levels of context manipulations across age groups and across groups of typically and atypically developing children. Overall, results support the suggestion that children recruit both dorsal and ventral prefrontal cortex when required to inhibit infrequent responses, while adults recruit predominantly ventral prefrontal cortex, as in the original go/nogo study (Casey et al., 1997).

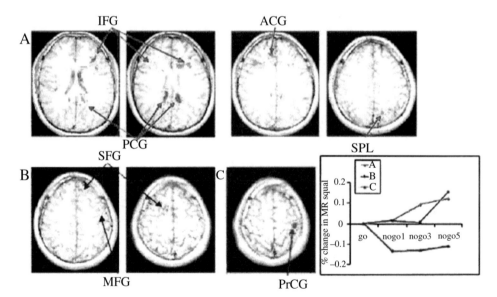

Figure 11.1
Differential patterns of activation in a parametric manipulation of the number of go trials preceding nogo trials. (*A*) Brain regions showing the context effect. (*B*) Brain regions showing an increase in activation only to nogo trials following five go trials. (*C*) Brain regions showing a response to the go trials. (*D*) Three patterns observed for the comparison of go trials with nogo trials after one, three, or five preceding go trials. (Adapted with permission from Durston, Thomas et al., 2002.) See plate 18 for color version.

Parametric manipulations do not work with all tasks. For example, in the n-back task, the approach introduces a potential confound. In other words, when behavioral performance on a task is not a simple monotonic function of task difficulty, but instead requires differential cognitive processes at different levels of difficulty (e.g., a certain type of rehearsal strategy at higher load as opposed to simple visual matching to a previously presented stimulus at a lower load), comparing children and adults who perform at the same level of accuracy may actually be comparing activity recruited by different processes. It would therefore be crucial to ascertain that the cognitive processes underlying monotonic changes in performance do not differ at different levels of the parametric manipulation.

A third approach in assessing performance and age-related contributions to functional differences involves post hoc grouping of participants on the basis of their performance (Schlaggar et al., 2002; Kang et al., 2003). Children (7–10 years old) and adults (18–35 years old) were required to generate a single-word verbal response to single words presented visually. Children were on average slower and less accurate than adults but, given the nature of the task, there was a substantial overlap between child and adult performance measures. Children and adults showed a similar pattern of activation in areas of left frontal and left extrastriate cortex that appeared to be performance driven, while extensions of these regions appeared to be age-dependent.

In order to understand whether these differences reflected developmental differences in the functional neuroanatomy of the task, as opposed to performance-related differences, the authors subdivided the child and adult data into one group in which child and adult performances were similar in terms of speed and accuracy ("matched" adults and children), and one in which there were clear differences between adult and child performances ("nonmatched" adults and children). Activity in one left frontal region (more anterior and ventral to the above regions) and one left extrastriate region (the most posterior) was related to performance, being greater in children in the nonmatched compared with the matched group. A region in which activity is affected by the age of the person irrespective of performance would have dissimilar activity between adults and children for both the matched and the nonmatched groups. One left frontal and one left extrastriate region were found to show this pattern. The left extrastriate region showed more robust activation in children than in adults, whereas the frontal region showed greater activation in adults than in children, due to the fact that children (in both subgroups) did not show activation in this area (although the bulk of the lateral frontal cortex was activated, and similarly so for children and adults). Figure 11.2 (plate 19) illustrates these comparisons and the related patterns of activation. These careful analyses highlight the importance of teasing apart performance and age-related differences. Age-related differences suggest that children and adults use both overlapping and

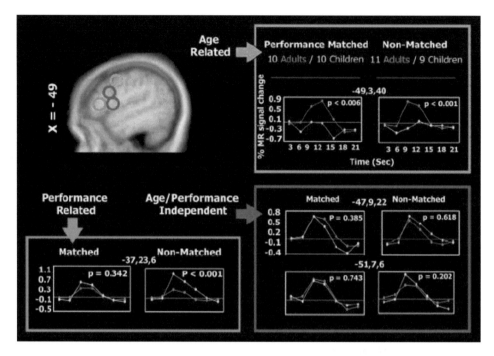

Figure 11.2
One of the alternatives available to developmental cognitive neuroscientists to distinguish activation differences that are performance-, as opposed to age-related, involves separating groups of adults and children in terms of their performance on a task. Schlaggar et al. employed this approach in a simple word-reading task. "Matched" groups of adults and children produced equivalent behavioral performances, in contrast to "nonmatched" groups. Frontal and extrastriate foci displayed activity that was either (1) performance- and age-independent, with adults and children producing similar activation in both the matched and the nonmatched group; (2) performance-dependent, with adults and children producing similar activation in the matched but not the nonmatched group; and (3) age-dependent, with dissimilar activity in adults and children for both the matched and the nonmatched group. (Adapted with permission from Schlaggar et al., 2002.) See plate 19 for color version.

distinct functional areas when engaged in word generation, and in turn that functional neuroanatomy varies at least partially through development.

Despite its merits, even this third approach has its limitations. While it allows for direct comparisons between adults and children, it effectively results in comparing high-functioning children with low-functioning adults. This potentially introduces differential effects related to overall level of intelligence, regardless of the age of participants. Critically, comparisons should also report demographic information on the adults included in the task, to ensure that matched children and adults did not differ substantially in terms of general intelligence. This would strengthen the interpretation of age-related over performance-related differences in functional anatomy. Furthermore, when isolating age-related differences, it remains difficult to tease apart differential influences of experience with the task from brain maturational changes. Finally, designing tasks that result in equivalent performance in adults and children may considerably limit the number of possible constructs that can be tested in this fashion. These three approaches are currently used to tease apart age-related and performance-related differences in activation between adults and children: correlations between signal, age, and performance; parametric manipulations of behavioral performance; and group matching on the basis of age and performance. How should developmental neuroscientists choose among these approaches? The solution will depend on the type of cognitive construct of interest and on whether particular behavioral paradigms can be modified to take these difficulties into account.

But what about assessing functional activity associated with cognitive functioning in even younger age groups? The level of deformation that needs to be imposed on images to move to a common stereotactic space may not undermine conclusions drawn from studies of children older than 7 or 8 years of age (Burgund et al., 2002; Kang et al., 2003), but inclusion of even younger children (infants) may not be possible because of the greater differences between these younger children and adults (Muzik et al., 2000). Other important variables, such as the ratio of gray to white matter, do not begin to approximate adult levels until later than 7 years of age (Courchesne et al., 2000). This difference may limit our ability to draw direct quantitative comparisons between adults, younger children, and infants, and thus extensive studies comparing younger children's brains with those of adults may be necessary before moving to a common stereotactic space for these age groups. Critically, behavioral measures should be recorded even for very young infants to assess whether changes in activation foci are task specific. Recording such responses while scanning is certainly a challenge for the youngest participants, but may be feasible by collecting simple measures (such as eye movements or looking times) either during or immediately after scanning (e.g., habituation to test compared with control stimuli). This is relatively easier to implement when using techniques other than functional imaging. Furthermore, important limitations to the temporal resolution of fMRI and the difficulties in recording MRI from the youngest children have meant that researchers interested in neurocognitive development from infancy have generally employed another technique, event-related potentials, as their recording methodology of choice.

Event-Related Potentials

Electrophysiology has historically been used to address questions about cognitive and brain development. With this technique, brain electrical activity can be recorded by attaching electrodes to the human scalp at various locations and connecting them to a differential amplifier. The output of the amplifier reveals a pattern of voltage variation over time known as the *electroencephalogram* (EEG). An extension of this procedure is to define a short period of time, or epoch, that is time-locked to the presentation of a particular stimulus or event to a subject or to the production of a response while recording the EEG. All voltage changes observed within this epoch are referred to as *event-related potentials* (ERPs). In contrast to other neuroimaging techniques, ERPs do not require the use of any radioactive substances (used in positron emission tomography, PET) or that the participants remain absolutely motionless during testing (as required in fMRI and magnetoencephalography). The noninvasive nature of ERPs makes them ideal to use with awake, behaving infants or young children, and therefore help to examine changes in brain and cognitive development from its outset into adulthood.

Both the temporal characteristics of waveforms and their topography in response to various visual or auditory stimuli have highlighted intriguing similarities and differences in the processing of auditory and visual stimuli in infants compared with adults. For example, Dehaene-Lambertz (2000) investigated phonetic and acoustic mismatch detection and discrimination in 4-month-olds, using high-density ERPs. She discovered that while the topography of the resulting waveforms indicated a degree of intrahemispheric specialization in the areas involved in discriminating acoustic and phonemic differences, the left hemisphere of 4-month-olds seemed equally involved in the processing of both types of stimuli, in contrast with the adult left-hemispheric advantage for phoneme processing. More recently, specific focus on phoneme processing in neonates, infants, and adults highlighted very similar ERPs across age groups (Dehaene-Lambertz & Pena, 2001; Dehaene-Lambertz & Gliga, 2004). Studies testing the mismatch negativity (MMN) to changes in vowels in newborns showed activity similar to that found in adults, but not the adult modulation in the ERP component during sleep compared with the awake state (Martynova et al., 2003). Later in childhood (between 3 and 6 years of age), the MMN is modulated by prolonged exposure to a foreign language (Cheour et al., 2002). Taken together, these findings highlight both stable and changing aspects in the neural correlates of auditory processing from infancy to adulthood. These findings suggest increasing specialization of cognitive processes through development, as well as differences in recruitment of (not always completely overlapping) functional circuits across age groups.

A number of studies have shown considerable change and stability in ERPs from the very first few months of life, measured in terms of the components associated with the encoding of faces (de Haan et al., 2002; Halit et al., 2003; and others, reviewed in de Haan et al., 2003), with the recognition of familiar stimuli (e.g., Snyder et al., 2002) and with the attentional control to guide eye-movements (Richards, 2002). For example, Johnson, Csibra, and colleagues (Csibra, 1998, 2000) investigated the development of ERPs locked to the onset of saccades by manipulating the offset of fixation preceding the appearance of interesting peripheral stimuli (the "gap effect"). Findings demonstrated a gradual development of the saccadic spike potential, a parietal marker of saccade planning in adults (Csibra et al.,1997). Six-month-olds did not show clear evidence of this component, but did show a left frontal positivity, probably a marker of cortical disinhibition of the colliculus initiated by stimulus offset. Although 12-month-old infants exhibited the spike potential, this had smaller amplitude than the potential found in adults, suggesting gradual development of cortical processes leading to saccade generation.

Using ERPs, the electrical changes that take place within the brain can be measured at the scalp almost simultaneously. Measures derived from brain electrical activity are typically recorded in the millisecond domain. Therefore, ERPs are considered to be the "gold standard" in terms of temporal resolution for cognitive neuroscience. This property makes ERP measures ideal for linking with behavior those electrophysiological changes which take place over short periods of time. In contrast, neither PET nor fMRI can provide satisfactory temporal information about the chronometry of mental events. The inherent temporal delay between the time that a neuronal change occurs and a detectable metabolic response, as measured by PET, or hemodynamic response, as measured by fMRI, limits the temporal resolution of these measures of brain activity. As a consequence, ERP measures are ideally suited for tracking the neural changes that coincide with rapid phasic changes in the behavioral state (Davidson et al., 2000).

The precision of ERP is invaluable to developmental scientists because it provides us with the tools to ask when, in ontogenetic time, various ERP components are modulated in a way that resembles adulthood, rather than relying solely on behavioral measures. Although vital, these measures are only the end product of multiple processes that could develop along differential developmental trajectories. To illustrate this point, Grossi et al. (2001) investigated the priming of rhymes, a process thought to be important for the development of reading, from 7 to 23 years of age. Two ERP effects associated with the task in adults were present at all ages, but they showed different time courses. A negative slow wave, which was larger over anterior regions of the left hemisphere and associated with rehearsal of the primes, increased with age and its asymmetry was correlated with reading ability. In contrast, the effects on a negative deflection to targets that was maximal over more posterior temporoparietal areas (in adults larger for nonrhyming than rhyming patterns and associated with phonological matching) showed a very stable time course across age groups.

Similarly, Davis et al. (2003) compared ERPs with go/nogo trials in 6-year-old children and adults, using a task similar to that used by Casey et al. (1997) in an fMRI environment described above. Modulation of the anterior N2 component did not differ greatly in children and adults, but modulation of the centroparietal P3 differed in its amplitude and scalp topography. This is intriguing because fMRI findings pointed to developmental changes in recruitment for *both* frontal and parietal areas (Bunge et al., 2002), whereas these ERP findings suggest that the temporal characteristics and spatial distribution of frontal neural activity did not vary greatly. Clearly, linking these methodologies by obtaining similar sets of data from the same participants will further constrain the interpretations of such findings.

Again, as with fMRI, although there are strengths of using ERPs to investigate the neural bases of developing cognitive processes, there are challenges that are specific to their application to the study of development (Johnson et al., 2001; de Haan & Thomas, 2002; Taylor & Baldeweg, 2002). In particular, a number of issues complicate comparing ERPs across age groups, from data acquisition to analysis and interpretation. With regard to recording EEG, unlike fMRI, motion is not as significant a drawback for ERPs, so greater motion in younger children does not normally completely compromise recordings. However, eye movements, blinks, and other motion artifacts, which can be more common in younger participants, increase the noise of the recorded signal. This is partially addressed by using algorithms that identify and eliminate channels that have recorded such artifacts and replace them by interpolating data from other channels. However, the use of such algorithms for interpolating missing data needs to rely on realistic models of infants' heads and scalp conductance. Furthermore, ERPs depend on averaging across a large number of trials, and this means that populations producing fewer trials of interest (as is most often the case with typically and atypically developing infants and children) will provide noisier average waveforms and less reliable condition differences.

Both from a statistical point of view and from an empirical one, the issue of variable numbers of trials and increased variability across age groups in ERP studies is not a trivial one. Snyder et al. (2002) examined the effects of the number of completed trials on ERPs to familiar or novel faces in a large sample of 6-month-old infants. Individual differences in the total number of completed trials influenced both the amplitude and the latency of ERP components associated with encoding, attention, and/or recognition (the negative component, Nc, and the slow wave). This finding is consistent with a large body of evidence indicating large individual differences in infant behavioral measures indexing these processes. These findings have implications for developmental ERP studies beyond infancy. The total number of trials that an individual completes may reflect, to some degree, individual differences in the rate or the extent of stimulus encoding or attention allocation to the stimulus for which researchers are hoping to extract an averaged ERP. Thus, age differences in the total number of trials obtained, could confound age differences in the ERP components of interest and should therefore be considered as a potential covariate in statistical analyses.

A number of characteristics in electrophysiological responses further complicate inferences about development. First, gross changes in skull conductancy across age groups suggest that only data from individuals in restricted age ranges should be combined when averaging waveforms. These noncognitive influences on age-related differences mean that in some cases only qualitative comparisons can be applied across groups, in terms of both the latency and the amplitude of ERP components of interest. For example, in the infant N290 a central/posterior negative deflection decreases in peak latency from 350 to 290 msec between 3 and 12 months of age. It is thought to be a developmental precursor to the adult N170, because at 12 months it is modulated by stimulus inversion in qualitatively the same way as in the adult N170, but there are also substantial differences in its characteristics compared with N170 (Halit et al., 2003; and reviewed in de Haan and Thomas, 2002; de Haan et al., 2003). As seen from fMRI studies, difficulties in incorporating age groups into a common analysis limit the inferences that can be made about similarities and differences in components, making a solution to this problem a priority for the future of developmental ERP work.

As with fMRI, teasing apart differences that depend on performance from those that are age-related is an important consideration. Thus, it is recommended that behavioral measures of performance be collected across age groups that allow for relationships between behavior and electrophysiology to be examined (Picton et al., 2000). This is even more important because of the noncognitive differences in ERP that are due to differences in scalp conductance which we discussed above: without behavioral performance, it would be difficult to disentangle cognitive and noncognitive reasons for age-related differences in ERP modulations. However, many developmental neuroscientists using ERPs to investigate developmental change rely on ERP recordings during passive viewing or listening tasks (e.g., as in the case of studies of face processing, reviewed in de Haan et al., 2003). This approach, although necessary in a number of cases (active responses cannot always be obtained easily in infants), precludes firm conclusions on whether differences in component latency and amplitude across age groups depend on differences in general processing of the stimuli or on more specific age-related changes. When behavioral measures (e.g., eye movements, reaction times, and accuracy) are obtained, approaches similar to those described above for functional imaging could be used to tease apart performance and age differences: correlating performance with individual differences in components of interest (e.g., Casey et al., 1997), employing parametric manipulations of task difficulty (e.g., Durston, Thomas, Worden, et al., 2002), and creating performance- and age-matched groups of participants (e.g., Schlaggar et al., 2002).

Although the temporal resolution of ERPs is a major advantage of this method, ERPs have relatively poor spatial resolution. Even with high-density arrays, their spatial resolution will always be inferior to techniques such as PET or fMRI. Because of its highly resistive properties, the skull acts as a spatial low-pass filter and smears the electrical activity over relatively large areas of the scalp (Davidson et al., 2000). As a result, the spatial distribution of neuronal potentials measured at the scalp's surface is relatively distorted. Accordingly, it is incorrect to assume that the neural generators of a signal are located under the scalp area where the signal is maximal: for any given distribution detected at the scalp, there may be more than one possible configuration of neural generators within the brain that could produce the identical response. The challenge of inferring the neural generators of scalp-recorded activity is also referred to as the *inverse problem*. From this perspective, combining ERPs with fMRI can be very useful in order to constrain the solution of source localization analysis of ERP data. With regard to development, this is not a trivial point. In cases in which waveforms differ across age groups, this could conceivably depend on identical neural sources being activated to a different extent. On the other hand, similarities in waveforms across age groups could be associated with distinct generators. Information about functional activation foci in identical tasks could be critical to distinguish these possibilities and the inferences that can be made about the neural correlates of developmental change.

Combining ERPs and fMRI

Both ERPs and fMRI are useful tools for developmental cognitive neuroscience. Because of their complementary nature, combining these methods would seem to be the best solution in gaining both temporal and spatial insight into the neural bases of cognitive processes. Together these methods can provide valuable insights regarding the sequencing and timing of activation of particular brain areas. Crucially for developmental neuroscientists, combining the two techniques would enable testing whether the activation foci measured with fMRI can be modeled as the generators in the ERP components across age groups, or whether identical ERP components may be accounted for by different functional foci across development. In other words, changes in the temporal and spatial dynamics of interactions across multiple cortical areas will be more easily assessed with imaging and electrophysiological recordings obtained from the same participants.

In practice, the approach of using ERP and fMRI simultaneously is not so straightforward. The application of magnetic fields while using fMRI can introduce electric currents, and electric currents can cause magnetic lines of force, possibly leading to artifacts in both BOLD and EEG signals (Allen et al., 1998). In addition, there are issues of the participant's safety to be considered: during an fMRI study, very small electrical currents can be induced in the body that may result in a certain amount of tissue heating. If, in addition, metallic elements are present (such as recording electrodes used for ERPs), conducting loops can concentrate in those elements, leading to shock or burning (Lemieux et al., 1997).

Several different approaches have been described for how to effectively combine ERPs and fMRI in one session. For example, during *EEG-triggered fMRI*, fMRI data are acquired at fixed intervals following events of interest in the EEG and during periods of rest. This approach is most appropriate when a definable event in the EEG can be reliably reproduced in the scanner. A second example is the *interleaved EEG/fMRI approach*, in which both ERP and fMRI data are collected while the participant is in the scanner, with periods of acquiring MR data being interleaved with periods of acquiring EEG data. In both of these approaches fMRI and ERP data are acquired serially. Alternatively, the *simultaneous EEG-fMRI* approach uses special recording equipment and data-processing algorithms that reduce or remove artifacts associated with the combined measurement of the two signals (Allen et al., 2000). Each of these approaches is used less frequently than the alternative of recording ERPs and fMRI in distinct, but temporally close, sessions. The latter approach may be more feasible when studying developmental populations.

A number of challenges face researchers attempting to combine functional imaging methods to study development, whether recording occurs simultaneously or in separate sessions. In the adult, paradigms often need to be modified to allow for coregistration, but this may compromise optimal experimental design for each of the techniques to be integrated. For example, short and jittered intertial intervals and rapid mixed-trial designs are the most commonly used when recording ERPs. Although these approaches are used in fMRI studies too, reliable percent signal change in the BOLD response often benefits from mini blocks of trials or longer intertrial intervals. Integrating these two types of design cannot always be accomplished successfully, and it may limit the types of empirical questions that researchers can ask in combined studies. Another problematic issue is the difficulty of controlling for order effects, especially in tasks designed to investigate attentional control. These tasks are often demanding and difficult, so administering them consecutively to the same participants may introduce order effects in the type of activity measured. Therefore, adult designs require careful counterbalancing.

All of the above issues are magnified in the context of developmental research because the number of trials that can be attained with a given task is generally reduced with young children, and especially in infants, compared with adult participants. Order effects are also complicated by the fact that children fatigue more easily. All of the previous solutions require extra trials or time on task that are not conducive when working with pediatric populations. Analysis tools that are available for coregistering data across methodologies (for example, EEG source localization packages) build models on assumptions that are accurate for adult brains. These tools are not adequate for developmental studies because they are based on adult models of skull conductance and thickness. Alternative tools for examining developmental EEG are becoming available (e.g., Richards, 2002) and could be used in the same way as in the adult case.

Although rare in developmental studies, more and more frequently in adult imaging studies, researchers are combining the two techniques to investigate, in more depth, the temporal dynamics, as well as the localization, of circuits involved in attentional control and selection (Di Russo et al., 2002; Di Russo et al., 2003; Martínez et al., 2001). For example, Martínez et al. (2001) investigated the cortical mechanisms of visual-spatial attentional selection using both fMRI and ERP recordings. Enhanced neural activity was recorded in both extrastriate and primary visual cortical areas. Importantly, ERP recordings indicated that the initial sensory components associated with this activation were not modulated by attention. In contrast, later components, also originating in visual cortex, were modulated by attention. The authors suggested that activity in primary visual cortex may be modulated by delayed reentrant feedback connections from higher visual areas. These findings also underscore how the long-lasting changes in the BOLD response, as measured by fMRI, may mask multiple (feedforward and feedback) processes that are apparent when imaging findings are combined with electrophysiological ones.

In order to better understand both the functional neuroanatomy of cognitive control and its temporal dynamics we have recently adapted a stimulus-response compatibility task, the "flanker task" (Eriksen and Eriksen, 1974), to record both functional images and ERPs in separate but temporally close sessions, initially in adults (Scerif et al., in press). Subjects were required to respond to a central arrow and to ignore potentially conflicting ("incompatible") information from flanking arrows. Preceding context (i.e., whether the trial of interest was preceded by "compatible" or "incompatible" trials) was used to manipulate top-down expectancy both prior to and immediately after the presentation of targets. As in other electrophysiological studies, late response-related components were most strongly modulated in high-conflict trials (incompatible trials preceded by compatible ones). However, we also found evidence of much earlier modulation of stimulus processing by previous context: the early visual P1 component was enhanced in the incompatible context only when an incompatible flanker array was presented (as illustrated in figure 11.3, and plate 20).

We interpret these early effects as partly related to an increased attentional focus on the target arrow, a consequence of exposure to repeated incompatible trials. This interpretation is consistent with imaging results, suggesting that parietal cortices are involved in the control of the focus of visuospatial attention (Casey et al., 2000). However, increased attentional focus alone is not sufficient to account for the fact that visual P1 is enhanced for incompatible trials of interest only. This result therefore suggests a very early interaction between attentional control mechanisms and stimulus features. fMRI alone would not have revealed such early and transient effects on stimulus processing. Combining the information on the electrophysiological markers of activation with the functional activation foci in the complementary fMRI experiment (run with the same participants) will strengthen the inferences that we can draw from the sources of this modulation.

From a developmental perspective, these findings are particularly intriguing. A number of published studies have shown that late or response-related components (such as the N200, the P3, or the error-related negativity) change with age as markers of improved endogenous control on responses across development (e.g., Ridderinkhof and van der Molen, 1995). What predictions can we make about these early markers of interactions between featural processing and attentional control? In children 7–8 years old, featural processing may well have developed to adult levels, but poorer control of the attentional focus may or may not result in modulation of visual P1 equivalent to adults. Yet another picture may emerge in infants, for whom both featural processing and control of the attentional focus may be developing rapidly. The developmental time course of the early attentional modulation effects and of the later response-related effects need not be identical, because they may depend on feedback from distinct parietal and frontal areas. At present these can only be speculative predictions, but we are in the process of testing them directly.

In sum, considerable efforts are still necessary to allow for the combination of fMRI and other techniques within a developmental context. Despite all these challenges, multitechnique approaches are very promising for developmental research because they allow us to enhance our understanding of the dynamics of neural activity underlying perceptual and cognitive development.

Issues and Future Directions

We have described two techniques used to examine cognitive and brain development and important issues and difficulties with using these techniques with pediatric populations. Despite these difficulties, the field promises exciting improvements in methodology and image analyses when applied to development. So what is in store for the future? A very important future step will be to examine longer developmental trajectories, extending earlier, perhaps into infancy for certain developmental questions, and later for others. To date, functional imaging studies rarely include children younger than 7 or 8 years of age, even though significant and extensive changes in cognitive abilities have already occurred. Many of the dynamic changes in brain development occur earlier than the period normally tested with fMRI at the moment (see Huttenlocher, 2002, for a comprehensive review). As we outlined

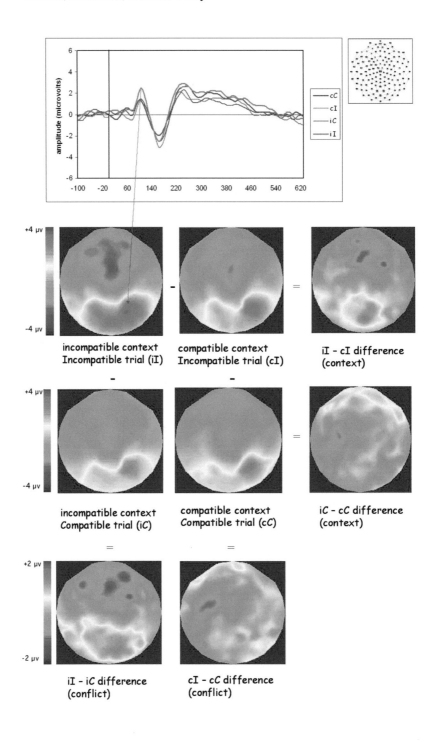

incompatible context
Incompatible trial (iI)

compatible context
Incompatible trial (cI)

iI – cI difference
(context)

incompatible context
Compatible trial (iC)

compatible context
Compatible trial (cC)

iC – cC difference
(context)

iI – iC difference
(conflict)

cI – cC difference
(conflict)

above, some researchers are now modifying scanning protocols to test infants and neonates. If younger children are to be imaged with fMRI more routinely, then we will have to reconsider the appropriateness of a common stereotactic space when comparing different age groups. An alternative future avenue of research is building an atlas of the developing brain from early in infancy through to childhood on which functional changes can be more reliably mapped, but this will require building statistical tools that will allow meaningful comparisons across atlases at different ages. These in turn may require controlling for yet unresolved potential differences in the shape of the hemodynamic response for neonates and infants and up to 6–7 years of age.

Besides the tracing of developmental trajectories for younger age groups, multiple issues remain open, especially for researchers interested in the dynamics of cognitive processes and their developmental emergence. As we mentioned earlier, individual imaging techniques address distinct developmental questions centered on the issue of functional specialization and localization. Therefore, converging method approaches are crucial in formulating and constraining our theories of developmental change (Casey and de Haan, 2002). We believe that a crucial component of these future developments will be the integration of fMRI with other techniques. This is because theoretical accounts (e.g., Casey et al., 2001) and empirical papers (e.g., Luna et al., 2001; Bunge et al., 2002; Klingberg et al., 2002) increasingly stress the importance of investigating distributed neural circuits instead of focusing on isolated brain regions, as has been more traditionally the case for functional imaging studies. For example, Klingberg and colleagues (2002) highlight functional correlations between frontal and parietal areas of activation during working memory tasks. Indeed, recordings of electrical activity show that frontal and posterior cortices increase coherence during the delay period (Sarnthein et al., 1998). These findings suggest that improvements in the functions of long-range connections across these areas may also be instrumental in development.

The importance of examining neural circuitry, as well as the functioning of individual cortical areas, is underscored by the disruption of neural circuitry in a number

Figure 11.3
Event-related potentials are locked to stimulus presentation in an adaptation of the flanker task (Eriksen and Eriksen, 1974) designed to investigate effects of previous response context (compatible or incompatible flanker arrays) on early stimulus processing of compatible and incompatible flanker arrays. Averaged waveforms across a number of posterior channels and scalp topographies across conditions at 112 msec post stimulus onset indicate an interaction between previous context and current stimulus array on very early stimulus processing, as indexed by a positive deflection in the visual P1 for incompatible flanker arrays preceded by incompatible flanker arrays only. (Reprinted with permission.) cI, incompatible trial preceded by compatible context; iI, incompatible trial preceded by incompatible context; iC, compatible trial preceded by incompatible context; cC, compatible trial preceded by compatible context. (Adapted from Scerif et al., in press) See plate 20 for color version.

of childhood disorders. For example, the inability to inhibit or suppress inappropriate thoughts or behaviors characterizes multiple atypically developing populations, such as attention deficit/hyperactivity disorder (ADHD), obsessive-compulsive disorder and Tourette's syndrome. Although the neurobiological etiology of these disorders is unresolved, increasing evidence points to the implication of prefrontal cortex and basal ganglia in all of them. Interesting dissociations in the pattern of behavioral performance that characterize each of these disorders seem to suggest the involvement of different basal ganglia thalamocortical circuits in each (reviewed in Casey et al., 2001), stressing the need to focus on differences in circuitry as well as on dysfunctions of individual areas. In the case of ADHD, dopaminergic hypofunction in frontostriatal connections has been implicated (e.g., Castellanos et al., 1996, Vaidya et al., 1998; Rubia et al., 1999).

Using the previously described parametric manipulation of go and no go trials, Durston, Thomas, Yang, et al. (2003) found that children with the condition did not activate frontostriatal circuits and anterior cingulate as children without ADHD did. In contrast, they activated posterior regions of parietal and occipital cortex more than typically developing children, as well as prefrontal regions previously shown not to correlate with performance on this task. This suggests the recruitment of a more diffuse network of neural systems when performing tasks that require cognitive control. These findings underscore the importance of combined work on normative populations and on children who are developing atypically. All together, the integration of both typical and atypical pediatric imaging stresses the future need to investigate changes in structural and functional connectivity across areas.

Another methodology that should be considered is that of diffusion tensor imaging (DTI). This is a relatively new technique that has been applied to questions of neural connectivity and development. It can detect changes in white matter microstructure based on properties of diffusion. Diffusion of water in white matter tracts is restricted by myelin and the regularity of fibers. Water diffuses more readily in parallel to a tract than perpendicular to it, a property termed anisotropic diffusion. Magnetic resonance imaging can be sensitized to water diffusion to quantify myelination and white matter microstructure in vivo, and has already been linked with brain development and individual differences in certain fiber tracts. Recently, DTI has been used to investigate typical developmental changes in myelination for specific cortical areas and wider networks. Klingberg et al. (1999) studied prefrontal white matter in 10-year-old children and adults, and found both age-related differences and stable patterns of organization. Lower myelination, as indexed by greater diffusion, characterized prefrontal white matter in children, but greater coherence of axonal organization in the right compared with the left frontal lobe was common to both adults and children. The time course of age differences in myelination is strikingly similar to the protracted development of prefrontal cortex functions, suggesting that the two may be related, although this hypothesis could be tested more directly by combining DTI and fMRI. This is precisely what Olesen and colleagues (2003) did, by measuring both functional activation and anisotropy during a working memory task performed by children and adolescents between 8 and 18 years of age. Working memory scores, fMRI activity, and anisotropy correlated independently in several regions. However, and most critically, anisotropy values in frontoparietal white matter correlated with BOLD response in closely located gray matter in the superior frontal sulcus and inferior parietal lobe, suggesting a much tighter link between the two than had previously been found.

DTI may also have invaluable applications to the study of developmental disorders. Klingberg et al. (2000) compared adults with poor and normal reading abilities and found that poor readers exhibited decreased anisotropy bilaterally in temporoparietal white matter. Furthermore, white matter anisotropy in the left hemisphere correlated with reading scores for both poor and normal readers, suggesting that it may be a marker of the efficiency of communications between visual, auditory, and language-processing areas of the brain.

What about combining DTI and fMRI to assess infants as well as children? As for the application of fMRI to the study of development, this approach has currently been used primarily in pediatric populations (for example, infants with perinatal stroke; Seghier et al., 2004). A more research-driven application of DTI to the study of development will require infant- and child-friendly adaptations to the scanning environment that are similar to those used for standard functional imaging of gray matter activation: control of motion artifacts, reduced noise levels, and careful habituation to the novelty of the scanning environment. The heightened levels of noise that characterize DTI scanning sequences, compared with standard structural and functional ones, may cause further problems with sound attenuation.

Optical topography (OT) or optical imaging is another technique enabling the investigation of neural functioning from infancy. OT devices are relatively small and much less invasive than a scanning environment. They emit infrared light at different wavelengths over the scalp, and changes in the reflected wavelengths allow one to estimate changes in oxyhemoglobin, deoxyhemoglobin, and total hemoglobin, and thus infer changes in cerebral blood volume and blood saturation in a manner comparable with the BOLD response in fMRI (Strangman et al., 2002). The silent and noninvasive nature of recording means that the technique can be used successfully with neonates, as has been demonstrated in a study testing phoneme discrimination in sleeping newborns (Pena et al., 2003). Due to space limitations, this technique cannot be reviewed here at length, but we refer the reader to an article describing it in detail (Maki et al., 1995). A particularly problematic factor is the fact that OT is mostly limited to recording from superficial cortical areas 2–3 cm below the scalp.

All of the previously described methods can provide both structural and functional information about the developing human brain. Combining these techniques with carefully designed assays of cognition can help constrain theories on what neural processes change with cognitive development.

To date, fMRI, DTI, and OT have not been able to capture the temporal dynamics of interacting brain areas precisely, nor how these dynamical interchanges vary with development. The millisecond-by-millisecond resolution of ERPs allows tracking the temporal dynamics of cognitive processes very precisely from the onset of each trial, rather than relying on slow changes in the BOLD response that are most likely not to reflect the faster and more transient components of cognitive processes. We believe that the combination of these techniques will strongly enhance our ability to understand neural and cognitive development and constrain current developmental theories.

Conclusions

We have described two functional imaging methods for use with developmental populations. Since "development" implies the study of change and not just the study of real-time processing within steady-state systems, the notion of a dynamic exchange of information (and hence corticocortical projections, temporal dynamics, etc.) should be central to any developmental investigation seeking to understand how an organism grows and develops. The focus of researchers in the area is indeed gradually moving from an interest in isolated parts of the brain to the circuitry and the distributed networks involved. Importantly, no single functional neuroimaging method can fully address developmental questions centered on the issue of dynamic interactions across areas. Therefore, converging method approaches are crucial in formulating and constraining our theories of neurocognitive development.

References

Allen, P. J., Josephs, O., & Turner, R. (2000). A method for removing imaging artifact from continuous EEG recorded during functional MRI. *NeuroReport* 12, 230–239.

Allen, P. J., Polizzi, G., Krakow, K., Fish, D. R., & Lemieux, L. (1998). Identification of EEG events in the MR scanner: The problem of pulse artifact and a method for its subtraction. *NeuroImage* 8, 229–239.

Braver, T. S., Cohen, J. D., Nystrom, L. E., Jonides, J., Smith, E. E., & Noll, D. C. (1997). A parametric study of prefrontal cortex involvement in human working memory. *NeuroImage* 5, 49–62.

Bunge, S. A., Hazeltine, E., Scanlon, M. D., Rosen, A. C., & Gabrieli, J. D. (2002). Dissociable contributions of prefrontal and parietal cortices to response selection. *NeuroImage* 5, 49–62.

Burgund, E. D., Kang, H. C., Kelly, J. E., Buckner, R. L., Snyder, A. Z., Petersen, S. E., & Schlaggar, B. L. (2002). The feasibility of a common stereotactic space for children and adults in fMRI studies of development. *NeuroImage* 17(1), 184–200.

Casey, B. J., Cohen, J. D., Jezzard, P., Turner, R., Noll, D. C., Trainor, R. J., Giedd, J., Kaysen, D., Hertz-Pannier, L., & Rapoport, J. L. (1995). Activation of prefrontal cortex in children during a nonspatial working memory task with functional MRI. *NeuroImage* 2(3), 221–229.

Casey, B. J., Cohen, J. D., O'Craven, K., Davidson, R. J., Irwin, W., Nelson, C. A., Noll, D. C., Hu, X., Lowe, M. J., Rosen, B. R., Truwitt, C. L., & Turski, P. A. (1998). Reproducibility of fMRI results across four institutions using a spatial working memory task. *NeuroImage* 8(3), 249–261.

Casey, B. J., & de Haan, M. (2002). Imaging methods in developmental science. *Developmental Science* 5, 265–267 (spec. iss.).

Casey, B. J., Durston, S., & Fossella, J. A. (2001). Evidence for a mechanistic model of cognitive control. *Clinical Neuroscience Research* 1, 267–282.

Casey, B. J., & Munakata, Y. (2002). Converging methods approach to developmental science. *Developmental Psychobiology* 40, 197–199.

Casey, B. J., Thomas, K. M., Welsh, T. F., Badgaiyan, R. D., Eccard, C. H., Jennings, J. R., & Crone, E. A. (2000). Dissociation of response conflict, attentional selection, and expectancy with functional magnetic resonance imaging. *Proceedings of the National Academy Sciences USA* 97, 8728–8733.

Casey, B. J., Trainor, R. J., Orendi, J. L., Schubert, A. B., Nystrom, L. E., Giedd, J. N., Castellanos, F. X., Haxby, J. V., Noll, D. C., Cohen, J. D., Forman, S. D., Dahl, R. E., & Rapoport, J. L. (1997). A developmental functional MRI study of prefrontal activation during performance of a Go-No-Go task. *Journal of Cognitive Neuroscience* 9, 835–847.

Castellanos, F. X., Giedd, J. N., Marsh, W. L., Hamburger, S. D., Vaituzis, A. C., Dickstein, D. P., Sarfatti, S. E., Vauss, Y. C., Snell, J. W., Lange, N., Kaysen, D., Krain, A. L., Ritchie, G. F., Rajapakse, J. C., & Rapoport, J. L. (1996). Quantitative brain magnetic resonance imaging in attention-deficit hyperactivity disorder. *Archives of General Psychiatry* 53(7), 607–616.

Cheour, M., Shestakova, A., Alku, P., Ceponiene, R., & Naatanen, R. (2002). Mismatch negativity shows that 3–6-year-old children can learn to discriminate non-native speech sounds within two months. *Neuroscience Letters* 325, 187–190.

Cohen, J. D., Forman, S. D., Braver, T. S., Casey, B. J., Servan-Schreiber, D., & Noll, D. C. (1994). Activation of prefrontal cortex in a nonspatial working memory task with functional MRI. *Human Brain Mapping* 1, 293–304.

Courchesne, E., Chisum, H. J., Townsend, J., Cowles, A., Covington, J., Egaas, B., Harwood, M., Hinds, S., & Press, G. A. (2000). Normal brain development and aging: Quantitative analysis at *in vivo* MR imaging in healthy volunteers. *Neuroradiology* 216, 672–682.

Csibra, G., Johnson, M. H., & Tucker, L. A. (1997). Attention and oculomotor control: A high-density ERP study of the gap effect. *Neuropsychologia* 35, 855–865.

Csibra, G., Tucker, L. A., & Johnson, M. H. (1998). Neural correlates of saccade planning in infants: A high-density ERP study. *International Journal of Psychophysiology* 29, 201–215.

Csibra, G., Tucker, L. A., Volein, A., & Johnson, M. H. (2000). Cortical development and saccade planning: The ontogeny of the spike potential. *NeuroReport* 11, 1069–1073.

Davidson, R. J., Jackson, D., & Larson, C. L. (2000). Human electroencephalography. In J. T. Cacioppo, G. Bernston, & L. Tassinary (Eds.), *Principles of Psychophysiology* 2nd ed., 27–52. New York: Cambridge University Press.

Davis, E. P., Bruce, J., Snyder, K., & Nelson, C. A. (2003). The X-trials: Neural correlates of an inhibitory control task in children and adults. *Journal of Cognitive Neuroscience* 15, 432–443.

de Haan, M., Johnson, M. H., & Halit, H. (2003). Development of face-sensitive event-related potentials during infancy: A review. *International Journal of Psychophysiology* 51, 45–58.

de Haan, M., Pascalis, O., & Johnson, M. H. (2002). Specialization of neural mechanisms underlying face recognition in human infants. *Journal of Cognitive Neuroscience* 14, 199–209.

de Haan, M., & Thomas, K. M. (2002). Applications of ERP and fMRI techniques to developmental science. *Developmental Science* 5, 335–343.

Dehaene-Lambertz, G. (2000). Cerebral specialization for speech and non-speech stimuli in infants. *Journal of Cognitive Neuroscience* 12, 449–460.

Dehaene-Lambertz, G., Dehaene, S., & Hertz-Pannier, L. (2002). Functional neuroimaging of speech perception in infants. *Science* 298(5600), 2013–2015.

Dehaene-Lambertz, G., & Gliga, T. (2004). Common neural basis for phoneme processing in infants and adults. *Journal of Cognitive Neuroscience* 16, 1375–1387.

Dehaene-Lambertz, G., & Pena, M. (2001). Electrophysiological evidence for automatic phonetic processing in neonates. *NeuroReport* 12, 3155–3158.

Di Russo, F., Martínez, A., & Hillyard, S. A. (2003). Source analysis of event-related cortical activity during visuo-spatial attention. *Cerebral Cortex* 13, 486–499.

Di Russo, F., Martínez, A., Sereno, M. I., Pitzalis, S., & Hillyard, S. A. (2002). Cortical sources of the early components of the visual evoked potential. *Human Brain Mapping* 15, 95–111.

Durston, S., Davidson, M. C., Thomas, K. M., Worden, M. S., Tottenham, N., Martínez, A., Watts, R., Ulug, A. M., & Casey, B. J. (2003). Parametric manipulation of conflict and response competition using rapid mixed-trial event-related fMRI. *NeuroImage* 20, 2135–2141.

Durston, S., Thomas, K. M., Worden, M. S., Yang, Y., & Casey, B. J. (2002). The effect of preceding context on inhibition: An event-related fMRI study. *NeuroImage* 16(2), 449–453.

Durston, S., Thomas, K. M., Yang, Y., Ulug, A. M., Zimmerman, R., & Casey, B. J. (2002). A neural basis for development of inhibitory control. *Developmental Science* 5(4), 9–16.

Durston, S., Tottenham, N. T., Thomas, K. M., Davidson, M. C., Eigsti, I. M., Yang, Y., Ulug, A. M., & Casey, B. J. (2003). Differential patterns of striatal activation in young children with and without ADHD. *Biological Psychiatry* 53(10), 871–878.

Eriksen, B. A., & Eriksen, C. W. (1974). Effect of noise letters upon the identification of a target letter in a nonsearch task. *Perception and Psychophysics* 16, 143–149.

Gaillard, W. D., Grandin, C. B., & Xu, B. (2001). Developmental aspects of paediatric fMRI: Considerations for image acquisition, analysis, and interpretation. *NeuroImage* 13(2), 239–249.

Grossi, G., Coch, D., Coffey-Corina, S., Holcomb, P. J., & Neville, H. J. (2001). Phonological processing in visual rhyming: A developmental ERP study. *Journal of Cognitve Neuroscience* 13, 610–625.

Hajnal, J. V., Myers, R., Oatridge, A., Schwieso, J. E., Young, I. R., & Bydder, G. M. (1994). Artifacts due to stimulus correlated motion in functional imaging of the brain. *Magnetic Resonance in Medicine* 31(3), 283–291.

Halit, H., de Haan, M., & Johnson, M. H. (2003). Cortical specialisation for face processing: Face-sensitive event-related potential components in 3- and 12-month-old infants. *NeuroImage* 19, 1180–1193.

Huttenlocher, P. R. (2002). *Neural Plasticity: The Effects of the Environment on the Development of the Cerebral Cortex.* Cambridge, MA: Harvard University Press.

Johnson, M. H., de Haan, M., Oliver, A., Smith, W., Hatzakis, H., Tucker, L. A., & Csibra, G. (2001). Recording and analyzing high density ERPs with infants using the Geodesic Sensor Net. *Developmental Neuropsychology* 19, 295–323.

Kang, H. C., Burgund, E. D., Lugar, H. M., Petersen, S. E., & Schlaggar, B. L. (2003). Comparison of functional activation foci in children and adults using a common stereotactic space. *NeuroImage* 19(1), 16–28.

Klingberg, T., Forssberg, H., & Westerberg, H. (2002). Increased brain activity in frontal and parietal cortex underlies the development of visuo-spatial working memory capacity during childhood. *Journal of Cognitive Neuroscience* 14(1), 1–10.

Klingberg, T., Hedehus, M., Temple, E., Salz, T., Gabrieli, J. D., Moseley, M. E., & Poldrack, R. A. (2000). Microstructure of temporo-parietal white matter as a basis for reading ability: Evidence from diffusion tensor magnetic resonance imaging. *Neuron* 25, 493–500.

Klingberg, T., Vaidya, C. J., Gabrieli, J. D., Moseley, M. E., & Hedehus, M. (1999), Myelination and organization of the frontal white matter in children: A diffusion tensor MRI study. *NeuroReport* 10, 2817–2821.

Kwong, K. K., Belliveau, J. W., Chesler, D. A., Goldberg, I. E., Weisskoff, R. M., Poncelet, B. P., Kennedy, D. N., Hoppel, B. E., Cohen, M. S., Turner, R., Cheng, H.-M., Brady, T. J., & Rosen, B. R. (1992). Dynamic magnetic resonance imaging of human brain activity during primary sensory stimulation. *Proceedings of the National Academy of Sciences USA* 89, 5675–5679.

Lemieux, L., Allen, P. J., Franconi, F., Symms, M. R., & Fish, D. R. (1997). Recording of EEG during fMRI experiments: Patient safety. *Magnetic Resonance in Medicine* 38, 943–952.

Liegeois, F., Connelly, A., Cross, J. H., Boyd, S. G., Gadian, D. G., Vargha-Khadem, F., & Baldeweg, T. (2004). Language reorganization in children with early-onset lesions of the left hemisphere: An fMRI study. *Brain* 127, 1229–1236.

Luna, B., Thulborn, K. R., Munoz, D. P., Merriam, E. P., Garver, K. E., Minshew, N. J., Keshavan, M. S., Genovese, C. R., Eddy, W. F., & Sweeney, J. A. (2001). Maturation of widely distributed brain function subserves cognitive development. *NeuroImage* 13, 786–793.

Maki, A., Yamashita, Y., Ito, Y., Watanabe, E., Mayanagi, Y., & Koizumi, H. (1995). Spatial and temporal analysis of human motor activity using noninvasive NIR topography. *Medical Physics* 22, 1997–2005.

Martínez, A., DiRusso, F., Anllo-Vento, L., Sereno, M. I., Buxton, R. B., & Hillyard, S. A. (2001). Putting spatial attention on the map: Timing and localization of stimulus selection processes in striate and extrastriate visual areas. *Vision Research* 41(10–11), 1437–1457.

Martynova, O., Kirjavainen, J., & Cheour, M. (2003). Mismatch negativity and late discriminative negativity in sleeping human newborns. *Neuroscience Letters* 340, 75–78.

Muzik, O., Chugani, D. C., Juhasz, C., Shen, C., & Chugani, H. T. (2000). Statistical parametric mapping: Assessment of application in children. *NeuroImage* 12(5), 538–549.

Nelson, C. A., Monk, C. S., Lin, J., Carver, L. J., Thomas, K. M., & Truwit, C. L. (2000). Functional neuro-anatomy of spatial working memory in children. *Developmental Psychobiology* 36(1), 109–116.

Ogawa, S., Tank, D. W., Menon, R., Ellermann, J. M., Kim, S. G., Merkle, H., & Ugurbil, K. (1992). Intrinsic signal changes accompanying sensory stimulation: Functional brain mapping using MRI. *Proceedings of the National Academy of Sciences USA* 89(13), 5951–5955.

Olesen, P. J., Nagy, Z., Westerberg, H., & Klingberg, T. (2003). Combined analysis of DTI and fMRI data reveals a joint maturation of white and grey matter in a fronto-parietal network. *Cognitive Brain Research* 18, 48–57.

Pena, M., Maki, A., Kovacic, D., Dehaene-Lambertz, G., Koizumi, H., Bouquet, F., & Mehler, J. (2003). Sounds and silence: An optical topography study of language recognition at birth. *Proceedings of the National Academy of Sciences USA* 100, 11702–11705.

Peterson, B. S. (2003). Brain imaging studies of the anatomical and functional consequences of preterm birth for human brain development. *Annals of the New York Academy of Science* 1008, 219–237.

Picton, T. W., Bentin, S., Berg, P., Donchin, E., Hillyard, S. A., Johnson, S. A., Johnson, R., Miller, G. R., Ritter, W., Ruchkin, D. S., Rugg, M. D., & Taylor, M. J. (2000). Guidelines for using human event-related potentials to study cognition: Recording standards and publication criteria. *Psychophysiology* 37, 127–152.

Richards, J. E. (2002). Cortical sources of ERP for infants' recognition of briefly presented visual stimuli. *Psychophysiology* 39, S70–S70.

Ridderinkhof, K. R., & van der Molen, M. W. (1995). A psychophysiological analysis of developmental differences in the ability to resist interference. *Child Development* 66, 1040–1056.

Rosen, B. R., Buckner, R. L., & Dale, A. M. (1998). Event-related functional MRI: Past, present, and future. *Proceedings of the National Academy of Sciences USA* 95, 773–780.

Rubia, K., Overmeyer, S., Taylor, E., Brammer, M., Williams, S. C., Simmons, A., & Bullmore, E. T. (1999). Hypofrontality in attention deficit hyperactivity disorder during higher-order motor control: A study with functional MRI. *American Journal of Psychiatry* 156(6), 891–896.

Sarnthein, J., Petsche, H., Rappelsberger, P., Shaw, G. L., & von Stein, A. (1998). Synchronization between prefrontal and posterior association cortex during human working memory. *Proceedings of the National Academy of Sciences USA* 95(12), 7092–7096.

Scerif, G., Worden, M. S., Seiger, L., & Casey, B. J. (in press). Top-down expectancy modulates early stimulus feature processing to resolve stimulus conflict. *Journal of Cognitive Neuroscience*.

Schlaggar, B. L., Brown, T. T., Lugar, H. M., Visscher, K. M., Miezin, F. M., & Petersen, S. E. (2002). Functional neuroanatomical differences between adults and school-age children in the processing of single words. *Science* 296(5572), 1476–1479.

Seghier, M. L., Lazeyras, F., Zimine, S., Maier, S. E., Hanquinet, S., Delavelle, J., Volpe, J. J., & Huppi, P. S. (2004). Combination of event-related fMRI and diffusion tensor imaging in an infant with perinatal stroke. *NeuroImage* 21, 463–472.

Snyder, K., Webb, S. J., & Nelson, C. A. (2002). Theoretical and methodological implications of variability in infant brain response during a recognition memory paradigm. *Infant Behavior and Development* 25, 466–494.

Strangman, G., Culver, J. P., Thompson, J. H., & Boas, D. A. (2002). A quantitative comparison of simultaneous BOLD fMRI and NIRS recordings during functional brain activation. *NeuroImage* 17, 719–731.

Talairach, J., & Tournoux, P. (1988). *Co-Planar Stereotaxic Atlas of the Human Brain*. New York: Thieme Medical Publishers.

Taylor, M. J., & Baldeweg, T. (2002). Application of EEG, ERP and intracranial recordings to the investigation of cognitive functions in children. *Developmental Science* 5(3), 318–334.

Thomas, K. M., King, S. W., Franzen, P. L., Welsh, T. F., Berkowitz, A. L., Noll, D. C., Birmaher, V., & Casey, B. J. (1999). A developmental functional MRI study of spatial working memory. *NeuroImage* 10, 327–338.

Vaidya, C. J., Austin, G., Kirkorian, G., Ridlehuber, H. W. Q., Desmond, J. E., Glover, G. H., & Gabrieli, D. E. (1998). Selective effects of methylphenidate in attention deficit hyperactivity disorder: A functional magnetic resonance study. *Proceedings of the National Academy of Sciences USA* 95, 14494–14499.

12 Functional Neuroimaging of Cognitive Aging

Sander M. Daselaar, Jeffrey Browndyke, and Roberto Cabeza

As we age, the anatomy and physiology of our brain decline, and so do our cognitive abilities. As our brain shrivels and its functions dwindle, cognitive processes slow down and fail. Yet, brain and cognitive systems do not endure the assaults of aging passively; they respond plastically to these attacks by reorganizing their functions. Functional neuroimaging techniques, such as positron emission tomography (PET) and functional MRI (fMRI), provide ideal methods to investigate patterns of neurocognitive decline and compensation in older adults. During cognitive performance, older adults (OAs) often fail to activate some of the brain regions recruited by young adults (YAs), and instead recruit other brain regions. These age-related changes in brain activity can be linked directly to the effects of aging on behavioral measures, providing a bridge between cerebral aging and cognitive aging. For this reason, the field of functional neuroimaging of cognitive aging has grown very fast since the mid-1990s. The goal of this chapter is to provide a concise introduction to this new and exiting field. As an introduction, we briefly describe two consistent patterns of age-related changes in brain activity. Then we review PET and fMRI studies of aging in various cognitive domains. Finally, we discuss some current issues and future directions.

Introduction

Functional neuroimaging studies have revealed at least two consistent patterns of age-related changes in brain activity during cognitive performance. First, several studies, particularly in the visual perception domain, have found an age-related decrease in occipital activity coupled with an age-related increase in PFC activity. Grady et al. (1994) were the first to describe this occipital-decrease/frontal-increase (ODFI) pattern, and they suggested that OAs compensated for visual processing deficits (occipital decrease) by recruiting higher-order cognitive processes (PFC increase). In this study OAs and YAs were matched in accuracy but differed in reaction times (RTs), so the authors further suggested that additional recruitment of PFC functions allows OAs to maintain a good accuracy level at the expense of slower reaction times. Most subsequent studies that found OFDI endorsed Grady et al.'s compensatory account of age-related PFC increases.

A second consistent finding is a tendency of OAs to show more bilateral (less asymmetric) PFC activations than YAs. This pattern was conceptualized as a *Hemispheric Asymmetry Reduction in Older Adults* (HAROLD) model (Cabeza, 2002), and a sample of studies supporting the model are listed in table 12.1. The HAROLD pattern was originally described by Cabeza, Grady et al. (1997) and attributed to a compensatory mechanism. This *compensation account* is consistent with evidence that bilateral activity in OAs is positively correlated with successful cognitive performance (Reuter-Lorenz et al., 2000), and is found in high-performing

Table 12.1
PET/fMRI activity in left and right PFC in younger and older adults

Cognitive Domain	Younger		Older	
Imaging Technique: Materials/Task (Reference)	Left	Right	Left	Right
Visual Perception				
PET: Face Matching (Grady et al., 1994, exp. 2)	−	+	++	++
PET: Face Matching (Grady et al., 2000)	+	+++	++	++
Language/Semantic Retrieval				
fMRI: Verb Generation (Persson et al., 2004)	+	−	+	+
Working Memory/Executive Functions				
PET: Letter DR (Reuter-Lorenz et al., 2000)	+	−	+	+
PET: Location DR (Reuter-Lorenz et al., 2000)	−	+	+	+
PET: Number N-Back: (Dixit et al., 2000)	+	+++	++	++
fMRI: No-Go Trials (Nielson et al., 2002)	−	+	+	+
Episodic Encoding/Semantic Retrieval				
PET: Word-pair—intentional (Cabeza et al., 1997)	++	+	+	+
fMRI: Word—incidental (Stebbins et al., 2002)	++	+	+	+
fMRI: Word—intentional (Logan et al., 2002)	++	+	+	+
fMRI: Word—incidental (Logan et al., 2002)	++	+	++	++
fMRI: Word—SME (Morcom et al., 2003)	++	+	++	++
Episodic Retrieval				
PET: Word Pair Cued-Recall (Cabeza et al., 1997)	−	++	+	+
PET: Word Stem Cued-Recall (Bäckman et al., 1997)	−	+	+	+
PET: Word Recognition (Madden et al., 1999)	−	+	++	++
PET: Face Recognition (Grady et al., 2002)	−	++	+	+

Note: Plus signs indicate significant activity in the left or right PFC, and minus signs indicate nonsignificant activity. The number of pluses is an approximate index of the relative amount of activity in left and right PFC in each study, and it cannot be compared across studies. DR, delayed response task; SME, subsequent memory effect.

rather than in low-performing OAs (Cabeza et al., 2002; Rosen et al., 2002). However, an alternative account is that a more widespread activation pattern reflects an age-related difficulty in engaging specialized neural mechanisms (e.g., Li & Lindenberger, 1999; Logan et al., 2002). This *dedifferentiation account* is consistent with an age-related increase in correlations across tasks (Lindenberger & Baltes, 1994). In general, available evidence tends to be more consistent with the compensation than with the dedifferentiation account (Daselaar & Cabeza, 2005), but further research is certainly required.

Functional Neuroimaging of Cognitive Aging

Table 12.2 displays Brodmann areas (BAs) and other regions showing age-related increases or decreases in activation during PET and fMRI studies of various cognitive functions. Some studies are reviewed in the text but are not included in the table because they focused on a few regions of interest (ROI) and/or reported complex interactions among several conditions rather than pairwise contrasts. As we consider each study, we will note the aforementioned consistent age-related activity changes, ODFI and HAROLD.

Visual Perception

Perception was the first domain where activation imaging was applied to investigate the neural correlates of cognitive aging. To date, all studies in this area have focused on the visual modality, and most on the perception of facial features and/or affective expressions.

The first activation study in the area of visual perception was a PET study by Grady et al. (1994) investigating face and location matching tasks. Consistent with the ventral/dorsal pathway distinction, both YAs and OAs showed occipitotemporal activations during face matching, and occipitoparietal activations during location matching. In both conditions, OAs showed decreased occipital activity but increased frontal activity (ODFI pattern). As noted before, Grady et al. proposed that OAs are less efficient in recruiting visual areas before the ventral-dorsal bifurcation, and compensate by relying more on anterior regions including PFC.

The ODFI pattern was replicated by two subsequent studies: Grady et al. (2000) and Levine et al. (2000). Grady et al. investigated perception of degraded and non-degraded faces and found an ODFI similar to Grady et al. (1994), with the difference that the age-related PFC increase was left-lateralized. Additionally, degraded face matching performance (accuracy and RTs) correlated with fusiform regions in YAs but with thalamic and hippocampal regions in OAs. These latter two regions were recruited during nondegraded face matching only by OAs, suggesting a

Table 12.2

Results of functional neuroimaging studies of cognitive aging

Column groupings — Per form: Ac, RT. LEFT HEMISPHERE: Subcort (cb, th, bg); Occip (17, 18, 19); Temporal (37, 20, 21, 22, 42, ins, 38); Parietal (39, 40, 7); MTL (PHG, Am, HC); Midline (Pre, PC, 24, 32, 4, 8).

Study	Contrast	Ac	RT	cb	th	bg	17	18	19	37	20	21	22	42	ins	38	39	40	7	PHG	Am	HC	Pre	PC	24	32	4	8
VISUAL PERCEPTION																												
P Grady 94	face: matching—bl									○					○													
P Grady 94	location: match—bl							●	○	○					○													○
P Grady 00	face-ndgr. match—bl				○			●		○	○				○		○	●				○	○					
P Levine 00	form perception—bl			●				○	●	●														●	○			
F GunningDixon 03	face expression: discrim.—bl						●	●	●	●									●	○						○	○	
F Iidaka 02	face expression: perception—bl					●		●									●					●						
ATTENTION																												
P Madden 97	visual search: divided-central	≠	≠					●																	○			
P Madden 02	visual srch: covariate w/ perform								●																			
F Cabeza 04	visual sustained attention—base	≈	≈	○				●	●									○				●	●				●	
F Thomsen 04	dichot. listening: attend-left		≠	●				●	○				●													●		●
LANGUAGE/SEMANTIC PROCESSING																												
P Madden 96	word: lex dec—Enc							●																				
P Madden 02	word: lex dec—bl	≈	≠	✤			●	✤												●							●	
F Johnson 01	word pairs: semantic dec—bl	≈						●					✤															
F Persson 04	word: verb gen. high demand—bl		≈			○					●																●	
F Grossman 02	sentence compreh.—bl	≈	≠														●	●	●				●					
WORKING MEMORY																												
Verbal																												
P Reuter-L. 00	letter: WM—bl (VOIs)	≠	≠																				●	○	●			
F Rypma 01	letter: WM: 6–1 letter load	≠	≈			●			●						○		●	●					●	○	●			
F Rypma 00	letter: WM Enc, main, retr	≈	≠																									
F Cabeza 04	word: WM—base			○			●	●	●								○	○				●	●					●
P Haut 00	number: self-ordering > ctrl	≈																	●									
P Haut 00	number: ext.-ordered > ctrl	≈									○		○															
F Johnson 04	word: refresh > repeat/read																											
Visuospatial																												
P Grady 98	face: WM—bl	≈	≠											●														
P Grady 98	incr w/ long delays								○															●				
P Reuter-L. 00	locat: WM—bl (VOIs)	≈	≠																					●				○
F Mitchell 00	objects.: combo > obj / loc	≠																						●				
F Park 03	scenes: maint or probe	≈	≠																					●				
F Lamar 04	DMTS—ctrl.	≠		●			●		●						○								●			●	●	●
F Lamar 04	DNMTS—ctrl.	≠		○												○								○		●	●	●
EXECUTIVE FUNCTIONS																												
F Nielsen 02	no-go > base	≠	≠			○											○	○										
F Milham 02	Stroop: incong > others	≈	≈					○	○				○	○					●									
F Langenecker 04	Stroop: incong > neutral	≠	≈																							○		
P Nagahama 97	WCST—bl	≠	≠	●				●	●								●	●					●					
P Esposito 99	WCST (corr w/ age)			●				○									●	●										
P Esposito 99	RPM (corr w/ age)			●							●		●	○				●						○				

Table 12.2
(continued)

	RIGHT HEMISPHERE																																							
Frontal								Frontal										Midline				MTL			Parietal			Temporal							Occip			Subcort		
6	44	45	47	11	46	9	10	10	9	46	11	47	45	44	6	8	4	32	24	PC	Pre	HC	Am	PHG	7	40	39	38	ins	42	22	21	20	37	19	18	17	bg	th	cb
		○	○		○			○		○		○○														○								○○○	○	●●			
○		○		○	○	○	○				●	●			●				●	●						●●	●●				●●			●	●	●			
						○	○						○					○					●	●		○○					○	○		●	●	●	●			●
	○				●							●		○				○						●			●						●	●		●				
○									○						●					●															●				
○		○			○					○			○	○	●			●	●		●	●													●				●
			●		●							●																											
	❖	❖				❖		❖											❖						●	●					○❖				●				
●			●		●								○																	○							○		
○	○					○	○	○	○					●	●												○				○○				●				
●					●	●	○	●	○○		●	●	○	●	●			●		●	●						●							●			●		
					●	●			●●	●			●●				●	●●		●	●				○	○								●		●			●
○					○	○			○●				○	○				●																						
						○																																		
						●																																		
○		●				○					●		●																				○					●	
○					○	○		●					○	○						●						●				○		○○	●	○			●	○	
	○	○				○			●			●	○		●																			●	○		○	●
○	○	○		○		○						○	○		●	○		●													●		○	●	○			
●						●																								●			○	●	○			
○			○			○						○	○			○	○				○				○													
	●				●	●	●	○	○		○	○						●		●	●			●		●							○	●	●		●	●
						●	○	○																						○			●		○	●	○			●

Table 12.2
(continued)

		Per form		Subcort			Occip			Temporal							Parietal			MTL			Midline					
Cognitive function Study	Contrast	Ac	RT	cb	th	bg	17	18	19	37	20	21	22	42	ins	38	39	40	7	PHG	Am	HC	Pre	PC	24	32	4	8
IMPLICIT MEMORY																												
P Bäckman 97	word stem priming																											
F Daselaar 05	word stem priming: nov—rep	≠													●													
F Lustig 04	semantic repetition priming: rep—bl	≈	≠																									
F Daselaar 03	skill learning	≈	≠																									
EPISODIC MEMORY ENCODING																												
Intentional encoding																												
P Cabeza 97	word pair: Enc—Rn/Rc	≈							●				○										○					●
P Madden 99	words: Enc—bl	≠	≈		○																							
P Anders 00	word pairs: FA Enc—FA Rc	≠								○	○	○			●			○										
F Logan 02 exp 1	words: intent enc—bl	≠																										
P Grady 95	face: Enc—2 bl	≠								●																	●	
P Grady 02	face: Enc—Rn	≠	≠	●						●	●	●			●	●								●	●			●	
P Schiavetto 02	obj ident Enc > obj loc Enc	≠																				●						
F Iidaka 01	object pairs: abstract Enc—bl	≠								●							●	●	●									
F Meulenbroek 04	route enc—Rn	≠							●	●			○				●	○					○	○			○	●
Incidental encoding																												
F Stebbins 02	word: deep—shallow																											●
F Logan 02 exp 2	word: deep—shallow	≈	≈																									
F Rosen 02	Old-high, word: deep—shallow	≈																										
F Daselaar 03b	word: deep—shallow		≈											●								●						
Subsequent memory																												
F Morcom 03	words Dm: Y long delay—O short delay	≈	≈									●						○										
F Daselaar 03c	Old-low, word: rem—bl	≠	≈																			●	●					
F Gutchess 05	picture Dm	≠						●	●									○				●					○	○
EPISODIC MEMORY RETRIEVAL																												
Recognition																												
P Cabeza 97	word pair: Rn—Enc	≈											○															
P Madden 99	word: Rn—bl	≠	≈		●																							○
P Cabeza 00	word: Rn—recEncy	≠	≈	○										●														
F Daselaar 03c	Old-high, word: Rn—bl	≈	≈																									
F Daselaar 03c	Old-low, word: Rn—bl	≠	≈	○								○			○													
F Cabeza 04	Rn—bl	≠		○				●	●			○						○		○			●	●	●		●	
F Daselaar 05	Rn: parametric high/low confidence	≈	≠															○				●						
P Grady 95	face: Rn—2 bl	≠																										
P Grady 02	face: Rn—Enc	≠							●									○					○		○			
Recall																												
P Schacter 96	stem Rc: low—high	≠																										
P Schacter 96	stem Rc: high—low	≠										○																
P Bäckman 97	stem Rc: Rc—bl	≠		●								●												○				
P Cabeza 97	pair Rc: Rc—Enc	≈										○																
P Anders 00	pair Rc: FA—FA Enc	≠			●			●	○														○	●			○	
P Cabeza 02	word Rc: Rc-bl, OA-high	≈																										
Context memory																												
P Cabeza 00	word: Context—Rn	≠							●																			
P Cabeza 02	Old-high, word: Context—Recall	≈																										
P Schiavetto 02	object: loc Rn > obj Rn	≠																				○						
F Meulenbroek 04	route Rn—enc	≠						○	○				●				○	●					●	●	●			○
F Maguire 03	autobio events—publ event	≈																										

Symbols: ● = regions more activated or activated only by young adults; ○ = regions more activated or activated only by old adults; ❖ = regions similarly activated in young and old groups.

Table 12.2
(continued)

	RIGHT HEMISPHERE																																							
Frontal								Frontal										Midline				MTL			Parietal			Temporal							Occip			Subcort		
6	44	45	47	11	46	9	10	10	9	46	11	47	45	44	6	8	4	32	24	PC	Pre	HC	Am	PHG	7	40	39	38	ins	42	22	21	20	37	19	18	17	bg	th	cb
											●	●																								●				
●					●																															○				
●	●	●	●		●			○	○	○				●	●		●									○					●	●				●				
		●	●						○					○	○			●				●											○							
		●	●																																●	●				
			●																					●		●	●								●	●	●	○		
○																		○	○																●					
	●	●	●		●									○	○																				○	○				
							○	○			●																													
○							○									○								●		○									●			○	○	
○		○					○	○	○		●					○		○			○						●											●		
			○				○	○																											○					
○							○							○	○			●	●		●	●	●											○	○	●				●
							○																		○										●					
																									●															
								●	●																●															
		○			○		○														○						●												●	
		○	○		○		●	●	●	●				○				○	○		○																		●	
							●	●	○																									●	●	●				
							●	●	○				○														●								●					
			●																																●			●		
●																		●	●					○		○	○					○		○	○	○		●		

Abbreviations: Anders = Anderson; bg = basal ganglia; bl = baseline; cb = cerebellum; corr = correlation; cpc = cuneus/precuneus; DA = divided attention; Enc = Encoding; FA = full attention; ins = insula; lex dec = lexical decision; mt = medial temporal; mtch = matching; ndgr = nondegraded; pass = passive; Rc = recall; Reuter-L = Reuter-Lorenz; Rn = recognition; sem = semantic; sm = sensorimotor; th = thalamus.

compensatory mechanism. Levine et al. investigated perception of simple visual textures. In addition to ODFI, this study showed an age-related decrease in right parahippocampal gyrus (PHG) activity and an age-related increase in anterior cingulate activity.

ODFI was also found in two studies investigating the perception of facial expressions of emotion: Gunning-Dixon et al. (2003) and Iidaka et al. (2002). In the emotion discrimination condition of Gunning-Dixon et al.'s study, OAs showed ODFI as well as decreases in amygdala activity and increases in anterior cingulate, temporal, and parietal activity. According to the authors, OAs compensated for deficits in visual/limbic regions by recruiting other brain regions including PFC. Iidaka et al. manipulated the emotions of faces during an age discrimination task. Activity in the left amygdala in response to negative facial affect was significantly reduced in OA. Age-related reductions were also observed in right PHG for positive facial affect, and in bilateral lingual gyrus regions for both positive and neutral facial affect. Some PFC regions were recruited by OAs but not by YAs. Thus, the two studies found ODFI as well as age-related decreases and increases in other brain regions.

Finally, the study by Park et al. (2004) investigated the effects of aging on ventral visual cortex activity during the perception of faces, places, and words. Compared with YAs, OAs showed more shared voxels across stimulus categories and greater dedifferentiation scores (e.g., the probability that a peak for one category is above threshold for other categories). The authors suggest that age-related functional dedifferentiation occurs in high-level visual sensory cortex and that these changes may partly account for age-related decreases in perceptual speed noted by Grady et al. (1994) and others.

To summarize visual perception studies, most studies showed the ODFI pattern as well as other age-related activation differences. In addition to the age-related decreases in occipital activity, several studies found decreases in medial temporal lobe (MTL) activity: two studies found decreases in right PHG (Iidaka et al., 2002; Levine et al., 2000), and two studies on emotional processing found decreases in the amygdala (Gunning-Dixon et al., 2003; Iidaka et al., 2002). MTL decreases may reflect an extension of occipital decreases into more anterior regions of the ventral pathway, or they may reflect specific memory-related or emotion-related mechanisms. Instead of an overall decrease in visual cortex activity, Park et al. (2004) found evidence of an age-related dedifferentiation in stimulus-specific activation patterns. Finally, age-related increases in activation were found not only in PFC but also in lateral temporal and parietal regions. These increases may be consistent with a compensatory interpretation, but they highlight the problem of determining what specific cognitive operations engage each of the regions differentially recruited by OAs.

Attention

As with visual perception, most attention and aging studies have been within the visual modality, with the notable exception of one study that investigated auditory attention. Two studies by Madden and collaborators investigated selective attention during visual search. In Madden et al.'s (1997) study, selective attention was cued by spatial locations. Participants had to indicate which of two target letters occurred within a matrix of letters. In the Central condition, the target always occurred in the center of the matrix, whereas in the Divided condition, it could appear in any matrix location. Extending ODFI to the visual attention domain, in the Divided-Central contrast OAs showed weaker activity in occipital regions but stronger activity in PFC regions. As in perception studies, the age-related PFC recruitment was interpreted as compensatory.

In Madden et al.'s (2002) study, selective attention was cued by color information. Participants had to detect whether a single upright L occurred among 17 rotated L distractors, and the difficulty of the search was varied by manipulating the number of letters presented in a different color: only the target (feature search), the target and 2 distractors (guided search), and the target and 8 distractors (conjunction search). OAs were less accurate in detecting the target, but they were as successful as YAs in using color information to guide attention to a subset of display items. Occipitotemporal activity increased as a function of difficulty, but more so in YAs. This difference reflected greater activity in OAs in the easier task conditions. According to the authors, this last finding may reflect a compensatory mechanism that does not involve the recruitment of brain regions outside the ventral occipito-temporal pathway, as previously found in other studies (i.e., ODFI). The ODFI pattern was also found in the sustained attention study by Cabeza et al. (2004), which is reviewed in the final summary section.

A third study by Madden et al. (2004, not in table 12.2) did not investigate selective attention during a visual search task but target/novelty detection during an oddball task. Participants pressed one key for frequent standard stimuli (squares: 87%) and infrequent novel stimuli (object pictures: 6%), and another key for infrequent target stimuli (circles: 7%). Activity was measured in frontal, occipital, and deep gray matter (striatum, thalamus, insula) ROIs. Targets activated PFC regions similarly for YAs and OAs, and deep gray matter regions to a greater extent in OAs. Novels activated occipital regions, and this activity was weaker in OAs. Interestingly, occipital activity was more bilateral in OAs (cf. HAROLD). Regression analyses relating activations to RTs identified the strongest relationship for YAs in PFC (middle frontal gyrus) and for OAs in deep gray matter (putamen and thalamus). According to the authors, OAs may emphasize attentional control of response regulation, in compensation for the age-related decline in visual processing efficiency.

Whereas the attention studies focused on the visual modality, the study by Thomsen et al. (2004) investigated the effects of aging on auditory attention. In each trial, two different consonant-vowel syllables were presented to each ear (dichotic listening) with the instruction to attend to and report either the left- or right-ear stimulus. Without attentional biasing, there is a right-ear advantage in this task, but this advantage can be shifted to the left ear by the attend-left instruction. OAs had difficulty with this top-down attentional biasing. The attend-left condition yielded a left dorsal PFC (BA 8/9) activation, which was reduced in OAs. Cortical thickness in this region was also reduced in OAs, suggesting that both functional and structural changes underlie age-related attentional deficits.

To summarize attention studies, whereas the selective attention study by Madden et al. (1997) and the sustained attention study by Cabeza et al. (2004) found the typical ODFI pattern, other studies found forms of compensation in OAs that did not involve greater PFC recruitment. The visual search study by Madden et al. (2002) found an age-related increase in visual cortex for easier search conditions, and the target detection study by Madden et al. (2004) found an age-related increase in deep gray matter regions. Age-related decreases in PFC activity are more noticeable in Thomsen et al.'s (2004) auditory attention study, but it is unclear if this is related to modality or to the behavioral performance, which was quite different in OAs and YAs.

Language/Semantic Processing

With the exception of two studies on sentence comprehension, most of the studies in the language/semantic processing domain investigated simple linguistic and semantic processes using words as stimuli. Three studies by Madden and collaborators investigated lexical decision (word/nonword). The first study (Madden et al., 1996) found that, consistent with visual perception studies, ventral pathway activity during lexical decision was weaker in OAs than in YAs. In a follow-up study that controlled for potential confounds (Madden, Langley et al., 2002), both groups activated left inferior PFC and left occipitotemporal regions, and again OAs showed weaker ventral pathway activity. OAs did not show greater PFC activity (i.e., ODFI) than YAs, suggesting that semantic retrieval does not lead to compensatory PFC recruitment, as other tasks do. Finally, a reanalysis of the previous data set (Whiting et al., 2003, not in table 12.2) distinguished the effects of lexical (word frequency) and sublexical (word length) factors on visual word identification. Activity in the left occipitotemporal pathway was a significant predictor of the effect of word frequency in OAs, such that increased activation in these regions was associated with a greater degree of word identification slowing. This finding suggests that some of the age-related variance in lexical decision making processes could be due to perceptual encoding difficulties rather than lexical access problems, and may reflect OAs' greater reliance on neural architecture for lexical-based processing to correctly and quickly identify words.

S. C. Johnson et al. (2001) investigated semantic decisions and phonological decisions about auditorily presented word pairs. During phonological tasks, OAs showed as much activity as YAs in superior temporal regions but reduced activity in the right angular gyrus and other regions. The results did not change when entering atrophy as a covariate, suggesting that they cannot be explained by anatomical differences. During semantic tasks, OAs and YAs showed similar activity in bilateral ventral PFC. Thus, like Madden, Langley et al. (2002), the results of this study emphasize the preservation of semantic processing in older adults.

Persson et al. (2004) investigated verb generation and manipulated selection demands by comparing nouns with few and many verb associations (e.g., scissors: cut vs. ball: throw, bounce, kick, etc.). During high-demand selection (Many condition), OAs showed weaker activity in left ventrolateral PFC but greater activity in right ventrolateral PFC. As a result, OAs showed a more bilateral pattern of PFC activity (i.e., HAROLD). An age-related reduction in activity was also found in the anterior cingulate cortex. Whereas the age-related decrease in left PFC was exclusive to the Many condition and suggests underrecruitment, the decrease in anterior cingulate also affected the Few condition and, hence, suggests a more general absence of resources. Inferior temporal activity showed an age-related decrease only in the Many condition, possibly reflecting semantic retrieval deficits. Finally, the basal ganglia showed an age-related increase in activity that, like the age-related increase in right ventrolateral PFC, could reflect a compensatory mechanism.

Whereas previous studies focused on simple language or semantic processes and used words as stimuli, Grossman and collaborators conducted two studies on sentence comprehension. One study (Grossman et al., 2002b) found that healthy OAs with poor sentence comprehension did not recruit a core network of left perisylvian brain regions to the same degree as YAs and OAs with good sentence comprehension. Greater PFC activity was not detected in the OAs with good sentence comprehension, but it was noted in the OAs with poor comprehension. Grossman et al. (2002b) suggest that the additional activity associated with poor comprehension in OAs may reflect the recruitment of nongrammatical problem-solving strategies to understand complex sentences.

The other study by Grossman and collaborators investigated comprehension of sentences involving different working memory demands (Grossman et al., 2002a). Common activation areas in YAs and OAs for all sentences independent of working memory load included the left temporal and ventrolateral PFC regions, and bilateral occipital cortex. Additional common activation associated with increased working memory load was noted in left ventrolateral PFC. For all sentences, OAs showed weaker activity in parietal cortex but greater activity in dorsal left PFC, right temporal, and bilateral anteromedial PFC regions. According to the authors, the latter age-related increases reflect upregulation of portions of rehearsal (Broca's area) and material-specific (right temporoparietal cortex) aspects of a large-scale working memory in order to support complex sentence comprehension.

To summarize language studies, when secondary processing demands in areas sensitive to age-related change are kept to a minimum, it can be seen that core language functions, such as semantic retrieval and sentence comprehension, may indeed be resistant to age-related change. As evidence, S. C. Johnson et al. (2001) note that the lack of greater task-related activity in their OA sample suggests that simple auditory semantic and phonological decisions may not require PFC compensatory activity, and the Madden et al. (1996) results seem to indicate that PFC activity may actually be reduced in OA under certain language task conditions. Additionally, the work of Persson et al. (2004) and Grossman et al. in high/low verb generation and sentence comprehension demands, respectively, suggests that age-related changes are minimal when the demands for mediating age-sensitive cognitive functions are low. The preservation of cortical regions mediating core language functions in YAs and OAs appears robust enough to posit that healthy aging is not associated with cortical reorganization or compensation of language abilities. It is the enhanced need for, or decline of, working memory and visual perceptual skills in OA that accounts for age-related differences detected to date.

Working Memory

Working memory (WM) processes comprise a variety of operations, from the simple maintenance of information over a brief delay, to the manipulation and monitoring of working memory contents, to the executive processes required by problem solving and reasoning tasks. Studies investigating executive processes are reviewed in the next section, whereas this section focuses on studies investigating relatively simpler verbal and visuospatial working memory processes.

Verbal Working Memory

Reuter-Lorenz et al. (2000) investigated a task in which participants maintained four letters in WM and then compared them with a probe letter. The main finding was that PFC activity was left-lateralized in YAs but bilateral in OAs. Like Cabeza, Grady et al. (1997), Reuter-Lorenz et al. interpreted this HAROLD pattern as compensatory. Consistent with this interpretation, OAs who showed the bilateral activation pattern were faster in the verbal WM task than those who did not. A follow-up study including additional participants (Reuter-Lorenz et al., 2001) found bilateral activations in OAs not only in PFC but also in parietal regions.

Also using letters, Rypma et al. (2001) examined verbal WM for different memory loads (1 vs. 6 letters). The 6 vs. 1 contrast yielded three main findings. First, left-lateralized ventrolateral PFC activity was similar in YAs and OAs. Second, right-lateralized dorsolateral PFC activity was weaker in OAs than in YAs. Finally, a left anterior PFC region was more activated in OAs than in YAs. The authors suggested that aging impairs executive aspects of WM mediated by dorsolateral PFC but not maintenance operations (e.g., phonological loop) mediated by left ventrolateral PFC. Additionally, the age-related increase in left PFC activity was attributed to functional compensation.

Using event-related fMRI, Rypma and D'Esposito (2000) differentiated the effects of aging on encoding, maintenance, and retrieval phases of WM. The main result was that dorsolateral PFC activity was reduced by aging during the retrieval phase, whereas ventrolateral PFC activity was not affected by aging during any phase. These results are consistent with the aforementioned dissociation between dorsolateral and ventrolateral PFC, and additionally suggest that the retrieval phase of WM is more sensitive to aging than the encoding and maintenance phases.

Haut et al. (2000) investigated self-ordering and externally ordered number gene-ration tasks. Compared with YAs, OAs showed reduced right PFC activity during the self-ordering task but increased left PFC activity during the externally ordered task. According to the authors, the decrease in right PFC may reflect reduced reliance on number visualization, whereas the increase in left PFC may reflect func-tional compensation.

Whereas the foregoing WM studies investigated relatively complex tasks, the study by M. K. Johnson et al. (2004) examined an extremely simple one. Participants silently read words presented one by one on the screen. Sometimes a word was repeated and sometimes a cue signaled participants to think about the previous word, a process dubbed "refreshing." Compared with Read and Repeat conditions, the Refresh condition activated left PFC, parietal, temporal, and anterior cingulate regions. Refreshing-related activity was mostly similar in the two groups, but a left PFC activation was significantly reduced in OAs. Given that refreshing is a compo-nent of many cognitive tasks, an age-related deficit in this basic process could have a widespread effect on cognitive functioning.

Visuospatial Working Memory

Grady et al. (1998) investigated a face WM task and varied the maintenance interval between 1 and 21 sec. There were three interesting findings. First, activity in right PFC area 45 was greater in YAs than in OAs, and increased with longer delays only for YAs, which suggests that YAs were better able to engage this region as task dif-ficulty increased. Second, OAs showed greater activity in left frontal BA 9/45, pos-sibly reflecting a compensatory mechanism or increased task demands. Finally, as delay extended from 1 to 6 sec, left MTL activity increased in YAs but decreased in OAs, which implies that OAs have difficulties initiating memory strategies mediated by MTL or sustaining MTL activity beyond very short retention intervals.

In McIntosh et al.'s (1999, not included in table 12.2) study, subjects maintained a target sine wave grating in visual short-term memory for either 0.4 or 4 sec, and then compared its spatial frequency with a probe grating. The difference in spatial frequency between targets and probes was adjusted for each subject, thereby matching performance across subjects. Despite equivalent performance, OAs showed weaker interactions among the regions underlying task performance. Conversely, they recruited unique PFC and MTL regions, which were related to task performance only in OAs. These results suggest that OAs compensated for reduced network interactions by recruiting additional brain regions. Moreover, some regions whose activity was not affected by aging, such as the right hippocampus, interacted with a different network of regions in the two groups (Della Maggiore et al., 2000). Taken together with the results of Cabeza, Grady et al. (1997) and Grady et al. (1999), this finding supports the idea that aging affects not only the activity of various brain regions but also the interactions between these regions.

In addition to a verbal WM condition, the aforementioned PET study by Reuter-Lorenz et al. (2000) included a spatial WM task. As reviewed above, during the verbal task, YAs activated right PFC and OAs additionally recruited left PFC. The spatial task yielded converse findings: YAs activated left PFC and OAs additionally recruited right PFC. Thus, even though the age-related increase was in opposite hemispheres, the outcome was in both cases the HAROLD pattern. This result supports the generalizability of the HAROLD model for different kinds of stimuli (see above).

Mitchell et al. (2000) investigated a WM paradigm with an important episodic encoding component. In each trial, participants were presented an object in a particular screen location and had to hold in WM the object, its location, or both (combination trials). Combination trials can be assumed to involve not only WM maintenance but also the binding of different information into an integrated memory trace (relational memory encoding). OAs showed a deficit in accuracy in the combination condition but not in the object and location conditions. Two regions were differentially involved in the combination condition in YAs but not in OAs: a left anterior hippocampal region and an anteromedial PFC region (right BA 10). According to the authors, a disruption of a hippocampal-PFC circuit may underlie binding deficits in OAs.

Park et al. (2003) found a similar age-related reduction in hippocampal activity in a study involving processing of complex visual scenes. Participants maintained scenes in working memory or viewed them continuously. The study yielded two main findings. First, the left hippocampus was more activated in the Viewing than in the

Maintenance condition in YAs but not in OAs. Second, during the probe, OAs showed greater ventral PFC activity than YAs, bilaterally. Although there was a trend for PFC activity to be more bilateral in OAs (i.e., HAROLD), the difference was not significant. As in Mitchell et al.'s (2000) study, the age-related reduction in hippocampal activity was attributed to deficits in relational processing. The age-related increase in ventral PFC activity was attributed to compensation and/or retrieval effort.

Finally, the study by Lamar et al. (2004) investigated activity during delayed match to sample (DMTS) and delayed nonmatch to sample (DNMTS) of figures varying in shape and color. In each trial, a figure was shown and, after a 5-sec delay, two figures were presented. Participants' task was to select from the pair the previously seen figure (DMTS) or the new figure (DNMTS). The study focused on the orbito-frontal cortex (OFC), a region that shows considerable age-related anatomical decline but is rarely investigated using functional neuroimaging. In YAs, DMTS differentially engaged medial OFC (BA 25) and DNMTS, lateral OFC (BA 11). OAs did not show this difference, suggesting that age-related OFC decline is not only anatomical but also functional. Beyond OFC, the main finding was that YAs activated more PFC regions, which could mediate attentional and conflict resolution processes, whereas OAs relied more on posterior regions, including temporal and occipital areas.

To summarize the results of WM studies, OAs often showed reduced activity in PFC regions engaged by YAs but greater activity in other PFC regions, such as contralateral PFC regions (i.e., the PFC hemisphere less engaged by YAs). In some cases (e.g., Reuter-Lorenz et al., 2000) contralateral recruitment led to a more bilateral pattern of PFC activity in OAs (i.e., HAROLD). In general, age-related increases in PFC activity were attributed to compensatory mechanisms. Three nonverbal working memory studies (Grady et al., 1998; Mitchell et al., 2000; Park et al., 2003) found age-related decreases in hippocampus activity, whereas no verbal working memory study found such decreases. It is possible that nonverbal tasks were more dependent on hippocampal-mediated relational memory processing, and hence, more sensitive to age-related deficits in these regions. We will return to this issue in the cross-function section below.

Executive Functions

Several PET and fMRI studies investigated the effects of aging on brain activity associated with executive functions, such as inhibitory control, task switching, dual-task performance, and reasoning. The studies in the inhibitory control category investigated WM, go/nogo, and Stroop tasks. Jonides et al. (2000, not included in table 12.2) investigated the effects of interference on the same letter maintenance

WM task used by Reuter-Lorenz et al. (2000; see above). Compared with the control condition, the interference condition yielded a left ventrolateral PFC activation, which was significantly weaker in OAs. This result suggests that aging diminishes the efficacy of the left ventrolateral PFC in resolving conflict among responses or among representations in WM.

Nielson et al. (2002) investigated the effects of aging on inhibitory control using a go/nogo task. Unlike the paradigm used by Jonides et al., inhibitory control in this task is associated with right frontal and parietal activations in YAs (Garavan et al., 1999). Nielson et al. found an age-related increase in left PFC and parietal regions, which resulted in a more bilateral frontoparietal activation pattern in OAs than in YAs. This HAROLD pattern was interpreted as compensatory.

Two studies investigated the Stroop task: Milham et al. (2002) and Langenecker et al. (2004). In the incongruent condition of the Milham et al. study, OAs showed reduced activity in left dorsolateral PFC and left parietal regions, but greater activity in bilateral ventral temporal and ventrolateral PFC regions. According to the authors, attentional control processes were deficient in OAs (decreases in dorsolateral PFC and parietal activity), allowing irrelevant verbal information to receive further processing (increases in ventral temporal activity) and to gain access to WM (increases in ventrolateral PFC activity). The study by Langenecker et al. replicated the age-related increase in ventrolateral PFC activity but not the age-related decreases in dorsolateral PFC and parietal regions. Langenecker et al. suggested that the discrepancies between the two studies reflect differences in task difficulty (greater in Milham et al.'s study).

DiGirolamo et al. (2001, not in table 12.2) investigated task switching. In YAs, several PFC and posterior brain regions were more activated for switching than nonswitching blocks, whereas in OAs, no difference was found. Contrasts with fixation indicated that OAs activated similar brain regions to YAs during switching blocks but that they also activated these regions during nonswitching blocks (i.e., no difference between conditions). According to the authors, OAs compensated for deficits in basic cognitive processes by recruiting executive functions even during relatively simple tasks, which do not require executive functions in YAs.

The study by Smith et al. (2001, not in table 12.2) investigated task switching during dual-task performance (arithmetic + working memory). Given that activations in YAs varied with level of performance, separate analyses were done for good and poor YAs. OAs and poor YAs showed greater left PFC activity (BA 9) during the dual task than during its constituent tasks, whereas good YAs did not show additional PFC activity during the dual task. The authors suggest that selective attention functions mediated by left PFC may be required by those who found the dual task more demanding: OAs and poor YAs.

Finally, two studies investigated problem-solving tasks dependent on executive functions, Nagahama et al. (1997) and Esposito et al. (1999). Nagahama et al. examined a modified version of the Wisconsin Card Sorting Test (WCST). Many regions, including left PFC and bilateral parietal and occipital regions, were more activated in YAs than in OAs. Left PFC regions tended to be more activated in OAs than in YAs, but the difference was nonsignificant. Nagahama et al. suggested that this activation could reflect greater effort to maintain selective attention. The age-related decrease in left PFC, coupled with the age-related increase in right PFC, suggests a more bilateral pattern of PFC activity in OAs than in YAs (i.e., HAROLD).

Esposito et al. (1999) examined the WCST and the Raven's Progressive Matrices (RPM) test on a relatively large group of subjects evenly distributed from 18 to 80 years of age. During RPM, regions activated in YAs (e.g., parahippocampal, fusiform, and parietal regions) were less activated in OAs, whereas regions deactivated in YAs (e.g., frontopolar and superior temporal regions) were less deactivated in OAs. The authors suggested that this attenuation of activation/deactivation patterns could reflect an age-related reduction in mental flexibility. During WCST, however, OAs showed activations (e.g., anterior PFC, cuneus, MTL) and deactivations (e.g., left PFC, anterior cingulate, and cerebellar regions) not shown by the YAs. According to Esposito et al., these age-related differences may reflect a failure to engage appropriate networks and suppress inappropriate networks, or a compensatory use of alternative networks. PFC-parietal interactions within the working-memory system and temporal-parietal-hippocampal interactions within posterior visuospatial processing systems were altered in OAs, suggesting disconnectivity and systems failure.

To summarize executive function studies, the most consistent findings were age-related increases in PFC activation. They occurred more frequently than for simpler WM tasks (see table 12.2), possibly reflecting greater cognitive demands for executive function tasks. This idea fits well with the compensation account suggested in several studies. Also consistent with this account, PFC regions were differentially engaged by YAs with limited cognitive resources (Smith et al., 2001). However, in some cases, age-related increases in PFC activity may reflect not compensation but a failure to inhibit irrelevant information at earlier stages of processing (Milham et al., 2002). In several of the studies, age-related PFC increases led to bilateral PFC activations in OAs (HAROLD).

Implicit Memory

Only four neuroimaging studies have investigated effects of aging on implicit memory. Bäckman et al. (1997) investigated age effects on word-stem completion priming. YAs and OAs showed equivalent behavioral priming effects and corresponding activity reductions in right occipital cortex. These findings indicate that word-stem priming is preserved in healthy aging.

Daselaar et al. (2005) studied age effects on word-stem priming with event-related fMRI. To prevant motion artifacts associated with verbal responding, the word stems were completed in silence followed by a button-press. For this reason, they used reductions in response times as a behavioral measure of priming. Both YAs and OAs showed a significant reduction in response times with priming. However, the priming effect was greater for the YAs. Common priming-related activity reductions were seen in left frontal, temporal, anterior cingulate, and occipital regions. However, again YAs showed greater reductions in occipital and left anterior temporal regions. Contrary to the study by Bäckman et al., these findings suggest that aging affects both perceptual (occipital) and lexical/semantic (left anterior temporal) components of word-stem priming.

Daselaar, Rombouts et al. (2003) investigated age effects on the acquisition of a motor sequence. They used an adapted version of the serial reaction time task, which involves manually trailing an asterisk on the screen that serially appears in one of four spatial positions. The task included two alternating conditions. In the first condition, the asterisk appeared randomly in one of the four locations. In the second condition, the asterisk followed a fixed 12-item sequence—unknown to the subjects—that was repeated throughout the scan session. Both groups showed similar reductions in response times comparing the fixed with the random sequence. Moreover, YAs and OAs did not show any differences in brain activity during sequence learning, indicating that motor skill learning is relatively unaffected by the aging process.

Lustig and Buckner (2004) examined semantic repetition priming in YAs, OAs, and AD patients, using event-related fMRI. Subjects first completed a prescan study phase during which they made living/nonliving judgments about words. During subsequent scanning, semantic judgments of new words and words repeated from the study were randomly intermixed. All groups showed comparable repetition-based reductions in response times and left PFC activations. These results indicate that semantic repetition priming is well preserved in OAs and AD patients, although it is worth noting that post hoc analyses on the time course data did reveal a slight group difference for repeated items in the left prefrontal cortex (BA 45/47).

Overall, these four studies indicate that implicit memory functions are relatively preserved. In contrast to other cognitive domains, there is no evidence of age-related reorganization of neural networks supporting implicit learning. All four studies found that OAs show learning-related activity in the same brain regions as YAs. Hence, although two studies reported some differences in activation magnitude

(Daselaar et al., 2005; Lustig et al., 2004), available neuroimaging evidence is in line with behavioral findings indicating that age-related changes in implicit memory functions are minor.

Episodic Encoding

Episodic memory is one of the cognitive functions most affected by aging, and one of the richest domains of cognitive aging research. The popularity of episodic memory has spread to functional neuroimaging of cognitive aging (see table 12.2). One of the main advantages of using functional neuroimaging to investigate age-related changes in episodic memory is that this method provides separate measures of the effects of aging on encoding and retrieval. Whereas behavioral methods can measure encoding performance only via retrieval performance, thereby confounding both processes, functional neuroimaging can independently measure brain activity in each of the two phases. In fact, many brain imaging studies of aging and episodic memory have scanned only one of the two memory stages. Thus, we review these data in separate sections, focusing this section on encoding data and the next on retrieval data.

Behavioral studies have indicated that encoding is most impaired in OAs when there is little environmental support to guide encoding (Craik, 1986). For instance, several studies (Eysenck, 1974; Mason, 1979; Simon, 1979) have found that age differences are larger when subjects try to memorize information without any guidance (intentional encoding) than when an effective encoding strategy is provided to them in the form of a semantic orienting task (incidental encoding). Studies investigating intentional and incidental encoding are reviewed in separate subsections below. Afterward, a third subsection focuses on studies in which encoding activity was analyzed on the basis of subsequent memory performance.

Intentional Encoding

In the studies reviewed in this section, participants were scanned while attempting to memorize words, faces, objects, or spatial routes. Starting with verbal studies, Cabeza, Grady et al. (1997) investigated intentional encoding of word pairs. They found that OAs showed less activity in left PFC. Importantly, they also noted that the YAs selectively recruited the left PFC, whereas OAs showed equivalent activity in left and right PFC (i.e., HAROLD). Since YAs and OAs had similar memory scores, the investigators interpreted the additional recruitment of right PFC by OAs as compensatory.

Madden, Turkington et al. (1999) studied intentional word encoding. YAs did not show any significant activations during encoding, whereas OAs activated bilateral frontal regions as well as the MTL and the thalamus. Only the thalamic activation was found to be significantly different. The authors suggested that this difference reflected increased attention in the OAs during the encoding condition.

Anderson et al. (2000) studied intentional encoding under conditions of full and divided attention. During full attention, the OAs showed reduced activity in left PFC as well as increased activity in right PFC, leading to bilateral frontal activity in OAs (i.e., HAROLD). Interestingly, divided attention reduced performance equally in both groups.

In line with the PET studies by Cabeza, Grady et al. (1997) and Anderson et al. (2000), Logan et al. (2002) reported that OAs, compared with YAs, showed less activity in left PFC but greater activity in right PFC, resulting in a more bilateral activity pattern (HAROLD) during intentional encoding of words.

Turning to face encoding studies, Grady et al. (1995) found that OAs showed less activity in the left PFC and MTL than YAs. Furthermore, they found a highly significant correlation in YAs, but not in OAs, between MTL and left PFC activity. Based on these results, they concluded that encoding in OAs is accompanied by reduced neural activity and diminished connectivity between PFC and MTL areas.

In the object encoding group, the study by Schiavetto et al. (2002) compared encoding of object identity and object location. During encoding, YAs and OAs performed a perceptual matching task with spatial locations or line drawings of objects. During subsequent recognition, they retrieved the location or identity of the previously studied objects. YAs showed domain-specific activity in inferior temporal regions during the object memory task and in posterior parietal regions during the location memory task. The OAs showed decreased activation in these regions, but a task-independent increase in right PFC during encoding. In line with the findings by Park et al. (2004), these findings suggest a reduction in functional specialization with age.

In Iidaka et al. (2001), YAs and OAs encoded related, unrelated, and abstract pairs of line drawings. YAs showed bilateral PFC activity for both unrelated and abstract pairs. Additional activity was observed in the parietal lobe, but only for the abstract pictures. Surprisingly, no frontal or parietal activity was seen for the related pictures. Overall, the OAs showed less activity in temporal and parietal areas during encoding of unrelated and abstract picture pairs. In addition, OAs showed a weaker correlation between memory performance and MTL activity. These results are suggestive of an age-related deficit in visuospatial processing and picture encoding.

Meulenbroek et al. (2004) investigated age differences in the neural correlates of route encoding in a virtual environment. YAs and OAs viewed a video sequence of a virtual home while encoding the directions taken at specific decision points. During subsequent recognition, the same video sequence was shown, but this time the participants had to indicate the correct direction at the decision points. OAs performed slightly worse on this task than YAs. Furthermore, they showed reduced activity in ventral and dorsal processing streams during route encoding. In line with the studies by Schiavetto et al. and Iidaka et al., these findings indicate an age-related deficit in visuospatial processing associated with reduced activity in parietal regions.

Finally, Nyberg et al. (2003) investigated intentional encoding in YAs and OAs after training with the loci mnemonic. This method involves learning to visualize a series of mental landmarks. After participants have learned the landmarks, the information that is to be encoded is linked to the different loci at study. During retrieval, participants recapitulate each landmark in serial order, and the information associated with each locus is then retrieved. In line with previous behavioral studies, Nyberg et al. found that OAs benefited less from the memory training than YAs. Furthermore, in YAs training resulted in increased activity in occipitoparietal and PFC regions during encoding. In contrast, OAs did not show PFC activity and only those OAs who benefited from the mnemonic showed increased activity in occipital and parietal regions. These findings suggest that age-related differences in the ability to enhance memory performance after training with the loci mnemonic are related to frontal and visuospatial deficits.

Incidental Encoding

Grady and colleagues (1999) used PET to investigate the effects of intentional vs. incidental encoding conditions. They scanned YAs and OAs during shallow (upper-case/lowercase, picture size), deep (living/nonliving), and intentional encoding of words and pictures. They identified two main patterns. First, picture encoding resulted in greater activity in visual and MTL regions, while word encoding yielded greater activity in left PFC and left lateral temporal cortex. Second, deep encoding produced greater left PFC activity, while intentional encoding yielded greater right PFC activity. The OAs showed the same patterns, but the overall level of activity was reduced. Interestingly, the investigators did not find a difference in deep vs. intentional encoding of pictures, indicating that age differences were greater for words than for pictures.

The same research group performed another study comparing intentional and incidental encoding conditions, this time using faces as study items (Grady et al., 2002). Convergent with their initial intentional face encoding study (Grady et al., 1995), OAs showed decreased activity in left PFC compared to YAs and diminished connectivity between frontal and MTL areas during both encoding conditions.

Stebbins et al. (2002) also compared deep and shallow encoding of words. They reported greater activity in both YAs and OAs for the deep relative to the shallow encoding condition. However, in line with Grady et al. (2002), the OAs showed decreased activation in left PFC. Furthermore, they found a correlation between decreased performance on neuropsychological tests and reduced PFC activity. As a result of the reduced left PFC activity, PFC activity in OAs was more symmetric than in YAs (i.e., HAROLD).

Logan et al. (2002) reported similar left PFC activity during deep encoding of words. However, when the OAs were intentionally trying to memorize the words, they did show reduced left PFC activity relative to YAs. Logan et al. suggested that activity was restored by providing an efficient strategy to the OAs. Furthermore, in line with the study by Cabeza, Grady et al. (1997), the OAs showed the HAROLD pattern under both intentional and incidental encoding conditions. Interestingly, further exploratory analyses revealed that this pattern was present in a group of old OAs (mean age = 80), but not in a group of young OAs (mean age = 67), suggesting that contralateral recruitment occurs very late in life.

Rosen et al. (2002) also studied deep and shallow encoding of words in YAs and OAs. However, they distinguished between OAs with high and low memory scores based on a neuropsychological test battery. They reported equivalent left PFC activity and greater right PFC activity in the old-high group relative to YAs. In contrast, the old-low group showed reduced activity in both left and right PFC. As a result, the old-high group showed a more bilateral pattern of PFC activity than YAs (HAROLD). This finding extends to encoding a similar finding obtained during retrieval by Cabeza et al. (2002; see below).

Finally, similar to Logan and colleagues, Daselaar, Veltman et al. (2003b) reported equivalent activity in left PFC in YAs and OAs during deep encoding of words. However, contrary to that study, the OAs showed decreased activity in the left hippocampus. Based on these findings, they concluded that MTL dysfunction during encoding is an important factor in age-related memory decline.

Subsequent Memory

Morcom et al. (2003) used event-related fMRI to study subsequent memory for semantically encoded words. Recognition memory for these words was tested after a short and a longer delay. At the short delay, performance in OAs was equal to that of YAs at the long delay. Under these conditions, activity in left inferior PFC and left MTL was greater for subsequently recognized than for forgotten words in both age groups. However, YAs showed greater activity than OAs in left anterior inferior temporal cortex. Conversely, OAs showed greater right PFC activity than YAs, resulting in a more bilateral pattern of frontal activity (HAROLD).

Daselaar, Veltman et al. (2003a) conducted a comparable event-related study. However, due to an insufficient number of forgotten items, they compared remembered items against a sensorimotor baseline. Furthermore, similar to the study by

Rosen et al. (2002), they distinguished between OAs with high (old-high) and low (old-low) memory function as assessed by a subsequent recognition task. Unlike Morcom et al. (2003), they reported similar PFC activity in all the groups, although there was a trend for reduced asymmetry in the old-high group (HAROLD). The most interesting finding was that, in line with Daselaar, Veltman et al. (2003b), the old-low group showed less activity in the anterior part of the MTL compared with the other groups. These findings indicate that, in addition to PFC deficits, MTL dysfunction also plays an important role in age-related memory decline.

Gutchess et al. (2005) studied subsequent picture memory using a deep processing task. Similar to Daselaar, Veltman et al. (2003a), they observed reduced activity in the MTL for subsequently remembered items, even when OAs were not divided into high- and low-memory groups. Interestingly, the OAs also showed increased activity in the left PFC. Since picture encoding in YAs was associated with bilateral PFC activity, these findings suggest a selective recruitment of left PFC, which may be compensatory.

To summarize encoding studies, the most consistent finding was an age-related reduction in left PFC activity. This finding was more frequent for intentional than for incidental encoding studies (see table 12.2), suggesting that the environmental support provided by a deep semantic encoding task may attenuate the age-related decrease in left PFC activity. This effect was found within subjects in the study by Logan et al. (2002). The difference between intentional and incidental encoding conditions suggests an important strategic component in age-related memory decline. The reduction in left PFC activity was often coupled with an increase in right PFC activity, leading to a bilateral pattern of PFC activity in older adults (HAROLD). Importantly, extending to encoding a finding previously reported for retrieval (Cabeza et al., 2002), two studies that divided OAs into high and low performers found the HAROLD pattern only in the high-performing group (Daselaar, Veltman et al., 2003a; Rosen et al., 2002), These findings provide direct support for the compensation account of HAROLD.

In line with studies on visual perception (Iidaka et al., 2002; Levine et al., 2000; Gunning-Dixon et al., 2003) and working memory (Grady et al., 1998; Mitchell et al., 2000; Park et al., 2003; Cabeza et al., 2004), several encoding studies found age-related reductions in MTL activity (Gutchess et al., 2005; Daselaar, Veltman et al., 2003a,b; Grady et al., 1995; Schiavetto et al., 2002). In one study (Daselaar, Veltman et al., 2003a), these MTL reductions were directly linked to reduced memory performance. These findings indicate that, besides frontal changes, reduced MTL function also contributes to age-related memory decline. Finally, age deficits in encoding of visuospatial information have been associated with reduced activity in parietal regions. This suggests that attentional deficits may play a role in age-related decline of visuospatial memory.

Episodic Memory Retrieval

As noted before, age-related deficits in episodic retrieval tend to be more pronounced for recall and context memory tasks than for recognition tasks (Spencer
& Raz, 1995), which is consistent with the notion that recollection is more sensitive
to aging than familiarity is (Yonelinas, 2002). Recognition, recall, and context
memory studies are reviewed in separate sections.

Recognition

The face encoding study by Grady et al. (1995) included a face recognition test.
During this task, OAs showed reduced activity in parietal and occipital regions but
activity equivalent to YAs in right PFC. This last finding contrasts with the age-
related reduction in left PFC activity found in the same study during face encoding.
Based on these results, the authors suggested that age effects are more pronounced
on encoding than on retrieval. As noted below, however, many subsequent PET and
fMRI studies have found reliable age-related changes in PFC activity during episodic retrieval.

The encoding study by Cabeza, Grady et al. (1997) also investigated word pair
recognition and word pair cued recall. During recognition, OAs showed stronger
activations in the precuneus, left temporal, and anterior cingulate regions but weaker
activations in right parietal regions. However, as described in the next section, fewer
regions showed age differences in brain activity during recognition than during
recall. These results are in line with behavioral findings indicating that age deficits
are more pronounced on recall than on recognition tasks.

Madden, Turkington et al. (1999) studied recognition after deep encoding
of words. They reported more bilateral PFC activity in OAs relative to YAs.
Subsequently, they used a stepwise regression method that distinguished between
exponential (tau) and Gaussian (mu) components of RT distributions. YAs showed
a correlation between mu and right PFC activity, whereas the OAs showed correlations in left and right PFC regions related to both mu and tau. Since tau is associated
with task-specific decision processes, and mu, with residual sensory coding and
response processes, the authors concluded that attentional demands were greater
for OAs, leading to the recruitment of additional regions. These findings suggest that
the retrieval network is more widely distributed in OAs.

Daselaar, Veltman et al. (2003a) used event-related fMRI to study recognition of
words in YAs and OAs. Based on recognition performance in the scanner, OAs were
divided into old-high and old-low groups. During recognition compared with baseline, the old-low group showed much increased activity throughout the brain relative
to the other groups. In addition, the old-low group and YAs showed bilateral PFC
activity, whereas the old-high group showed a more left-lateralized pattern of frontal

activity. In other words, the old-low group showed a nonselective increase in global brain activity, whereas the old-high group showed a selective recruitment of left PFC. The authors interpreted these findings in terms of strategic retrieval differences. Interestingly, when correctly recognized old words were compared with correctly rejected new words, these group differences disappeared. The difference in activity between these two trial types is generally considered to be a correlate of retrieval success. Hence, these findings suggest that age differences in episodic recognition reflect strategic differences rather than a change in the processes supporting the actual recovery of information.

Stern and colleagues (2005) used PET to study the effects of cognitive reserve (CR) on brain activity during recognition of abstract shapes. CR refers to the ability of an individual to cope with advancing brain pathology in order to minimize symptoms. Stern et al. used a factor score summarizing years of education and scores on two IQ indices as a measure of CR. The memory task involved immediate recognition after study list presentation. Study list size was titrated so that performance was around 75% for all participants. A study list size of a single item was used as the baseline condition. A set of functionally connected regions, which were identified using the CR score and which included MTL, insula, thalamus, and PFC regions, was differentially activated in YAs and OAs. YAs with a high CR score showed greater activity in these regions, whereas OAs with a high CR score showed decreased activity in these regions. These results were interpreted to reflect compensation in these OAs by reorganizing the retrieval network used by YAs.

Cabeza et al. (2004) investigated the effects of aging on several tasks, including a verbal recognition task. During this task, they found age-related increases in PFC and decreases in parietal and visual regions. In the medial temporal lobes, they found a dissociation between a hippocampal region that showed weaker activity in OAs than in YAs and a parahippocampal region that showed the converse pattern (figure 12.1, plate 21). Given evidence that hippocampal and parahippocampal regions are respectively more involved in recollection and familiarity (for reviews, see Aggleton & Brown, 1999; Yonelinas, 2002), this finding is consistent with the notion that OAs are more impaired in recollection than in familiarity (e.g., J. M. Jennings & Jacoby, 1993; Parkin & Walter, 1992). Actually, the age-related increase in parahippocampal cortex suggests that OAs may be compensating for recollection deficits by relying more on familiarity. Supporting this idea, OAs had a larger number of Know responses than YAs, and these responses were positively correlated with the parahippocampal activation.

Deselaar et al. (2005) investigated the effects of retrieval confidence in recognition memory. YAs and OAs made old/new judgments about previously studied words, followed by a 4-point confidence judgment. Recognition performance was equated by testing the YAs after one exposure to the study list, whereas the OAs

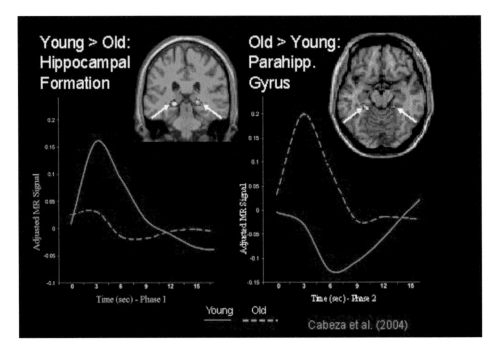

Figure 12.1
Dissociation between two medial temporal lobe regions. The hippocampal formation, bilaterally, was more activated in YAs than in OAs during all tasks (task-independent age effect), whereas the parahip-pocampal gyrus, bilaterally, was more activated in OAs than in YAs during the ER task (task-specific age effect). The age-related increase in parahippocampal gyrus was positively correlated with the number of Know responses, consistent with the idea that OAs rely more on familiarity during recognition (Cabeza et al., 2004). See plate 21 for color version.

encoded the words twice. OAs showed less activity in regions associated with recollection, including the left parietotemporal cortex, retrosplenial cortex, and hippocampus, as well as similar activity in regions that showed a familiarity pattern, including dorsal posterior cingulate, and left parietooccipital cortex. Finally, OAs showed increased familiarity-related activity in the rhinal area of anterior MTL. Consistent with their previous findings, these results suggest a greater reliance on familiarity-based recognition in OAs.

Recall
Schacter et al. (1996) scanned young and old subjects while they were recalling previously studied words. High and low levels of recall were produced by varying encoding conditions. In the High-minus-Low contrast both groups showed similar hippocampal activations. In the Low-minus-High contrast, bilateral anterior PFC regions were more activated in YAs than in OAs, whereas left posterior PFC areas

were more activated in OAs. These findings support the idea that elderly use different functional networks for retrieval than YAs do.

Bäckman et al. (1997) used a word-stem cued recall task similar to the one used by Schacter et al. (1996). Compared with YAs, OAs showed weaker activations in the cerebellum—possibly reflecting a deficit in self-initiated retrieval and processing speed—and in Wernicke's area—possibly reflecting a deficit in visual-auditory encoding. Surprisingly, MTL was more activated in OAs than in YAs. As in Cabeza, Grady et al. (1997), whereas PFC activity in YAs was right-lateralized, an age-related increase in left PFC activity made PFC activity in OAs bilateral (HAROLD).

In addition to the word pair recognition test described in the previous section, Cabeza, Grady et al. (1997) also investigated a cued recall test. Again, OAs showed weaker activity in the anterior cingulate and left temporal cortex. In addition, consistent with Schacter et al. (1996), OAs showed weaker activations in right PFC than the YAs. Conversely, OAs showed greater activity than YAs in left PFC. The net result was that PFC activity during recall was right-lateralized in YAs but bilateral in OAs (HAROLD). The authors noted this change in hemispheric asymmetry and interpreted it as compensatory.

Anderson et al. (2000) investigated the effects of divided attention on cued recall of word pairs. They reported negligible effects of divided attention in both groups. However, under full attention conditions, OAs showed weaker activations primarily in right PFC but stronger activations primarily in left PFC, suggesting an attenuation of the right-lateralized pattern shown by YAs (HAROLD).

Context Memory

Cabeza et al. (2000) investigated item and temporal-order memory tasks. In the item task, a word pair was presented consisting of one studied word and one new word, and participants indicated which word had been studied. In the temporal-order task, both words had been studied, and participants indicated which of the two words appeared later in the study list. Cabeza et al. reported that YAs showed increased activation in right PFC for temporal-order compared with item memory, whereas OAs did not. In contrast, the activations during item memory were relatively unaffected by age. These findings are in line with the hypothesis that memory deficits in OAs are due to PFC dysfunction, and that context memory is more heavily dependent on the frontal lobes than item memory.

In another study of context memory by Cabeza and colleagues (2002), YAs, high-performing OAs (old-high), and low-performing OAs (old-low) studied words presented auditorily or visually. During scanning, words were presented visually, and the subjects made either old/new decisions (item memory) or heard/seen decisions (context memory). Consistent with their previous results, YAs showed right PFC activity for context trials, whereas OAs showed bilateral PFC activity (HAROLD). Importantly, however, this pattern was seen only for the old-high adults, supporting a compensation account of the HAROLD pattern. As noted above, the finding of HAROLD for old-high, but not for old-low, was extended to the encoding domain by Rosen et al. (2002).

Schiavetto et al. (2002) investigated not only the encoding (see "Encoding") but also the retrieval of object identity and object location information. OAs showed a reduction in domain-specific regions, including the inferior temporal cortex, during object memory, and posterior parietal regions during location memory. During retrieval, they also showed an increase in right visual cortex, which was common to both types of stimuli. In line with the visual perception study by Park et al. (2004), these findings suggest an age-related shift from domain-specific to domain-general processes.

The route encoding study by Meulenbroek et al. (2004) included a recognition phase. During route recognition, YAs and OAs saw the same video sequence shown during encoding, and indicated the correct direction with a left or a right button-press. OAs performed slightly worse than YAs and showed greater anterior MTL activity. The authors suggested that, during navigational retrieval, OAs showed a diminished novelty signal originating from the anterior MTL. Since larger differences were observed during the encoding phase of this task, they also suggested that age-related deficits in navigational memory are primarily caused by encoding problems.

Maguire and Frith (2003) investigated the recall of autobiographical events gathered in a prescan interview. Although the groups activated largely the same regions, the authors observed a striking difference in the MTL. YAs showed left-lateralized MTL activity, whereas OAs showed bilateral activity in the MTL. These findings suggest that HAROLD extends beyond the PFC not only to other cortical regions (as shown by several studies) but also to subcortical areas.

Summarizing the studies on retrieval, the HAROLD pattern has been found more frequently in studies using more challenging, recall and context memory tasks than during simple item recognition. These findings suggest a three-way interaction between age, task difficulty, and frontal laterality. Importantly, by distinguishing between old-high and old-low adults, the study by Cabeza et al. (2002) provided direct evidence for the compensation account of HAROLD.

Retrieval studies of aging also revealed an intriguing difference from encoding studies. In agreement with perceptual and WM studies, encoding studies observed age-related reductions in MTL activity, whereas several retrieval studies reported increases in MTL activity with age (Cabeza et al., 2004; Daselaar et al., 2006; Maguire & Frith, 2003; Bäckman et al., 1997; Meulenbroek et al., 2004; Schiavetto et al., 2002). In keeping with behavioral findings, the results reported by Cabeza,

Daselaar, and colleagues suggest that these increases may reflect a greater reliance on familiarity-based retrieval in OAs (Cabeza et al., 2004; Daselaar et al., 2005).

Overall, neuroimaging studies of encoding and retrieval have identified common (HAROLD) as well as differential patterns (decrease vs. increase in MTL) of age-related changes in brain activity during the two memory phases. These findings exemplify one of the great strengths of functional neuroimaging in studying cognitive aging, the opportunity to obtain independent measures of brain activity during different stages of a cognitive task.

Direct Cross-Function Comparisons

This concise review of neuroimaging studies of cognitive aging has highlighted two task-independent patterns, HAROLD and ODFI, as well as task-specific effects, such as an age-related increase in MTL during episodic retrieval. However, these observations are based on cross-study comparisons, and thus it is unclear if these similarities and differences are truly related to aging or merely reflect similarities and differences of the tasks and stimuli employed. The only way in which one can ensure that age-related changes in activity are task-independent or task-specific is to compare the effects of aging on brain activity during different cognitive tasks directly within subjects.

This was the goal of a study recently conducted in our laboratory (Cabeza et al., 2004). Using event-related fMRI, we directly compared age-related changes in activity during working memory (WM), visual attention (VA), and episodic retrieval (ER). WM was investigated with a word delayed-response test, VA with a sustained attention task, and ER with a word recognition task. To identify task-independent age effects, we used a conjunction procedure that isolated age-related differences in activity that occurred in each and every cognitive task, and to identify task-specific age effects, we used a masking procedure that excluded from the age-related differences in activations of each task those previously identified as task-independent.

The main task-independent age effect on brain activity was a reduction in visual cortex activity coupled with an increase in PFC activity (figure 12.2, plate 22). The reduction in visual cortex activity fits well with the theory that an age-related decline in sensory processing is a common cause of cognitive aging (Baltes & Lindenberger, 1997). The increase in PFC activity suggests that some forms of functional compensation in OAs may be common across tasks. As noted in the "Perception" section, the shift from occipital activity to PFC activity in older adults was originally noted by Grady et al. (1994), who suggested that OAs compensated for deficits in visual processing by recruiting PFC regions (see also Madden et al., 1996). Consistent with this idea, we found a reliable negative correlation between the age-related decrease

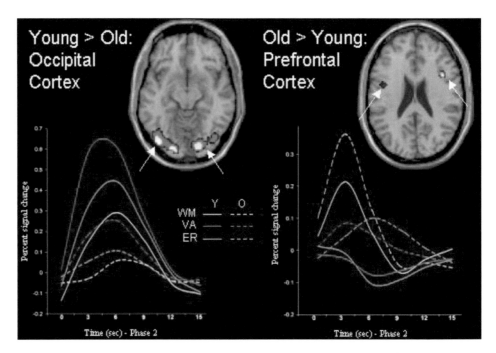

Figure 12.2
Task-independent age effects. Compared with YAs, OAs showed weaker activity in occipital cortex but greater activity in frontal regions (Cabeza et al., 2004). See plate 22 for color version.

in occipital activity and the age-related increase in PFC activity in the WM task (r = −0.5, p < 0.02).

Task-specific age effects included an age-related increase in MTL activity during ER, as well as a different lateralization of age-related PFC recruitment in WM and VA tasks. As illustrated by figure 12.3 (plate 23), in the case of WM, OAs showed greater activity than YAs in right PFC, whereas in the case of VA, OAs showed greater activity in left PFC. Since PFC activity during ER in YAs was largely bilateral, contralateral recruitment could not be observed. In contrast, in the case of WM and VA, some PFC regions were lateralized in YAs, and contralateral recruitment yielded a more bilateral pattern of activity in OAs than in YAs. This pattern has been found in variety of cognitive tasks, including perception, episodic memory, semantic memory, working memory, language, and inhibition tests (for a review, see Cabeza, 2002). These studies show that when PFC activity is left-lateralized in YAs, OAs may recruit additional activity in right PFC, and when PFC activity is right-lateralized in YAs, OAs may recruit additional activity in left PFC. As illustrated by figure 12.2, we found both forms of contralateral recruitment in the same experiment and within the same participants (see also Reuter-Lorenz et al., 2000). In sum,

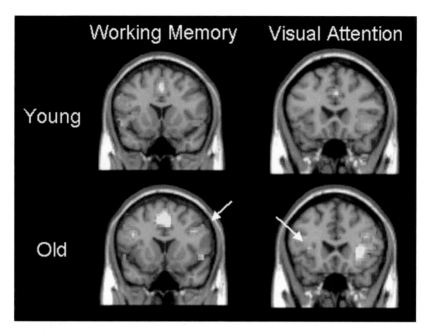

Figure 12.3
OAs showed contralateral recruitment in right PFC during WM and in left PFC during VA. As a result of these changes, activity in certain PFC regions was more bilateral in OAs than in YAs (Hemispheric Asymmetry Reduction in Older Adults, or HAROLD) (Cabeza et al., 2004). See plate 23 for color version.

using a cross-function approach in which we compared different cognitive tasks within the same study, we have replicated ODFI and HAROLD both within experiment and within participants.

Issues

This section discusses some of the main problems faced by researchers conducting activation imaging studies of cognitive aging, and considers some possible solutions. The issues are organized according to the four main components of a functional neuroimaging experiment: subjects, tasks and design, behavioral performance, and activations. Since these four elements are intimately related, many of the issues discussed below could be classified under a different heading.

Subjects

When selecting healthy OAs, one is faced with a dilemma. On one hand, one would like to select OAs who are perfectly healthy and who are matched to YAs in all possible variables except age. One the other hand, one would also like to investigate a sample of OAs that is representative of the general OA population. This is a general problem of cognitive aging research, but some aspects of it are particularly thorny in functional neuroimaging studies, such as screening criteria and the subpopulation of OAs investigated.

Regarding health screening, researchers agree about some inclusion/exclusion criteria but not others. Most researchers agree that participants with high blood pressure should be excluded; hypertension not only may alter blood flow measures but it is also associated with covert cerebrovascular damage (Skoog, 1998). Most studies exclude participants taking medications that could alter blood flow, but clear guidelines about which drugs do so is not available. Likewise, participants are usually excluded if they show pronounced atrophy or white-matter damage in MRI scans, but the boundary between normal and abnormal structural changes is not clear. Thus, there is an urgent need for studies assessing the effect of the various subject-related factors on hemodynamic measures. A good example is the study by Jennings et al. (1998), which found that, during a WM task, hypertensive OAs showed different activation patterns than normotensive OAs.

Regarding OA subpopulations, OAs may differ both quantitatively and qualitatively. Quantitatively, OAs may differ in level of cognitive performance, with some OAs performing as well as YAs and others performing significantly below. This variability in age-related cognitive decline difference may account for some inconsistencies in the imaging literature (see discussion about performance differences below). Qualitatively, OAs may differ regarding the particular neurocognitive component in which they are most impaired. As shown by Glisky and collaborators (1995, 2001), some OAs may be more affected on PFC-mediated executive functions, whereas other OAs may be more affected in MTL-mediated memory functions. Obviously, the proportions of these two patterns in the sample investigated are likely to affect what age effects one finds. Thus, future studies should try to characterize different levels of performance and aging patterns, and investigate their effect on brain activation patterns.

Tasks and Design

Cognitive tasks are never "pure"; they always involve a complex blend of different cognitive operations. Thus, when an age-related difference in activation is found, it is important to determine which component of the task is responsible for the difference. This type of task analysis could help explain some inconsistencies in the literature. For example, Cabeza, Grady et al. (1997) found a significant age-related reduction in PFC activity during verbal recognition, whereas Madden, Turkington et al. (1999) did not. Given that recognition memory involves both recollection and familiarity (Yonelinas, 2002), and that recollection is sensitive to aging (J. R. Jennings

& Jacoby, 1993), the inconsistent findings could reflect a greater recollection component in the recognition task investigated by Cabeza et al. (associative recognition) than in the one studied by Madden et al. (item recognition).

The standard solution to the problem of task complexity is the subtraction method, which compares target and control conditions assumed to differ primarily in the process of interest. There are two main problems with this method, and both are magnified by group contrasts. First, activations reflect both the target condition and the control condition employed. Thus, OAs may show weaker activations than YAs not because they did not engage a region during the target task but because they also engaged it during the control task (e.g., DiGirolamo et al., 2001). This problem is attenuated but not eliminated by using low-level baselines, such as the fixation period in event-related fMRI studies, because low-level baselines may also show age-related differences. For example, Lustig et al. (2003) scanned YAs and OAs during a semantic classification task, which was intermixed with blocks of passive rest. They found that OAs showed less activity during rest (task-related deactivation) in posterior midline regions. These regions are commonly activated in YAs during low-level baseline conditions (Daselaar et al., 2004; McKiernan et al., 2003; Shulman et al., 1997). Lustig et al. proposed that age differences in rest activity reflect a less efficient allocation in OAs of available resources to task-relevant processes.

Second, the subtraction method rests on the assumption that the extra component of the target condition does not affect the components shared with the control condition (pure insertion assumption; Friston et al., 1996). This assumption is problematic (e.g., J. M. Jennings et al., 1997), and may be further violated when the inserted task components interact with limitations in cognitive resources in OAs. To address this problem, future studies should complement subtraction analyses with other methods, such as parametric manipulations, multivariate analyses, and activity-performance correlations.

Performance

Brain activity can vary as a function of performance measures, such as accuracy (e.g., Prince et al., 2005) and reaction time (e.g., Rypma & D'Esposito, 2000). Therefore, in functional neuroimaging studies, if OAs perform more poorly than YAs, it is unclear whether differences in activation between OAs and YAs reflect the age effects or dissimilarities in performance. This is a typical "chicken and egg problem": Do OAs perform poorly because their brain activity is different, or is their brain activity different because they perform poorly?

One approach to this problem is to match performance in young and old groups by manipulating tasks (Cabeza et al., 2000; Morcom et al., 2003) or by scanning high-functioning elderly who naturally perform as well as young adults (e.g., Cabeza,

Grady et al., 1997). When cognitive performance is similar in the young and old groups, group differences in brain activity can be safely attributed to aging. The main problem of this approach is that when performance differences are eliminated, it becomes more difficult to relate activation findings to the cognitive deficits typically displayed by OAs. A possible solution to this problem is to have an "easy" and a "difficult" version of the task, and compare YAs and OAs both when performance is matched (e.g., YA-difficult vs. OA-easy) and when an age-related deficit is present (e.g., YA-difficult vs. OA-difficult or YA-easy vs. OA-easy) (Cabeza et al., 2000).

Another way to address the problem of performance differences is to use event-related fMRI designs and analyze only correct trials in both groups. This method does not eliminate differences in RTs, unless the number of trials is sufficiently large to allow selecting trials with similar RTs in the two groups. An alternative solution is to enter RTs as a covariate in the analyses, but this entails the risk of eliminating activity associated with processes of interest (which are usually correlated with RTs).

Activations

After subjects have been appropriately selected, task components suitably analyzed, and performance differences properly controlled, researchers are still faced with the fundamental problem of interpreting the age-related differences in activation they have found. The issues in this area can be divided into three groups: determining what kind of age-related activation differences were found; interpreting aging effects on a particular brain region; and evaluating global network changes.

Determining the kind of age-related activity difference found is not a trivial problem. First, one must determine whether YAs and OAs engage the same region to different degrees (quantitative difference) or different brain regions (qualitative difference). The interpretation of these two patterns is different, but distinguishing between them is not easy. For example, quantitative differences may appear to be qualitative due to threshold effects. Also, when YAs and OAs activate neighboring areas (e.g., BA 9 vs. BA 46), the finding may be described as the "same" activation in different locations or as "different" activations. Second, another knotty problem is whether age-related differences in activation reflect changes in neural architecture or changes in cognitive architecture (see chapter 14, in this volume). In other words, did YAs and OAs engage different regions to perform the same cognitive operations, or did they recruit different regions to perform different cognitive operations? If one wants to know if the neural correlates of process A change with age, it is critical that both groups engage process A to the same extent. At the same time, if aging is associated with a shift from process A to process B, then the neural correlates of *both* processes should be investigated in *both* groups. The main problem, of course, is how to determine exactly the processes engaged by human subjects, since cognitive tasks can be performed in many different ways and introspective reports provide very limited information about the actual operations performed by the subjects.

Interpreting age-related differences in activation is also complex. In general, age-related decreases in activation have been interpreted as detrimental and age-related increases as beneficial. Unfortunately, the relation between neural activity and cognitive performance is not so simple; less activity may reflect more efficient processing (Karni et al., 1995; Raichle et al., 1994), and more activity may reflect unnecessary or even disruptive processes (Cabeza, Grady et al., 1997). Correlations could help interpret activation differences if one assumes that activations positively correlated with performance are beneficial and those negatively correlated with performance are detrimental. However, an activation may be beneficial for performance but be negatively correlated with performance *across subjects* when the region is recruited by participants who have difficulty with the task. To explain by using an analogy, a walking stick helps walking performance but its use is negatively correlated with walking performance (because is used by those who have difficulty walking). Event-related designs can also help distinguish between beneficial and detrimental interpretations if one assumes that activity during successful trials is beneficial and activity during unsuccessful trials is detrimental. Yet, again, a region may be beneficial for performance but only for demanding trials, which have a greater chance of being unsuccessful.

Finally, although most studies have interpreted age-related differences in terms of local changes (e.g., PFC dysfunction), these differences may also reflect global network changes. For example, using structural equation modeling, we have found that age-related changes in the activity of a left PFC region during episodic encoding and retrieval were partly due to age-related changes in the interactions between this region and other components of the episodic memory network (Cabeza, McIntosh et al., 1997). Thus, one of the main challenges for future imaging studies of cognitive aging is to investigate not only local changes but also changes in functional connectivity.

Conclusions

In this chapter we reviewed PET and fMRI studies of aging in the domains of visual perception, attention, language, working memory, implicit memory, and episodic memory encoding and retrieval. In addition to many task-specific differences, these studies revealed two consistent patterns of age-related changes in brain activity: an occipital decrease coupled with an increase in frontal regions (ODFI), and a general reduction in the asymmetry of brain activity (HAROLD). ODFI has been attributed to compensation for visual deficits by recruiting higher-order cognitive processes mediated by PFC. HAROLD has been attributed to compensation for age-related neural decline by means of contralateral recruitment. As discussed, direct support for the compensation accounts of ODFI and HAROLD has come from functional neuroimaging studies that correlated individual activation patterns with performance, or that directly compared high- and low-performing OAs.

However, although ODFI and HAROLD have consistently been reported in many different studies and across several cognitive domains, the identification of the patterns has been based primarily on cross-experiment comparisons. Accordingly, it is not clear if these similarities and differences are truly related to aging or merely reflect similarities and differences of the tasks and stimuli employed. More controlled observations are required in future functional neuroimaging studies of aging—for instance, by comparing the effects of aging on brain activity during different cognitive tasks directly within subjects. A good example of such an approach is the study by Cabeza et al. (2004) that replicated both ODFI and HAROLD across three different cognitive domains within the same study and within the same participants.

In the final section of the chapter, we discussed several issues in functional neuroimaging of aging regarding subjects, task design, performance, and the interpretation of activations. Probably the most important issue relates to performance differences between YAs and OAs. If OAs perform more poorly in functional neuroimaging studies, it is unclear if differences in activation reflect true age effects or simply differences in task performance. Several approaches have been discussed to deal with performance differences, including selection of high-performing OAs, manipulations of task difficulty, and the exclusion of incorrect responses using event-related fMRI. Since none of these alternatives are completely satisfactory, the best solution may be to try to characterize the specific relation between brain activity, age, individual differences, and task difficulty, using correlational and parametric approaches.

Acknowledgments

This work was supported by grants from the National Institute of Aging (R01AG19731; R. Cabeza, primary investigator) and Duke Bryan ADRC (P50AG05128; J. Browndyke).

References

Aggleton, J. P., & Brown, M. W. (1999). Episodic memory, amnesia, and the hippocampal-anterior thalamic axis. *Behavioral and Brain Sciences* 22, 425–489.

Anderson, N. D., Iidaka, T., McIntosh, A. R., Kapur, S., Cabeza, R., & Craik, F. I. M. (2000). The effects of divided attention on encoding- and retrieval-related brain activity: A PET study of yournger and older adults. *Journal of Cognitive Neuroscience* 12, 775–792.

Bäckman, L., Almkvist, O., Andersson, J., Nordberg, A., Windblad, B., Rineck, R., et al. (1997). Brain activation in young and older adults during implicit and explicit retrieval. *Journal of Cognitive Neuroscience* 9(3), 378–391.

Baltes, P. B., & Lindenberger, U. (1997). Emergence of a powerful connection between sensory and cognitive functions across the adult life span: A new window to the study of cognitive aging? *Psychology and Aging* 12, 12–21.

Cabeza, R. (2002). Hemispheric asymmetry reduction in old adults: The HAROLD model. *Psychology and Aging* 17, 85–100.

Cabeza, R., Anderson, N. D., Houle, S., Mangels, J. A., & Nyberg, L. (2000). Age-related differences in neural activity during item and temporal-order memory retrieval: A positron emission tomography study. *Journal of Cognitive Neuroscience* 12, 197–206.

Cabeza, R., Anderson, N. D., Locantore, J. K., & McIntosh, A. R. (2002). Aging gracefully: Compensatory brain activity in high-performing older adults. *NeuroImage* 17, 1394–1402.

Cabeza, R., Daselaar, S. M., Dolcos, F., Prince, S., Budde, M., & Nyberg, L. (2004). Age-related changes in brain activity during working memory, attention, and episodic memory: Task-independent vs. task-specific effects. *Cerebral Cortex* 14, 365–375.

Cabeza, R., Grady, C. L., Nyberg, L., McIntosh, A. R., Tulving, E., Kapur, S., et al. (1997). Age-related differences in neural activity during memory encoding and retrieval: A positron emission tomography study. *Journal of Neuroscience* 17, 391–400.

Cabeza, R., McIntosh, A. R., Tulving, E., Nyberg, L., & Grady, C. L. (1997). Age-related differences in effective neural connectivity during encoding and recall. *NeuroReport* 8, 3479–3483.

Craik, F. I. M. (1986). A functional account of age differences in memory. In F. Lix & H. Hagendorf (Eds.), *Human Memory and Cognitive Capabilities, Mechanisms, and Performances*, 499–422. Amsterdam: Elsevier Science.

Daselaar, S. M., & Cabeza, R. (2005). Age-related changes in hemispheric organization. In R. Cabeza, L. Nyberg, & D. C. Park (Eds.), *Cognitive Neuroscience of Aging*, 325–353. New York: Oxford University Press.

Daselaar, S. M., Fleck, M., Dobbins, I. G., Madden, D. J., Cabeza, R. (2006). Effects of healthy aging on hippocampal and rhinal memory functions: An event-related fMRI study. *Cerebral Cortex*, in press.

Daselaar, S. M., Prince, S. E., & Cabeza, R. (2004). When less means more: Deactivations during encoding that predict subsequent memory. *NeuroImage* 23(3), 921–927.

Daselaar, S. M., Rombouts, S. A., Veltman, D. J., Raaijmakers, J. G., & Jonker, C. (2003). Similar network activated in young and elderly adults during the acquisition of a motor sequence. *Neurobiology of Aging* 24, 1013–1019.

Daselaar, S. M., Veltman, D. J., Rombouts, S. A., Lazeron, R. H., Raaijmakers, J. G., & Jonker, C. (2003a). Neuroanatomical correlates of episodic encoding and retrieval in young and elderly subjects. *Brain* 126, 43–56.

Daselaar, S. M., Veltman, D. J., Rombouts, S. A., Raaijmakers, J. G., & Jonker, C. (2003b). Deep processing activates the medial temporal lobe in young but not in elderly adults. *Neurobiology of Aging* 24, 1005–1011.

Daselaar, S. M., Veltman, D. J., Rombouts, S. A. R. B., Raaijmakers, J. G. W., & Jonker, C. (2005). Aging affects both perceptual and lexical/semantic components of word stem priming. *Neurobiology of Learning & Memory* 83, 251–252.

Della Maggiore, V., Sekuler, A. B., Grady, C. L., Bennett, P. J., Sekuler, R., & McIntosh, A. R. (2000). Corticolimbic interactions associated with performance on a short-term memory task are modified by age. *Journal of Neuroscience* 20, 8410–8416.

DiGirolamo, G. J., Kramer, A. F., Barad, V., Cepeda, N. J., Weissman, D. H., Milham, M. P., et al. (2001). General and task-specific frontal lobe recruitment in older adults during executive processes: A fMRI investigation of task-switching. *NeuroReport* 12(9), 2065–2071.

Dixit, N. K., Gerton, B. K., Dohn, P., Meyer-Lindenberg, A., & Berman, K. F. (2000). *Age-related changes in rCBF activation during an N-Back working memory paradigm occur prior to age 50.* Paper presented at the Neuroimage Human Brain Mapping.

Esposito, G., Kirby, G. S., Van Horn, J. D., Ellmore, T. M., & Faith Berman, K. (1999). Context-dependent, neural system-specific neurophysiological concomitants of ageing: Mapping PET correlates during cognitive activation. *Brain* 122, 963–979.

Eysenck, M. W. (1974). Age differences in incidental learning. *Developmental Psychology* 10, 936–941.

Friston, K. J., Price, C. J., Fletcher, P., Moore, C., Frackowiak, R. S. J., & Dolan, R. J. (1996). The trouble with cognitive subtraction. *NeuroImage* 4, 97–104.

Garavan, H., Ross, T. J., & Stein, E. A. (1999). Right hemispheric dominance of inhibitory control: An event-related functional MRI study. *Proceedings of the National Academy of Sciences* USA 96(14), 8301–8306.

Glisky, E. L., Polster, M. R., & Routhieaux, B. C. (1995). Double dissociation between item and source memory. *Neuropsychology* 9, 229–235.

Glisky, E. L., Rubin, S. R., & Davidson, P. S. R. (2001). Source memory in older adults: An encoding or retrieval problem? *Journal of Experimental Psychology: Learning, Memory, and Cognition* 27, 1131–1146.

Grady, C. L., Bernstein, L. J., Beig, S., & Siegenthaler, A. L. (2002). The effects of encoding strategy on age-related changes in the functional neuroanatomy of face memory. *Psychology and Aging* 17, 7–23.

Grady, C. L., Maisog, J. M., Horwitz, B., Ungerleider, L. G., Mentis, M. J., Salerno, J. A., et al. (1994). Age-related changes in cortical blood flow activation during visual processing of faces and location. *Journal of Neuroscience* 14(3, pt. 2), 1450–1462.

Grady, C. L., McIntosh, A. R., Bookstein, F., Horwitz, B., Rapoport, S. I., & Haxby, J. V. (1998). Age-related changes in regional cerebral blood flow during working memory for faces. *NeuroImage* 8, 409–425.

Grady, C. L., McIntosh, A. R., Horwitz, B., Maisog, J. M., Ungerleider, L. G., Mentis, M. J., et al. (1995). Age-related reductions in human recognition memory due to impaired encoding. *Science* 269(5221), 218–221.

Grady, C. L., McIntosh, A. R., Horwitz, B., & Rapoport, S. I. (2000). Age-related changes in the neural correlates of degraded and nondegraded face processing. *Cognitive Neuropsychology* 217, 165–186.

Grady, C. L., McIntosh, A. R., Raja, M. N., Beig, S., & Craik, F. I. M. (1999). The effects of age on the neural correlates of episodic encoding. *Cerebral Cortex* 9, 805–814.

Grossman, M., Cooke, A., DeVita, C., Alsop, D., Detre, J., Chen, W., et al. (2002a). Age-related changes in working memory during sentence comprehension: An fMRI study. *NeuroImage* 15(2), 302–317.

Grossman, M., Cooke, A., DeVita, C., Chen, W., Moore, P., Detre, J., et al. (2002b). Sentence processing strategies in healthy seniors with poor comprehension: An fMRI study. *Brain & Language* 80(3), 296–313.

Gunning-Dixon, F. M., Gur, R. C., Perkins, A. C., Schroeder, L., Turner, T., Turetsky, B. I., et al. (2003). Age-related differences in brain activation during emotional face processing. *Neurobiology of Aging* 24(2), 285–295.

Gutchess, A. H., Welsh, R. C., Hedden, T., Bangert, A., Minear, M., Liu, L. L., et al. (2005). Aging and the neural correlates of successful picture encoding: Frontal activations compensate for decreased medial-temporal activity. *Journal of Cognitive Neuroscience* 17(1), 84–96.

Haut, M. W., Kuwabara, H., Leach, S., & Callahan, T. (2000). Age-related changes in neural activation during working memory performance. *Aging, Neuropsychology and Cognition* 7(2), 119–129.

Iidaka, T., Okada, T., Murata, T., Omori, M., Kosaka, H., Sadato, N., et al. (2002). Age-related differences in the medial temporal lobe responses to emotional faces as revealed by fMRI. *Hippocampus* 12(3), 352–362.

Iidaka, T., Sadato, N., Yamada, H., Murata, T., Omori, M., & Yonekura, Y. (2001). An fMRI study of the functional neuroanatomy of picture encoding in younger and older adults. *Cognitive Brain Research* 11(1), 1–11.

Jennings, J. M., & Jacoby, L. L. (1993). Automatic versus intentional uses of memory: Aging, attention, and control. *Psychology and Aging* 8(2), 283–293.

Jennings, J. M., McIntosh, A. R., Kapur, S., Tulving, E., & Houle, S. (1997). Cognitive subtractions may not add up: The interaction between semantic processing and response mode. *NeuroImage* 5(3), 229–239.

Jennings, J. R., Muldoon, M. F., Ryan, C. M., Mintun, M. A., Meltzer, C. C., Townsend, D. W., et al. (1998). Cerebral blood flow in hypertensive patients: An initial report of reduced and compensatory blood flow responses during performance of two cognitive tasks. *Hypertension* 31, 1216–1222.

Johnson, M. K., Mitchell, K. J., Raye, C. L., & Greene, E. J. (2004). An age-related deficit in prefrontal cortical function associated with refreshing information. *Psychological Science* 15(2), 127–132.

Johnson, S. C., Saykin, A. J., Flashman, L. A., McAllister, T. W., O'Jile, J. R., Sparling, M. B., et al. (2001). Similarities and differences in semantic and phonological processing with age: Patterns of functional MRI activation. *Aging, Neuropsychology & Cognition* 8(4), 307–320.

Jonides, J., Marshuetz, C., Smith, E. E., Reuter-Lorenz, P. A., Koeppe, R. A., & Hartley, A. (2000). Brain activation reveals changes with age in resolving interference in verbal working memory. *Journal of Cognitive Neuroscience* 12, 188–196.

Karni, A., Meyer, G., Jezzard, P., Adams, M. M., & et al. (1995). Functional MRI evidence for adult motor cortex plasticity during motor skill learning. *Nature* 377(6545), 155–158.

Lamar, M., Yousem, D. M., & Resnick, S. M. (2004). Age differences in orbitofrontal activation: An fMRI investigation of delayed match and nonmatch to sample. *NeuroImage* 21(4), 1368–1376.

Langenecker, S. A., Nielson, K. A., & Rao, S. M. (2004). fMRI of healthy older adults during Stroop interference. *NeuroImage* 21(1), 192–200.

Levine, B. K., Beason-Held, L. L., Purpura, K. P., Aronchick, D. M., Optican, L. M., Alexander, G. E., et al. (2000). Age-related differences in visual perception: A PET study. *Neurobiology of Aging* 21(4), 577–584.

Li, S.-C., & Lindenberger, U. (1999). Cross-level unification: A computational exploration of the link between deterioration of neurotransmitter systems and dedifferentiation of cognitive abilities in old age. In L.-G. Nilsson & H. J. Markowitsch (Eds.), *Cognitive Neuroscience of Memory*, 103–146. Seattle, WA: Hogrefe & Huber.

Lindenberger, U., & Baltes, P. B. (1994). Sensory functioning and intelligence in old age: A strong connection. *Psychology and Aging* 9, 339–355.

Logan, J. M., Sanders, A. L., Snyder, A. Z., Morris, J. C., & Buckner, R. L. (2002). Under-recruitment and nonselective recruitment: Dissociable neural mechanisms associated with aging. *Neuron* 33, 827–840.

Lustig, C., & Buckner, R. L. (2004). Preserved neural correlates of priming in old age and dementia. *Neuron* 42(5), 865–875.

Lustig, C., Snyder, A. Z., Bhakta, M., O'Brien, K. C., McAvoy, M., Raichle, M. E., et al. (2003). Functional deactivations: Change with age and dementia of the Alzheimer type. *Proceedings of the National Academy of Sciences USA* 100(24), 14504–14509.

Madden, D. J., Gottlob, L. R., Denny, L. L., Turkington, T. G., Provenzale, J. M., Hawk, T. C., et al. (1999). Aging and recognition memory: Changes in regional cerebral blood flow associated with components of reaction time distributions. *Journal of Cognitive Neuroscience* 11(5), 511–520.

Madden, D. J., Langley, L. K., Denny, L. L., Turkington, T. G., Provenzale, J. M., Hawk, T. C., et al. (2002). Adult age differences in visual word identification: Functional neuroanatomy by positron emission tomography. *Brain & Cognition* 49(3), 297–321.

Madden, D. J., Turkington, T. G., Coleman, R. E., Provenzale, J. M., DeGrado, T. R., & Hoffman, J. M. (1996). Adult age differences in regional cerebral blood flow during visual word identification: Evidence from $H_2^{15}O$ PET. *NeuroImage* 3, 127–142.

Madden, D. J., Turkington, T. G., Provenzale, J. M., Denny, L. L., Hawk, T. C., Gottlob, L. R., et al. (1999). Adult age differences in functional neuroanatomy of verbal recognition memory. *Human Brain Mapping* 7, 115–135.

Madden, D. J., Turkington, T. G., Provenzale, J. M., Denny, L. L., Langley, L. K., Hawk, T. C., et al. (2002). Aging and attentional guidance during visual search: Functional neuroanatomy by positron emission tomography. *Psychology and Aging* 17, 24–43.

Madden, D. J., Turkington, T. G., Provenzale, J. M., Hawk, T. C., Hoffman, J. M., & Coleman, R. E. (1997). Selective and divided visual attention: Age-related changes in regional cerebral blood flow measured by H$_2^{15}$O PET. *Human Brain Mapping* 5, 389–409.

Madden, D. J., Whiting, W. L., Provenzale, J. M., & Huettel, S. A. (2004). Age-related changes in neural activity during visual target detection measured by fMRI. *Cerebral Cortex* 14(2), 143–155.

Maguire, E. A., & Frith, C. D. (2003). Aging affects the engagement of the hippocampus during autobiographical memory retrieval. *Brain* 126, 1–13.

Mason, S. E. (1979). Effects of orienting tasks on the recall and recognition performance of subjects differing in age. *Developmental Psychology* 15, 467–469.

McIntosh, A. R., Sekuler, A. B., Penpeci, C., Rajah, M. N., Grady, C. L., Sekuler, R., et al. (1999). Recruitment of unique neural systems to support visual memory in normal aging. *Current Biology* 9, 1275–1278.

McKiernan, K. A., Kaufman, J. N., Kucera-Thompson, J., & Binder, J. R. (2003). A parametric manipulation of factors affecting task-induced deactivation in functional neuroimaging. *Journal of Cognitive Neuroscience* 15(3), 394–408.

Meulenbroek, O., Petersson, K. M., Voermans, N., Weber, B., & Fernandez, G. (2004). Age differences in neural correlates of route encoding and route recognition. *NeuroImage* 22(4), 1503–1514.

Milham, M. P., Erickson, K. I., Banich, M. T., Kramer, A. F., Webb, A., Wszalek, T., et al. (2002). Attentional control in the aging brain: Insights from an fMRI study of the Stroop task. *Brain & Cognition* 49(3), 277–296.

Mitchell, K. J., Johnson, M. K., Raye, C. L., & D'Esposito, M. (2000). fMRI evidence of age-related hippocampal dysfunction in feature binding in working memory. *Cognitive Brain Research* 10, 197–206.

Morcom, A. M., Good, C. D., Frackowiak, R. S., & Rugg, M. D. (2003). Age effects on the neural correlates of successful memory encoding. *Brain* 126(1), 213–229.

Nagahama, Y., Fukuyama, H., Yamaguchi, H., Katsumi, Y., Magata, Y., Shibasaki, H., et al. (1997). Age-related changes in cerebral blood flow activation during a card sorting test. *Experimental Brain Research* 114, 571–577.

Nielson, K. A., Langenecker, S. A., & Garavan, H. P. (2002). Differences in the functional neuroanatomy of inhibitory control across the adult lifespan. *Psychology and Aging* 17, 56–71.

Nyberg, L., Sandblom, J., Jones, S., Neely, A. S., Petersson, K. M., Ingvar, M., et al. (2003). Neural correlates of training-related memory improvement in adulthood and aging. *Proceedings of the National Academy of Sciences USA* 100(23), 13728–13733.

Park, D. C., Polk, T. A., Park, R., Minear, M., Savage, A., & Smith, M. R. (2004). Aging reduces neural specialization in ventral visual cortex. *Proceedings of the National Academy of Sciences USA* 101(35), 13091–13095.

Park, D. C., Welsh, R. C., Marshuetz, C., Gutchess, A. H., Mikels, J., Polk, T. A., et al. (2003). Working memory for complex scenes: Age differences in frontal and hippocampal activations. *Journal of Cognitive Neuroscience* 15(8), 1122–1134.

Parkin, A. J., & Walter, B. M. (1992). Recollective experience, normal aging, and frontal dysfunction. *Psychology and Aging* 7, 290–298.

Persson, J., Sylvester, C. Y., Nelson, J. K., Welsh, K. M., Jonides, J., & Reuter-Lorenz, P. A. (2004). Selection requirements during verb generation: Differential recruitment in older and younger adults. *NeuroImage* 23(4), 1382–1390.

Prince, S. E., Daselaar, S. M., & Cabeza, R. (2005). Neural correlates of relational memory: Successful encoding and retrieval of semantic and perceptual associations. *Journal of Neuroscience* 25, 1203–1210.

Raichle, M. E., Fiez, J. A., Videen, T. O., MacLeod, A.-M. K., Pardo, J. V., Fox, P. T., et al. (1994). Practice-related changes in human brain functional anatomy during nonmotor learning. *Cerebral Cortex* 4(1), 8–26.

Reuter-Lorenz, P., Jonides, J., Smith, E. S., Hartley, A., Miller, A., Marshuetz, C., et al. (2000). Age differences in the frontal lateralization of verbal and spatial working memory revealed by PET. *Journal of Cognitive Neuroscience* 12, 174–187.

Reuter-Lorenz, P., Marshuetz, C., Jonides, J., Smith, E. S., Hartley, A., & Koeppe, R. A. (2001). Neurocognitive ageing of storage and executive processes. *European Journal of Cognitive Psychology* 13, 257–278.

Rosen, A. C., Prull, M. W., O'Hara, R., Race, E. A., Desmond, J. E., Glover, G. H., et al. (2002). Variable effects of aging on frontal lobe contributions to memory. *NeuroReport* 13, 2425–2428.

Rypma, B., & D'Esposito, M. (2000). Isolating the neural mechanisms of age-related changes in human working memory. *Nature Neuroscience* 3, 509–515.

Rypma, B., Prabhakaran, V., Desmond, J. E., & Gabrieli, J. D. E. (2001). Age differences in prefrontal cortical activity in working memory. *Psychology and Aging* 16, 371–384.

Schacter, D. L., Savage, C. R., Alpert, N. M., Rauch, S. L., & Albert, M. S. (1996). The role of hippocampus and frontal cortex in age-related memory changes: A PET study. *NeuroReport* 7, 1165–1169.

Schiavetto, A., Kohler, S., Grady, C. L., Winocur, G., & Moscovitch, M. (2002). Neural correlates of memory for object identity and object location: Effects of aging. *Neuropsychologia* 40(8), 1428–1442.

Shulman, G. L., Corbetta, M., Buckner, R. L., Fiez, J. A., Miezin, F. M., Raichle, M. E., et al. (1997). Common blood flow changes across visual tasks. 1. Increases in subcortical structures and cerebellum but not in nonvisual cortex. *Journal of Cognitive Neuroscience* 9(5), 624–647.

Simon, E. (1979). Depth and elaboration of processing in relation to age. *Journal of Experimental Psychology: Humam Learning and Cognition* 5, 115–124.

Skoog, I. (1998). Status of risk factors for vascular dementia. *Neuroepidemiology* 17, 2–9.

Smith, E. E., Geva, A., Jonides, J., Miller, A., Reuter-Lorenz, P., & Koeppe, R. A. (2001). The neural basis of task-switching in working memory: Effects of performance and aging. *Proceedings of the National Academy of Sciences USA* 98(4), 2095–2100.

Spencer, W. D., & Raz, N. (1995). Differential effects of aging on memory for content and context: A meta-analysis. *Psychology and Aging* 10(4), 527–539.

Stebbins, G. T., Carrillo, M. C., Dorman, J., Dirksen, C., Desond, J., Turner, D. A., et al. (2002). Aging effects on memory encoding in the frontal lobes. *Psychology and Aging* 17, 44–55.

Stern, Y., Habeck, C., Moeller, J., Scarmeas, N., Anderson, K. E., Hilton, H. J., et al. (2005). Brain networks associated with cognitive reserve in healthy young and old adults. *Cerebral Cortex* 15, 394–402.

Thomsen, T., Specht, K., Hammar, A., Nyttingnes, J., Ersland, L., & Hugdahl, K. (2004). Brain localization of attentional control in different age groups by combining functional and structural MRI. *NeuroImage* 22(2), 912–919.

Whiting, W. L., Madden, D. J., Langley, L. K., Denny, L. L., Turkington, T. G., Provenzale, J. M., et al. (2003). Lexical and sublexical components of age-related changes in neural activation during visual word identification. *Journal of Cognitive Neuroscience* 15(3), 475–487.

Yonelinas, A. P. (2002). The nature of recollection and familiarity: A review of 30 years of research. *Memory and Language* 46, 441–517.

13 Functional Neuroimaging of Emotion and Social Cognition

Elizabeth A. Phelps and Kevin S. LaBar

Introduction

Our current understanding of the representation of emotion in the human brain has been largely driven by research on nonhuman animals demonstrating that some brain regions seem to be specialized for emotion processing. One of the earliest findings of an "emotional" brain region was a study by Kluver and Bucy (1937) in which monkeys with large medial temporal lobe lesions displayed a range of odd emotional responses, such as approaching objects that are normally feared (e.g., snakes), orally exploring nonedible objects, and changes in sexual behavior, a constellation of social/emotional deficits termed "psychic blindness." The original Kluver-Bucy lesion included a number of medial temporal lobe structures; however, Weiskrantz (1956) later isolated the amygdala as the critical structure whose lesion led to psychic blindness. Since that time, the amygdala has been considered a primary component of the neural circuits of emotion (Davidson & Irwin, 1999; LeDoux, 1996). Although there are several other brain structures that have been identified as important for normal emotional and social processing and responses (Papez, 1937; Damasio, 1999), early research in the cognitive neuroscience of emotion—often motivated by animal models—has emphasized the importance of the amygdala.

In this chapter, we review what has been learned about the human amygdala using functional imaging. We start with an assessment of functional imaging methods. We then proceed with a review of current research on the role of the human amygdala in emotional learning and memory, attention and perception, and social cognition.

Methods for Assessing Amygdala Function

The functions of the human amygdala have been historically difficult to assess, despite the prominence of this brain region in animal models of emotion and motivation. This has been due in part to methodological issues associated with emotion in general and the amygdala in particular. Some of the measurement problems in functional imaging investigations of amygdala function are discussed below. Because of the limitations of each technique in isolation, convergence of information across multiple methods is critical for advancing an understanding of cognitive-emotional interactions and their neural substrates.

Behavioral Paradigms

We note at the outset that neuroscientific approaches are only as good as the experimental paradigms used to probe brain function. In this regard, assessment of emotion has lagged behind other mental faculties. Several factors have contributed to the neglect of emotional paradigm development, including (1) the "cognitive revolution" of mid-twentieth-century psychology, which advocated analysis of "pure" cognition in the absence of motivational and emotional influences; (2) the "fuzziness" of emotion as a construct and debates centering around the fundamental structure of affective space (Scherer, 2000); (3) the tripartite nature of emotional response systems—behavior, physiology, and verbal report—that are loosely coupled (Lang, 1993); (4) intra- and interindividual variability; and (5) ethical limitations in procuring emotional responses in the laboratory. The availability of standardized stimulus sets has improved the ability to systematically probe emotional processes with brain imaging and in patient populations. These include standard sets of emotional facial expressions (Ekman & Friesen, 1975), pictures (Lang et al., 1999), words (Bradley & Lang, 1999a), and environmental sounds (Bradley & Lang, 1999b). Some domains of emotion have also benefited by adaptations of experimental paradigms from animal models, such as those related to fear learning and reward processing. Continued efforts in developing dynamic emotional stimuli and interactive socio-emotional contexts using computer morphing and virtual reality software (e.g., LaBar et al., 2003; Rizzo et al., 2001) will facilitate brain imaging of more complex affective processes in parallel with technical advances that improve simultaneous detection of behavioral and physiological responses.

Functional Brain Imaging

Neurophysiological and psychological aspects of amygdala function present several challenges for applying cognitive neuroscience tools to study emotional processes. Several advantages and disadvantages of common brain imaging techniques are summarized below.

Event-Related Potentials (ERPs)   Amygdala neurons are arranged in largely closed-field configurations (Halgren, 1992). For this reason, electrical potentials do not propagate to the scalp, and the only means to directly observe electrical responses from the amygdala is by intracranial recordings of epileptic patients. Scalp ERP studies of amygdala-lesioned patients, however, would be informative to examine the impact of amygdala damage on emotion-related ERPs generated by other brain regions.

Magnetoencephalography (MEG)   MEG does not suffer from the signal propagation limitations of ERPs, so it is possible to measure magnetic fields eminating from the amygdala. Unfortunately, there are few research centers available to conduct such studies. Localizing MEG effects to the amygdala can be difficult, given its small size and location deep within the temporal lobe, as well as the relatively broad distributions of emotion-related potentials.

PET   Initial positron emission tomography studies provided important insights into emotional functions of the amygdala. Recording physiological and verbal responses is more straightforward with this technique than with functional magnetic resonance imaging (fMRI). However, analysis of typical PET data requires a degree of spatial smoothing that is larger than the width of the amygdala itself, potentially recruiting brain signals from adjacent regions. In addition, the temporal parameters of PET studies are limited by the half-life of the radioisotope injected into the participant (e.g., data is typically accumulated across 60 sec time periods with 150), as well as the limited repeatability of the experiment within subjects due to ethical considerations concerning repeated exposure to radioactive substances (George et al., 2000). For studies of sustained mood, PET may be particularly useful, but for investigations of emotional influences lasting shorter durations, trial blocking is required.

   In addition to untoward effects on cognitive functions (e.g., changing cognitive "set"), blocking trials by emotional category confounds emotional processing with mood induction and may miss transient amygdala activation that habituates over repeated trials (e.g., Breiter et al., 1996; Wright et al., 2001). Recent advances in PET technology have improved some of these issues, but this technique has been largely supplanted in cognitive activation studies by fMRI due to its superior spatial and temporal resolution as well as other advantages (cost, noninvasiveness, etc.). PET nonetheless remains a powerful tool for examining pharmacological effects in the amygdala—radioisotopes can be designed that bind to specific receptor molecules to provide a unique view into the anatomical distribution of neurotransmitter subtypes in healthy and psychiatric populations.

fMRI   Functional magnetic resonance imaging has become the main tool for brain imaging of amygdala function, although not without its challenges. Because the amygdala is bounded medially by sinuses and ventrolaterally by the lateral ventricle,

424 Elizabeth A. Phelps and Kevin S. LaBar

it is situated in a region characterized by magnetic susceptibility-induced signal loss. Quantitative analysis of signal-to-noise in the vicinity of the amygdala shows that the signal losses contribute to intersubject and interhemispheric variability in amygdala activation during emotional encoding (figure 13.1, plate 24; LaBar et al., 2001). These issues are more difficult to resolve at high field strengths and are particularly critical for voxelwise statistical analyses that require precise spatial registration of signal changes across subjects (but see Posse et al., 2003; Wang et al., 2005). Although current methods do not allow resolution of individual amygdaloid subnuclei, it is possible to segregate signals grossly into anterior-posterior, medial-lateral, and dorsal-ventral subdivisions (e.g., Anderson et al., 2003a; Whalen, Rausch, et al., 1998; Dolcos et al., 2004b).

Further complicating the interpretation of amygdala activation to emotional stimuli is the role of individual differences. Amygdala activity has been shown to vary across individuals according to several personality, social, and genetic factors. These include gender (Cahill et al., 2004; Canli, Desmond, et al., 2002; Hamann et al., 2004), age (Mather et al., 2004), extraversion (Canli, Sivers, et al., 2002), implicit measures of racial bias (Phelps et al., 2000), motivational regulatory focus (prevention/promotion) (Cunningham et al., 2005), and genetic variation in serotonin receptor function (Hariri et al., 2002). Thus, standard group-averaged analytic approaches may mask amygdala activity and contribute to the lack of replicability across population samples. For this reason, comprehensive characterization of personality and demographic characteristics of the participants is becoming critical, as well as complementary statistical analyses that include assessment of individual differences.

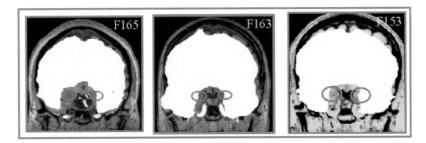

Figure 13.1
Signal voids in the vicinity of the amygdala due to magnetic susceptibility artifacts. Images depict thresholded signal-to-noise maps overlaid onto each subject's structural scan in a coronal section through the amygdala (outlined in red). For all three subjects, the medial aspect of the left and right amygdalae are located outside the sensitivity map, indicating insufficient signal-to-noise for a *t*-test comparison based on an expected 1% peak signal change. None of these participants showed significant amygdala activation during the encoding of emotionally aversive complex scenes. Data were acquired from a 1.5 T Siemens Vision scanner using conventional whole-brain gradient-echo echoplanar imaging. (Adapted from LaBar et al., 2001.) See plate 24 for color version.

Volumetry   Structural MRI scans provide an opportunity to examine volumetric changes in the amygdala as a function of neurologic or psychiatric illness, as well as healthy development and aging. As with fMRI, volumetric measurements are currently limited to gross differentiation of the amygdala from adjacent medial temporal lobe structures, and individual subnuclei cannot be resolved. A major difficulty with amygdala volumetry is the delineation of anatomic borders, particularly the caudoventral border between the amygdala and hippocampus, the rostrodorsal border with the basal forebrain, and the medial border with the subjacent periamygdaloid/perirhinal cortices. Differences in volumetric methodologies can contribute to variation in results across studies (Brierly et al., 2002). Precise measurements using anatomic landmarks, high-resolution images, interactive viewing in three orthogonal planes, and spatial reorientation of images onto a common axis are required (Brierly et al., 2002; Convit et al., 1999).

TMS   Repetitive transcranial magnetic stimulation is a relatively new technique that enables reversible interruption or stimulation of brain activity due to a focused magnetic pulse train delivered from a coil placed on the scalp (Fitzpatrick & Rothman, 2000). Currently, the spatial spread and limited depth of the signal pulses make TMS unavailable for the study of amygdala function.

Summary

Each functional neuroimaging method has its relative advantages and disadvantages. The study of emotional information processing and amygdala function poses specific challenges above and beyond other aspects of brain function. Some of these challenges will be circumvented with future technological improvements, but others will not. Because neuroimaging data are inherently correlational, studies of neurologic patients are important to reveal cognitive-emotional interactions for which the integrity of the amygdala is essential, although lesion studies also have unique limitations (e.g., lack of anatomical specificity, the presence of underlying neurological disorders, poor temporal resolution). Converging evidence across multiple measures is therefore critical. As we discuss the role of the amygdala in various cognitive-emotional interactions, it is important to keep these issues in mind so that results across different methodologies can be interpreted appropriately.

Functional Neuorimaging of Emotion and Social Cognition

Emotional Learning and Memory

One of the fundamental lessons of cognitive neuroscience since the mid-1990s is the distribution of learning and memory functions across multiple intersecting systems in the brain (Gabrieli, 1998; Squire & Zola, 1996; Tulving & Schacter, 1990). Two primary modes or expressions of memory have been identified—explicit (declarative) and implicit (nondeclarative). Explicit memory refers to the conscious recollection of facts or events from one's past that rely on the integrity of the hippocampus and related medial temporal lobe-diencephalic structures. Implicit memory refers to nonconscious behavioral changes to previously encountered stimuli that are mediated outside the hippocampal-diencephalic system. Rather than reflecting a unitary construct, implicit memory encompasses a constellation of unconscious processes that have different neural correlates and operating characteristics.

Emotionally salient events can be encoded and retrieved through the engagement of either of these modes of memory. Since the construct of "emotion" is as complex as that of "memory," mnemonic aspects of emotion processing are likely mediated by interactions among multiple brain regions and neurotransmitter systems. The analysis below synthesizes the human amygdala's contributions to emotional memory but does not constitute a comprehensive neurobiological account. Other neural structures are not considered in detail, and there is only limited information regarding the amygdala itself. The available evidence indicates that the amygdala's role in memory transcends the implicit-explicit distinction. However, its functions may be limited to specific regions of affective space dissociated across arousal and valence dimensions (LaBar, 2003).

Implicit Emotional Memory

The amygdala's role in implicit emotional memory has been readily studied using tasks adapted from the animal literature. In particular, a convergence of information across methods supports its central prominence in conditioned emotional learning. Conditioning paradigms provide a valuable means to investigate how innocuous stimuli acquire and retain emotional significance. The amygdala's contribution to other forms of implicit emotional memory (e.g., preference formation) have not been well established.

Fear conditioning paradigms have provided a useful starting point for investigating emotional memory in the implicit domain. The neural circuitry and cellular mechanisms contributing to this form of learning have been exquisitely detailed in animal studies and are conserved across the phyla (Davis, 1994; Fendt & Fanselow, 1999; LaBar & LeDoux, 2001). In a typical fear conditioning task, an innocuous stimulus (the conditioned stimulus, CS) is presented in association with an aversive event (the unconditioned stimulus, US). After several CS-US pairings, physiological indices of fear emerge in reaction to the CS alone. These responses can be extinguished by subsequently presenting the CS without reinforcement.

The amygdala's central role in fear conditioning has been demonstrated in both lesion and imaging studies in humans. Patients with unilateral (LaBar et al., 1995) and bilateral amygdala damage (Bechara et al., 1995) fail to show physiological evidence of conditioned fear, in spite of the ability to explicitly report that the CS predicts the US. Declarative knowledge of stimulus contingencies is thus insufficient for generating conditioned fear physiologically (see LaBar & Disterhoft, 1998). Amnesic patients without amygdala damage show the converse effect. They cannot state the stimulus contingencies but nonetheless show intact skin conductance responses on simple fear conditioning tasks (Bechara et al., 1995; LaBar & Phelps, 2005). Interestingly, amnesics who initially acquire conditioned fear fail to recover their skin conductance responses when the fearfulness of the spatial context is reinstated after extinction (LaBar & Phelps, 2005). As in other species, the hippocampus may play a selective role in contextual modulation of emotional memory even though it is not required for learning simple emotional associations (Kim & Fanselow, 1992; Phillips & LeDoux, 1992; Wilson et al., 1995).

The role of the human amygdala in fear conditioning has been confirmed in neuroimaging studies. Healthy participants show amygdala activation during the acquisition (Büchel et al., 1998; LaBar et al., 1998) and extinction (LaBar et al., 1998; Phelps et al., 2004) phases of conditioned fear learning. The extent of amygdala activation correlates with conditioned skin conductance amplitudes in individual subjects, a finding that does not generalize to paralimbic regions (Cheng et al., 2003; Furmark et al., 1997; LaBar et al., 1998). The amygdala's response is maximal on early acquisition and extinction trials, when the predictive associations between the CS and US are initially changed. Similar temporal dynamics have been reported in a subset of lateral amygdala neurons in electrophysiological studies in the rat (Quirk et al., 1995; Repa et al., 2001). In rats, amygdala plasticity occurs very rapidly after CS onset, implicating the involvement of direct thalamic inputs. In humans, fear-relevant stimuli that were previously conditioned engage the amygdala even when presented unconsciously (Morris, Öhman, et al., 1998). Amygdala processing during fear learning thus signals rapid detection of changes in emotional salience that *can* (but does not *always*) occur outside of awareness (LaBar & Disterhoft, 1998).

Despite the utility of fear conditioning as a hallmark test of emotional associative learning, there is considerable variability across participants in the magnitude of their conditionability. These individual differences are reliable across repeated testing sessions (Fredrikson et al., 1993) and involve multiple influences of personality traits (Eysenck & Kelley, 1987), stress hormones and gender (Shors, 2004; Zorawski et al., 2005), aging and contingency awareness (LaBar et al., 2004), and genetic factors (Garpenstrand et al., 2001; Hettema et al., 2003). Additional studies are needed to determine the extent to which these variables modulate amygdala engagement during different phases of conditioned fear learning.

Explicit Emotional Memory

The amygdala, which has the primary role in implicit emotional memory as assessed with physiological measures in fear conditioning, has also been shown to have a modulatory role on explicit memory. Research with nonhuman animals indicates that the amygdala may modulate the storage, or consolidation, of hippocampal-dependent memory through activation of beta-adrenergic receptors in the amygdala, which is a component of the arousal response (see McGaugh, 2000, for a review). In addition, the amygdala may modulate the encoding of explicit memory through altering attention and perception for emotional stimuli (see "Attention and Perception," below).

Functional imaging has sufficient spatial and temporal resolution to differentiate the role of medial temporal lobe structures across distinct stages of memory processing in the healthy brain (but see the section "Methods for Assessing Amygdala Function," above, for some caveats). Therefore functional neuroimaging in healthy subjects is particularly useful for assessing emotional influences across distinct stages of memory processing. Initial PET studies had implicated a relationship between the degree of amygdala activation during emotional stimulus encoding and later memory performance (Cahill et al., 1996; Hamann et al., 1999). Given the limitations of PET described above, more definitive evidence regarding this relationship awaited the development of event-related fMRI techniques in which item-based analyses became possible and signal changes from adjacent medial temporal lobe regions could be distinguished more readily.

"Subsequent memory" paradigms are now commonly used to identify brain regions whose degree of activation during encoding predicts later recollection for individual study items (reviewed in Wagner et al., 1999). In subsequent memory paradigms, data are binned according to whether individual items are later remembered or forgotten by each participant, and the "difference in memory" (Dm) effect is calculated by subtracting activity indexing the encoding of forgotten items from remembered items. Canli et al. (2000) showed that the Dm effect in the amygdala was larger for aversive than for neutral pictures, and that the degree of activation varied according to self-reported arousal. Subsequent studies extended these emotional Dm effects to positively valent stimuli (figure 13.2; Dolcos et al., 2004b) and showed that the amygdala interacts with other medial temporal lobe regions, including the hippocampus and entorhinal cortex, to promote the encoding of emotional items into long-term memory (Dolcos et al., 2004b; Kensinger & Corkin, 2004; Richardson et al., 2004).

Although the amygdala has been emphasized in these reports, subsequent memory effects for emotional stimuli are also found in prefrontal cortex (Dolcos et al., 2004a; Kensinger & Corkin, 2004), and the relative roles of the prefrontal and medial temporal lobe compartments have not yet been delineated.

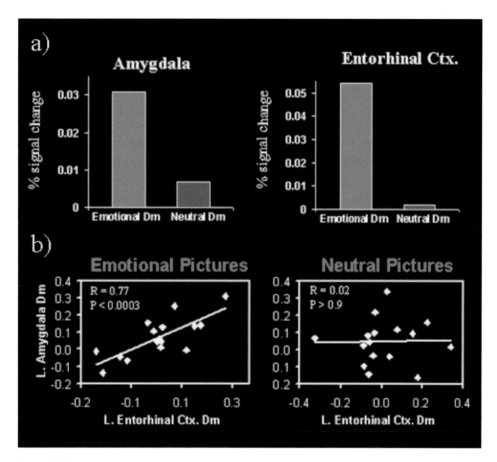

Figure 13.2
Enhancement of the subsequent memory (Dm) effect by emotional arousal in the basolateral amygdale and entorhinal cortex. (*a*) Percent signal change is extracted from anatomical regions of interest drawn on each participant's coronal scan and averaged across participants. The bar graphs compare brain activity during encoding that differentiates remembered from forgotten items for emotional (positive and negative combined) and neutral pictures. (*b*) The activity in these two regions is correlated more strongly for the emotional Dm effect (*left*) than for the neutral Dm effect (*right*). Data are shown for the left hemisphere, although similar correlations were found in the right hemisphere. These data indicate both greater activity and a tighter functional coupling of activity in the two regions during successful encoding of emotional items compared to successful encoding of neutral items. (Adapted from Dolcos et al., 2004b.)

It is important to note that these emotional memory effects are more selective than emotional perception effects, which recruit a much broader network of ventral brain regions (e.g., Taylor et al., 1998; Yamasaki et al., 2002; Wang et al., 2005). This may explain why patients with amygdala lesions often have intact arousal responses and ratings to emotional stimuli during encoding but fail to show arousal-mediated memory effects. One must bear in mind that subsequent memory paradigms do not capture *all* relevant processes involved in emotional memory formation, since they do not measure postencoding effects, including rumination, rehearsal, and consequences of stress hormone release, which also contribute to long-term emotional memory (K. A. Ochsner & Schacter, 2000).

Although classic views of emotional memory emphasize the amygdala's role in encoding and consolidation processes (McGaugh, 2000), there is now evidence that the amygdala also contributes to emotional memory retrieval (Nader et al., 2000). In humans, this has been examined with functional neuroimaging using both laboratory-based emotional memory tasks and retrieval of autobiographical memories. In laboratory-based studies, positive and negative scenes encoded just prior to PET scanning selectively activate the amygdala during recognition memory test blocks containing a high density of studied items (Dolan et al., 2000). Using fMRI, negative scenes that were retrieved with a subjective sense of recollection ("remember") vs. familiarity ("know") showed enhanced activation of the amygdala. In contrast, this effect was observed in the parahippocampus for neutral scenes (Sharot et al., 2004). Dolcos et al. (2005) extended these findings to examine retrieval of emotionally arousing and neutral scenes after a retention interval of one year. They showed greater activation in the amygdala, hippocampus, and entorhinal cortex during the successful retrieval of emotionally arousing scenes compared with neutral ones. In addition, activity in the amygdala and hippocampus differentiated emotional retrieval associated with a sense of recollection from that associated only with a sense of familiarity.

In this line of research, it is important to differentiate the signaling of memory retrieval operations from emotional perceptual processes, physiological responses, or feeling states generated by the retrieval cue itself. The above studies handled this issue by including emotional stimuli in the baseline condition and by characterizing responses as an interaction between retrieval success (e.g., hits vs. misses; "remember" vs. "know") and emotional content (e.g., emotionally arousing vs. neutral). An alternative logic involves emotional paired associate learning tasks in which subjects learn to associate neutral cues with either emotional or neutral contexts, and then retrieval is tested by presentation of the neutral cues. Using this design, Maratos et al. (2001) reported amygdala activation in response to neutral words that cued negatively valent sentences studied prior to fMRI scanning. However, amygdala-lesioned patients perform normally on tasks in which neutral words are associated with emotional sentence contexts (Phelps et al., 1998), so this result must be interpreted with caution.

Functional imaging studies have also revealed amygdala activation during the retrieval of autobiographical memories, though not always (reviewed in Maguire, 2001). Autobiographical events provide an interesting and relevant domain to examine emotional memory because the emotions elicited can be strong in comparison with standard laboratory stimuli, the memories are personally salient, and more remote time periods can be probed. However, the study of autobiographical memory poses additional procedural issues since the encoding situation is not controlled, it is hard to verify what is being retrieved in the scanning environment, and it is difficult to come up with appropriate control tasks and retrieval cues. Markowitsch (1995) proposed that the retrieval of memories from the personal past depends on the connections between medial temporal and inferior frontal lobe structures, particularly those which course through the frontotemporal junction in the right hemisphere. Some studies have shown coactivation of the amygdala, hippocampus/ parahippocampal cortex, and inferior frontal regions during autobiographical retrieval (e.g., Fink et al., 1996; Greenberg et al., 2005; Maguire & Frith, 2003; Markowitsch et al., 2000). However, the relative contributions of these regions have not been well established. For example, studies that have manipulated the emotional content of the memories have not seen clear modulation of the amygdala (Damasio et al., 2000; Lane et al., 1997; Maguire & Frith, 2003; Piefke et al., 2003). Although the emotional arousal associated with autobiographical memories predicts many of the phenomenological characteristics of the memory, such as its vividness and sense of recollection (Bluck & Li, 2001; Reisberg et al., 1988; Talarico et al., 2004), future work is needed to determine if these effects are associated with amygdala activation during autobiographical retrieval.

Summary

Affective space is conceptually parsed according to two principal factors or underlying dimensions—arousal and valence (Bradley et al., 1992; Russell, 1980). The foregoing analysis supports a basic dissociation between the amygdala's contribution to arousal and valence functions in memory. Whereas the amygdala mediates arousal effects across various stages of explicit memory processing (encoding, consolidation, and retrieval) and during conditioned emotional learning, implicit and explicit memory effects that are linked to affective valence independent of arousal, such as preference formation (Elliott & Dolan, 1998; Tranel & Damasio, 1993) and semantic categorization of valent words (Phelps et al., 1997; 1998), occur outside the amygdaloid system, perhaps involving frontotemporal interactions. Unlike its sister structure, the hippocampus, the amygdala's role in memory cuts across the implicit-explicit dichotomy. Arousal systems are especially linked to survival functions, including defensive, reproductive, and maternal behaviors, which may account for the amygdala's participation in certain domains of emotional memory over others. Our understanding of these functions will be further refined with improved neuroscientific methodologies and paradigm development. In particular, future studies should characterize the amygdala's role in other forms of implicit memory and clarify the scope of its influence beyond emotional learning situations related to survival functions such as fear.

Attention and Perception

A fundamental characteristic of emotional stimuli is that they represent value or importance to the perceiver. Given that emotion signals value, it is perhaps not surprising that neural circuitry has developed to facilitate learning and remembering of emotionally salient events. In order for an organism to respond optimally to a stimulus with an emotional content, it would also be adaptive for emotional stimuli to receive priority in attentional and perceptual processing. This is especially important when stimuli signal potential threat that may require heightened vigilance or fast action. Although the amygdala has primarily been described as important in emotional learning, a growing body of evidence suggests that a secondary role for the amygdala is to allow for the rapid detection of threat by interacting with attention and perception (Davis & Whalen, 2001).

Emotion has been proposed to facilitate attentional processing, resulting in the capture of attention (e.g., J. M. G. Williams et al., 1996) and enhanced awareness of emotional stimuli (e.g., Anderson, 2005). For instance the classic "cocktail party effect" demonstrated that meaningful stimuli, such as your name, are more likely to break through an attentional bottleneck to reach awareness (Cherry, 1953). Similarly, it has been found that faces with emotional expressions, particularly threatening expressions such as anger, are detected more quickly in an array of faces (Hansen & Hansen, 1988). In addition, patients with unilateral neglect are more likely to detect fear faces in the neglected field (Vuilleumier & Schwartz, 2001). Finally, there is enhanced detection of arousing words during an attentional blink paradigm, which highlights the temporal limitations of attention (Anderson, 2005). In all of these situations where attentional resources are limited, emotional stimuli reach awareness more readily, thus receiving priority in stimulus processing. It is proposed that the amygdala plays a key role in emotion's modulation of attention.

The Amygdala and Automaticity
In order to facilitate attention and awareness of emotional stimuli, the amygdala must detect these stimuli prior to awareness and independent of attentional focus. Stimuli that are processed without attentional resources are often referred to as

being processed with "automaticity" (Medin et al., 2005). Although there are situations where attention does influence the amygdala response (described below), in most tasks it has been found that the amygdala can respond to emotional events outside of awareness and attentional focus.

The first demonstration that the amygdala responds without awareness came from studies examining responses to faces with emotional expressions. In an early fMRI study using the standardized Ekman & Frisen faces (1975), Breiter and colleagues (1996) found enhanced amygdala activation to faces with a fear expression, relative to neutral faces. In an extension of this work, Whalen, Rausch, et al. (1998) presented neutral and fear faces that were masked to prevent awareness. In this task, the face stimuli were presented for 30 msec, followed by a mask of another, neutral face. In this condition, subjects are unaware of the presence of the fear face stimuli. Nevertheless, the amygdala response to the fear faces was as robust as the earlier Breiter et al. (1996) study, although there much less of a cortical response to the masked faces.

Later studies examined the interaction of attention and amygdala activation more directly. A study by Vuilleumier and colleagues (2001) presented pictures of two faces, with either neutral or fear expressions, along with two houses and asked subjects to attend to (and match) the faces or houses on different trials. Activation of the amydgala was observed to fear vs. neutral faces whether subjects were attending to faces or houses, whereas activation in the fusiform face area (FFA), although modulated by emotion, was dependent on whether or not the faces were the attended target. Additional studies by Anderson, Christoff, Panitz, et al. (2003), using overlapping images of places and faces, and M. A. Williams et al. (2004), using binocular rivalry, found similar results—amygdala activation to fear vs. neutral faces was not modulated by attention, whereas activation in other regions (parahippocampal place area and FFA, for places and faces, respectively) depended on attention.

It has been suggested that amygdala activation to fear faces irrespective of attention and awareness may be due, in part, to the existence of both a cortical and a subcortical pathway for the detection of emotional stimuli by the amygdala (Morris et al., 1999; M. A. Williams et al., 2004). Studies of auditory fear conditioning in rats have shown that lesions to auditory cortex do not prevent the acquisition of auditory fear conditioning. However, if both the auditory cortex and a subcortical pathway involving thalamic nuclei are damaged, then auditory fear conditioning is impaired (Romanski & LeDoux, 1993). This subcortical pathway can detect crude auditory signals that bypass auditory cortex. It has been proposed that this subcortical pathway is an "early warning system" that enables the quick detection of emotional, and potentially threatening, stimuli (LeDoux, 1996).

In humans, there have been a few attempts to find support for a subcortical visual pathway for the detection of stimuli by the amygdala. A study by Vuilleumier et al.

(2003) took advantage of the fact that a visual subcortical pathway would be more sensitive to low spatial frequency information, whereas ventral visual cortex should respond preferentially to high spatial frequency information. When presenting both intact fear and neutral faces along with faces that contained either high or low spatial frequency information, they found the amygdala, pulvinar, and superior colliculus (components of a subcortical pathway) responded to intact and low spatial frequency fear vs. neutral faces, whereas the fusiform cortex showed greater activation to intact and high-spatial frequency faces. Additional evidence for a subcortical pathway for the automatic detection of threat by the amygdala comes from fMRI studies of patients with "blindsight"—they have damage to the extrastriate cortex and suffer from cortical blindness. When fear vs. neutral faces were presented to these patients, amygdala activation was observed even though the stimuli were not consciously detected. The findings of these studies combining lesion and functional imaging techniques are consistent with a subcortical pathway for detection of fear faces by the amygdala (Morris, DeGelder, et al., 2001; Pegna et al., 2005).

Although there is strong evidence that the amygdala can respond to emotional stimuli, primarily faces, irrespective of attentional focus, there are a few studies that have shown some modulation of the amygdala with attention. For instance, the studies by Anderson et al. (2003a) and M. A. Williams et al. (2004) that found similar amygdala activation to fear faces irrespective of attentional focus, also examined responses to faces with expressions of disgust and happiness, respectively. For these other facial expressions, amygdala activation was observed, but only when the faces were unattended. Attention to the disgust and happy faces diminished the amygdala response, suggesting a top-down modulation of amygdala activation with awareness. These results demonstrate that attention and awareness can influence amygdala activation. Although the amygdala does respond automatically to these emotional faces (i.e., without attentional focus), these responses are inhibited when they are the focus of attention.

In a study designed to test the limits of the amygdala's automatic response to fear faces, Pessoa and colleagues (2002) designed a demanding attention task in which subjects were required to attend to either a face presented at fixation or two bars in the periphery. In this task, drawing attention away from a fear face eliminated any observable amygdala BOLD response. These results are especially important, because they suggest that although amygdala activation to fear (vs. neutral) faces may appear to be automatic and independent of attention in most circumstances, there are situations where the attentional manipulation is so demanding that the principles of automacity are not an accurate description of the amygdala's response to emotional events.

The Pessoa et al. (2002) study, in which lack of attentional focus eliminates observed amygdala activation, has led to questions as to whether a subcortical pathway for detection of visual stimuli exists in humans. The authors argue that if a subcortical pathway can be used to detect a fear face, then activation of the amygdala should *never* be dependent on whether or not the face is the focus of attention. Although Pessoa and colleagues have clearly shown that the amygdala response to fear faces is modulated by attentional focus in a very demanding task, one of the limitations of fMRI is that the BOLD signal is not assessed as an absolute response, but as a relative response between conditions that are considered significantly different only if certain criteria are met. For this reason, it is not possible to say that there is no amygdala BOLD response to the fear faces without attentional focus; rather, one can say that no significant differential amygdala activation was observed.

Of course, the same criticism can be applied to fMRI studies that propose to support the existence of a subcortical pathway by claiming to find amygdala activation to fear faces in the absence of a visual cortex response (M. A. Williams et al., 2004) or to some specific properties of the visual stimulus and not others (Vuilleumier et al., 2003). In these cases, it can only be concluded that responses inconsistent with the claim of a subcortical pathway for detection by the amygdala were not observed using the statistical standards applied. There is still significant debate as to whether there is a subcortical pathway for the amygdala's detection of visual stimuli in humans, and it is unclear whether functional imaging techniques, when used without other methodologies, will be able to address this question fully.

However, regardless of whether the amygdala receives information about the emotional significance of a face by a cortical or a subcortical pathway, the amygdala's response to fear faces meets most of the principles of automaticity: is it is independent of attention and awareness, with certain limitations for highly demanding attention tasks.

The Facilitation of Attention

The amygdala's response to fear faces prior to awareness and, mostly, irrespective of attentional focus is thought to be the basis of its ability to facilitate attentional and perceptual processing. It has been shown in monkeys that the amygdala has reciprocal connections with visual cortex (Amaral et al., 1992; see figure 13.3). It is hypothesized that the amygdala receives input about the emotional properties of a stimulus early in processing and, through feedback to the visual cortex, modulates further attentional and perceptual processes. Consistent with this hypothesis, a PET study by Morris, Friston, et al. (1998) reported that responses of the amygdala to fear vs. neutral faces were correlated with a similar modulation in the extrastriate cortex. In addition, Anderson and Phelps (2001) used the attentional blink paradigm, in which subjects are asked to identify two target words from a stream of words presented in rapid succession, to examine the amygdala's modulation of

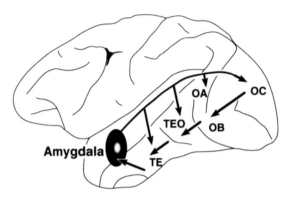

Figure 13.3
Schematic illustration of the reciprocal connectivity of the amygdala and visual cortices in the temporal and occipital lobes. (Adapted from Amaral et al., 1992.)

attention. In this task, subjects show a decrement in the ability to report the second target word when it is presented soon after the first target word, indicating a temporal attentional refractory period—as if attention "blinked" (Chun & Potter, 1995). When Anderson and Phelps changed the arousing properties of the second target word, they found an attenuation of the attentional blink effect. In other words, arousal facilitated the identification of the word during the "blink" interval, and patients with damage to the left amygdala failed to show the normal emotional attenuation of the attentional blink effect.

The Anderson and Phelps (2001) study provides strong support for the conclusion that the amygdala plays a critical role in the facilitation of the attention with emotion, but it does not indicate the mechanism by which this occurs. In an effort to find evidence for the hypothesized feedback mechanism underlying the modulation of attention and perception with emotion, Vuilleumier and colleagues (2004) combined functional imaging and lesion methodologies. They examined activation of visual areas to fear vs. neutral faces in patients with amygdala and hippocampal damage, and found that lesions to the amygdala resulted in the elimination of differential activation to fear vs. neutral faces in visual cortical areas, whereas damage to the hippocampus alone did not (see figure 13.4, plate 25). By combining methodologies, Vuilleumier et al. were able to find strong support of a modulatory role the amygdala in visual processing regions with emotional stimuli.

However, the visual cortex regions identified by Vuilleumier et al. (2004) are generally thought to support perceptual processes, not necessarily the allocation of attention (see chapter 4 in this volume). A growing body of evidence suggests that many observed effects of attention are linked to enhanced perception (Carrasco,

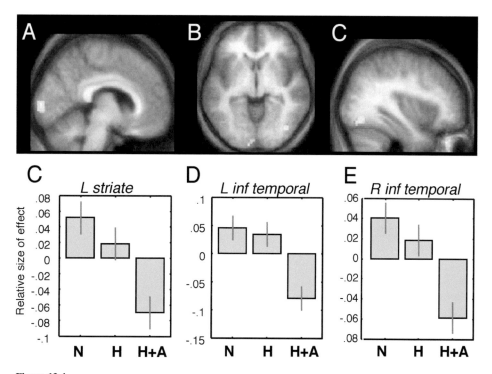

Figure 13.4

Statistical parametric maps of emotion x group interaction (*A–C*) across the whole brain showing the main effect for fearful vs. neutral faces differed between patient groups in the left striate cortex (*A*), left and right inferior temporal lobe (*B*), and right inferior temporal lobe (*C*). Parameter estimates for the relative size of effect in this ANOVA (arbitrary units, mean centered) for peaks in left striate cortex, left inferior temporal lobe, and right inferior temporal lobe show increased activation to fearful faces in both normal controls (N) and patients with damage confined to the hippocampus (H), but not patients with both hippocampal and amygdala damage (A + H). (Adapted from Vuilleumier et al., 2004.) See plate 25 for color version.

2004) and activation of visual, perceptual regions that occur with attention (Polonsky et al., 2000). Consistent with the notion that emotion enhances activation in visual processing regions, thus facilitating awareness and identification of emotional stimuli, a recent study found enhanced contrast sensitivity for stimuli cued with a fear face (Phelps et al., in press). Contrast sensitivity is an early visual process that is known to be coded by primary visual areas (Carrasco, 2004). These results suggest that emotion actually enhances how well we see. Combined with the imaging and lesions results cited above, there appears to be strong support for the proposal that the amygdala modulates processing in visual regions and facilitates attention and perception for emotional events.

Summary

Through research using a convergence of methodologies, there is considerable evidence for the hypotheses that the amygdala, by providing feedback to sensory cortical areas, modulates attention and perception for emotional stimuli, thus giving it priority in stimulus processing. However, the literature examining the interaction of awareness, attentional focus, perception, and amygdala function has almost exclusively examined responses to fear faces (although see Anderson, Christoff, et al. 2003; Morris, Öhman, et al. 1998; M. A. Williams et al., 2004). This stimulus has been suggested to be an especially potent signal of potential threat (see "Social Cognition," below). Future studies will need to further explore the limitations of the amygdala's automatic response to emotional stimuli and its modulation of visual processes by using both different stimulus types and a wider range of attention and perception tasks.

Social Cognition

As mentioned above, the research on the amygdala's role in attention and perception has largely relied on social stimuli (i.e., faces) that convey emotions, which could be a considered a limitation in the generality of these findings. At the same time, this research highlights the amygdala's importance in the social communication of emotion, particularly fear or threat. One of the early deficits reported by Kluver and Bucy (1937) following amygdala lesions in monkeys was odd social interactions. Since these initial findings, a wide range of studies have indicated that the amygdala may be a component of the neural systems underlying social interaction. Functional imaging research has highlighted the amygdala's involvement in two aspects of social behavior: the social communication and social learning of threat or fear.

Social Communication

As the functional imaging studies cited above indicate, the amygdala appears to show a preferential response to fear faces. Consistent with these data, patients with amygdala damage have a specific impairment in their ability to rate the intensity of fear expression while their ability to rate other expressions is relatively intact (Adolphs et al., 1999). This begs the question: What is special about fear faces? Although there is no clear answer, it has been proposed by Whalen (1998) that a primary adaptive role for the amygdala is the detection of threat in the environment to allow for increased vigilance, and fear in another's face may be an optimal signal of potential threat. Of course, one might also consider anger in another's face to be a good indication of threat. However, anger, unlike fear, is a direct indication of threat, in that anger indicates exactly where the threat is coming from (i.e., the angry person). Fear in another's face, on the other hand, suggests that there is a threat, but the immediate source of that threat is unclear. This added ambiguity in the source of threat would require greater vigilance by the perceiver. This suggests that the amygdala, if it is a component of a general threat detection mechanism used to trigger increased vigilance, should be most engaged in response to fear. In an effort to test this hypothesis, Whalen et al. (2001) compared amygdala activation to anger vs. fear vs. neutral facial expressions. They found greater amygdala activation to anger vs. neutral faces, but also greater activation to fear vs. anger faces. In other words, the amygdala does respond to the threat present in an angry face, but the added ambiguity of the source of threat in a fear face engages the amygdala even more.

A facial expression, such as fear, conveys a great deal of information. As the work of Ekman and Friesen (1975) and others has shown, different expressions engage specific patterns of musculature in the face, including around the eyes, mouth, forehead, and eyebrow areas. Although all of these aspects of facial expression are potentially useful in identifying specific expressions, recent research has suggested that the eyes may be particularly important for the detection of fear by the amygdala. Using fMRI, Whalen et al. (2004) presented just the eyes of fear vs. happy expressions. The eyes were presented briefly and masked so that subjects were unaware that they were viewing impoverished emotional stimuli. Simply viewing fearful vs. happy eyes resulted in greater activation of the amygdala. Consistent with this imaging data, a recent study by Adolphs et al. (2005) found that when freely viewing fear vs. neutral faces, the facial feature that normal subjects fixated on the most was the eyes, and this feature was also the most critical for identifying fear expressions. However, a patient with bilateral amygdala damage rarely fixated on the eyes when asked to judge fear faces and needed more overall facial information to identify expressions. When this patient was explicitly told to fixate on the eyes, her identification of fear expressions improved, but she failed to adapt this strategy without explicit instruction. These results suggest that the amygdala may also be important for engaging in the behaviors that are most helpful in the detection of fear in facial expressions.

Although there is extensive evidence that the amygdala responds preferentially to fear expressions, there are other social signals that can indicate threat. A recent study by De Gelder et al. (2004) found that presenting scenes of body movements consistent with fear vs. happiness resulted in activation of the amygdala. In addition, fMRI (Winston et al., 2002) and lesion (Adolphs et al., 1998) studies have found that the amygdala may also be important in judging whether an individual is trustworthy from face stimuli. Individuals who are not trustworthy may be more likely to be a potential threat. Patients with amygdala lesions tend to give higher trustworthiness and approachability ratings to unfamiliar faces than normal subjects are (Adolphs et al., 1998). In addition, faces rated as untrustworthy are shown to lead

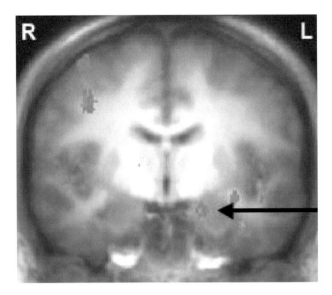

Figure 13.5
A statistical map presented in the coronal plane showing significant signal increases in the left amygdala (arrow) for the contrast of negative vs. positively cues surprise faces. (Adapted from Kim et al., 2004.) See plate 26 for color version.

males presented to white American subjects elicited amygdala activation in most, but not all, of the subjects. The magnitude of amygdala activation across subjects was correlated with the strength of the implicit, negative attitudes expressed. That is, those white American subjects who showed a greater negative implicit social bias toward blacks also showed greater amygdala activation to unfamiliar black vs. white faces (see figure 13.6, plate 27; Phelps et al., 2000).

Similar results have been observed in black American subjects, who show greater amygdala activation to black vs. white unfamiliar faces (Hart et al., 2000). However, personal experience with specific members of a social group can change the pattern of amygdala response. When pictures of familiar black and white individuals who have positive cultural images were presented to white American subjects (e.g., Martin Luther King, John F. Kennedy, Denzel Washington, Harrison Ford), there was no consistent pattern of amygdala activation to the black vs. white familiar faces, and no relationship between measures of race bias and amygdala activation. These results suggest that learned cultural stereotypes, whose expression varies across individuals, can bias amygdala activation to a face of another race, and that positive experience with an individual can alter this amygdala response.

The studies examining changes in amygdala activation to ambiguous social stimuli based on the social context in which they are presented, highlights the amygdala's

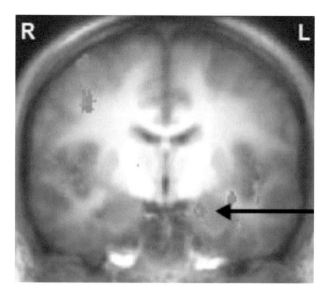

Figure 13.5
A statistical map presented in the coronal plane showing significant signal increases in the left amygdala (arrow) for the contrast of negative vs. positively cues surprise faces. (Adapted from Kim et al., 2004.) See plate 26 for color version.

males presented to white American subjects elicited amygdala activation in most, but not all, of the subjects. The magnitude of amygdala activation across subjects was correlated with the strength of the implicit, negative attitudes expressed. That is, those white American subjects who showed a greater negative implicit social bias toward blacks also showed greater amygdala activation to unfamiliar black vs. white faces (see figure 13.6, plate 27; Phelps et al., 2000).

Similar results have been observed in black American subjects, who show greater amygdala activation to black vs. white unfamiliar faces (Hart et al., 2000). However, personal experience with specific members of a social group can change the pattern of amygdala response. When pictures of familiar black and white individuals who have positive cultural images were presented to white American subjects (e.g., Martin Luther King, John F. Kennedy, Denzel Washington, Harrison Ford), there was no consistent pattern of amygdala activation to the black vs. white familiar faces, and no relationship between measures of race bias and amygdala activation. These results suggest that learned cultural stereotypes, whose expression varies across individuals, can bias amygdala activation to a face of another race, and that positive experience with an individual can alter this amygdala response.

The studies examining changes in amygdala activation to ambiguous social stimuli based on the social context in which they are presented, highlights the amygdala's

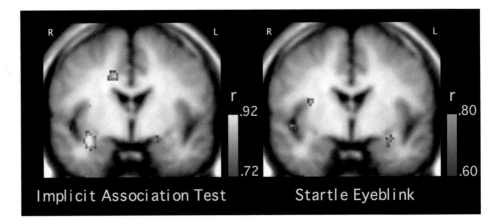

Figure 13.6
Correlation maps indicating brain regions where the relative differential BOLD response to black vs. white unfamiliar faces is significantly correlated with implicit measures of race bias for white American subjects. The implicit measures are (*left*) the Implicit Association Test (IAT), a reaction time measurement designed to measure conflict in evaluative judgments (Greenwald et al., 1998) and startle eyeblink (*right*) a physiological measure that assesses the strength of the startle reflex as it is modulated by emotional valence (Grillon et al., 1991). For both implicit measures of race bias, negative bias toward black is correlated with differential BOLD responses in the right amygdala. (Adapted from Phelps et al., 2000.) See plate 27 for color version.

dynamic role in assigning emotional value to stimuli. However, the amygdala's involvement in social learning extends beyond responses to face stimuli in negative contexts, to social learning concerning inanimate objects.

Social Learning
The studies on fear conditioning (see section "Implicit Memory," above) emphasize that the amygdala is critical for learning the relation between neutral and aversive stimuli. In fear conditioning, a neutral stimulus acquires aversive properties by being paired with an aversive event. However, there are other means by which neutral stimuli can acquire aversive properties. For example, one could learn that a neighborhood dog is potentially dangerous by being bitten. This is example of fear conditioning. However, simply being told that the dog is mean and might bite would also result in a negative, fear response to the dog. Learning symbolically by verbal instruction is a primary means of social learning in humans. In addition, watching the dog bite someone else might result in a fear response to the dog. Observation is another means of emotional, social learning. In everyday life, it is not uncommon to learn the emotional properties of stimuli through social interaction. Social learning of fear might be considered a more efficient form of emotional learning, since the direct experience of an aversive event is not necessary. Recent research suggests that the amygdala may play a role in the social learning of fear.

In a study designed to assess the amygdala's involvement in the symbolic communication of fear, called Instructed Fear, subjects were told that presentation of a square of a specific color might be paired with a mild shock to the wrist (the "threat" condition), while presentations of a square of another color would never be paired with a shock (the "safe" condition). None of the subjects actually received a shock in this study. Nevertheless, all of the subjects indicated they believed a shock would be presented with the "threat" stimulus, and showed an increased skin conductance response (SCR) to it presentation. Activation of the left amygdala was observed to presentations of the "threat" vs. "safe" stimulus (see figure 13.7, plate 28; Phelps et al., 2001). As in fear conditioning (LaBar et al, 1998), the magnitude of this amygdala activation was correlated with the strength of the fear response as measured with SCR. This BOLD response to a threat stimulus suggests that the amygdala responds to learned fears which are symbolically represented, and imagined and anticipated, but never actually experienced. However, these imaging results do not indicate a critical role for the amygdala. A follow-up study found that patients with damage to the left amygdala failed to show any physiological expression of instructed fear (Funayama et al., 2001), indicating that the amygdala plays a critical role in the expression of instructed fears.

Although the amygdala is critical for the expression of instructed fear, it is unlikely that it is involved in the acquisition of these fears. As research on fear conditioning in humans indicates, learning to consciously recollect that a

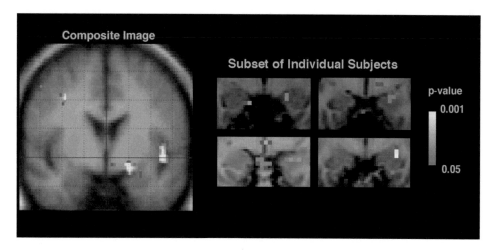

Figure 13.7
Group composite (*left*) and selected individual (*right*) statistical maps showing left amygdala activation to a colored square verbally linked to the possibility of a mild shock ("threat") versus another colored square not linked to shock ("safe"), demonstrating left amygdala involvement in instructed fear. (Adapted from Phelps et al., 2001.) See plate 28 for color version.

stimulus predicts an aversive event depends on the hippocampus, not the amygdala (Bechara et al., 1995). During instructed fear, subjects have only this abstract representation of the aversive properties of the stimulus, and patients with amygdala damage can readily report the aversive nature of a threat stimulus when asked (Funayama et al., 2001). It is likely that the amygdala is important for the expression of instructed fear but, unlike fear conditioning, it is not critical for its acquisition and storage. Research on the expression of learned fears with and without awareness supports the notion that the amygdala's role may differ between these two types of learning. Unlike conditioned fear, instructed fears are not expressed unless the subject is aware of the presentation of the CS or threat stimulus (Olsson & Phelps, 2004). Instructed fear also requires only the left amygdala for expression, whereas the expression of fear conditioning is impaired following right or left amygdala damage (LaBar et al., 1995). These results suggests that there are differences in the neural circuitry underlying these two types of fear learning, even though both conditioned fear and instructed fear require the amygdala for expression.

In contrast to instructed fear, social learning through observation can be expressed without awareness (Olsson & Phelps, 2004). In observational fear learning, the subject watches a confederate undergo fear conditioning in which a neutral stimulus is paired with an aversive event (e.g., shock to the wrist). The subject is then given the same procedure that was just observed, although, unknown to subject, no shocks are actually presented. The similarity in expression of observational and conditioned fear without awareness suggests that the vicarious experience of watching someone's reaction to an aversive event may engage similar neural mechanisms as actually experiencing the event. Indeed, there is evidence for observational fear learning across species (Mineka et al., 1984), suggesting that this type of social learning may depend on evolutionarily shared neural mechanisms. Olsson et al. (2004) examined amygdala activation to the observation of a confederate undergoing fear conditioning. They found significant bilateral amygdala activation when observing the confederate receiving a shock. When subjects were then told they would participate in the experiment themselves, similar activation was found to the observed CS+ (vs. the observed CS-) even though no shocks were presented. These results indicate that the amygdala is involved in both the acquisition and the expression of fears learned through social observation, much like fear conditioning (LeDoux, 1996).

Research on the social learning of fear indicates that socially acquired fears rely on neural systems that overlap with those identified in animal models of fear conditioning, perhaps even more so for social observation than verbal instruction. These results are important in that they suggest that these detailed animal models may be applicable to everyday social learning situations that are common in human experience. For humans, a large portion of fears are imagined and anticipated, but not based on any direct aversive experience. The amygdala's involvement in socially acquired fears suggests that it is a general mechanism for emotional learning which is important across learning methods.

Summary

Research on the amygdala's role in social cognition has extended animal models of emotional responding to complex social situations in humans. The evidence to date emphasizes the amygdala's role in the social communication and learning of threat or fear. Using functional imaging to understanding the representation of social information is relatively new, but this type of research is rapidly expanding. This emerging interest in social behavior and the brain is bringing investigators with interests in a wide range of topics to functional imaging methodologies—such as philosophers studying moral judgments; social psychologists interested in social bias; and economists studying economic decisions. Like cognitive psychologists before them, researchers in these fields are beginning recognize the value of neuroscience and functional imaging tools in their efforts to understand complex human behaviors.

Issues

Studies examining the cognitive neuroscience of emotion and social cognition have highlighted the importance of a number of neural structures, including the orbitofrontal cortex (e.g., Damasio, 1999), the medial prefrontal cortex (e.g., Mitchell et al., 2002), regions of the anterior cingulate (e.g., Whalen Bush, et al., 1998), the striatum (e.g., Delgado et al., 2000), the insular cortex (e.g., Critchley et al., 2004), and the superior temporal sulcus (see Adolphs, 2001). In this chapter, we chose to focus on the amygdala because of its prominence in functional imaging studies of emotion, but it is only a piece of an ongoing story (see, e.g., Drevets, 1998, for the amygdala's involvement in psychopathology). Indeed, there are exciting literatures emerging on individual differences (e.g., Canli, Sivers, et al., 2002) and the modulation of amygdala function through emotion regulation strategies (e.g., K. N. Ochsner et al., 2002).

Even with these limitations, our present chapter indicates that a rich literature on the functional imaging of emotion and social cognition is beginning to emerge. The amygdala has been identified as critical for implicit emotional learning, as assessed with fear conditioning, and for some aspects of appetitive conditioning. The amygdala also plays a role in the modulation of hippocampal-dependent memories for emotional events. This modulation seems to depend on the arousal response to an emotional stimulus, irrespective of its valence. The studies demonstrating a role for the amygdala in the modulation of attention and perception have, thus far, mostly investigated fearful or threatening stimuli, although there are some exceptions.

Finally, the amygdala's role in social cognition has been linked primarily to the social comminication and learning of threat. Although there is functional imaging evidence that the amygdala responds preferentially to arousing stimuli that are both positive and negative (Anderson, Christoff, Stappen, et al., 2003), research in some domains (i.e., attention and perception, social cognition) suggests that a subset of its functions may be specific to negative or fearful stimuli. Future research will need to further clarify the multiple, interacting roles of the amygdala across different behavioral domains and characteristics of emotional stimuli.

Throughout this chapter, we have highlighted the need for convergent methods. By relying on detailed animal models as a starting point, our understanding of the representation of emotion in the human brain has benefited tremendously. However, as we try to extend these neural circuits to emotional and social behaviors that are more complex and uniquely human, functional imaging techniques will need to be combined with other techniques, such as lesion studies and pharmacological manipulations, to provide insight into structure-function relationships in humans. Finally, as we move forward, it will become increasingly important to understand not only the function of specific structures but also the operation of networks of neural systems that underlie human emotion and social cognition. Functional connectivity analyses and computational approaches will become more critical as we begin to explore these complex interactions. Combining a broad range of functional imaging methodologies with other neuroscience techniques and sophisticated behavioral paradigms will enable a more complete understanding of the neural systems of emotion and social cognition.

References

Adolphs, R. (2001). The neurobiology of social cognition. *Current Opinion in Neurobiology* 11, 231–239.

Adolphs, R., Gosselin, F., Buchanan, T. W., Tranel, D., Schyns, P., & Damasio, A. R. (2005). A mechanism for impaired fear recognition after amygdala damage. *Nature* 433, 68–72.

Adolphs, R., Tranel, D., & Damasio, A. R. (1998). The human amygdala and social judgment. *Nature* 393, 417–418.

Adolphs, R., Tranel, D., Hamann, S., Young, A. W., Calder, A. J., Phelps, E. A., Anderson, A., Lee, G. P., & Damasio, A. R. (1999). Recognition of facial emotion in nine individuals with bilateral amygdala damage. *Neuropsychologia* 37, 1111–1117.

Amaral, D. G., Behniea, H., & Kelly, J. L. (2003). Topographic organization of projections from the amygdala to the visual cortex in the macaque monkey. *Neuroscience* 118, 1099–1120.

Amaral D. G., Price, J. L., Pitkanen A., & Carmichael, S. T. (1992). Anatomical organization of the primate amygdaloid complex. In J. P. Aggleton, (Ed.), *The amygdala: Neurobiological aspects of emotion, memory, and mental dysfunction*, 1–65, New York: Wiley-Liss.

Anderson, A. K. (2005). Affective influences on the attentional dynamics supporting awareness. *Journal of Experimental Psychology: General* 134, 258–281.

Anderson, A. K., Christoff, K., Panitz, D., De Rosa, E., & Gabrieli, J. D. (2003). Neural correlates of the automatic processing of threat facial signals. *Journal of Neuroscience* 23, 5627–5633.

Anderson, A. K., Christoff, K., Stappen, I., Panitz, D., Ghahremani, G. C., Glover, G., et al. (2003). Dissociated neural representations of intensity and valence in human olfaction. *Nature Neuroscience* 6, 196–202.

Anderson, A. K., & Phelps, E. A. (2001). The human amygdala supports affective modulatory influences on visual awareness. *Nature* 411, 305–309.

Bechara, A., Tranel, D., Damasio, H., Adolphs, R., Rockland, C., & Damasio, A. R. (1995). Double dissociation of conditioning and declarative knowledge relative to the amygdala and hippocampus in humans. *Science* 269, 1115–1118.

Biernat, M., & Crandall, C. S. (1999). Racial attitudes. In J. P. Robinson, P. H. Shaver, & L. S. Wrightsman (Eds.), *Measures of political attitudes*, 291–412. San Diego: Academic Press.

Bluck, S., & Li, K. Z. H. (2001). Predicting memory completeness and accuracy: Emotion and exposure in repeated autobiographical recall. *Applied Cognitive Psychology* 15, 145–158.

Bradley, M. M., Greenwald, M. K., Petry, M. C., & Lang, P. J. (1992). Remembering pictures: Pleasure and arousal in memory. *Journal of Experimental Psychology: Learning, Memory, & Cognition* 18, 379–390.

Bradley, M. M., & Lang, P. J. (1999a). *Affective Norms for English Words (ANEW)*. Gainesville: NIMH Center for the Study of Emotion and Attention, University of Florida.

Bradley, M. M., & Lang, P. J. (1999b). *International Affective Digitized Sounds (IADS): Stimuli, Instruction Manual and Affective Ratings*. Gainesville: Center for Research in Psychophysiology, University of Florida.

Breiter, H. C., Etcoff, N. L., Whalen, P. J., Kennedy, W. A., Rauch, S. L., Buckner, R. L., et al. (1996). Response and habituation of the human amygdala during visual processing of facial expression. *Neuron* 17, 875–887.

Brierly, B., Shaw, P., & David, A. S. (2002). The human amygdala: A systematic review and meta-analysis of volumetric magnetic resonance imaging. *Brain Research Reviews* 39, 84–105.

Büchel, C., Morris, J., Dolan, R. J., & Friston, K. J. (1998). Brain systems mediating aversive conditioning: An event-related fMRI study. *Neuron* 20, 947–957.

Cahill, L., Babinsky, R., Markowitsch, H. J., & McGaugh, J. L. (1995). The amygdala and emotional memory. *Nature* 377, 295–296.

Cahill, L., Haier, R. J., Fallon, J., Alkire, M., Tang, C., Keator, D., et al. (1996). Amygdala activity at encoding correlated with long-term, free recall of emotional information. *Proceedings of the National Academy of Sciences USA* 93, 8016–8021.

Cahill, L., Prins, B., Weber, M., & McGaugh, J. L. (1994). β-adrenergic activation and memory for emotional events. *Nature* 371, 702–704.

Cahill, L., Uncapher, M., Kilpatrick, L., Alkire, M. T., & Turner, J. (2004). Sex-related hemispheric lateralization of amygdala function in emotionally influenced memory: An fMRI investigation. *Learning & Memory* 11, 261–266.

Canli, T., Desmond, J. E., Zhao, Z., & Gabrieli, J. D. E. (2002). Sex differences in the neural basis of emotional memories. *Proceedings of the National Academy of Sciences USA* 99, 10789–10794.

Canli, T., Sivers, H., Whitfield, S. L., Gotlib, I. H., & Gabrieli, J. D. E. (2002). Amygdala response to happy faces as a function of extraversion. *Science* 296, 2191.

Canli, T., Zhao, Z., Brewer, J., Gabrieli, J. D. E., & Cahill, L. (2000). Event-related activation in the human amygdala associates with later memory for individual emotional experience. *Journal of Neuroscience* 20, RC99(1–5).

Carrasco, M. (2004) Covert transient attention increases contrast sensitivity and spatial resolution: Support for signal enhancement. In L. Itti, G. Rees, & J. Tsotsos (Eds.), *Neurobiology of Attention*, San Diego: Elsevier.

Cheng, D. T., Knight, D. C., Smith, C. N., Stein, E. A., & Helmstetter, F. J. (2003). Functional MRI of human amygdala activity during Pavlovian fear conditioning: Stimulus processing versus response expression. *Behavioral Neuroscience* 117, 3–10.

Cherry, E. C. (1953). Some experiments on the recognition of speech, with one and two ears. *Journal of the Acoustical Society of America* 25, 975–979.

Chun, M. M., & Potter, M. C. (1995). A two-stage model for multiple target detection in rapid serial visual presentation. *Journal of Experimental Psychology: Human Perception and Performance* 21, 109–127.

Convit, A., McHugh, P., Wolf, O. T., de Leon, M. J., Bobinski, M., De Santi, S., et al. (1999). MRI volume of the amygdala: A reliable method allowing separation from the hippocampal formation. *Psychiatry Research: Neuroimaging* 90, 113–123.

Critchley, H. D., Wiens, S., Rorstein, P., Ohman, A., & Dolan, R. J. (2004). Neural systems supporting interoceptive awareness. *Nature Neuroscience* 7, 102–103.

Cunningham, W. A., Raye, C. L., & Johnson, M. K. (2005). Neural correlates of evaluation associated with promotion and prevention regulatory focus. *Cognitive, Affective, and Behavioral Neuroscience*, 5, 202–211.

Damasio, A. (1999). *The Feeling of What Happens*. New York: Harcourt Brace.

Damasio, A. R., Grabowski, T. J., Bechara, A., Damasio, H., Ponto, L. L. B., Parvizi, J., et al. (2000). Subcortical and cortical brain activity during the feeling of self-generated emotions. *Nature Neuroscience* 3, 1049–1056.

Davidson, R. J., & Irwin, W. (1999). The functional neuroanatomy of emotion and affective style. *Trends in Cognitive Science* 3, 11–21.

Davis, M. (1994). The role of the amygdala in emotional learning. *International Review of Neurobiology* 36, 225–266.

Davis, M., & Whalen, P. J. (2001). The amygdala: Vigilance and emotion. *Molecular Psychiatry* 6, 13–34.

De Gelder, B., Snyder, J., Greve, D., Gerard, G., & Hadjikhani, N. (2004). Fear fosters flight: A mechanism for fear contagion when perceiving emotion expressed by a whole body. *Proceedings of the National Academy of Sciences USA* 101, 195–203.

Delgado, M. R., Nystrom, L. E., Fissell, C., Noll, D. C., & Fiez, J. A. (2000). Tracking the hemodynamic responses to reward and punishment in the striatum. *Journal of Neurophysiology* 84, 3072–3077.

Dolan, R. J., Lane, R., Chua, P., & Fletcher, P. (2000). Dissociable temporal lobe activation during emotional episodic memory retrieval. *NeuroImage* 11, 203–209.

Dolcos, F., LaBar, K. S., & Cabeza, R. (2004a). Dissociable effects of arousal and valence on prefrontal activity indexing emotional evaluation and subsequent memory: An event-related fMRI study. *NeuroImage* 23, 64–74.

Dolcos, F., LaBar, K. S., & Cabeza, R. (2004b). Interaction between the amygdala and the medial temporal lobe memory system predicts better memory for emotional events. *Neuron* 42, 855–863.

Dolcos, F., LaBar, K. S., & Cabeza, R. (2005). Remembering one year later: Role of the amygdala and medial temporal lobe memory system in retrieving emotional memories. *Proceedings of the National Academy of Sciences USA* 102, 2626–2631.

Drevets, W. C. (1998). Functional neuroimaging studies of depression: The anatomy of melancholia. *Annual Review of Medicine* 49, 341–361.

Ekman. P., & Friesen, W. V. (1975). *Unmasking the Face*. Englewood Cliffs, NJ: Prentice-Hall.

Elliott, R., & Dolan, R. J. (1998). Neural response during preference and memory judgments for subliminally presented stimuli: A functional neuroimaging study. *Journal of Neuroscience* 18, 4697–4704.

Eysenck, H. J., & Kelley, M. J. (1987). The interaction of neurohormones with Pavlovian A and Pavlovian B conditioning in the causation of neurosis, extinction, and incubation of anxiety. In G. Davey (Ed.), *Cognitive Processes and Pavlovian Conditioning in Humans*, 251–287. New York: John Wiley.

Fendt, M., & Fanselow, M. S. (1999). The neuroanatomical and neurochemical basis of conditioned fear. *Neuroscience and Biobehavioral Reviews* 23, 743–760.

Fink, G. R., Markowitsch, H. J., Reinkemeir, M., et al. (1996). Cerebral representation of one's own past: Neural networks involved in autobiographical memory. *Journal of Neuroscience* 16, 4275–4282.

Fitzpatrick, S. M., & Rothman, D. L. (2000). Meeting report: Transcranial magnetic stimulation and studies of human cognition. *Journal of Cognitive Neuroscience* 12, 704–709.

Fredrikson, M., Annas, P., Georgiades, A., Hursti, T., & Tersman, Z. (1993). Internal consistency and temporal stability of classically conditioned skin conductance responses. *Biological Psychology* 35, 153–163.

Funayama, E. S., Grillon, C. G., Davis, M., & Phelps, E. A. (2001). A double dissociation in the affective modulation of startle in humans: Effects of unilateral temporal lobectomy. *Journal of Cognitive Neuroscience* 13, 721–729.

Furmark, T., Fischer, H., Wik, G., Larsson, M., & Fredrikson, M. (1997). The amygdala and individual differences in human fear conditioning. *NeuroReport* 8, 3957–3960.

Gabrieli, J. D. E. (1998). Cognitive neuroscience of human memory. *Annual Review of Psychology* 49, 87–115.

Garpenstrand, H., Annas, P., Ekblom, J., Oreland, L., & Fredrikson, M. (2001). Human fear conditioning is related to dopaminergic and serotonergic biological markers. *Behavioral Neuroscience* 115, 358–364.

George, M. S., Ketter, T. A., Kimbrell, T. A., Speer, A. M., Lorberbaum, J., Liberatos, C. C., et al. (2000). Neuroimaging approaches to the study of emotion. In J. C. Borod (Ed.), *Neuropsychology of Emotion*, 106–134. New York: Oxford University Press.

Greenberg, D. L., Rice, H. J., Cooper, J. J., Cabeza, R., Rubin, D. C., & LaBar, K. S. (2005). Co-activation of the amygdala, hippocampus, and inferior frontal gyrus during autobiographical memory retrieval. *Neuropsychologia* 43, 659–674.

Greenwald, A. G., McGhee, J. L., & Schwartz, J. L. (1998). Measuring individual differences in social cognition: The Implicit Association Test. *Journal of Personality and Social Psychology* 74, 1464–1480.

Grillon, C., Rezvan, A., Woods, S. W., Marikangas, K., & Davis, M. (1991). Fear-potentiated startle in humans: Effects of anticipatory anxiety on the acoustic blink reflex. *Psychophysiology* 28, 588–595.

Halgren, E. (1992). Emotional neurophysiology of the amygdala within the context of human cognition. In J. P. Aggleton (Ed.), *The Amygdala: Neurobiological Aspects of Emotion, Memory, and Mental Dysfunction*, 191–228. New York: Wiley-Liss.

Hamann, S. B., Ely, T. D., Grafton, S. T., & Kilts, C. D. (1999). Amygdala activity related to enhanced memory for pleasant and aversive stimuli. *Nature Neuroscience* 2, 289–293.

Hamann, S. B., Herman, R. A., Nolan, C. L., & Wallen, K. (2004). Men and women differ in amygdala response to visual sexual stimuli. *Nature Neuroscience* 7, 411–416.

Hansen, C. H., & Hansen, R. D. (1988). Finding the face in the crowd: An anger superiority effect. *Journal of Personality and Social Psychology* 54, 917–924.

Hariri, A. R., Mattay, V. S., Tessitore, A., Kolachana, B., Fera, F., Goldman, D., et al. (2002). Serotonin transporter genetic variation and the response of the human amygdala. *Science* 297, 400–403.

Hart, A. J., Whalen, P. J., Shin, L. M., McInerney, S. C., Fischer, H., & Rauch, S. L. (2000). Differential response in the human amygdala to racial outgroup vs ingroup face stimuli. *NeuroReport* 11, 2351–2355.

Hettema, J. M., Annas, P., Neale, M. C., Kendler, K. S., & Fredrikson, M. (2003). A twin study of the genetics of fear conditioning. *Archives of General Psychiatry* 60, 702–708.

Kensinger, E. A., & Corkin, S. (2004). Two routes to emotional memory: Distinct neural processes for valence and arousal. *Proceedings of the National Academy of Sciences USA* 101, 3310–3315.

Kim, H., Sommerville, L. H., Johnstone, T., Polis, S., Alexander, A. L., Shin, L. M., & Whalen, P. J. (2004). Contextual modulation of amygdala responsivity to surprised faces. *Journal of Cognitive Neuroscience* 16, 1730–1745.

Kim, J. J., & Fanselow, M. S. (1992). Modality-specific retrograde amnesia of fear. *Science* 256, 675–677.

Kluver, H., & Bucy, P. C. (1937). "Psychic blindness" and other symptoms following bilateral temporal lobectomy in rhesus monkeys. *American Journal of Physiology* 119, 352–353.

LaBar, K. S. (2003). Emotional memory functions of the human amygdala. *Current Neurology and Neuroscience Reports* 3, 363–364.

LaBar, K. S., Cook, C. A., Torpey, D. C., & Welsh-Bohmer, K. A. (2004). Impact of healthy aging on awareness and fear conditioning. *Behavioral Neuroscience* 118, 905–915.

LaBar, K. S., Crupain, M. J., Voyvodic, J. B., & McCarthy, G. (2003). Dynamic perception of facial affect and identity in the human brain. *Cerebral Cortex* 13, 1023–1033.

LaBar, K. S., & Disterhoft, J. F. (1998). Conditioning, awareness, and the hippocampus. *Hippocampus* 8, 620–626.

LaBar, K. S., Gatenby, J. C., Gore, J. C., LeDoux, J. E., & Phelps, E. A. (1998). Human amygdala activation during conditioned fear acquisition and extinction: A mixed-trial fMRI study. *Neuron* 20, 937–945.

LaBar, K. S., Gitelman, D. R., Mesulam, M.-M., & Parrish, T. B. (2001). Impact of signal-to-noise on functional MRI of the human amygdala. *NeuroReport* 12, 3461–3464.

LaBar, K. S., & LeDoux, J. E. (2001). Coping with danger: The neural basis of defensive behaviors and fearful feelings. In B. S. McEwen (Ed.), *Handbook of Physiology, Sec. 7, The Endocrine System*, vol. 4, *Coping with the Environment: Neural and Endocrine Mechanisms*, 139–154. New York: Oxford University Press.

LaBar, K. S., LeDoux, J. E., Spencer, D. D., & Phelps, E. A. (1995). Impaired fear conditioning following unilateral temporal lobectomy in humans. *Journal of Neuroscience* 15, 6846–6855.

LaBar, K. S., & Phelps, E. A. (1998). Arousal-mediated memory consolidation: Role of the medial temporal lobe in humans. *Psychological Science* 9, 490–493.

LaBar, K. S., & Phelps, E. A. (2005). Reinstatement of conditioned fear in humans is context-dependent and impaired in amnesia. *Behavioral Neuroscience* 119, 677–686.

Lane, R. D., Reiman, E. M., Bradley, M. M., Lang, P. J., Ahern, G. L., Davidson, R. J., et al. (1997). Neuroanatomical correlates of pleasant and unpleasant emotion. *Neuropsychologia* 35, 1437–1444.

Lang, P. J. (1993). The three system approach to emotion. In N. Birbaumer & A. Öhman (Eds.), *The Organization of Emotion*, 18–30. Toronto: Hogrefe-Huber.

Lang, P. J., Bradley, M. M., & Cuthbert, B. N. (1999). *International Affective Picture System (IAPS): Technical Manual and Affective Ratings*. Gainesville: Center for Research in Psychophysiology, University of Florida.

LeDoux, J. E. (1996). *The Emotional Brain*. New York: Simon and Schuster.

Maguire, E. A. (2001). Neuroimaging studies of autobiographical event memory. *Philosophical Transactions of the Royal Society of London* B356, 1441–1451.

Maguire, E. A., & Frith, C. D. (2003). Lateral asymmetry in the hippocampal response to the remoteness of autobiographical memories. *Journal of Neuroscience* 23, 5302–5307.

Maratos, E. J., Dolan, R. J., Morris, J. S., Henson, R. N. A., & Rugg, M. D. (2001). Neural activity associated with episodic memory for emotional context. *Neuropsychologia* 39, 910–920.

Markowitsch, H. J. (1995). Which brain regions are critically involved in the retrieval of old episodic memory? *Brain Research Reviews* 21, 117–127.

Markowitsch, H. J., Calabrese, P., Würker, M., Durwen, H. F., Kessler, J., Babinsky, R., et al. (1994). The amygdala's contribution to memory—a study on two patients with Urbach-Wiethe disease. *NeuroReport* 5, 1349–1352.

Markowitsch, H. J., Thiel, A., Rinkemeier, M., Kessler, J., Koyuncu, A., & Heiss, W. (2000). Right amygdalar and temporofrontal activation during autobiographic, but not during fictitious memory retrieval. *Behavioural Neurology* 12, 181–190.

Mather, M., Canli, T., English, T., Whitfield, S., Wais, P., Ochsner, K., et al. (2004). Amygdala responses to emotionally valenced stimuli in older and younger adults. *Psychological Science* 15, 259–263.

McGaugh, J. L. (2000). Memory—a century of consolidation. *Science* 287, 248–251.

Medin, B. L., Ross, B. H., & Markman, A. B. (2005). *Cognitive Psychology*, 4th ed. Hoboken, NJ: Wiley.

Mineka, S., Davidson, M., Cook, M., & Keir, R. (1984). Observational conditioning of snake fear in rhesus monkeys. *Journal of Abnormal Psychology* 93, 355–372.

Mitchell, J. P., Heathorton, T. F., & Macrae, C. N. (2002). Distinct neural systems subserve person and object knowledge. *Proceedings of the National Academy of Sciences USA* 100, 2157–2162.

Morris, J. S., Buchel, C., & Dolan, R. J. (2001). Parallel neural responses in amygdala subregions and sensory cortex during implicit fear conditioning. *NeuroImage* 13, 1044–1052.

Morris, J. S., DeGelder, B., Weiskrantz, L. & Dolan, R. J. (2001). Differential extrageniculostriate and amygdala responses to presentation of emotional faces in a cortically blind field. *Brain* 124, 1241–1252.

Morris, J. S., Friston, K. J., Buchel, C., Frith, C. D., Young, A. W., Calder, A. J., & Dolan, R. J. (1998). A neuromodulatory role for the human amygdala in processing emotional facial expressions. *Brain* 121, 47–57.

Morris, J. S., Öhman, A., & Dolan, R. J. (1998). Conscious and unconscious emotional learning in the human amygdala. *Nature* 393, 467–470.

Morris, J. S., Öhman, A., & Dolan, R. J. (1999). A subcortical pathway to the right amygdala mediating "unseen" fear. *Proceedings of the National Academy of Sciences USA* 96, 1680–1685.

Nader, K., Schafe, G. E., & LeDoux, J. E. (2000). Fear memories require protein synthesis in the amygdala for reconsolidation after retrieval. *Nature* 406, 722–726.

Nosek, B. A., Cunningham, W. A., Banaji, M. R., & Greenwald, A. G. (2000). *Measuring implicit attitudes on the Internet.* Abstract presented at the Society for Personality and Social Psychology, Nashville, TN.

Ochsner, K. A., & Schacter, D. L. (2000). A social cognitive neuroscience approach to emotion and memory. In J. C. Borod (Ed.), *The Neuropsychology of Emotion*, 163–193. New York: Oxford University Press.

Ochsner, K. N., Bunge, S. A., Gross, J. J., & Gabrielli, J. D. E. (2002). Rethinking feelings: An fMRI study of the cognitive regulation of emotion. *Journal of Cognitive Neuroscience* 14, 1215–1229.

Olsson, A., Nearing, K., Zheng, J., & Phelps, E. A. (2004). *Learning by observing: neural correlates of fear learning through social observation.* Paper presented at 34th Annual Meeting of the Society for Neuroscience, San Diego.

Olsson, A., & Phelps, E. A. (2004). Learned fear of "unseen" faces after Pavlovian, observational and instructed fear. *Psychological Science* 15, 822–828.

Papez, J. W. (1937) A proposed mechanism of emotion. *Archives of Neurology and Psychiatry* 79, 217–224.

Pegna, A. J., Khateb, A., Lazeyras, F., & Seghier, M. L. (2005). Discriminating emotional faces without primary visual cortices involves the right amygdala. *Nature Neuroscience* 8, 24–25.

Pessoa, L., McKenna, M., Gutierrez, E., & Ungerleider, L. G. (2002). Neural processing of emotional faces requires attention. *Proceedings of the National Academy of Sciences USA* 99, 11458–11463.

Phelps, E. A., Delgado, M. R., Nearing, K. I., & LeDoux, J. E. (2004). Extinction learning in humans: Role of the amygdala and vmPFC. *Neuron* 43, 897–905.

Phelps, E. A., LaBar, K. S., Anderson, A. K., O'Connor, K. J., Fulbright, R. K., & Spencer, D. D. (1998). Specifying the contribution of the human amygdala to emotional memory: A case study. *Neurocase* 4, 527–540.

Phelps, E. A., LaBar, K. S., & Spencer, D. D. (1997). Memory for emotional words following unilateral temporal lobectomy. *Brain & Cognition* 34, 512–521.

Phelps, E. A., Ling, S., & Carrasco, M. (in press). Emotion facilitates perception and potentiates the perceptual benefit of attention. *Psychological Science.*

Phelps, E. A., O'Connor, K. F., Cunningham, W. A., Funayama, E. S., Gatenby, J. C., Gore, J. C., & Banaji, M. R. (2000). Performance on indirect measures of race evaluation predicts amygdala activation. *Journal of Cognitive Neuroscience* 12, 729–738.

Phillips, R. G., & LeDoux, J. E. (1992). Differential contribution of amygdala and hippocampus to cued and contextual fear conditioning. *Behavioral Neuroscience* 106, 274–285.

Piefke, M., Weiss, P. H., Zilles, K., Markowitsch, H. J., & Fink, G. (2003). Differential remoteness and emotional tone modulate the neural correlates of autobiographical memory. *Brain* 126, 650–668.

Polonsky, A., Blake, R., Braun, J., & Heeger, D. J. (2000) Neuronal activity in human primary visual cortex correlates with perception during binocular rivalry. *Nature Neuroscience* 3, 1153–1159.

Posse, S., Fitzgerald, D., Gao, K., Habel, U., Rosenberg, D., Moore, G. J., et al. (2003). Real-time fMRI of temporolimbic regions detects amygdala activation during single-trial self-induced sadness. *NeuroImage* 18, 760–768.

Quirk, G. J., Repa, J. C., & LeDoux, J. E. (1995). Fear conditioning enhances short-latency auditory responses of lateral amygdala neurons: Parallel recordings in the freely behaving rat. *Neuron* 15, 1029–1039.

Reisberg, D., Heuer, F., McLean, J., & O'Shaughnessy, M. (1988). The quantity, not the quality, of affect predicts memory vividness. *Bulletin of the Psychonomic Society* 26, 100–103.

Repa, J. C., Muller, J., Apergis, J., et al. (2001). Two different lateral amygdala cell populations contribute to the initiation and storage of memory. *Nature Neuroscience* 4, 724–731.

Richardson, M. P., Strange, B. A., & Dolan, R. J. (2004). Encoding of emotional memories depends on amygdala and hippocampus and their interactions. *Nature Neuroscience* 7, 278–285.

Rizzo, A. A., Neumann, U., Enciso, R., Fidaleo, D., & Noh, J. Y. (2001). Performance-driven facial animation: Basic research on human judgments of emotional state in facial avatars. *Cyberpsychology & Behavior* 4, 471–487.

Romanski, L. M., & LeDoux, J. E. (1993). Information cascade from auditory cortex to the amygdala: Corticocortical and corticoamygdaloid projections of the temporal cortex in rat. *Cerebral Cortex* 3, 515–532.

Russell, J. A. (1980). A circumplex model of affect. *Journal of Personality and Social Psychology* 39, 1161–1178.

Scherer, K. R. (2000). Psychological models of emotion. In J. C. Borod (Ed.), *The Neuropsychology of Emotion*, 137–162. New York: Oxford University Press.

Sharot, T., Delgado, M. R., & Phelps, E. A. (2004). How emotion enhances the feeling of remembering. *Nature Neuroscience* 7, 1376–1380.

Shors, T. J. (2004). Learning during stressful times. *Learning & Memory* 11, 137–144.

Singer, T., Kiebel, S. J., Winston, J. S., Dolan, R. J., & Frith, C. D. (2004). Brain responses to the acquired moral status of faces. *Neuron* 19, 653–662.

Squire, L. R., & Zola, S. M. (1996). Structure and function of declarative and nondeclarative memory systems. *Proceedings of the National Academy of Sciences USA* 93, 13515–13522.

Talarico, J. M., LaBar, K. S., & Rubin, D. C. (2004). Emotional intensity predicts autobiographical memory experience. *Memory & Cognition* 32, 1118–1132.

Taylor, S. F., Liberzon, I., Fig, L. M., Decker, L. R., Minoshima, S., & Koeppe, R. A. (1998). The effect of emotional content on visual recognition memory: A PET activation study. *NeuroImage* 8, 188–197.

Tranel, D., & Damasio, A. R. (1993). The covert learning of affective valence does not require structures in hippocampal system or amygdala. *Journal of Cognitive Neuroscience* 5, 79–88.

Tranel, D., & Hyman, B. T. (1990). Neuropsychological correlates of bilateral amygdala damage. *Archives of Neurology* 47, 349–355.

Tulving, E., & Schacter, D. L. (1990). Priming and human memory systems. *Science* 247, 301–306.

Vuilleumier, P., Armony, J. L., Driver, J., and Dolan, R. J. (2001). Effects of attention and emotion on face processing in the human brain: An event-related fMRI study. *Neuron* 30, 829–841.

Vuilleumier, P., Armony, J. L., Driver, J., and Dolan, R. J. (2003). Distinct spatial frequency sensitivities for processing faces and emotional expressions. *Nature Neuroscience* 6, 624–631.

Vuilleumier, P., Richardson, M. P., Armony, J. L., Driver, J., & Dolan, R. J. (2004). Distant influences of amygdala lesion on visual cortical activation during emotional face processing. *Nature Neuroscience* 7, 1271–1278.

Vuilleimier, P., & Schwartz, S. (2001). Beware and be aware: Capture of spatial attention by fear-related stimuli in neglect. *NeuroReport* 12, 1119–1122.

Wagner, A. D., Koutstaal, W., & Schacter, D. L. (1999). When encoding yields remembering: Insights from event-related neuroimaging. *Philosophical Transactions of the Royal Society of London* B354, 1307–1324.

Wang, L., McCarthy, G., Song, A. W., & LaBar, K. S. (2005). Amygdala activation to sad pictures during high-field (4 Tesla) functional magnetic resonance imaging. *Emotion* 5, 12–22.

Weiskrantz, L. (1956). Behavioral changes associated with ablation of the amygdaloid complex in monkeys. *Journal of Comparitive Physiology and Psychology* 49, 381–391.

Whalen, P. J. (1998). Fear, vigilance, and ambiguity: Initial neuroimaging studies of the human amygdala. *Current Directions in Psychological Science* 7, 177–188.

Whalen, P. J., Bush, G., McNally, R. J., Wilhelm, S., McInerney, S. C., Jenike, M. A., et al. (1998). The emotional counting Stroop paradigm: A functional magnetic resonance imaging probe of the anterior cingulate affective division. *Biological Psychiatry* 44, 1219–1228.

Whalen, P. J., Kagan, J., Cook, R. G., Davis, F. C., Kim, H., Plois, S., McLaren, D. G., Somervilles, L. H., McLean, A. A., Maxwell, J. S., & Johnstone, T. (2004). Human amygdala responsivity to masked fearful eye whites. *Science* 306, 2061.

Whalen, P. J., Rausch, S. L., Etcoff, N. L., McInerney, S. C., Lee, M. B., & Jenike, M. A. (1998). Masked presentations of emotional facial expressions modulate amygdala activity without explicit knowledge. *Journal of Neuroscience* 18, 411–418.

Whalen, P. J., Shin, L. M., McInerney, S. C., Fischer, H., Wright, C. I., & Rauch, S. L. (2001). A functional MRI study of human amygdala responses to facial expressions of fear vs. anger. *Emotion* 1, 70–83.

Williams, J. M. G., MacLeod, C., & Mathews, A. (1996). The emotional Stroop task and psychopathology. *Psychological Bulletin* 120, 3–24.

Williams, M. A., Morris, A. P., McGlone, F., Abbott, D. F., & Mattingly, J. B. (2004). Amygdala responses to fearful and happy facial expressions under conditions of binocular suppression. *Journal of Neuroscience* 24, 2898–2904.

Wilson, A., Brooks, D. C., & Bouton, M. E. (1995). The role of the rat hippocampal system in several effects of context in extinction. *Behavioral Neuroscience* 109, 828–836.

Winston, J. S., Strange, B. A., O'Doherty, J. O., & Dolan, R. J. (2002). Automatic and intentional brain responses during evaluation of trustworthiness of faces. *Nature Neuroscience* 5, 277–283.

Wright, C. I., Fischer, H., Whalen, P. J., McInerney, S. C., Shin, L. M., & Rauch, S. L. (2001). Differential prefrontal cortex and amygdala habituation to repeatedly presented emotional stimuli. *NeuroReport* 12, 379–383.

Yamasaki, H., LaBar, K. S., & McCarthy, G. (2002). Dissociable prefrontal brain systems for attention and emotion. *Proceedings of the National Academy of Sciences USA* 99, 11447–11451.

Zorawski, M., Cook, C. A., Kuhn, C. M., & LaBar, K. S. (2005). Sex, stress, and fear: Individual differences in conditioned learning. *Cognitive, Affective, and Behavioral Neuroscience* 5, 191–201.

Functional Neuroimaging of Neuropsychologically Impaired Patients

Cathy J. Price, Uta Noppeney, and Karl J. Friston

Introduction

This chapter addresses some key issues that arise when performing brain imaging experiments on patients with neurological insult and psychological impairment. Since the mid-1990s, neuropsychology has been fundamentally augmented by neurophysiological measures of cognitive processing. This has led to a revision of some cognitive models and a shift in emphasis from cognitive science to cognitive neuroscience. In this chapter, we consider how functional neuroimaging of neuropsychological patients can be applied to understand structure-function relationships in the human brain and the mechanisms that underlie recovery of function following brain damage. The chapter is divided into four sections. The first reviews the aims and limitations of neuropsychological studies, with an emphasis on the lesion-deficit model. The second focuses on functional imaging studies of patients and how they can overcome the difficulties that confound the lesion deficit model. The third, under "Issues," highlights the limitations of functional neuroimaging studies and how these problems can be resolved by reference to the lesion-deficit model. A systematic approach for combining functional imaging and neuropsychological studies is presented that allows one to identify the neuronal structures sustaining functional recovery following brain damage.

Neuropsychological Studies of Brain-Damaged Patients

Neuropsychology is the study of patients with functional deficits where the pathology is known to a lesser or greater extent. Neuropsychological investigations have contributed to our understanding of normal brain function by informing models of cognition and functional neuroanatomy. Typically, models of cognition are engendered or modified by neuropsychological studies when patients demonstrate a double dissociation in the impairment of selective functions. For instance, different types of dyslexia point to a double dissociation in reading processes: Some patients (surface dyslexics) retain the ability to read words with regular spelling-to-sound correspondence but fail to read words that do not comply with spelling rules. In contrast, other patients (phonological dyslexics) suffer from the reverse dissociation: they are able to read familiar words irrespective of their spelling but have difficulty reading novel words that rely on spelling-to-sound correspondences. Together, these behavioral deficits constitute a double dissociation in function. This particular double dissociation has been taken to imply the independence of two routes to reading (Coltheart, 1980; Coltheart et al., 1993; Marshall & Newcombe, 1973), one that relies on spelling-to-sound correspondences, and another that relies on prior lexical knowledge.

With respect to functional anatomy, the inferences that can be drawn from brain-damaged patients are based on the lesion-deficit model. To be informative, the lesion-deficit model requires a patient with a selective brain lesion and a selective cognitive deficit. Lesion studies are based on the rationale that a lesion-induced decline in a particular cognitive function demonstrates that the lesioned area was necessary or made an important contribution to this cognitive function. In other words, the function of the damaged brain region is simply equated with the impaired cognitive skill. Some classic examples of the lesion-deficit model, as applied to neuropsychological patients, were documented by nineteenth-century neurologists. For instance, postmortem studies demonstrated that a patient who had been impaired at articulating language had damage encompassing the third frontal convolution (Broca, 1861) and that a patient with a deficit in speech comprehension had damage to the left posterior temporal cortex (Wernicke, 1874).

By deduction, Broca's area was associated with speech production and Wernicke's area was associated with speech comprehension. Wernicke developed the model further to predict that patients could have intact speech comprehension (indicating intact responses in Wernicke's area) and intact speech production (indicating intact responses in Broca's area) but a deficit in auditory repetition due to a disconnection between Broca's and Wernicke's areas. This type of disconnection syndrome, referred to as conduction aphasia, was demonstrated by Lichtheim (1885) in a patient who had damage to the white matter tract that connects Broca's area with Wernicke's area (the arcuate fasciculus). Through clinical descriptions and localization of lesions, Wernicke and Lichtheim were able to demonstrate that disorders of language arose either from damage to the "centers of memory images" or to disconnections between the so-called centers. In other words, patients may behave abnormally following damage either to a cortical region with a particular functional specialization (e.g., Broca's area or Wernicke's area) or to the white matter that connects cortical regions (e.g., the arcuate fasciculus).

Limitations of the Lesion-Deficit Model

The shortcomings of the lesion-deficit model are well appreciated (Shallice, 1988). Perhaps the most obvious is that pathological (as opposed to experimental) lesions seldom conform to functionally homogeneous neuroanatomical systems or cortical tissue. Damage to a selected area may disrupt anatomical connections and, therefore, the responsiveness of remote undamaged areas. For example, in the case of diaschisis (Feeney & Baron, 1986), a reduction in metabolism can occur in brain areas that are remote from the injured region but are connected to it. Indeed, it is impossible to distinguish between the impact of lesion due to the loss of neuronal tissue per se and the more pervasive dysfunction that the lesion has on distributed undamaged regions (Goltz, 1881).

The second profound limitation is that the lesion-deficit model is confounded by the fact that similar lesions are associated with different behavioral impairments in different subjects. Conversely, different lesions can result in similar behavioral deficits. Thus, a lesion-deficit association can not be used to infer that a region is either sufficient for, or uniquely identifiable with, the function in question. Indeed, there may be different neuronal systems that sustain the same task in different subjects, or the same task before and after brain damage. To explain these inconsistencies, various holistic theories of brain function were developed (Goldstein, 1934), including the concept of cortical equipotentiality (Lashley, 1929). However, idiosyncratic behavioral manifestations of brain injury could also be due to the fact that most (if not all) cognitive tasks are multifactorial in their demands, which profoundly complicates any attempt at pinpointing a specific lesion-deficit relationship.

Third, the lesion-deficit model can reveal structure-function relationships only in the context of impaired function (the deficit). It cannot tell us anything about the structural basis of intact functions. Thus, if damage to an area impairs task A but not task B, we can say only that the area is necessary for task A. However, we cannot say that the area was not involved in task B, because performance on task B might be maintained by an alternative system that compensates for the damaged area. In summary, all that can be concluded from a lesion-deficit study is that a lesioned area, or the connections passing through the lesioned area, were necessary for a lost cognitive function.

Given these well-recognized difficulties in applying the lesion-deficit model to neuropsychological patients, current neuropsychological practice, with a few notable exceptions (e.g., the use of the WADA test in temporal lobe epilepsy patients for preneurosurgical assessment), does not hold a strict adherence to the lesion-deficit model. With the advent of CT and MRI, the role of neuropsychological practice moved from the tenuous position of inferring discrete lesion location from cognitive assessment results to one of diagnostic consultation, treatment planning, and objective characterization of the patients' functional capacities. Likewise, practicing neuropsychologists are currently using fMRI in a clinical setting to gain a better understanding of diagnostic etiology, disease progression, and the efficacy of rehabilitative efforts post brain injury.

Functional Imaging Studies of Neuropsychologically Impaired Patients

Functional neuroimaging studies of patients have the potential to overcome many of the limitations associated with the lesion-deficit model. Specifically, unlike the lesion-deficit model, functional imaging is not limited to a particular region of the brain that has been damaged; rather, the system of distributed cortical areas that sustain sensory, motor, or cognitive tasks can be identified. Functional imaging of patients can therefore be used to examine the responsiveness of both damaged and undamaged regions; and, most critically, it can be used to investigate the neuronal mechanisms that sustain recovery. Below we discuss how functional imaging of patients can be used to counter the limitations of the lesion-deficit model.

Structural and Functional Disconnections

There are many examples of structural disconnection syndromes that have been described in the neuropsychological literature. In the previous section, we referred to conduction aphasia that was thought to result from damage to the white matter tracts that connect Broca's and Wernicke's areas (Lichtheim, 1885). This is an example of an anatomical disconnection inferred by using structural (postmortem) and functional (behavior) indices. In most cases, however, structural damage includes both gray and white matter, and functional uncoupling may not be mediated by a simple anatomical disconnection. Take, for example, the classical interpretation of pure alexia as a disconnection between visual processing in occipitotemporal cortex and word-form processing in the left angular gyrus (Damasio & Damasio, 1983). The argument here is that visual processing must be intact because the patients can recognize letters and objects. Likewise, word-form processing must be preserved because the patients can write the words they cannot read. Therefore the problem must be in the integration of visual and word-form processing. However, to posit an anatomical disconnection assumes that reading does not depend on any intermediate processing stage in cortical areas that are damaged in pure alexics.

If conduction aphasia and pure alexia are indeed examples of anatomical disconnection syndromes, then functional imaging of the patients should reveal task-dependent activation in undamaged brain regions. For example, the conduction aphasia hypothesis could be tested directly with functional neuroimaging by demonstrating that Broca's area responds normally during self-generated speech tasks but abnormally during repetition. Similarly, Wernicke's area should respond normally during comprehension tasks but not during repetition. In other words, abnormal regional responses would be observed when, and only when, Broca's and Wernicke's areas interact directly during repetition. Likewise, the pure alexia hypothesis could be tested with functional neuroimaging by demonstrating that the left angular gyrus performs normally during written word output but abnormally during reading. To our knowledge, these functional imaging experiments have not been conducted, but see Paulesu et al. (1996) and Horwitz et al. (1998) for implementation of the same rationale with dyslexic subjects.

Functional disconnections can also be as a consequence of cortical (synaptic) damage rather than white matter (axonal) damage. The classic example is crossed cerebellar diaschisis, which refers to the reduced metabolism and blood flow in the cerebellar hemipshere contralateral to the cerebral lesion (Feeney & Baron, 1986). Crossed cerebellar diaschisis is thought to occur because each cerebellar hemisphere is intimately connected to the contralateral cerebral cortex through feedback circuits. Indeed, damage to the cerebellum can also cause cortical diaschisis (Hausen et al., 1997), and the effect of diaschisis can also be observed as changes in the structure of the affected area (Chakravarty, 2002; Price et al., 2001).

Diaschisis can also be context-sensitive or task-dependent. In this case it is referred to as dynamic diaschisis (Price et al., 2001). Dynamic diaschisis occurs because responses in any activated region depend on the inputs to that area. In Price et al., we used functional neuroimaging to investigate how lesions to Broca's area impair neuronal responses in remote undamaged cortical regions. Four patients with speech output problems, but relatively preserved comprehension, were scanned while viewing words (relative to consonant letter strings). In normal subjects, this results in left-lateralized activation in the posterior inferior frontal, middle temporal, and posterior inferior temporal cortices. Each patient activated abnormally in the undamaged posterior inferior temporal cortex: Rather than showing increased activation (as in normals), the patients showed decreased activation relative to the baseline condition. The reversal of responses in the left posterior inferior temporal region, and the observation that the same area responded normally during a semantic task, illustrate the context-sensitive nature of this diaschistic abnormality. In other words, the posterior temporal responses were abnormal only when they depended upon interactions with the damaged inferior frontal cortex. Dynamic diaschisis is thus a reflection of abnormalities in functional integration among distributed brain regions.

In the last few years, there has been an increasing interest in functional integration (how changes in the way regions interact with one another produce new functions). One approach for characterizing functional interactions involves assessing the temporal correlations between activity in distant cortical regions, which may be expressed during some tasks but not others. In electrophysiological studies, which record spike trains of neural activity or changes in the resulting potentials, the temporal scale is on the order of milliseconds. In functional neuroimaging, which measures hemodynamic changes, the temporal scale is on the order of seconds, and a significant correlation simply implies that activity (pooled over the time scale) goes up and down together in distant regions. Such temporal correlations imply functional connectivity that could reflect either direct connections between the correlated regions (i.e., activity changes in one region cause activity changes in another region) or indirect connections whereby the correlated regions share connections from a region that is the source of the correlated activity. For the purposes of this chapter, the point is that functional connectivity techniques can be applied to the study of patients with the hypothesis that brain damage will profoundly affect the way that different brain regions interact together (Maguire et al., 2001; Rowe et al., 2002; Vuilleumier et al., 2001).

To summarize, functional neuroimaging provides a potential means to test directly the disconnection syndromes described by the nineteenth-century neurologists. The critical observation is to show that the responsiveness of an undamaged region is context dependent, where the context is determined by task-dependent activity in other connected regions. In other words, a region shows differential responses depending on the task and which cortical inputs are being used. In patients, we might expect to see a nondamaged region perform normally on some tasks and abnormally on other tasks, depending on whether input from a disconnected region is required. Functional imaging studies of patients therefore need to distinguish abnormal functional segregation (i.e., the function of a discrete cortical area is abnormal) from abnormal functional integration (i.e., abnormal interactions among different brain regions).

Inconsistent Structure-Function Relationships

As discussed in a previous section, lesion-deficit associations are confounded by observations that similar lesions are associated with different behavioural impairments in different subjects; and different lesions can result in similar behavioral deficits. How can this inconsistency be explained? Since no two lesions are ever the same, one simple explanation is that different lesions damage different functional components. A damaged area may also retain a degree of responsiveness (perilesional activity) that is sufficient to maintain performance. More controversial are theories which propose that the same task can be sustained by different neuronal systems. Such theories are based on concepts of equipotentiality (Lashley, 1929), redundancy, and degeneracy. In the following, we discuss how functional neuroimaging of the patient can help us to understand the inconsistent results from neuropsychological studies.

Peri-infarct Activity

Peri-infarct activity refers to residual functional responsiveness at the site of damage and indicates that the damaged area may retain some functionality. Structural indices of lesions (from conventional CT and MRI) do not necessarily imply a complete loss of function, and peri-infarct activity can sometimes explain why a patient with a large lesion makes an unexpectedly good recovery. Recovery of a lost function results either from the reactivation of tissue that was initially incapacitated (e.g., due to a reduction in edema), or from plasticity in viable tissue which supports the function that was originally executed by lost cells. Thus a degree of functionality may reemerge during the acute stages of recovery when edema is controlled and circulation is reestablished in areas subject to partial ischemia.

Functional imaging studies can detect areas where a degree of functional responsiveness is retained even in areas that appear damaged on structural images. Typically these areas are around the region of insult (e.g., peri-infarct tissue) and sometimes within the lesion. Activation may even look normal everywhere except at the lesion site, where it appears "patchy" (Heiss et al., 1997; Warburton et al., 1999). Patchy or incomplete activations suggest that fewer cells are capable of responding. Functional imaging has an important role to play in revealing peri-infarct activation. However, since it inevitably varies from patient to patient, depending on the size and location of the lesion, it will not be detected in group comparisons. The search for peri-infarct activity therefore relies on studies where each subject is analyzed individually. It is necessary for a functional validation of the designated "lesion," but apart from this, the demonstration of peri-infarct responsiveness is not useful for the identification of structure-function relationships.

Multiple Neuronal Systems for the Same Task

The remarkable resilience of cognitive functions to focal brain damage suggests that there might not be a one-to-one mapping between neuronal structures and cognitive functions. Instead, multiple neuronal systems might be capable of producing the same behavioral response. We refer to many-to-one structure function relationships as "degenerate." The term "degeneracy" has been defined as "the ability of elements that are structurally different to perform the same function or yield the same output" (Edelman & Gally, 2001). At the level of cognitive anatomy, degeneracy means that multiple sets of brain regions can sustain the same cognitive task.

Many cognitive models even postulate multiple processes (or strategies) that can yield the same output. For instance, based on neuropsychological data, it has been suggested that the appropriate action for an object can be retrieved either directly from visual structural features or indirectly by accessing semantic (contextual, associative) knowledge (Rumiati, 1998, #1334; Phillips, 2002, #518). Similarly, reading familiar, regularly spelled words might be accomplished via either spelling-sound relationships or lexical semantic processes (Coltheart et al., 1993; Plaut et al., 1996). These models demonstrate that cognitive functions—like structural elements—can, in principle, be characterized at multiple levels of description. This is important, because the number of disjoint elements that can perform the same operation can change with either the structural or the functional level of description; see figure 14.1. Furthermore, it should be noted that degeneracy does not necessarily involve completely dissociable systems. In the example illustrated in figure 14.1, there is degeneracy at several levels of the task description (visual input to left or right visual field; motor response with left or right hand), but there are other components that are not degenerate (e.g., the hypothetical example of the motor engrams in figure 14.1). Thus, degenerate systems may be spatially disjoint (e.g. one system in the left hemisphere and another in the right hemisphere) or they may share common areas (see figure 14.2 for examples of disjoint and overlapping systems).

Functional neuroimaging can be used to investigate whether the same task engages different sets of regions in different subjects (individual variability) or even different sets of regions at different times within the same subject. Moreover, functional imaging studies of patients provide a unique source of data because they can reveal neuronal systems that are not activated in normal subjects. Not many functional imaging studies, to date, have explored individual variability within or between subjects. To the contrary, most functional imaging studies are primarily concerned with the neuronal systems that activate in common to all subjects. This is characteristically revealed using statistical models that treat intersubject variability as noise, thereby allowing inferences to be drawn at the population level—an approach that is not suited to the exploration of degeneracy. Take, for example, a task that can be performed by one of two disjoint systems (A and B). If half the subjects activate System A and the other half activate System B, statistical inference at the population level would be insensitive to activation in either system. In contrast, a fixed effect analysis (where error variance is low and degrees of freedom are high) would show concurrent activation in both systems, but it would not be able to determine whether the activated areas were part of one or more systems. Segregating different neuronal systems for the same task therefore rests on a series of individual case studies in both normal subjects and brain-damaged patients.

Degeneracy as a Mechanism for Recovery

Critically, functional recovery in patients with focal brain lesions can, in many cases, be explained in terms of degenerate structure-function mappings. In children recovering from brain damage, abnormal neuronal systems might emerge during neurodevelopment by virtue of long-term potentiation, axonal regeneration, and sprouting

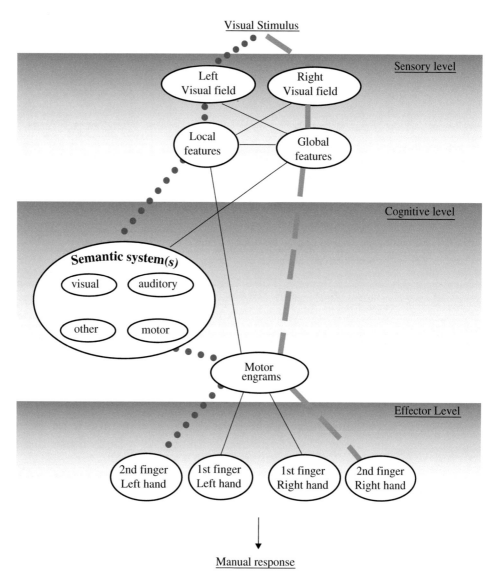

Figure 14.1
Levels of degeneracy.

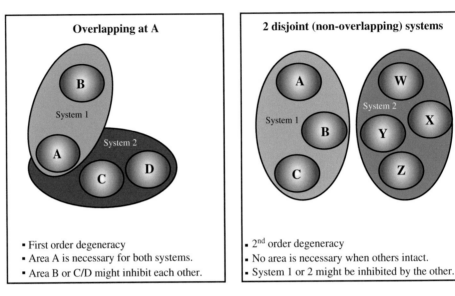

Figure 14.2
Overlapping and disjoint degenerate systems.

(Chen et al., 2002). However, in adulthood, the degenerate structures available for recovery must have been present in the patient's brain prior to neurological damage. Indeed, it is highly unlikely that adult patients would generate new neuronal systems (not present in the normal brain). This is because long-range extrinsic axonal connections are not thought to be able to form de novo in the mature brain, despite the ability of some mitotically competent cells to divide and create new cells (Barinaga, 1998; Gross, 2000).

Degenerate systems that sustain recovery in adulthood could be expressed in different ways. For example, there may be the following:

1. Multiple neuronal systems that normally respond in parallel to produce the same output. In this case, recovery following damage to only one of these systems would be reflected by patient activation in a subset of the normal areas. For example, if reading written words activates systems involved in applying spelling-to-sound correspondences as well as whole word recognition, then damage to one of these systems may simply result in activation limited to the other system (see Price et al., 2003).

2. Only one prepotent degenerate neuronal system may activate in neurologically normal subjects, with other neuronal systems remaining latent or inhibited. Following damage to the prepotent system, recovery occurs because the undamaged latent system can be engaged. In this case, functional imaging would reveal activation in

areas that are not observed in normal subjects. For example, Blank et al. (2003) observed that damage to the left inferior frontal area that is normally engaged during speech production tasks results in activation of the right inferior frontal cortex even though right inferior frontal activation is "inhibited" in control subjects.

3. There may be several degenerate neuronal systems that are each capable of performing the task in neurologically normal subjects. For example, subjects might sometimes activate the neuronal system involved in reading by spelling-to-sound correspondences, but after adaptation, activate the system involved in reading by whole word recognition. Recovery following damage to only one of the systems would force the patient to use the intact system. In this case, patient activation would resemble some, but not all, of the patterns observed in neurologically normal subjects.

In each of the above cases, damage to only one system does not disable task performance because alternative systems are available to take over the function of the damaged system. How do recovery mechanisms, described here in terms of degeneracy, correspond to those used in the clinical literature (Hallett, 2000; Kertesz, 1993)? Below, we will briefly review terms such as "plasticity," "functional reorganization," "redundancy," "vicariation," "unmasking," and "contralateral vs. ipsilateral compensation."

Plasticity refers to neuronal reorganization that takes place during learning or relearning in the normal or damaged brain. During neuronal reorganization, functions previously performed by the ischemic area are assumed by other ipsilateral or contralateral brain areas (Green, 2003). A key distinction can be made between long-term plasticity and short-term plasticity. Long-term plasticity is enduring, with a time course that varies from minutes to years. Short-term plasticity is "dynamic," with a time course that ranges from several milliseconds to seconds. In the postdevelopmental period, both long- and short-term plasticity are mediated by changes in the strength of preexisting connections (i.e., the efficacy of existing synapses is altered). The point that neuronal reorganization results from changes in a preexisting system is important because it suggests that degenerate brain systems are already established prior to brain damage. This point is sometimes lost in discussions of functional recovery in adults, because much of the work on "plasticity" and in humans has been derived from brain injury in children, where the concepts have more empirical support.

Another important point is that dynamic or short-term plasticity can be expressed in many natural and experimental contexts ranging from changes that underlie attentional modulation to profound changes in the organization of somatosensory fields shortly after deafferentation of inhibiting inputs (Buonomano & Merzenich,

1998). It follows that it would be incorrect to ascribe changes in attentional set to substantial remodeling of the anatomical connections. Similarly, rapid neuronal reorganization that occurs when a system is disinhibited (see below) does not necessarily represent a rewiring of the system. In summary, acknowledging the contribution of dynamic plasticity to neuronal reorganization is crucial for the interpretation of neuroimaging studies of patients recovering a lost function.

Functional reorganization takes place when a patient uses a different set of cognitive processes to implement the same task; for instance, when patients learn a new strategy to recover the ability to perform a lost function. A specific example is provided by dyslexic patients who adopt a serial letter-by-letter reading strategy to compensate for a deficit in parallel word processing (Patterson & Kay, 1982). Critically, however, cognitive reorganization is unlikely to occur in the absence of neuronal reorganization because learning a new cognitive strategy will involve short-term plasticity. To demonstrate cognitive reorganization in the absence of neuronal reorganization would require an experiment that forced normal subjects to adopt the same cognitive strategy as the patients. In the letter-by-letter reading example, normals and patients would need to perform two types of task: one involving parallel reading and one involving serial reading. A differential activation pattern between parallel and serial reading for normals but not for patients would be consistent with evidence for a serial reading strategy being implemented in the absence of neuronal change. In contrast, to demonstrate neuronal reorganization in the absence of cognitive reorganization, it is necessary to show that the cognitive architecture (including the attentional set and performance level) is the same in both patients and normal subjects.

This may not be possible, particularly since the cognitive architecture is likely to change as the neuronal implementation changes. There may, for example, be small changes in cognitive processing (e.g., attentional demands) that cannot be detected by behavioral measures even when they elicit significant changes in neuronal responses. In summary, cognitive and neuronal reorganization are tightly linked. Cognitive reorganization is likely to engender neuronal reorganization, and neuronal reorganization is likely to result in changes in the cognitive set. Degenerate systems will thus vary from one another in terms of both their neuronal structure and their cognitive function, but with different structures and functions being able to sustain the same task.

Redundancy has been used to describe compensation for brain damage by activation of intact areas that may or may not be engaged by neurologically normal subjects. Redundancy thus implies degenerate systems that can function redundantly in the normal brain. Redundancy can be distinguished from degeneracy as follows. Degeneracy characterizes structure-function relationships, but redundancy refers to how the systems are functioning. For example, if two degenerate systems coactivate to perform the same function, this would be redundant or inefficient because activation of one structure would suffice. Degenerate systems can nevertheless be considered efficient (i.e., not redundant) because each brain structure also contributes to other tasks. In other words, degeneracy assumes not just a many-to-one structure-function relationship but also a many-to-many structure-function relationship.

As an analogy, consider the function of the hands. Both hands are normally used to lift a table, play the piano, or use a knife and fork. This is efficient because, with only one hand, piano playing is limited, there is less strength for lifting a table, and you cannot cut and spear your food with a fork simultaneously. However, there are other tasks, such as waving or writing, that require only one hand. Therefore, damage to one hand does not prevent waving or writing with the undamaged hand. Waving could be accomplished with the undamaged hand with very little relearning, whereas writing with the nondominant hand would require substantial relearning. The point is that it is not redundant to have two hands, because many tasks require two hands. It is, however, redundant to use two hands if only one would suffice. In summary, degenerate structural sets in biological systems are not simply duplicates but structurally different (i.e., nonisomorphic) elements that provide the necessary variability for selection processes to operate on. This contrasts with the notion of "redundancy." Critically, redundant use of multiple structural configurations necessitates degeneracy (Friston & Price, 2003).

Vicariation has been used to describe the rather implausible scenario that the functional takeover is enacted by regions with previously unrelated functional descriptions (Zahn et al., 2004; Zahn et al., 2002). To return to the analogy of hand function: if both hands are lost, people can learn to write and paint with their feet. Although feet perform functions that are not associated with hands, they also share functions such as gripping. Thus, it is not correct to say that writing with your feet is an example of vicariation. At the neuronal level, it is highly unlikely that recovery would occur by recruiting brain areas that have functions unrelated to the damaged area because this would imply the growth of new neuronal processes (cellular plasticity/neurogenesis). As discussed above, it is generally accepted that the gross schema of extrinsic connectivity is fixed in the mature brain. In short, like equipotentiality, vicariation is a concept that is encountered in the literature but not in the brain.

Unmasking is used to describe activation in areas that are not activated in normals but become activated because brain damage has "disinhibited" preexisting connections. In contrast to vicariation, the assumption is that the system was present but latent prior to damage. Unmasking/disinhibition is usually used in relation to rapid changes (e.g., in motor representations) that occur within minutes (e.g., by modulation of GABAergic inhibition). Functional imaging should be able to distinguish disinhibition from learning-related plasticity on the basis that "disinhibition" occurs earlier in the reorganization process than learning-related plasticity and will be less dependent on rehabilitation therapy. The questions raised by unmasking concern the functional significance of the disinhibited system. Do the disinhibited areas play a necessary role in recovery? Or do they reflect maladaptive disinhibition (Johansen-Berg et al., 2002)?

Contralateral vs Ipsilateral compensation. The degenerate systems most likely to be disinhibited are those in the contralateral hemisphere that are homologous to the damaged areas. This is because the functional role played by any brain component (cortical area, subarea, neuronal population, or neuron) is defined by the connections and interactions it has with other cortical areas. Therefore, functional similarities between neuronal systems depend on the similarity in their connection profiles, which is likely to be greatest within a cytoarchitectonic region or in the homologous area of the contralateral hemisphere (by virtue of transcallosal inter-hemispheric connections). Several functional imaging studies have demonstrated that language or motor recovery is associated with activation in contralateral homologous areas (Blank et al., 2003; Blasi et al., 2002; Calvert et al., 2000; Gold & Kertesz, 2000; Kertesz, 1988; Leff et al., 2000; Mimura et al., 1998; Thulborn et al., 1999; Weiller et al., 1995). In contrast, other studies have emphasized that recovery depends on restored activation in unaffected regions of the damaged hemisphere (Heiss et al., 1999; Karbe et al., 1998) or that early involvement of the contralateral hemisphere is followed by later involvement of the ipsilateral hemisphere (Fernandez et al., 2004; Foltys et al., 2003).

These discrepant results suggest that lesion location and extension, as well as the onset and time course of the pathological process, determine the reorganization pattern. Assessing the relative importance of each of these mechanisms rests in part on determining which areas are necessary for recovery and which areas reflect maladaptive disinhibition triggered by the lesion (Johansen-Berg et al., 2002; Ward et al., 2003). For instance, Ward et al. have demonstrated a negative correlation between recovery and the degree of task-related activation in both contralateral and ipsilateral areas. Thus, patients with poor recovery were more likely to activate novel brain regions that are not observed in the control group, while patients with complete recovery were more likely to reproduce a "normal" pattern of activation.

Summary of How Functional Imaging Studies of Patients Can Be Applied

The systems-level approach that functional neuroimaging offers has several important implications for understanding neuropsychologically impaired patients. First, unlike the lesion-deficit model, it does not assume that cognitive processes or operations are localized in discrete anatomical modules, but allows for functional specialization that is embedded in the interactions among two or more areas. In relation to patient studies, the systems-level approach enables one to identify where there is abnormal function in the absence of structural damage and where the responsiveness of an undamaged region is context dependent (i.e., responds normally in some tasks and abnormally in others). Functional imaging also allows inferences about changes in functional connectivity and interactions among distributed regions.

Second, the systems-level approach that functional imaging offers can be used to explore the neuronal mechanisms that sustain recovery or maintenance of a function following brain damage. This includes the identification of neuronal systems that compensate for damage, and peri-infarct activation that indicates where functional responsiveness has been maintained in areas that appear damaged on structural images (e.g., structural MRI or CT scans). Understanding the mechanisms of recovery should reveal why the effect of lesion site has variable consequences in different individuals. We will return to the issue of how functional imaging of patients can provide insights into the neuronal systems that enable the recovery of function following brain damage. First, however, we turn to some of the profound difficulties that are encountered when trying to conduct functional imaging studies of brain-damaged patients.

Issues

Limitations of Functional Neuroimaging Studies of Patients

Despite the insights provided by functional imaging studies of patients, there are several potential limitations. Perhaps the most counterintuitive is that to make inferences about abnormal neuronal responses, the patient needs to perform the task correctly. If the patient cannot perform the task, then the corresponding neuronal correlates will not be expressed, and reduced activation could simply reflect a failure to engage processes that were not impaired. Take, for example, the case of a patient who could comprehend speech but not produce it. A functional imaging study of speech production would show areas of reduced activation for the patient relative to control subjects. Although it is tempting to infer that reduced activation, relative to normals, is a consequence of neuronal reorganization, reduced activation may also occur because unimpaired processes (e.g., semantic and perceptual) are not engaged normally when the task is not performed and the appropriate cognitive and attentional set is not maintained.

Another limitation of functional imaging studies is that even if the patient can perform the task, functional imaging cannot detect activation in latent systems that are not engaged when the prepotent system is available. Nor can it distinguish which of the areas that do activate are necessary for task performance. For example, during object recognition, some objects might evoke activation in areas involved in emotional processing or name retrieval even though these processes are not necessary for recognition. Activation may also be evoked by the processes of interest but be redundant because other areas are also carrying out the same function. Thus, functional imaging studies cannot deduce which of the activated areas are "critical" for performance; or how many neuronal systems are capable of sustaining the task.

Functional activations in patients with brain damage or other neurological conditions also need to be viewed with caution because there may be changes in the neurovascular coupling, $CMRO_2$ rate, rCBF, or rCBV, which in turn could produce spurious effects in the neuroimaging results. For instance, reduced BOLD signal surrounding an area of tissue damage could be the result of neuronal dysfunction, but could also arise from a reduced BOLD ratio secondary to arterial stenosis or hypometabolic states. Such artifacts may also depend on the age of the subject. Hence there may be age-by-injury interactions in functional neuroimaging data, where the predicates of the BOLD response are doubly affected. Finally, there are practical limitations on using functional neuroimaging with patients that need to be considered. Patients may have more difficulty understanding the scanning conditions, remaining still, and complying with the task demands. The approach outlined in the next section is therefore applicable only in the case of patients who are able to comply with the scanning conditions and can produce accurate responses to the tasks under investigation.

Combining Functional Imaging and Neuropsychological Studies

Critically, the advantages and limitations of functional imaging studies complement the advantages and disadvantages of lesion studies. As we argued above, one of the limitations of lesion studies—in a single patient—is that they are limited to inferences concerning brain damage and impaired task performance, but they tell us nothing about the relationship between the damaged area and intact cognitive functions because of the compensatory measures adopted by patients to overcome their deficits. In contrast, functional imaging can reveal activation that maintains task performance, but it is limited with respect to interpretations regarding impaired performance. In other words, lesions tell us what areas are necessary (but not sufficient), whereas functional imaging identifies sufficient sets of areas for one task relative to another, but not whether these areas are necessary. The limitations of these two techniques are therefore complementary and can be partially overcome by systematically harnessing the relative advantages of each.

This section describes how normal and abnormal structure-function relationships in the human brain can be determined by systematically combining functional imaging and neuropsychological data. The approach is applicable to multiple tasks, but here we refer only to generic "task performance" that can be either intact (task is completed correctly) or impaired (response errors). In other words, the aim is to identify the full set of regions for a task, and to partition these regions into sets of necessary and sufficient brain systems that are each capable of sustaining task performance. To this end, we start with some definitions of what we mean by necessary and sufficient.

A *sufficient system* refers to the minimal set of brain areas that need to be engaged to perform one task relative to another. There are two parts to this definition—"the performance of one task relative to another" and the "minimal set." With respect to the former, the point is that the set of areas which are sufficient will obviously change with the tasks. Thus, the sufficient set for reading aloud, relative to viewing a fixation point, will be larger than the set for reading aloud relative to reading silently. With respect to the minimal set of brain areas, this will depend on the order of degeneracy, which is defined as the number of disjoint sufficient systems. Functional imaging should, in principle, be able to identify the sets of areas that are activated for one task relative to another (assuming all activations are detected). However, as we have already acknowledged, functional imaging cannot determine how many sufficient systems are coactivated. Moreover, functional imaging studies cannot exclude the possibility that parts of the engaged system have not been activated—this depends on the sensitivity of the imaging technique and the acceptance of the null hypothesis.

A *necessary brain area* is a region that is critical for task performance. We use the term "necessary" to imply that the task could not be performed if the area was damaged. Furthermore, we define "performance" in terms of correct responses because errorful performance suggests that there is no degeneracy available to compensate for the lost function. Performance can also be defined in terms of efficiency and the speed of correct responses, but this is not particularly informative for characterizing degenerate brain systems because it could emerge in the context of degeneracy (a less efficient system has been engaged) or no degeneracy ("peri-infarct" activation). Critically, the claim "necessary for correct responses" depends on neuropsychological measures. Other methods, such as TMS, typically show only a "slowing" in task performance rather than a qualitative change in task performance, and therefore can only make inferences concerning the efficiency of the response. Likewise, functional imaging cannot be used to establish that activation is necessary. Furthermore, the designation of an area as necessary will be different in patients and neurologically normal subjects. If degenerate systems are available, an area may not be necessary in normal subjects but may become necessary following damage to one of the systems. This has been demonstrated using the WADA test following lesions to the right hemisphere in the context of a previous lesion to the left hemisphere. For example, injection of sodium amytal in the right hemisphere does not normally disrupt language; but Kinsbourne (1971) reported impaired language capabilities in patients who had recovered from aphasia following a left hemisphere lesion. In summary, necessity can be established only by lesioning an area or system. Functional neuroimaging has no role in this context.

Harnessing Functional Imaging and Neuropsychological Data

As indicated in the previous section, the roles of functional imaging and neuropsychological studies are complementary. Lesions tell us which areas are necessary (but not sufficient), whereas functional imaging identifies sufficient sets of areas but not whether these areas are necessary. However, neither technique alone can identify the minimum number of sufficient systems for sustaining the task. For example, the identification of degenerate neuronal systems on the basis of neuropsychological studies would require the effects from a vast variety of lesions to be investigated over a wide range of tasks. However, the number of patients required can be dramatically reduced by harnessing the neuropsychological study to functional imaging data and focusing only on the effect of damage to areas that activate in response to the task. In other words, guided by functional imaging data, lesion studies can test whether damage to a component of the system impairs performance or not. To our knowledge, the first report of a neuropsychologically based study that was constrained by functional imaging results was an investigation of a patient with a right cerebellar infarct (Fiez et al., 1992) motivated by the observation that functional imaging studies show activity in the right cerebellum during verbal fluency (Petersen et al., 1988). On nonmotor tasks, the patient showed deficits completing and learning a word generation task but had normal or above normal behavior when performing standardized language tasks. In this instance, a neuroimaging study motivated a neuropsychological study and the neuropsychological study allowed inferences to be made regarding a subcomponent of the language system.

Functional imaging of normal subjects and neuropsychological studies of patients with damage to the normal system are not by themselves able to dissociate all possible degenerate systems for a task. Patients may perform well using a latent system, not observed in the normals, that compensates for the damaged areas (figure 14.3A). Indeed, even after lesioning all the normal regions, the patient might still be able to perform that task. This is where functional imaging of the brain-damaged patients plays a critical role in identifying latent systems. Thus, to classify regions as belonging to type B, C, or D in figure 14.3A, we need functional imaging of the patients who have damage to the normal system (e.g., region B or C in figure 14.3A) but intact performance. This slightly counterintuitive fact follows from degeneracy: with degeneracy there may be no necessary areas until all but one sufficient set has been

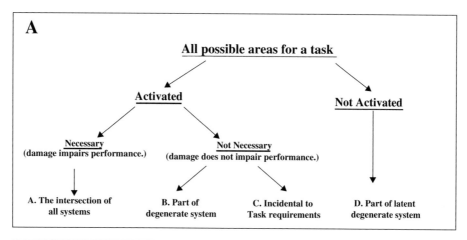

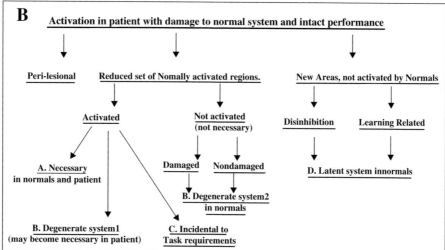

Figure 14.3
(*A*) Types of activation in normal subjects. (*B*) Types of activation in patients when task performance is intact.

lesioned. Therefore, patients can be used to identify latent systems, even if they do not tell which ones are necessary.

Functional imaging of the patient will determine whether performance was maintained by activation in the damaged area (peri-infarct activation), a reduced set of the normal areas; or in latent areas (figure 14.3B). Peri-infarct activation in the damaged area means that we cannot say that the intact performance occurred in the absence of the damaged area. Thus, if the only difference between patient and normals was in the damaged area, this patient cannot tell us anything about degenerate organization. The second possibility is that the patient performs the task by activating a reduced set of the normally activated regions. This observation provides information on how the areas activated by control subjects might dissociate into different systems. For example, reduced activation in undamaged areas suggests that these areas were part of the same (dysfunctional) system that included the damaged area but also part of a different system to the activated areas. The third possibility is that the patient activates areas that are not observed in normal subjects. In this case the new areas become candidates for latent systems that can be detected only following brain damage. As discussed above, activation in new areas may result from "disinhibition" or be learning related. Disinhibition is more likely to emerge in the early stages after brain damage, with learning-related effects emerging weeks or months after brain damage. Thus, dissociating disinhibition and learning-related effects requires longitudinal imaging studies of the patient's recovery (on tasks that the patient is able to perform).

Although functional imaging of a single patient can provide important clues to structure-function relationships, a full understanding requires reference to further neuropsychological studies. For example, if a patient activates areas not observed in normal subjects, we need to determine whether these activations in latent areas are necessary for patient performance. This would require neuropsychological studies of patients who have damage to areas identified as latent in addition to damage in the normal system. Thus, the investigation of structure-function relationships becomes an iterative procedure of combining imaging and lesion data (figure 14.4).

The logistic steps for delineating two or three neuronal systems are summarized schematically in figure 14.4. Step I involves functional imaging of normal subjects to identify the set of regions that activate for one task relative to another. We take the example of activation in two regions only, areas A and B. Even with this simple example, there are at least ten plausible combinations of regions that are each sufficient for task performance. For instance, the task may require both areas, only one area, or either. It is also possible, that neither A nor B is necessary if the function can be taken over by latent areas (e.g., C in figure 14.4) that are not activated (perhaps inhibited) in normal subjects. Degeneracy is indicated whenever the task

Step I. Functional Imaging of Normals reveal normal system for one task relative to another.

Example: Normals activate areas A & B. What is the necessary and sufficient set of regions?

Possibilities:	Sufficient for Task	Necessary	Order of Deneracy
Solution 1:	A & B	A & B	1
Solution 2:	A or B	-	2
Solution 3:	A only	A	1
Solution 4:	B only	B	1
If a latent system C can replace function of A and B:			
Solution 5:	[A & B] or C	-	2
If a latent system C can replace function of A or B:			
Solution 6:	A & [B or C]	A	1
Solution 7:	B & [A or C]	B	1
Solution 8:	B or C	-	2
Solution 9:	A or C	-	2
Solution 10:	A or B or C	-	3

Step II. Neuropsychological studies of patients with lesions to normal system reveal necessary areas

	Patients with Lesions to:				
	Area A	Area B	Areas A and B		
If Performance:	Impaired	Impaired	Impaired	*then*	Solution 1
" "	Intact	Intact	Impaired	"	Solution 2
" "	Impaired	Intact	Impaired	"	Solution 3 or 6
" "	Intact	Impaired	Impaired	"	Solution 4 or 7
" "	Intact	Intact	Intact	"	Solution 5,8,9 or 10

Step III. Functional imaging studies of padients with lesions to normal system reveal alterativve system C

No latent system

Performance impaired after	Lesion to A not B & patient with Lesion to B activates A only	*then*	Solution 3
" "	Lesion to B not A & patient with Lesion to A activates B only	"	Solution 4

Latent system C

Performance impaired after	Lesion to A not B & patient with Lesion to B activates A and C	*then*	Solution 6
" "	Lesion to B not A & patient with Lesion to A activates B and C	"	Solution 7
Performance intact after	Lesion to A &/or B & patient reveals alternative system C	*then*	Solution 5,8,9 or 10

Step IV. Neuropsychological studies of patients with lesions to C

	Patients with Lesions to:				
	Area C	Areas A & C	Areas B & C	Areas A, B & C	
If Performance:	Intact	Impaired	Impaired	Impaired	*then*
" "	Intact	Intact	Impaired	Impaired	" Solution 8
" "	Intact	Impaired	Intact	Impaired	" Solution 9
" "	Intact	Intact	Intact	Impaired	" Solution 10

Figure 14.4
Delineating degenerate neural systems: A theoretical example.

can be performed by one set *or* another. Activation in C is an example of degeneracy in latent areas that are not observed in normal subjects. Competence in A or B is an example of degeneracy in systems that normally activate redundantly.

Step II of figure 14.4 illustrates the important role that neuropsychological studies play in establishing the necessity of a region. Functional competence in C is an important prelude to neuroimaging studies, since only those patients who retain intact performance need to be scanned. The point to note is that even if patients with every possible combination of lesions were available for testing, neuropsychological studies still could not resolve the differential roles of the different regions, unless the data are combined with that from neuroimaging. Step III of figure 14.4 illustrates how imaging patients with selective lesions and intact performance can determine whether task performance is being maintained by a reduced set of regions or activation in areas not observed in normals (i.e., C in figure 14.4). The latter case indicates degeneracy and motivates step IV, which involves behavioral studies of patients with lesions to areas C, A, and B.

Figure 14.5 illustrates the iterative nature of the approach and how the order of degeneracy can be established. The order of degeneracy corresponds to the number of disjoint sets of areas that are sufficient for task performance. It can be operationally defined as the minimum number of areas that have to be removed before the function is lost (i.e., one area for first-order degeneracy, two areas for second-order degeneracy). Note that first-order degeneracy is the same as no degeneracy. Degeneracy enforces a subtle shift in the objectives of identifying structure—function relationships. The aim is no longer to find a necessary and sufficient system because there may not be a necessary system. The aim is now to identify the disjoint sufficient sets of regions.

Limitations of This Approach

Although it is theoretically possible that the combination of imaging and lesion studies, as illustrated in figures 14.4 and 14.5, could delineate all the sufficient system(s) for one task relative to another, it is not so simple in practice. Lesion studies are inherently limited because selective damage to many brain regions, particularly specific combinations of brain regions, is rare. Therefore, there may be insufficient patients to test all combinations of regional lesions. Studies with transcranial magnetic stimulation (TMS), that simulate transient brain lesions, may represent an alternative way forward. The procedures described in figures 14.4 and 14.5 also entail two more assumptions. One is that the lesions have no residual viability (i.e., no peri-infarct activity). The other is that the task activates an identical set of cognitive or neuronal systems for all subjects prior to brain damage. Both these assumptions can be tested, the former by excluding patients with peri-infarct activation and the latter by exploring intersubject variability in the normal subjects.

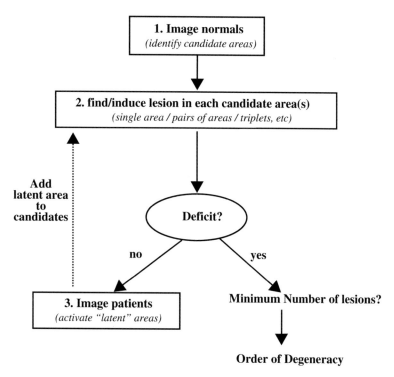

Figure 14.5
Combining techniques to establish the order of degeneracy.

In summary, the joint and complementary use of functional neuroimaging and neuropsychology offers a fundamental advantage over either technique in isolation. Neuroimaging in normal subjects defines the sufficient set of regions for performing one task relative to another. Neuropsychology establishes the necessity of component brain areas. Functional imaging of the patients themselves identifies the latent degenerate systems. Identifying degenerate neuronal systems that are each sufficient to perform a task therefore requires an iterative approach integrating information from functional imaging and behavioral studies of normals and patients (Price & Friston, 2002).

Conclusions

Functional imaging studies of neuropsychologically impaired patients have not enjoyed the immediate success that was attained by functional imaging studies of normal subjects. This is largely because it has taken time to appreciate some of the deeper issues surrounding study design, analysis, and interpretation. Nevertheless, functional imaging studies of brain-damaged patients who retain task competence can provide information that is not available from structural imaging, behavioral assessments, or functional imaging with normal subjects. This is because intact task performance following a brain lesion does not necessarily entail normal neuronal responses in undamaged cortical areas. Abnormal neuronal responses, in the context of normal performance, can indicate alternative neuronal and cognitive mechanisms for supporting the same task. This, in turn, has important implications for understanding the mechanisms that mediate recovery and the organizational principles that underlie functional architectures in the human brain.

References

Barinaga, M. (1998). No-new-neurons dogma loses ground. *Science* 279(5359), 2041–2042.

Blank, S. C., Bird, H., Turkheimer, F., & Wise, R. J. (2003). Speech production after stroke: The role of the right pars opercularis. *Annals of Neurology* 54(3), 310–320.

Blasi, V., Young, A. C., Tansy, A. P., Petersen, S. E., Snyder, A. Z., & Corbetta, M. (2002). Word retrieval learning modulates right frontal cortex in patients with left frontal damage. *Neuron* 36(1), 159–170.

Broca, P. (1861). Remarques sur le siège de la faculté du langage articulé: Suivies d'une observation d'aphémie. *Bulletin de la Société Anatomique de Paris* 6, 330–357, 398–407. Translated in R. Herrnstein & Boring E. G. (1965). *A Sourcel Book in the History of Psychology*. Cambridge, MA: Harvard University Press.

Buonomano, D. V., & Merzenich, M. M. (1998). Cortical plasticity: From synapses to maps. *Annual Review of Neuroscience* 21, 149–186.

Calvert, G. A., Brammer, M. J., Morris, R. G., Williams, S. C., King, N., & Matthews, P. M. (2000). Using fMRI to study recovery from acquired dysphasia. *Brain and Language* 71(3), 391–399.

Chakravarty, A. (2002). Crossed cerebral-cerebellar diaschisis: MRI evaluation. *Neurology India* 50(3), 322–325.

Chen, R., Cohen, L. G., & Hallett, M. (2002). Nervous system reorganization following injury. *Neuroscience* 111(4), 761–773.

Coltheart, M. (1980). Deep dyslexia: A review of the syndrome. In M. Coltheart, K. Patterson, & J. Marshall (Eds.), *Deep Dyslexia*. London: Routledge and Kegan Paul.

Coltheart, M., Curtis, B., Atkins, P., & Haller, M. (1993). Models of reading aloud: Dual-route and parallel-distributed-processing approaches. *Psychological Review* 100, 589–608.

Damasio, A., & Damasio, H. (1983). The anatomic basis of pure alexia. *Neurology* 33, 1573–1583.

Edelman, G. M., & Gally, J. A. (2001). Degeneracy and complexity in biological systems. *Proceedings of the National Academy of Sciences USA* 98(24), 13763–13768.

Feeney, D. M., & Baron, J. C. (1986). Diaschisis. *Stroke* 17(5), 817–830.

Fernandez, B., Cardebat, D., Demonet, J. F., Joseph, P. A., Mazaux, J. M., Barat, M., & Allard, M. (2004). Functional MRI follow-up study of language processes in healthy subjects and during recovery in a case of aphasia. *Stroke* 35(9), 2171–2176.

Fiez, J. A., Petersen, S. E., Cheney, M. K., & Raichle, M. E. (1992). Impaired non-motor learning and error detection associated with cerebellar damage. A single case study. *Brain* 115(1), 155–178.

Foltys, H., Krings, T., Meister, I. G., Sparing, R., Boroojerdi, B., Thron, A., & Topper, R. (2003). Motor representation in patients rapidly recovering after stroke: A functional magnetic resonance imaging and transcranial magnetic stimulation study. *Clinical Neurophysiology* 114(12), 2404–2415.

Friston, K. J., & Price, C. J. (2003). Degeneracy and redundancy in cognitive anatomy. *Trends in Cognitive Sciences* 7(4), 151–152.

Gold, B. T., & Kertesz, A. (2000). Right hemisphere semantic processing of visual words in an aphasic patient: An fMRI study. *Brain and Language* 73(3), 456–465.

Goldstein, K. (1934). *Der Aufbau des Organismus. Einführung in die Biologie unter besonderer Berücksichtigung der Erfahrungen am Kranken Menschen.* The Hague: Nijhoff.

Goltz, F. L. (1881). Discussion on the Localizaion of Function in the Cortex Cerebri. In W. MacCormac (Ed.), Transactions of the International Medical Congress, 7th session, vol. I, 218–228, 234–237. London: Kolkmann.

Green, J. B. (2003). Brain reorganization after stroke. *Topics in Stroke Rehabilitation* 10(3), 1–20.

Gross, C. (2000). Coding for visual categories in the human brain. *Nature Neuroscience* 3(9), 855–856.

Hallett, M. (2000). Plasticity. In R. Frackowiak, J. C. Mazziotta, & A. Toga (Eds.), *Mapping: The Disorders*, 569–585. San Diego: Academic Press.

Hausen, H. S., Lachmann, E. A., & Nagler, W. (1997). Cerebral diaschisis following cerebellar hemorrhage. *Archives of Physical Medicine and Rehabilitation* 78(5), 546–549.

Heiss, W. D., Karbe, H., Weber-Luxenburger, G., Herholz, K., Kessler, J., Pietrzyk, U., & Pawlik, G. (1997). Speech-induced cerebral metabolic activation reflects recovery from aphasia. *Journal of the Neurological Sciences* 145(2), 213–217.

Heiss, W. D., Kessler, J., Thiel, A., Ghaemi, M., & Karbe, H. (1999). Differential capacity of left and right hemispheric areas for compensation of poststroke aphasia. *Annals of Neurology* 45(4), 430–438.

Horwitz, B., Rumsey, J. M., & Donohue, B. C. (1998). Functional connectivity of the angular gyrus in normal reading and dyslexia. *Proceedings of the National Academy of Sciences USA* 95(15), 8939–8944.

Johansen-Berg, H., Dawes, H., Guy, C., Smith, S. M., Wade, D. T., & Matthews, P. M. (2002). Correlation between motor improvements and altered fMRI activity after rehabilitative therapy. *Brain* 125(12), 2731–2742.

Karbe, H., Thiel, A., Weber-Luxenburger, G., Herholz, K., Kessler, J., & Heiss, W. D. (1998). Brain plasticity in poststroke aphasia: What is the contribution of the right hemisphere? *Brain and Language* 64(2), 215–230.

Kertesz, A. (1988). What do we learn from recovery from aphasia? *Advances in Neurology* 47, 277–292.

Kertesz, A. (1993). Recovery and treatment. In K. M. Heilman & E. Valenstein (Eds.), *Clinical Neuropsychology*, 3rd ed. Oxford: Oxford University Press.

Kinsbourne, M. (1971). The minor cerebral hemisphere as a source of aphasic speech. *Archives of Neurology* 15, 530–535.

Lashley, K. S. (1929). *Brain Mechanisms and Intelligence.* Chicago: University of Chicago Press.

Leff, A. P., Scott, S. K., Crewes, H., Hodgson, T. L., Cowey, A., Howard, D., & Wise, R. J. (2000). Impaired reading in patients with right hemianopia. *Annals of Neurology* 47(2), 171–178.

Lichtheim, L. (1885). On aphasia. *Brain* 7, 433–484.

Maguire, E. A., Vargha-Khadem, F., & Mishkin, M. (2001). The effects of bilateral hippocampal damage on fMRI regional activations and interactions during memory retrieval. *Brain* 124(6), 1156–1170.

Marshall, J. C., & Newcombe, F. (1973). Patterns of paralexia: A psycholinguistic approach. *Journal of Psycholinguistic Research* 2, 175–199.

Mimura, M., Kato, M., Sano, Y., Kojima, T., Naeser, M., & Kashima, H. (1998). Prospective and retrospective studies of recovery in aphasia: Changes in cerebral blood flow and language functions. *Brain* 121(11), 2083–2094.

Patterson, K., & Kay, J. (1982). Letter-by-letter reading: Psychological descriptions of a neurological syndrome. *Quarterly Journal of Experimental Psychology A* 34(3), 411–441.

Paulesu, E., Frith, U., Snowling, M., Gallagher, A., Morton, J., Frackowiak, R. S., & Frith, C. D. (1996). Is developmental dyslexia a disconnection syndrome? Evidence from PET scanning. *Brain* 119(1), 143–157.

Petersen, S. E., Fox, P. T., Posner, M. I., Mintun, M., I., & Raichle, M. E. (1988). Positron emission tomographic studies of the cortical anatomy of single-word processing. *Nature* 331(6157), 585–589.

Phillips, J. A., Humphreys, G. W., Noppeney, U., & Price, C. J. (2002). The neural substrates of action retrieval: A examination of semantic and visual routes to action. *Visual Cognition* 9, 662–684.

Plaut, D., McClelland, J., Seidenberg, M., & Patterson, K. (1996). Understanding normal and impaired word reading: Computational principles in quasi-regular domains. *Psychological Review* 103, 56–115.

Price, C. J., & Friston, K. J. (2002). Degeneracy and cognitive anatomy. *Trends in Cognitive Sciences* 6(10), 416–421.

Price, C. J., Gorno-Tempini, M-L., Graham, K., Biggio, N., Mechelli, A., Patterson K., & Noppeney, U. (2003). Normal and pathological reading: Converging data from lesion and imaging studies. *NeuroImage* 20(1), S30–S41.

Price, C. J., Warburton, E. A., Moore, C. J., Frackowiak, R. S., & Friston, K. J. (2001). Dynamic diaschisis: Anatomically remote and context-sensitive human brain lesions. *Journal of Cognitive Neuroscience* 13(4), 419–429.

Rowe, J., Stephan, K. E., Friston, K., Frackowiak, R., Lees, A., & Passingham, R. (2002). Attention to action in Parkinson's disease: Impaired effective connectivity among frontal cortical regions. *Brain* 125(2), 276–289.

Rumiati, R. I., & Humphreys, G. W. (1998). Recognition by action: Dissociating visual and semantic routes to action in normal observers. *Journal of Experimental Psychology. Human Perception and Performance* 24, 631–647.

Shallice, T. (1988). *From Neuropsychology to Mental Structure*. New York: Cambridge University Press.

Thulborn, K. R., Carpenter, P. A., & Just, M. A. (1999). Plasticity of language-related brain function during recovery from stroke. *Stroke* 30(4), 749–754.

Vuilleumier, P., Sagiv, N., Hazeltine, E., Poldrack, R. A., Swick, D., Rafal, R. D., & Gabrieli, J. D. (2001). Neural fate of seen and unseen faces in visuospatial neglect: A combined event-related functional MRI and event-related potential study. *Proceedings of the National Academy of Sciences USA* 98(6), 3495–3500.

Warburton, E., Price, C. J., Swinburn, K., & Wise, R. J. S. (1999). Mechanisms of recovery from aphasia: Evidence from positron emission tomography studies. *Journal of Neurology, Neurosurgery and Psychiatry* 66(2), 155–161.

Ward, N. S., Brown, M. M., Thompson, A. J., & Frackowiak, R. S. (2003). Neural correlates of outcome after stroke: A cross-sectional fMRI study. *Brain* 126(6), 1430–1448.

Weiller, C., Isensee, C., Rijntjes, M. et al. (1995). Recovery from Wernicke's aphasia: A positron emission tomography study. *Annals of Neurology* 37, 723–732.

Wernicke, C. (1874). *Der aphasische Symptomenkomplex*. Breslau, Poland: Cohen & Weigert.

Zahn, R., Drews, E., Specht, K., Kemeny, S., Reith, W., Willmes, K., Schwarz, M., & Huber, W. (2004). Recovery of semantic word processing in global aphasia: A functional MRI study. *Cognitive Brain Research* 18(3), 322–336.

Zahn, R., Huber, W., Drews, E., Specht, K., Kemeny, S., Reith, W., Willmes, K., & Schwarz, M. (2002). Recovery of semantic word processing in transcortical sensory aphasia: A functional magnetic resonance imaging study. *Neurocase* 8(5), 376–386.

Contributors

Todd S. Braver
Department of Psychology
Washington University
St. Louis, Missouri

Jeffrey Browndyke
Bryan Alzheimer's Disease Research
Center
Duke University Medical Center
Durham, North Carolina

Roberto Cabeza
Center for Cognitive Neuroscience
Duke University
Durham, North Carolina

B. J. Casey
Sackler Institute for Developmental
Psychobiology
Weill Medical College of Cornell
University
New York, New York

Jody C. Culham
Department of Psychology
University of Western Ontario
London, Ontario, Canada

Clayton E. Curtis
Center for Neural Science
Department of Psychology
New York University
New York, New York

Mark D'Esposito
Helen Wills Neuroscience Institute
Department of Psychology
University of California
Berkeley, California

Sander M. Daselaar
Center for Cognitive Neuroscience
Duke University
Durham, North Carolina

Lila Davachi
Department of Psychology
New York University
New York, New York

Ian G. Dobbins
Department of Psychological & Brain
Sciences
Duke University
Durham, North Carolina

Karl J. Friston
Wellcome Department of Cognitive
Neurology
Institute of Neurology
London, United Kingdom

Barry Giesbrecht
Department of Psychology
University of California at Santa
Barbara
Santa Barbara, California

Todd C. Handy
Department of Psychology
University of British Columbia
Vancouver, British Columbia, Canada

Joseph B. Hopfinger
Department of Psychology
University of North Carolina at Chapel
Hill
Chapel Hill, North Carolina

Scott A. Huettel
Brain Imaging and Analysis Center
Duke University Medical Center
Durham, North Carolina

Irene P. Kan
Department of Psychology
University of Pennsylvania
Philadelphia, Pennsylvania

Alan Kingstone
Department of Psychology
University of British Columbia
Vancouver, British Columbia, Canada

Eleni Kotsoni
Centre for Brain and Cognitive
Development
Birkbeck College
London, United Kingdom

Kevin S. LaBar
Center for Cognitive Neuroscience
Duke University
Durham, North Carolina

George R. Mangun
Center for Mind and Brain
University of California at Davis
Davis, California

Gregory McCarthy
Brain Imaging and Analysis Center
Duke University Medical Center
Durham, North Carolina

Uta Noppeney
Wellcome Department of Cognitive
Neurology
Institute of Neurology
London, United Kingdom

Robyn T. Oliver
Department of Psychology
University of Pennsylvania
Philadelphia, Pennsylvania

Elizabeth A. Phelps
The Phelps Laboratory
New York University
New York, New York

Russell A. Poldrack
Brain Research Institute
Department of Psychology
University of California-Los Angeles
Los Angeles, California

Cathy J. Price
Wellcome Department of Cognitive
Neurology
Institute of Neurology
London, United Kingdom

Marcus E. Raichle
Departments of Radiology, Neurology,
Anatomy, and Neurobiology
Washington University School of
Medicine
St Louis, Missouri

Hannes Ruge
Department of Psychology
Washington University
St. Louis, Missouri

Gaia Scerif
School of Psychology
University of Nottingham
Nottingham, United Kingdom

Allen W. Song
Brain Imaging and Analysis Center
Duke University Medical Center
Durham, North Carolina

Sharon L. Thompson-Schill
Department of Psychology
University of Pennsylvania
Philadelphia, Pennsylvania

Daniel T. Willingham
Department of Psychology
University of Virginia
Charlottesville, Virginia

Richard J. S. Wise
MRC Clinical Sciences Centre
Hammersmith Hospital
London, United Kingdom

Index

Printed in the United States
by Baker & Taylor Publisher Services